Chapman & Hall/CRC Biostatistics Series

# Sample Size Calculations in Clinical Research

## Second Edition

# Chapman & Hall/CRC Biostatistics Series

Editor-in-Chief

**Shein-Chung Chow, Ph.D.**
Professor
Department of Biostatistics and Bioinformatics
Duke University School of Medicine
Durham, North Carolina, U.S.A.

Series Editors

**Byron Jones**
Senior Director
Statistical Research and Consulting Centre
(IPC 193)
Pfizer Global Research and Development
Sandwich, Kent, UK

**Jen-pei Liu**
Professor
Division of Biometry
Department of Agronomy
National Taiwan University
Taipei, Taiwan

**Karl E. Peace**
Director, Karl E. Peace Center for Biostatistics
Professor of Biostatistics
Georgia Cancer Coalition Distinguished Cancer Scholar
Georgia Southern University, Statesboro, GA

# Chapman & Hall/CRC Biostatistics Series

## Published Titles

1. *Design and Analysis of Animal Studies in Pharmaceutical Development,* Shein-Chung Chow and Jen-pei Liu
2. *Basic Statistics and Pharmaceutical Statistical Applications,* James E. De Muth
3. *Design and Analysis of Bioavailability and Bioequivalence Studies, Second Edition, Revised and Expanded,* Shein-Chung Chow and Jen-pei Liu
4. *Meta-Analysis in Medicine and Health Policy,* Dalene K. Stangl and Donald A. Berry
5. *Generalized Linear Models: A Bayesian Perspective,* Dipak K. Dey, Sujit K. Ghosh, and Bani K. Mallick
6. *Difference Equations with Public Health Applications,* Lemuel A. Moyé and Asha Seth Kapadia
7. *Medical Biostatistics,* Abhaya Indrayan and Sanjeev B. Sarmukaddam
8. *Statistical Methods for Clinical Trials,* Mark X. Norleans
9. *Causal Analysis in Biomedicine and Epidemiology: Based on Minimal Sufficient Causation,* Mikel Aickin
10. *Statistics in Drug Research: Methodologies and Recent Developments,* Shein-Chung Chow and Jun Shao
11. *Sample Size Calculations in Clinical Research,* Shein-Chung Chow, Jun Shao, and Hansheng Wang
12. *Applied Statistical Design for the Researcher,* Daryl S. Paulson
13. *Advances in Clinical Trial Biostatistics,* Nancy L. Geller
14. *Statistics in the Pharmaceutical Industry, 3rd Edition,* Ralph Buncher and Jia-Yeong Tsay
15. *DNA Microarrays and Related Genomics Techniques: Design, Analysis, and Interpretation of Experiments,* David B. Allsion, Grier P. Page, T. Mark Beasley, and Jode W. Edwards
16. *Basic Statistics and Pharmaceutical Statistical Applications, Second Edition,* James E. De Muth
17. *Adaptive Design Methods in Clinical Trials,* Shein-Chung Chow and Mark Chang
18. *Handbook of Regression and Modeling: Applications for the Clinical and Pharmaceutical Industries,* Daryl S. Paulson
19. *Statistical Design and Analysis of Stability Studies,* Shein-Chung Chow
20. *Sample Size Calculations in Clinical Research, Second Edition,* Shein-Chung Chow, Jun Shao, and Hansheng Wang

**Chapman & Hall/CRC Biostatistics Series**

# Sample Size Calculations in Clinical Research
## Second Edition

**Shein-Chung Chow**
Duke University School of Medicine
Duham, North Carolina, U.S.A.

**Jun Shao**
University of Wisconsin
Madison, U.S.A.

**Hansheng Wang**
Peking University
Beijing, China

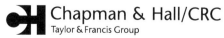

Chapman & Hall/CRC
Taylor & Francis Group
Boca Raton  London  New York

Chapman & Hall/CRC is an imprint of the
Taylor & Francis Group, an **informa** business

Chapman & Hall/CRC
Taylor & Francis Group
6000 Broken Sound Parkway NW, Suite 300
Boca Raton, FL 33487-2742

© 2008 by Taylor & Francis Group, LLC
Chapman & Hall/CRC is an imprint of Taylor & Francis Group, an Informa business

No claim to original U.S. Government works
Printed in the United States of America on acid-free paper
10 9 8 7 6 5 4 3 2 1

International Standard Book Number-13: 978-1-58488-982-3 (Hardcover)

This book contains information obtained from authentic and highly regarded sources. Reprinted material is quoted with permission, and sources are indicated. A wide variety of references are listed. Reasonable efforts have been made to publish reliable data and information, but the author and the publisher cannot assume responsibility for the validity of all materials or for the consequences of their use.

No part of this book may be reprinted, reproduced, transmitted, or utilized in any form by any electronic, mechanical, or other means, now known or hereafter invented, including photocopying, microfilming, and recording, or in any information storage or retrieval system, without written permission from the publishers.

For permission to photocopy or use material electronically from this work, please access www.copyright.com (http://www.copyright.com/) or contact the Copyright Clearance Center, Inc. (CCC) 222 Rosewood Drive, Danvers, MA 01923, 978-750-8400. CCC is a not-for-profit organization that provides licenses and registration for a variety of users. For organizations that have been granted a photocopy license by the CCC, a separate system of payment has been arranged.

**Trademark Notice:** Product or corporate names may be trademarks or registered trademarks, and are used only for identification and explanation without intent to infringe.

---

**Library of Congress Cataloging-in-Publication Data**

---

Sample size calculations in clinical research / [edited by] Shein-Chung Chow, Jun Shao, and Hansheng Wan. -- 2nd ed.
   p. ; cm. -- (Chapman & Hall/CRC biostatistics series ; 20)
"A CRC title."
Includes bibliographical references and index.
ISBN 978-1-58488-982-3 (alk. paper)
  1. Clinical medicine--Research--Statistical methods. 2. Drug development--Statistical methods. 3. Sampling (Statistics) I. Chow, Shein-Chung, 1955- II. Shao, Jun. III. Wang, Hansheng, 1977- IV. Title. V. Series.
  [DNLM: 1. Sample Size. 2. Biometry--methods. WA 950 S192 2008]

R853.S7S33 2008
615.5072'4--dc22
                                                                  2007009660

---

**Visit the Taylor & Francis Web site at**
http://www.taylorandfrancis.com

**and the CRC Press Web site at**
http://www.crcpress.com

# Series Introduction

The primary objectives of the *Biostatistics Book Series* are to provide useful reference books for researchers and scientists in academia, industry, and government, and also to offer textbooks for undergraduate and/or graduate courses in the area of biostatistics. This book series will provide comprehensive and unified presentations of statistical designs and analyses of important applications in biostatistics, such as those in biopharmaceuticals. A well-balanced summary will be given of current and recently developed statistical methods and interpretations for both statisticians and researchers/scientists with minimal statistical knowledge who are engaged in the field of applied biostatistics. The series is committed to providing easy-to-understand, state-of-the-art references and textbooks. In each volume, statistical concepts and methodologies will be illustrated through real world examples.

Clinical development is an integral part of pharmaceutical development. Sample size calculation plays an important role for providing accurate and reliable assessment of the efficacy and safety of the pharmaceutical entities under investigation. Sample size calculation is usually conducted based on a pre-study power analysis for achieving a desired power for detection of a clinically meaningful difference at a given level of significance. In practice, however, sample size required for an intended clinical trial is often obtained using inappropriate test statistic for correct hypotheses, appropriate test statistic for wrong hypotheses, or inappropriate test statistic for wrong hypotheses. Consequently, the validity and integrity of the clinical study is questionable. For good clinical practice (GCP), it is then required that sample size calculation be performed using appropriate statistics for correct hypotheses that will address the scientific/clinical questions regarding the pharmaceutical entities under investigation. Sample size calculation is one of the keys to the success of studies conducted at various phases of clinical development. It not only ensures the validity of the clinical trials, but also assures that the intended trials will have a desired power for correctly detecting a clinically meaningful difference of the pharmaceutical entity under study if such a difference truly exists.

This book provides a comprehensive and unified presentation of various test statistics and formulas/procedures for sample size calculation that are commonly employed at various phses of clinical development. It also provides a challenge to clinical scientists especially biostatisticians regarding current regulatory requirements, methodologies and recent developments for those issues that remain unsolved such as testing equivalence/non-inferiority in active control trials and comparing variabilities (or reproducibilities) in clinical development.

This second edition would be beneficial to biostatisticians, medical researchers, and pharmaceutical scientists who are engaged in the areas of medical and pharmaceutical research.

*Shein-Chung Chow*

# Preface

Clinical development is an integral part of pharmaceutical development, which is a lengthy and costly process for providing accurate and reliable assessment of the efficacy and safety of pharmaceutical entities under investigation. Sample size calculation plays an important role, which ensures the success of studies conducted at various phases of clinical development. It not only ensures the validity of the clinical trials, but also assures that the intended trials will have a desired power for correctly detecting a clinically meaningful difference of the pharmaceutical entity under study if such a difference truly exists.

Sample size calculation is usually conducted through a pre-study power analysis. The purpose is to select a sample size such that the selected sample size will achieve a desired power for correctly detecting a pre-specified clinically meaningful difference at a given level of significance. In clinical research, however, it is not uncommon to perform sample size calculation with inappropriate test statistics for wrong hypotheses regardless of the study design employed. This book provides formulas and/or procedures for determination of sample size required not only for testing equality, but also for testing non-inferiority/superiority, and equivalence (similarity) based on both untransformed (raw) data and log-transformed data under a parallel-group design or a crossover design with equal or unequal ratio of treatment allocations. It provides not only a comprehensive and unified presentation of various statistical procedures for sample size calculation that are commonly employed at various phases of clinical development, but also a well-balanced summary of current regulatory requirements, methodology for design and analysis in clinical research and recent developments in the area of clinical development.

This book is a useful reference for clinical scientists and biostatisticians in the pharmaceutical industry, regulatory agencies, and academia, and other scientists who are in the related fields of clinical development. The primary focus of this book is on statistical procedures for sample size calculation and/or justification that are commonly employed at various phases of clinical research and development. This book provides clear, illustrated explanations of how the derived formulas and/or statistical procedures for sample size calculation and/or justification can be used at various phases of clinical research and development.

The book contains 15 chapters, which cover various important topics in clinical research and development, such as comparing means, comparing proportions, comparing time-to-event data, tests for independence and goodness-of-fit in contingency tables, comparing variabilities in clinical research, sample size adjustment and/or re-estimation in interim analysis, procedures for sample size calculation for optimal or flexible multiple-stage designs for phase II cancer trials, sample size calculation based on rank statistics, sample size calculation for standard, higher-order, and replicated crossover designs, sample size calculation for dose response studies and microarray studies, Bayesian sample size calculation, and sample size calculation in other areas such as QT/QTc studies with time-dependent replicates, propensity score analysis in non-randomized studies, analysis of variance with repeated measures, quality of life studies, bridging studies, and vaccine clinical trials. Each chapter provides a brief history or background, regulatory requirements (if any), statistical design and methods for data analysis, recent development, and related references.

From Taylor & Francis, we thank Acquisitions Editor David Crubbs for providing us with the opportunity to work on this project, and the Production Editor for his/her outstanding efforts in preparing this book for publication. We are deeply indebted to Duke University and the University of Wisconsin for their support. We would like to express our gratitude to many friends from the academia, industry and government for their input, support and encouragement during the preparation of this edition.

Finally, we are fully responsible for any errors remaining in this book. The views expressed are those of the authors and are not necessarily those of their respective company and university. Any comments and suggestions that you may have are very much appreciated for the preparation of future editions of this book.

*Shein-Chung Chow*
*Jun Shao*
*Hansheng Wang*

# Contents

| 1 | **Introduction** | | **1** |
|---|---|---|---|
| | 1.1 | Regulatory Requirement | 2 |
| | 1.2 | Basic Considerations | 7 |
| | 1.3 | Procedures for Sample Size Calculation | 13 |
| | 1.4 | Aims and Structure of the Book | 21 |
| 2 | **Considerations Prior to Sample Size Calculation** | | **25** |
| | 2.1 | Confounding and Interaction | 26 |
| | 2.2 | One-Sided Test Versus Two-Sided Test | 28 |
| | 2.3 | Crossover Design Versus Parallel Design | 30 |
| | 2.4 | Subgroup/Interim Analyses | 32 |
| | 2.5 | Data Transformation | 36 |
| | 2.6 | Practical Issues | 38 |
| 3 | **Comparing Means** | | **49** |
| | 3.1 | One-Sample Design | 50 |
| | 3.2 | Two-Sample Parallel Design | 57 |
| | 3.3 | Two-Sample Crossover Design | 65 |
| | 3.4 | Multiple-Sample One-Way ANOVA | 70 |
| | 3.5 | Multiple-Sample Williams Design | 74 |
| | 3.6 | Practical Issues | 78 |
| 4 | **Large Sample Tests for Proportions** | | **83** |
| | 4.1 | One-Sample Design | 84 |
| | 4.2 | Two-Sample Parallel Design | 89 |
| | 4.3 | Two-Sample Crossover Design | 95 |
| | 4.4 | One-Way Analysis of Variance | 99 |
| | 4.5 | Williams Design | 101 |
| | 4.6 | Relative Risk—Parallel Design | 104 |
| | 4.7 | Relative Risk—Crossover Design | 109 |
| | 4.8 | Practical Issues | 111 |

## 5 Exact Tests for Proportions — 117
- 5.1 Binomial Test — 117
- 5.2 Fisher's Exact Test — 121
- 5.3 Optimal Multiple-Stage Designs for Single Arm Trials — 124
- 5.4 Flexible Designs for Multiple-Arm Trials — 141
- 5.5 Remarks — 143

## 6 Tests for Goodness-of-Fit and Contingency Tables — 145
- 6.1 Tests for Goodness-of-Fit — 146
- 6.2 Test for Independence—Single Stratum — 148
- 6.3 Test for Independence—Multiple Strata — 151
- 6.4 Test for Categorical Shift — 153
- 6.5 Carry-Over Effect Test — 158
- 6.6 Practical Issues — 161

## 7 Comparing Time-to-Event Data — 163
- 7.1 Basic Concepts — 164
- 7.2 Exponential Model — 166
- 7.3 Cox's Proportional Hazards Model — 174
- 7.4 Weighted Log-Rank Test — 179
- 7.5 Practical Issues — 185

## 8 Group Sequential Methods — 187
- 8.1 Pocock's Test — 188
- 8.2 O'Brien and Fleming's Test — 192
- 8.3 Wang and Tsiatis' Test — 193
- 8.4 Inner Wedge Test — 197
- 8.5 Binary Variables — 201
- 8.6 Time-to-Event Data — 202
- 8.7 Alpha Spending Function — 204
- 8.8 Sample Size Re-Estimation — 206
- 8.9 Conditional Power — 209
- 8.10 Practical Issues — 211

## 9 Comparing Variabilities — 215
- 9.1 Comparing Intra-Subject Variabilities — 216
- 9.2 Comparing Intra-Subject CVs — 224
- 9.3 Comparing Inter-Subject Variabilities — 233
- 9.4 Comparing Total Variabilities — 241
- 9.5 Practical Issues — 254

## 10 Bioequivalence Testing         257
   10.1 Bioequivalence Criteria . . . . . . . . . . . . . . . . . . . . . . 258
   10.2 Average Bioequivalence . . . . . . . . . . . . . . . . . . . . . 259
   10.3 Population Bioequivalence . . . . . . . . . . . . . . . . . . . . 263
   10.4 Individual Bioequivalence . . . . . . . . . . . . . . . . . . . . 265
   10.5 In Vitro Bioequivalence . . . . . . . . . . . . . . . . . . . . . 271

## 11 Dose Response Studies         279
   11.1 Continuous Response . . . . . . . . . . . . . . . . . . . . . . 280
   11.2 Binary Response . . . . . . . . . . . . . . . . . . . . . . . . 284
   11.3 Time-to-Event Endpoint . . . . . . . . . . . . . . . . . . . . . 285
   11.4 Williams' Test for Minimum Effective Dose (MED) . . . . . 287
   11.5 Cochran-Armitage's Test for Trend . . . . . . . . . . . . . . 293
   11.6 Dose Escalation Trials . . . . . . . . . . . . . . . . . . . . . 296
   11.7 Concluding Remarks . . . . . . . . . . . . . . . . . . . . . . 301

## 12 Microarray Studies         303
   12.1 Literature Review . . . . . . . . . . . . . . . . . . . . . . . 304
   12.2 False Discovery Rate (FDR) Control . . . . . . . . . . . . . 305
   12.3 Family-wise Error Rate (FWER) Control . . . . . . . . . . 315
   12.4 Concluding Remarks . . . . . . . . . . . . . . . . . . . . . . 324

## 13 Bayesian Sample Size Calculation         327
   13.1 Posterior Credible Interval Approach . . . . . . . . . . . . . 328
   13.2 Posterior Error Approach . . . . . . . . . . . . . . . . . . . 344
   13.3 The Bootstrap-Median Approach . . . . . . . . . . . . . . . 350
   13.4 Concluding Remarks . . . . . . . . . . . . . . . . . . . . . . 353

## 14 Nonparametrics         355
   14.1 Violation of Assumptions . . . . . . . . . . . . . . . . . . . 356
   14.2 One-Sample Location Problem . . . . . . . . . . . . . . . . 357
   14.3 Two-Sample Location Problem . . . . . . . . . . . . . . . . 361
   14.4 Test for Independence . . . . . . . . . . . . . . . . . . . . . 365
   14.5 Practical Issues . . . . . . . . . . . . . . . . . . . . . . . . . 369

## 15 Sample Size Calculation in Other Areas         373
   15.1 QT/QTc Studies with Time-Dependent Replicates . . . . . 374
   15.2 Propensity Analysis in Non-Randomized Studies . . . . . . 383
   15.3 ANOVA with Repeated Measures . . . . . . . . . . . . . . 389
   15.4 Quality of Life . . . . . . . . . . . . . . . . . . . . . . . . . 394
   15.5 Bridging Studies . . . . . . . . . . . . . . . . . . . . . . . . 399
   15.6 Vaccine Clinical Trials . . . . . . . . . . . . . . . . . . . . . 408

**Appendix: Tables of Quantiles** 417

**Bibliography** 427

**Index** 451

# Chapter 1

# Introduction

In clinical research, during the planning stage of a clinical study, the following questions are of particular interest to the investigators: (i) how many subjects are needed in order to have a desired power for detecting a clinically meaningful difference (e.g., an 80% chance of correctly detecting a clinically meaningful difference), and (ii) what's the *trade-off* between cost-effectiveness and power if only a small number of subjects are available for the study due to limited budget and/or some medical considerations. To address these questions, a statistical evaluation for sample size calculation is often performed based on some statistical inference of the primary study endpoint with certain assurance. In clinical research, sample size calculation plays an important role for assuring validity, accuracy, reliability, and integrity of the intended clinical study.

For a given study, sample size calculation is usually performed based on some statistical criteria controlling type I and/or type II errors. For example, we may choose sample size in such a way that there is a desired precision at a fixed confidence level (i.e., fixed type I error). This approach is referred to as *precision analysis* for sample size calculation. The method of precision analysis is simple and easy to perform and yet it may have a small chance of correctly detecting a true difference. As an alternative, the method of pre-study *power analysis* is usually conducted to estimate sample size. The concept of the pre-study power analysis is to select required sample size for achieving a desired power for detecting a clinically/scientifically meaningful difference at a fixed type I error rate. In clinical research, the pre-study power analysis is probably the most commonly used method for sample size calculation. In this book, we will focus on sample size calculation based on power analysis for various situations in clinical research.

In clinical research, to provide an accurate and reliable sample size calculation, an appropriate statistical test for the hypotheses of interest is necessarily derived under the study design. The hypotheses should be established to reflect the study objectives under the study design. In practice, it is not uncommon to observe discrepancies among study objective (hypotheses), study design, statistical analysis (test statistic), and sample size calculation. These discrepancies can certainly distort the validity and integrity of the intended clinical trial.

In the next section, regulatory requirement regarding the role of sample size calculation in clinical research is discussed. In Section 1.2, we provide some basic considerations for sample size calculation. These basic considerations include study objectives, design, hypotheses, primary study endpoint, and clinically meaningful difference. The concepts of type I and type II errors and procedures for sample size calculation based on precision analysis, power analysis, probability assessment, and reproducibility probability are given in Section 1.3. Aim and structure of the book is given in the last section.

## 1.1 Regulatory Requirement

As indicated in Chow and Liu (1998), the process of drug research and development is a lengthy and costly process. This lengthy and costly process is necessary not only to demonstrate the efficacy and safety of the drug product under investigation, but also to ensure the study drug product possesses good drug characteristics such as identity, strength, quality, purity, and stability after it is approved by the regulatory authority. This lengthy process includes drug discovery, formulation, animal study, laboratory development, clinical development, and regulatory submission. As a result, clinical development plays an important role in the process of drug research and development because all of the tests are conducted on humans. For approval of a drug product under investigation, the United States Food and Drug Administration (FDA) requires that at least two adequate and well-controlled clinical studies be conducted for providing substantial evidence regarding the efficacy and safety of the drug product (FDA, 1988). However, the following scientific/statistical questions are raised: (i) what is the definition of an adequate and well-controlled clinical study? (ii) what evidence is considered substantial? (iii) why do we need at least two studies? (iv) will a single large trial be sufficient to provide substantial evidence for approval? and (v) if a single large trial can provide substantial evidence for approval, how large is considered large? In what follows, we will address these questions.

## 1.1. Regulatory Requirement

Table 1.1.1: Characteristics of an Adequate and Well-Controlled Study

| Criteria | Characteristics |
|---|---|
| Objectives | Clear statement of investigation's purpose |
| Methods of analysis | Summary of proposed or actual methods of analysis |
| Design | Valid comparison with a control to provide a quantitative assessment of drug effect |
| Selection of subjects | Adequate assurance of the disease or conditions under study |
| Assignment of subjects | Minimization of bias and assurance of comparability of groups |
| Participants of studies | Minimization of bias on the part of subjects, observers, and analysis |
| Assessment of responses | Well-defined and reliable |
| Assessment of the effect | Requirement of appropriate statistical methods |

### 1.1.1 Adequate and Well-Controlled Clinical Trials

Section 314.126 of 21 CFR (Code of Federal Regulation) provides the definition of an adequate and well-controlled study, which is summarized in Table 1.1.1.

As can be seen from Table 1.1.1, an adequate and well-controlled study is judged by eight characteristics specified in the CFR. These characteristics include study objectives, methods of analysis, design, selection of subjects, assignment of subjects, participants of studies, assessment of responses, and assessment of the effect. For study objectives, it is required that the study objectives be clearly stated in the study protocol such that they can be formulated into statistical hypotheses. Under the hypotheses, appropriate statistical methods should be described in the study protocol. A clinical study is not considered adequate and well-controlled if the employed study design is not valid. A valid study design allows a quantitative assessment of drug effect with a valid comparison with a control. The selection of a *sufficient* number of subjects with the disease or conditions under study is one of the keys to the integrity of an adequate and well-controlled study. In an adequate and well-controlled clinical study, subjects should be randomly assigned to treatment groups to minimize potential bias by ensuring comparability between treatment groups with respect to demographic variables such as age, gender, race, height and weight, and other patient characteristics or prognostic factors such as medical history and disease severity. An adequate and well-controlled study requires that the primary study endpoint or response variable should be well-defined and assessed with a certain degree of accuracy and reliability. To achieve this goal, statistical inferences on the drug effect should be obtained based on the responses of the primary study endpoint observed from the sufficient number of subjects using appropriate statistical methods derived under the study design and objectives.

### 1.1.2 Substantial Evidence

The substantial evidence as required in the *Kefauver-Harris* amendments to the *Food and Drug and Cosmetics Act* in 1962 is defined as the evidence consisting of adequate and well-controlled investigations, including clinical investigations, by experts qualified by scientific training and experience to evaluate the effectiveness of the drug involved, on the basis of which it could fairly and responsibly be concluded by such experts that the drug will have the effect it purports to have under the conditions of use prescribed, recommended, or suggested in the labeling or proposed labeling thereof. Based on this amendment, the FDA requests that reports of adequate and well-controlled investigations provide the primary basis for determining whether there is substantial evidence to support the claims of new drugs and antibiotics.

### 1.1.3 Why at Least Two Studies?

As indicated earlier, the FDA requires at least two adequate and well-controlled clinical trials be conducted for providing substantial evidence regarding the effectiveness and safety of the test drug under investigation for regulatory review and approval. In practice, it is prudent to plan for more than one trial in the phase III study because of any or combination of the following reasons: (i) lack of pharmacological rationale, (ii) a new pharmacological principle, (iii) phase I and phase II data are limited or unconvincing, (iv) a therapeutic area with a history of failed studies or failures to confirm seemingly convincing results, (v) a need to demonstrate efficacy and/or tolerability in different sub-populations, with different co-medication or other interventions, relative to different competitors, and (vi) any other needs to address additional questions in the phase III program.

Shao and Chow (2002) and Chow, Shao and Hu (2002) pointed out that the purpose of requiring at least two clinical studies is not only to assure the *reproducibility* but also to provide valuable information regarding *generalizability*. Reproducibility is referred to as whether the clinical results are reproducible from location (e.g., study site) to location within

## 1.1. Regulatory Requirement

the same region or from region to region, while generalizability is referred to as whether the clinical results can be generalized to other similar patient populations within the same region or from region to region. When the sponsor of a newly developed or approved drug product is interested in getting the drug product into the marketplace from one region (e.g., where the drug product is developed and approved) to another region, it is a concern that differences in ethnic factors could alter the efficacy and safety of the drug product in the new region. As a result, it is recommended that a bridging study be conducted to generate a limited amount of clinical data in the new region in order to extrapolate the clinical data between the two regions (ICH, 1998a).

In practice, it is often of interest to determine whether a clinical trial that produced positive clinical results provides substantial evidence to assure reproducibility and generalizability of the clinical results. In this chapter, the reproducibility of a positive clinical result is studied by evaluating the probability of observing a positive result in a future clinical study with the same study protocol, given that a positive clinical result has been observed. The generalizability of clinical results observed from a clinical trial will be evaluated by means of a sensitivity analysis with respect to changes in mean and standard deviation of the primary clinical endpoints of the study.

### 1.1.4 Substantial Evidence with a Single Trial

Although the FDA requires that at least two adequate and well-controlled clinical trials be conducted for providing substantial evidence regarding the effectiveness of the drug product under investigation, a single trial may be accepted for regulatory approval under certain circumstances. In 1997, FDA published the *Modernization Act* (FDAMA), which includes a provision (Section 115 of FDAMA) to allow data from one adequate and well-controlled clinical trial investigation and confirmatory evidence to establish effectiveness for risk/benefit assessment of drug and biological candidates for approval under certain circumstances. This provision essentially codified an FDA policy that had existed for several years but whose application had been limited to some biological products approved by the Center for Biologic Evaluation and Research (CBER) of the FDA and a few pharmaceuticals, especially orphan drugs such as zidovudine and lamotrigine. As it can be seen from Table 1.1.2, a relatively strong significant result observed from a single clinical trial (say, p-value is less than 0.001) would have about 90% chance of reproducing the result in future clinical trials.

Consequently, a single clinical trial is sufficient to provide substantial evidence for demonstration of efficacy and safety of the medication under study. However, in 1998, FDA published a guidance which shed light on this

Table 1.1.2: Estimated Reproducibility Probability Based on Results from a Single Trial

| $t$-statistic | p-value | Reproducibility |
|---|---|---|
| 1.96 | 0.050 | 0.500 |
| 2.05 | 0.040 | 0.536 |
| 2.17 | 0.030 | 0.583 |
| 2.33 | 0.020 | 0.644 |
| 2.58 | 0.010 | 0.732 |
| 2.81 | 0.005 | 0.802 |
| 3.30 | 0.001 | 0.901 |

approach despite that the FDA has recognized that advances in sciences and practice of drug development may permit an expanded role for the single controlled trial in contemporary clinical development (FDA, 1998).

### 1.1.5 Sample Size

As the primary objective of most clinical trials is to demonstrate the effectiveness and safety of drug products under investigation, sample size calculation plays an important role at the planning stage to ensure that there are sufficient subjects for providing accurate and reliable assessment of the drug products with certain statistical assurance. In practice, hypotheses regarding medical or scientific questions of the study drug are usually formulated based on the primary study objectives. The hypotheses are then evaluated using appropriate statistical tests under a valid study design to ensure that the test results are accurate and reliable with certain statistical assurance. It should be noted that a valid sample size calculation can only be done based on appropriate statistical tests for the hypotheses that can reflect the study objectives under a valid study design. It is then suggested that the hypotheses be clearly stated when performing a sample size calculation. Each of the above hypotheses has different requirement for sample size in order to achieve a desired statistical assurance (e.g., 80% power or 95% assurance in precision).

Basically, sample size calculation can be classified into sample size estimation/determination, sample size justification, sample size adjustment, and sample size re-estimation. Sample size estimation/determination is referred to the calculation of required sample size for achieving some desired statistical assurance of accuracy and reliability such as an 80% power, while sample size justification is to provide statistical justification for a *selected* sample size, which is often a small number due to budget constraints and/or some medical considerations. In most clinical trials, sample size is necessarily adjusted for some factors such as dropouts or covariates in order to yield sufficient number of evaluable subjects for a valid statistical assessment of the study medicine. This type of sample size calculation is known as sample size adjustment. In many clinical trials, it may be desirable to conduct interim analyses (planned or unplanned) during the conduct of the trial. For clinical trials with planned or unplanned interim analyses, it is suggested that sample size be adjusted for controlling an overall type I error rate at the nominal significance level (e.g., 5%). In addition, when performing interim analyses, it is also desirable to perform sample size re-estimation based on cumulative information observed up to a specific time point to determine whether the selected sample size is sufficient to achieve a desired power at the end of the study. Sample size re-estimation may be performed in a blinded or unblinded fashion depending upon whether the process of sample size re-estimation will introduce bias to clinical evaluation of subjects beyond the time point at which the interim analysis or sample size re-estimation is performed. In this book, however, our emphasis will be placed on sample size estimation/determination. The concept can be easily applied to (i) sample size justification for a selected sample size, (ii) sample size adjustment with respect to some factors such as dropouts or covariates, and (iii) sample size re-estimation in clinical trials with planned or unplanned interim analyses.

## 1.2 Basic Considerations

In clinical research, sample size calculation may be performed based on precision analysis, power analysis, probability assessment, or other statistical inferences. To provide an accurate and reliable sample size calculation, it is suggested that an appropriate statistical test for the hypotheses of interest be derived under the study design. The hypotheses should be established to reflect the study objectives and should be able to address statistical/medical questions of interest under the study design. As a result, a typical procedure for sample size calculation is to determine or estimate sample size based on an appropriate statistical method or test, which is derived under the hypotheses and the study design, for testing the hypotheses in order to achieve a certain degree of statistical inference (e.g., 95% assurance or 80% power) on the effect of the test drug under investigation. As indicated earlier, in practice it is not uncommon to observe discrepancies among study objective (hypotheses), study design, statistical analysis (test statistic), and sample size calculation. These discrepancies certainly have an impact on sample size calculation in clinical research. Therefore, it is suggested that the following be carefully considered when performing sample size calculation: (i) the study objectives or the hypotheses of interest be clearly stated, (ii) a valid design with appropriate statistical tests be used, (iii) sample size be determined based on the test for the hypotheses of interest, and (iv) sample size be determined based on the primary study endpoint and (v) the clinically meaningful difference of the primary study endpoint that the clinical study is intended to detect.

### 1.2.1 Study Objectives

In clinical research, it is important to clearly state the study objectives of intended clinical trials. The objectives of clinical studies may include one or more of the following four objectives: (i) demonstrate/confirm efficacy, (ii) establish a safety profile, (iii) provide an adequate basis for assessing the benefit/risk relationship to support labeling, and (iv) establish the dose-response relationship (ICH, 1998b). Since most clinical studies are conducted for clinical evaluation of efficacy and safety of drug products under investigation, it is suggested that the following study objectives related to efficacy and safety be clarified before choosing an appropriate design strategy for the intended trial.

|  |  | Safety | | |
|---|---|---|---|---|
|  |  | Equivalence | Non-inferiority | Superiority |
| | Equivalence | E/E | E/N | E/S |
| Efficacy | Non-inferiority | N/E | N/N | N/S |
| | Superiority | S/E | S/N | S/S |

For example, if the intent of the planned clinical study is to develop an alternative therapy to the standard therapy that is quite toxic, then we may consider the strategy of E/S, which is to show that the test drug has equal efficacy but less toxicity (superior safety). The study objectives will certainly have an impact on the sample size calculation. Sample size calculation provides required sample size for achieving the study objectives.

### 1.2.2 Study Design

In clinical trials, different designs may be employed to achieve the study objectives. A valid study design is necessarily chosen to collect relevant clinical information for achieving the study objectives by addressing some statistical/medical hypotheses of interest, which are formulated to reflect the study objectives.

In clinical research, commonly employed study designs include parallel-group design, crossover design, enrichment design, and titration design (see,

## 1.2. Basic Considerations

e.g., Chow and Liu, 1998). The design strategy can certainly affect sample size calculation because statistical methods or tests are usually derived under the hypotheses and study design. As an example, Fleming (1990) discussed the following design strategies that are commonly used in clinical therapeutic equivalence/non-inferiority and superiority trials.

| Design | Description |
| --- | --- |
| Classical | STD + TEST versus STD |
| Active Control | TEST versus STD |
| Dual Purpose | TEST versus STD versus STD + TEST |

The classical design is to compare the combination of a test drug (TEST) and a standard therapy (STD) (i.e., STD + TEST) against STD to determine whether STD+TEST yields superior efficacy. When the intent is to determine whether a test drug could be used as an alternative to a standard therapy, one may consider an active control design involving direct randomization to either TEST or STD. This occurs frequently when STD is quite toxic and the intent is to develop an alternative therapy that is less toxic, yet equally efficacious. To achieve both objectives, a dual purpose design strategy is useful.

Note that in practice, a more complicated study design, which may consist of a combination of the above designs, may be chosen to address more complicated statistical/medical questions regarding the study drug. In this case, standard procedure for sample size calculation may not be directly applicable and a modification will be necessary.

### 1.2.3 Hypotheses

In most clinical trials, the primary study objective is usually related to the evaluation of the effectiveness and safety of a drug product. For example, it may be of interest to show that the study drug is effective and safe as compared to a placebo for some intended indications. In some cases, it may be of interest to show that the study drug is as effective as, superior to, or equivalent to an active control agent or a standard therapy. In practice, hypotheses regarding medical or scientific questions of the study drug are usually formulated based on the primary study objectives. The hypotheses are then evaluated using appropriate statistical tests under a valid study design.

In clinical trials, a hypothesis is usually referred to as a postulation, assumption, or statement that is made about the population regarding the effectiveness and safety of a drug under investigation. For example, the statement that there is a direct drug effect is a hypothesis regarding the treatment effect. For testing the hypotheses of interest, a random sample is usually drawn from the targeted population to evaluate hypotheses about the drug product. A statistical test is then performed to determine whether the null hypothesis would be rejected at a pre-specified significance level. Based on the test result, conclusion(s) regarding the hypotheses can be drawn. The selection of hypothesis depends upon the study objectives. In clinical research, commonly considered hypotheses include point hypotheses for testing equality and interval hypothesis for testing equivalence/non-inferiority and superiority, which are described below. A typical approach for demonstration of the efficacy and safety of a test drug under investigation is to test the following hypotheses

**Test for Equality**

$$H_0 : \mu_T = \mu_P \quad \text{versus} \quad H_a : \mu_T \neq \mu_P, \quad (1.2.1)$$

where $\mu_T$ and $\mu_P$ are the mean response of the outcome variable for the test drug and the placebo, respectively. We first show that there is a statistically significant difference between the test drug and the placebo by rejecting the null hypothesis, and then demonstrate that there is a high chance of correctly detecting a clinically meaningful difference if such difference truly exists.

**Test for Non-Inferiority**

In clinical trials, one may wish to show that the test drug is as effective as an active agent or a standard therapy. In this case, Blackwelder (1982) suggested testing the following hypotheses:

$$H_0 : \mu_S - \mu_T \geq \delta \quad \text{versus} \quad H_a : \mu_S - \mu_T < \delta, \quad (1.2.2)$$

where $\mu_S$ is the mean for a standard therapy and $\delta$ is a difference of clinical importance. The concept is to reject the null hypothesis and conclude that the difference between the test drug and the standard therapy is less than a clinically meaningful difference $\delta$ and hence the test drug is as effective as the standard therapy. This study objective is not uncommon in clinical trials especially when the test drug is considered to be less toxic, easier to administer, or less expensive than the established standard therapy.

**Test for Superiority**

To show superiority of a test drug over an active control agent or a standard therapy, we may consider the following hypotheses:

$$H_0 : \mu_T - \mu_S \leq \delta \quad \text{versus} \quad H_a : \mu_T - \mu_S > \delta. \quad (1.2.3)$$

## 1.2. Basic Considerations

The rejection of the above null hypothesis suggests that the difference between the test drug and the standard therapy is greater than a clinically meaningful difference. Therefore, we may conclude that the test drug is superior to the standard therapy by rejecting the null hypothesis of (1.2.3). Note that the above hypotheses are also known as hypotheses for testing *clinical* superiority. When $\delta = 0$, the above hypotheses are usually referred to as hypotheses for testing *statistical* superiority.

**Test for Equivalence**

In practice, unless there is some prior knowledge regarding the test drug, usually we do not know the performance of the test drug as compared to the standard therapy. Therefore, hypotheses (1.2.2) and (1.2.3) are not preferred because they have pre-determined the performance of the test drug as compared the standard therapy. As an alternative, the following hypotheses for therapeutic equivalence are usually considered:

$$H_0 : |\mu_T - \mu_S| \geq \delta \quad \text{versus} \quad H_a : |\mu_T - \mu_S| < \delta. \quad (1.2.4)$$

We then conclude that the difference between the test drug and the standard therapy is of no clinical importance if the null hypothesis of (1.2.4) is rejected.

It should be noted that a valid sample size calculation can only be done based on appropriate statistical tests for the hypotheses that can reflect the study objectives under a valid study design. It is then suggested that the hypotheses be clearly stated when performing a sample size calculation. Each of the above hypotheses has different requirement for sample size in order to achieve a desired power or precision of the corresponding tests.

### 1.2.4 Primary Study Endpoint

A study objective (hypotheses) will define what study variable is to be considered as the primary clinical endpoint and what comparisons or investigations are deemed most clinically relevant. The primary clinical endpoints depend upon therapeutic areas and the indications that the test drugs sought for. For example, for coronary artery disease/angina in cardiovascular system, patient mortality is the most important clinical endpoint in clinical trials assessing the beneficial effects of drugs on coronary artery disease. For congestive heart failure, patient mortality, exercise tolerance, the number of hospitalizations, and cardiovascular morbidity are common endpoints in trials assessing the effects of drugs in congestive heart failure, while mean change from baseline in systolic and diastolic blood pressure and cardiovascular mortality and morbidity are commonly used in hypertension trials. Other examples include change in forced expiratory volume in 1 second ($FEV_1$) for asthma in respiratory system, cognitive and functional scales specially designed to assess Alzheimer's disease and Parkinson's disease in central nervous system, tender joints and pain-function endpoints (e.g., Western Ontario and McMaster University Osteoarithritis Index) for osteoarthritis in musculoskeletal system, and the incidence of bone fracture for osteoporosis in the endocrine system.

It can be seen from the above that the efficacy of a test drug in treatment of a certain disease may be characterized through multiple clinical endpoints. Capizzi and Zhang (1996) classify the clinical endpoints into primary, secondary, and tertiary endpoints. Endpoints that satisfy the following criteria are considered primary endpoints: (i) should be of biological and/or clinical importance, (ii) should form the basis of the objectives of the trial, (iii) should not be highly correlated, (iv) should have sufficient power for the statistical hypotheses formulated from the objectives of the trial, and (v) should be relatively few (e.g., at most 4). Sample size calculation based on detecting a difference in some or all primary clinical endpoints may result in a high chance of false positive and false negative results for evaluation of the test drug. Thus, it is suggested that sample size calculation should be performed based on a single primary study endpoint under certain assumption of the single primary endpoint. More discussion regarding the issue of false positive and false negative rates caused by multiple primary endpoints can be found in Chow and Liu (1998).

## 1.2.5 Clinically Meaningful Difference

In clinical research, the determination of a clinically meaningful difference, denoted by $\delta$, is critical in clinical trials such as equivalence/non-inferiority trials. In therapeutic equivalence trials, $\delta$ is known as the equivalence limit, while $\delta$ is referred to as the non-inferiority margin in non-inferiority trials. The non-inferiority margin reflects the degree of inferiority of the test drug under investigation as compared to the standard therapy that the trials attempts to exclude.

A different choice of $\delta$ may affect the sample size calculation and may alter the conclusion of clinical results. Thus, the choice of $\delta$ is critical at the planning stage of a clinical study. In practice, there is no gold rule for determination of $\delta$ in clinical trials. As indicated in the ICH E10 Draft Guideline, the non-inferiority margin cannot be chosen to be greater than the smallest effect size that the active drug would be reliably expected to have compared with placebo in the setting of the planned trial, but may be smaller based on clinical judgment (ICH, 1999). The ICH E10 Guideline suggests that the non-inferiority margin be identified based on past experience in placebo control trials of adequate design under conditions similar to those planned for the new trial. In addition, the ICH E10 Guideline emphasizes that the determination of $\delta$ should be based on both statistical reasoning and clinical judgment, which should not only reflect uncertainties in the evidence on which the choice is based, but also be suitably conservative.

In some cases, regulatory agencies do provide clear guidelines for selection of an appropriate $\delta$ for clinical trials. For example, as indicated by Huque and Dubey (1990), the FDA proposed some non-inferiority margins for some clinical endpoints (binary responses) such as cure rate for anti-infective drug products (e.g., topical antifungals or vaginal antifungals). These limits are given in Table 1.2.1. For example, if the cure rate is between 80% and 90%, it is suggested that the non-inferiority margin or a clinically meaningful difference be chosen as $\delta = 15\%$.

On the other hand, for bioequivalence trials with healthy volunteers, the margin of $\delta = \log(1.25)$ for mean difference on log-transformed data such as area under the blood or plasma concentration-time curve (AUC) or maximum concentration $C_{\max}$ is considered (FDA, 2001).

In clinical trials, the choice of $\delta$ may depend upon absolute change, percent change, or effect size of the primary study endpoint. In practice, a standard effect size (i.e., effect size adjusted for standard deviation) between 0.25 and 0.5 is usually chosen as $\delta$ if no prior knowledge regarding clinical performance of the test drug is available. This recommendation is made based on the fact that the standard effect size of clinical importance observed from most clinical trials is within the range of 0.25 and 0.5.

## 1.3 Procedures for Sample Size Calculation

In practice, sample size may be determined based on either precision analysis or power analysis. Precision analysis and power analysis for sample size determination are usually performed by controlling type I error (or confi-

Table 1.2.1: Non-Inferiority Margins for Binary Responses

| $\delta$ (%) | Response Rate for the Active Control (%) |
|---|---|
| 20 | 50-80 |
| 15 | 80-90 |
| 10 | 90-95 |
| 5 | > 95 |

Source: FDA Anti-Infectives Drug Guideline

dence level) and type II error (or power), respectively. In what follows, we will first introduce the concepts of type I and type II errors.

### 1.3.1 Type I and Type II Errors

In practice, two kinds of errors occur when testing hypotheses. If the null hypothesis is rejected when it is true, then a type I error has occurred. If the null hypothesis is not rejected when it is false, then a type II error has been made. The probabilities of making type I and type II errors, denoted by $\alpha$ and $\beta$, respectively, are given below:

$$\alpha = P\{\text{type I error}\}$$
$$= P\{\text{reject } H_0 \text{ when } H_0 \text{ is true}\},$$
$$\beta = P\{\text{type II error}\}$$
$$= P\{\text{fail to reject } H_0 \text{ when } H_0 \text{ is false}\}.$$

An upper bound for $\alpha$ is a significance level of the test procedure. Power of the test is defined as the probability of correctly rejecting the null hypothesis when the null hypothesis is false, i.e.,

$$\text{Power} = 1 - \beta$$
$$= P\{\text{reject } H_0 \text{ when } H_0 \text{ is false}\}.$$

As an example, suppose one wishes to test the following hypotheses:

$$H_0 : \text{The drug is ineffective} \quad \text{versus} \quad H_a : \text{The drug is effective}.$$

Then, a type I error occurs if we conclude that the drug is effective when in fact it is not. On the other hand, a type II error occurs if we claim that the drug is ineffective when in fact it is effective. In clinical trials, none of these errors is desirable. With a fixed sample size a typical approach is to avoid a type I error but at the same time to decrease a type II error so that there is a high chance of correctly detecting a drug effect when the drug is indeed effective. Typically, when the sample size is fixed, $\alpha$ decreases as $\beta$ increases and $\alpha$ increases as $\beta$ decreases. The only approach to decrease both $\alpha$ and $\beta$ is to increase the sample size. Sample size is usually determined by controlling both type I error (or confidence level) and type II error (or power).

In what follows, we will introduce the concepts of precision analysis and power analysis for sample size determination based on type I error and type II error, respectively.

## 1.3.2  Precision Analysis

In practice, the maximum probability of committing a type I error that one can tolerate is usually considered as the level of significance. The confidence level, $1-\alpha$, then reflects the probability or confidence of not rejecting the true null hypothesis. Since the confidence interval approach is equivalent to the method of hypotheses testing, we may determine sample size required based on type I error rate using the confidence interval approach. For a $(1-\alpha)100\%$ confidence interval, the precision of the interval depends on its width. The narrower the interval is, the more precise the inference is. Therefore, the precision analysis for sample size determination is to consider the maximum half width of the $(1-\alpha)100\%$ confidence interval of the unknown parameter that one is willing to accept. Note that the maximum half width of the confidence interval is usually referred to as the *maximum error* of an estimate of the unknown parameter. For example, let $y_1, y_2, ..., y_n$ be independent and identically distributed normal random variables with mean $\mu$ and variance $\sigma^2$. When $\sigma^2$ is known, a $(1-\alpha)100\%$ confidence interval for $\mu$ can be obtained as

$$\bar{y} \pm z_{\alpha/2}\frac{\sigma}{\sqrt{n}},$$

where $z_{\alpha/2}$ is the upper $(\alpha/2)$th quantile of the standard normal distribution. The maximum error, denoted by $E$, in estimating the value of $\mu$ that one is willing to accept is then defined as

$$E = |\bar{y} - \mu| = z_{\alpha/2}\frac{\sigma}{\sqrt{n}}.$$

Thus, the sample size required can be chosen as

$$n = \frac{z_{\alpha/2}^2 \sigma^2}{E^2}. \qquad (1.3.1)$$

Note that the maximum error approach for choosing n is to attain a specified precision while estimating $\mu$ which is derived based only on the interest of type I error. A nonparametric approach can be obtained by using the following Chebyshev's inequality

$$P\{|\bar{y} - \mu| \leq E\} \geq 1 - \frac{\sigma^2}{nE^2},$$

and hence

$$n = \frac{\sigma^2}{\alpha E^2}. \qquad (1.3.2)$$

Note that the precision analysis for sample size determination is very easy to apply either based on (1.3.1) or (1.3.2). For example, suppose we wish to have a 95% assurance that the error in the estimated mean is less than 10% of the standard deviation (i.e., $0.1\sigma$). Thus

$$z_{\alpha/2}\frac{\sigma}{\sqrt{n}} = 0.1\sigma.$$

Hence

$$n = \frac{z_{\alpha/2}^2 \sigma^2}{E^2} = \frac{(1.96)^2 \sigma^2}{(0.1\sigma)^2} = 384.2 \approx 385.$$

The above concept can be applied to binary data (or proportions). In addition, it can be easily implemented for sample size determination when comparing two treatments.

### 1.3.3 Power Analysis

Since a type I error is usually considered to be a more important and/or serious error which one would like to avoid, a typical approach in hypothesis testing is to control $\alpha$ at an acceptable level and try to minimize $\beta$ by choosing an appropriate sample size. In other words, the null hypothesis can be tested at pre-determined level (or nominal level) of significance with a desired power. This concept for determination of sample size is usually referred to as *power analysis* for sample size determination.

For determination of sample size based on power analysis, the investigator is required to specify the following information. First of all, select a significance level at which the chance of wrongly concluding that a difference exists when in fact there is no real difference (type I error) one is willing to tolerate. Typically, a 5% level of significance is chosen to reflect a 95% confidence regarding the unknown parameter. Secondly, select a desired power at which the chance of correctly detecting a difference when the difference truly exists one wishes to achieve. A conventional choice of power is either 90% or 80%. Thirdly, specify a clinically meaningful difference. In most clinical trials, the objective is to demonstrate effectiveness and safety of a drug under study as compared to a placebo. Therefore, it is important to specify what difference in terms of the primary endpoint is considered of clinical or scientific importance. Denote such a difference by $\Delta$. If the investigator will settle for detecting only a large difference, then fewer subjects will be needed. If the difference is relatively small, a larger study group (i.e., a larger number of subjects) will be needed. Finally, the knowledge regarding the standard deviation (i.e., $\sigma$) of the primary endpoint considered in the study is also required for sample size determination. A very precise method of measurement (i.e., a small $\sigma$) will permit detection of any given difference with a much smaller sample size than would be required with a less precise measurement.

## 1.3. Procedures for Sample Size Calculation

Suppose there are two group of observations, namely $x_i, i = 1, ..., n_1$ (treatment) and $y_i, i = 1, ..., n_2$ (control). Assume that $x_i$ and $y_i$ are independent and normally distributed with means $\mu_1$ and $\mu_2$ and variances $\sigma_1^2$ and $\sigma_2^2$, respectively. Suppose the hypotheses of interest are

$$H_0 : \mu_1 = \mu_2 \quad \text{versus} \quad H_1 : \mu_1 \neq \mu_2.$$

For simplicity and illustration purpose, we assume (i) $\sigma_1^2$ and $\sigma_2^2$ are known, which may be estimated from pilot studies or historical data, and (ii) $n_1 = n_2 = n$. Under these assumptions, a Z-statistic can be used to test the mean difference. The Z-test is given by

$$Z = \frac{\bar{x} - \bar{y}}{\sqrt{\frac{\sigma_1^2}{n} + \frac{\sigma_2^2}{n}}}.$$

Under the null hypothesis of no treatment difference, $Z$ is distributed as $N(0, 1)$. Hence, we reject the null hypothesis when

$$|Z| > z_{\alpha/2}.$$

Under the alternative hypothesis that $\mu_1 = \mu_2 + \delta$ (without loss of generality we assume $\delta > 0$), a clinically meaningful difference, $Z$ is distributed as $N(\mu^*, 1)$, where

$$\mu^* = \frac{\delta}{\sqrt{\frac{\sigma_1^2}{n} + \frac{\sigma_2^2}{n}}} > 0.$$

The corresponding power is then given by

$$P\left\{|N(\mu^*, 1)| > z_{\alpha/2}\right\} \approx P\left\{N(\mu^*, 1) > z_{\alpha/2}\right\}$$
$$= P\left\{N(0, 1) > z_{\alpha/2} - \mu^*\right\}.$$

To achieve the desired power of $(1 - \beta)100\%$, we set

$$z_{\alpha/2} - \mu^* = -z_\beta.$$

This leads to

$$n = \frac{(\sigma_1^2 + \sigma_2^2)(z_{\alpha/2} + z_\beta)^2}{\delta^2}. \quad (1.3.3)$$

To apply the above formula for sample size calculation, consider a double-blind, placebo-controlled clinical trial. Suppose the objective of the study is to compare a test drug with a control and the standard deviation for the treatment group is 1 (i.e., $\sigma_1 = 1$) and the standard deviation of the control group is 2 (i.e., $\sigma_2 = 2$). Then, by choosing $\alpha = 5\%$, and $\beta = 10\%$, we have

$$n = \frac{(\sigma_1^2 + \sigma_2^2)(z_{\alpha/2} + z_\beta)^2}{\delta^2} = \frac{(1^2 + 2^2)(1.96 + 1.28)^2}{1^2} \approx 53.$$

Thus, a total of 106 subjects is required for achieving a 90% power for detection of a clinically meaningful difference of $\delta = 1$ at the 5% level of significance.

## 1.3.4 Probability Assessment

In practice, sample size calculation based on power analysis for detecting a small difference in the incidence rate of rare events (e.g., 3 per 10,000) may not be appropriate. In this case, a very large sample size is required to observe a single event, which is not practical. In addition, small difference in the incidence rate (e.g., 2 per 10,000 versus 3 per 10,000) may not be of practical/clinical interest. Alternatively, it may be of interest to justify the sample size based on a probability statement, e.g., there is a certain assurance (say $(1-\epsilon)100\%$) that the mean incidence rate of the treatment group is less than that of the control group with probability $(1-\alpha)100\%$.

Suppose there are two groups of observations, namely $x_i, i = 1, \cdots, n$ (treatment) and $y_i, i = 1, \cdots, n$ (control). Assume that $x_i$ and $y_i$ are independent and identically distributed as Bernoulli random variables with mean $p_1$ and $p_2$, i.e., $B(1, p_1)$ and $B(1, p_2)$, respectively, and that

$$P(\bar{x} \leq \bar{y}|n) + P(\bar{x} > \bar{y}|n) = 1$$

for large $n$. Then

$$P(\bar{x} < \bar{y}|n) = p.$$

The hypotheses of interest are

$$H_0 : p \notin (\epsilon, 1) \quad \text{versus} \quad H_1 : p \in (\epsilon, 1),$$

for some $\epsilon > 0$, where $p = P(\bar{x} = \bar{y}|n)$ for some $n$. A test for the hypothesis that $p \in (\epsilon, 1)$ is

$$\phi(x, y) = I(\bar{x} < \bar{y}).$$

We then reject the null hypothesis if $\phi(x, y) = 1$. Then, given $p_1 < p_2$, the power is given by

$$\begin{aligned}
\text{Power} &= P(\bar{x} < \bar{y}) \\
&= P\left( \frac{\bar{x} - \bar{y} - (p_1 - p_2)}{\sqrt{\frac{p_1(1-p_1)+p_2(1-p_2)}{n}}} < \frac{p_2 - p_1}{\sqrt{\frac{p_1(1-p_1)+p_2(1-p_2)}{n}}} \right) \\
&\approx \Phi\left( \frac{p_2 - p_1}{\sqrt{\frac{p_1(1-p_1)+p_2(1-p_2)}{n}}} \right).
\end{aligned}$$

Therefore, for a given power $1 - \beta$, the sample size, $n$, can be estimated by letting

$$\frac{(p_2 - p_1)}{\sqrt{\frac{p_1(1-p_1)+p_2(1-p_2)}{n}}} = z_\beta,$$

## 1.3. Procedures for Sample Size Calculation

which gives
$$n = \frac{z_\beta^2 [p_1(1-p_1) + p_2(1-p_2)]}{(p_2 - p_1)^2}.$$

To illustrate the above procedure, consider a double-blind, active-control trial. The objective of this trial is to compare a test drug with a reference drug (active control). Suppose the event rate of the reference drug is 0.075 and the event rate of the test drug is 0.030. Then, with $\beta = 10\%$, we have
$$n = \frac{1.28^2(0.075 \times (1 - 0.075) + 0.030 \times (1 - 0.030))}{(0.075 - 0.030)^2} \approx 80.$$

Thus, a total of 160 subjects is needed in order to achieve a 90% power for observing less accident rate in test drug group.

### 1.3.5 Reproducibility Probability

As indicated, current regulation for approval of a test drug under investigation requires at least two adequate and well-controlled clinical trials be conducted for proving substantial evidence regarding the effectiveness and safety of the drug product. Shao and Chow (2002) investigated the probability of reproducibility of the second trial and developed an estimated power approach. As a result, sample size calculation of the second clinical trial can be performed based on the concept of reproducibility probability. Suppose these are two group of observations obtained in the first trial, namely, $x_{1i}, i = 1, ..., n_1$ (treatment) and $x_{2i}, i = 1, ..., n_2$ (control). Assume that $x_{1i}$ and $x_{2i}$ are independent and normally distributed with means $\mu_1$ and $\mu_2$ and common variances $\sigma^2$, respectively. The hypotheses of interest are
$$H_0: \mu_1 = \mu_2 \quad \text{versus} \quad H_1: \mu_1 \neq \mu_2.$$

When $\sigma^2$ is known, we reject $H_0$ at the 5% level of significance if and only if $|T| > t_{n-2}$, where $t_{n-2}$ is the $(1-\alpha/2)$th percentile of the $t$-distribution with $n - 2$ degrees of freedom, $n = n_1 + n_2$,
$$T = \frac{\bar{x}_1 - \bar{x}_2}{\sqrt{\frac{(n_1-1)s_1^2 + (n_2-1)s_2^2}{n-2}} \sqrt{\frac{1}{n_1} + \frac{1}{n_2}}},$$

and $\bar{x}_i$ and $s_i^2$ are the sample means and variances calculated based on data from the $i$th group, respectively. Thus, the power of $T$ is given by
$$\begin{aligned} p(\theta) &= P(|T(y)| > t_{n-2}) \\ &= 1 - T_{n-2}(t_{n-2}|\theta) + T_{n-2}(-t_{n-2}|\theta), \end{aligned} \quad (1.3.4)$$

where

$$\theta = \frac{\mu_1 - \mu_2}{\sigma\sqrt{\frac{1}{n_1} + \frac{1}{n_2}}}$$

and $T_{n-2}(\cdot|\theta)$ denotes the distribution function of the $t$-distribution with $n-2$ degrees of freedom and the non-centrality parameter $\theta$. Let $x$ be the observed data from the first trial and $T(x)$ be the value of $T$ based on $x$. Replacing $\theta$ in the power in (1.3.4) by its estimate $T(x)$, the estimated power

$$\hat{P} = p(T(x)) = 1 - T_{n-2}(t_{n-2}|T(x)) + T_{n-2}(-t_{n-2}|T(x)),$$

is defined by Shao and Chow (2002) as a reproducibility probability for the second trial. Based on this concept, sample size calculation for the second trial can be obtained as

$$n^* = \frac{(T^*/\Delta T)^2}{\frac{1}{4n_1} + \frac{1}{4n_2}},$$

where $T^*$ is the value obtained such that a desired reproducibility probability is attained and $\Delta$ is given by

$$\Delta = \frac{1 + \epsilon/(\mu_1 - \mu_2)}{C},$$

where $\epsilon$ and $C$ reflect the population mean and variance changes in the second trial. In other words, in the second trial it is assumed that the population mean difference is changed from $\mu_1 - \mu_2$ to $\mu_1 - \mu_2 + \epsilon$ and the population variance is changed from $\sigma^2$ to $C^2\sigma^2$, where $C > 0$.

### 1.3.6 Sample Size Re-Estimation Without Unblinding

In clinical trials, it is desirable to perform a sample size re-estimation based on clinical data accumulated up to the time point. If the re-estimated sample size is bigger than the originally planned sample size, then it is necessary to increase the sample size in order to achieve the desired power at the end of the trial. On the other hand, if the re-estimated sample size is smaller than the originally planned sample size, a sample size reduction is justifiable. Basically, sample size re-estimation involves either unblinding or without unblinding of the treatment codes. In practice, it is undesirable to perform sample size re-estimation with unblinding of the treatment codes as even the significance level will be adjusted for potential statistical penalty for the unblinding. Thus, sample size re-estimation without unblinding the treatment codes has become very attractive. Shih (1993) and Shih and Zhao (1997) proposed some procedures without unblinding for sample size re-estimation within interim data for double-blinded clinical trials with binary outcomes. Detailed procedure for sample size re-estimation with unblinding will be given in Chapter 8.

In practice, it is suggested that a procedure for sample size re-estimation be specified in the study protocol and should be performed by an external statistician who is independent of the project team. It is also recommended that a data monitoring committee (DMC) be considered to maintain the scientific validity and integrity of the clinical trial when performing sample size re-estimation at the interim stage of the trial. More details regarding sample size re-estimation are provided in Chapter 8.

## 1.4 Aims and Structure of the Book

### 1.4.1 Aim of the Book

As indicated earlier, sample size calculation plays an important role in clinical research. Sample size calculation is usually performed using an appropriate statistical test for the hypotheses of interest to achieve a desired power for detection of a clinically meaningful difference. The hypotheses should be established to reflect the study objectives for clinical investigation under the study design. In practice, however, it is not uncommon to observe discrepancies among study objectives (or hypotheses), study design, statistical analysis (or test statistic), and sample size calculation. These inconsistencies often result in (i) wrong test for right hypotheses, (ii) right test for wrong hypotheses, (iii) wrong test for wrong hypotheses, or (iv) right test for right hypotheses with insufficient power. Therefore, the aim of this book is to provide a comprehensive and unified presentation of statistical concepts and methods for sample size calculation in various situations in clinical research. Moreover, the book will focus on the interactions between clinicians and biostatisticians that often occur during various phases of clinical research and development. This book is also intended to give a well-balanced summarization of current and emerging clinical issues and recently developed statistical methodologies in the area of sample size calculation in clinical research. Although this book is written from a viewpoint of clinical research and development, the principles and concepts presented in this book can also be applied to a non-clinical setting.

### 1.4.2 Structure of the Book

It is our goal to provide a comprehensive reference book for clinical researchers, pharmaceutical scientists, clinical or medical research associates, clinical programmers or data coordinators, and biostatisticians in the areas of clinical research and development, regulatory agencies, and academia.

The scope of this book covers sample size calculation for studies that may be conducted during various phases of clinical research and development. Basically, this book consists of eighteen chapters which are outlined below.

Chapter 1 provides a brief introduction and a review of regulatory requirement regarding sample size calculation in clinical research for drug development. Also included in this chapter are statistical procedures for sample size calculation based on precision analysis, power analysis, probability assessment, and reproducibility probability. Chapter 2 covers some statistical considerations such as the concept of confounding and interaction, a one-sided test versus or a two-sided test in clinical research, a crossover design versus a parallel design, subgroup/interim analysis, and data transformation. Also included in this chapter are unequal treatment allocation, adjustment for dropouts or covariates, the effect of mixed-up treatment codes, treatment or center imbalance, multiplicity, multiple-stage design for early stopping, and sample size calculation based on rare incidence rate.

Chapter 3 focuses on sample size calculation for comparing means with one sample, two samples, and multiple samples. Formulas are derived under different hypotheses testing for equality, superiority, non-inferiority, and equivalence with equal or unequal treatment allocation. In addition, sample size calculation based on Bayesian approach is also considered in this chapter. Chapter 4 deals with sample size calculation for comparing proportions based on large sample tests. Formulas for sample size calculation are derived under different hypotheses testing for equality, superiority, non-inferiority, and equivalence with equal or unequal treatment allocation. In addition, issues in sample size calculation based on the confidence interval of the relative risk and/or odds ratio between treatments are also examined.

Chapter 5 considers sample size calculation for binary responses based on exact tests such as the binomial test and Fisher's exact test. Also included in this chapter are optimal and flexible multiple-stage designs that are commonly employed in phase II cancer trials. The emphasis of Chapter 6 is placed on tests for contingency tables such as the goodness of fit test and test for independence. Procedures for sample size calculation are derived under different hypotheses for testing equality, superiority, non-inferiority, and equivalence with equal or unequal treatment allocation.

Chapter 7 provides sample size calculation for comparing time-to-event data using Cox's proportional hazards model and weighted log-rank test. Formulas are derived under different hypotheses testing for equality, superiority, non-inferiority, and equivalence with equal or unequal treatment allocation. Chapter 8 considers the problems of sample size estimation and re-estimation in group sequential trials with various alpha spending functions. Also included in this chapter are the study of conditional power for as-

## 1.4. Aims and Structure of the Book

sessment of futility and a proposed procedure for sample size re-estimation without unblinding.

Chapter 9 discusses statistical methods and the corresponding sample size calculation for comparing intra-subject variabilities, intra-subject coefficient of variations (CV), inter-subject variabilities, and total variabilities under replicated crossover designs and parallel-group designs with replicates. Chapter 10 summarizes sample size calculation for assessment of population bioequivalence, individual bioequivalence, and *in vitro* bioequivalence under replicated crossover designs as suggested in the FDA 2001 guidance (FDA, 2001).

Chapter 11 summarizes sample size calculation for dose ranging studies including the determination of minimum effective dose (MED) and maximum tolerable dose (MTD). Chapter 12 considers sample size calculation for microarray studies controlling false discovery rate (FDR) and family-wise error rate (FWER). Bayesian sample size calculation is discussed in Chapter 13. Sample size calculation based on nonparametrics for comparing means with one or two samples is discussed in Chapter 14. Chapter 15 includes sample size calculations in other areas of clinical research such as QT/QTc studies, the use of propensity score analysis in non-randomized or observational studies, analysis of variance with repeated measurements, quality of life assessment, bridging studies, and vaccine clinical trials.

For each chapter, whenever possible, real examples concerning clinical studies of various therapeutic areas are included to demonstrate the clinical and statistical concepts, interpretations, and their relationships and interactions. Comparisons regarding the relative merits and disadvantages of statistical methods for sample size calculation in various therapeutic areas are discussed whenever deem appropriate. In addition, if applicable, topics for future research development are provided.

# Chapter 2

# Considerations Prior to Sample Size Calculation

As indicated in the previous chapter, sample size calculation should be performed using appropriate statistical methods or tests for hypotheses which can reflect the study objectives under the study design based on the primary study endpoint of the intended trial. As a result, some information including study design, hypotheses, mean response and the associated variability of the primary study endpoint, and the desired power at a specified $\alpha$ level of significance are required when performing sample size calculation. For good statistics practice, some statistical considerations such as stratification with respect to possible confounding/interaction factors, the use of a one-sided test or a two-sided test, the choice of a parallel design or a crossover design, subgroup/interim analyses and data transformation are important for performing an accurate and reliable sample size calculation. In addition, some practical issues that are commonly encountered in clinical trials, which may have an impact on sample size calculation, should also be taken into consideration when performing sample size calculation. These practical issues include unequal treatment allocation, adjustment for dropouts or covariates, mixed-up treatment codes, treatment study center imbalance, multiplicity, multiple-stage for early stopping, and sample size calculation based on rare incidence rate.

In the next section, we introduce the concepts of confounding and interaction effects in clinical trials. Section 2.2 discusses the controversial issues between the use of a one-sided test and a two-sided test in clinical research. In Section 2.3, we summarize the difference in sample size calculation between a crossover design and a parallel design. The concepts of group sequential boundaries and alpha spending function in subgroup/interim analysis in clinical trials are discussed in Section 2.4. Section 2.5 clarifies some issues that are commonly seen in sample size calculation based on transformed data such as log-transformed data under a parallel design or a crossover design. Section 2.6 provides a discussion regarding some practical issues that have impact on sample size calculation in clinical trials. These issues include unequal treatment allocation in randomization, sample size adjustment for dropouts or covariates, the effect of mixed-up treatment codes during the conduct of clinical trials, the loss in power for treatment and/or center imbalance, the issue of multiplicity in multiple primary endpoints and/or multiple comparisons, multiple-stage design for early stopping, and sample size calculation based on rare incidence rate in safety assessment.

## 2.1 Confounding and Interaction

### 2.1.1 Confounding

Confounding effects are defined as effects contributed by various factors that cannot be separated by the design under study (Chow and Liu, 1998). *Confounding* is an important concept in clinical research. When confounding effects are observed in a clinical trial, the treatment effect cannot be assessed because it is contaminated by other effects contributed by various factors.

In clinical trials, there are many sources of variation that have an impact on the primary clinical endpoints for clinical evaluation of a test drug under investigation. If some of these variations are not identified and not properly controlled, they can become mixed in with the treatment effect that the trial is designed to demonstrate, in which case the treatment effect is said to be confounded by effects due to these variations. In clinical trials, there are many subtle, unrecognizable, and seemingly innocent confounding factors that can cause ruinous results of clinical trials. Moses (1992) gives the example of the devastating result in the confounder being the personal choice of a patient. The example concerns a polio-vaccine trial that was conducted on two million children worldwide to investigate the effect of Salk poliomyelitis vaccine. This trial reported that the incidence rate of polio was lower in the children whose parents refused injection than in those who received placebo after their parent gave permission (Meier, 1989). After an exhaustive examination of the data, it was found that susceptibility to poliomyelitis was related to the differences between families who gave the permission and those who did not. Therefore, it is not clear whether the effect of the incidence rate is due to the effect of Salk poliomyelitis vaccine or due to the difference between families giving permission.

### 2.1.2 Interaction

An interaction effect between factors is defined as a joint effect with one or more contributing factors (Chow and Liu, 1998). *Interaction* is also an important concept in clinical research. The objective of a statistical interaction investigation is to conclude whether the joint contribution of two or more factors is the same as the sum of the contributions from each factor when considered alone. When interactions among factors are observed, an overall assessment on the treatment effect is not appropriate. In this case, it is suggested that the treatment must be carefully evaluated for those effects contributed by the factors.

In clinical research, almost all adequate and well-controlled clinical trials are multicenter trials. For multicenter trials, the FDA requires that the treatment-by-center interaction be examined to evaluate whether the treatment effect is consistent across all centers. As a result, it is suggested that statistical tests for homogeneity across centers (i.e., for detecting treatment-by-center interaction) be provided. The significant level used to declare the significance of a given test for a treatment-by-center interaction should be considered in light of the sample size involved. Gail and Simon (1985) classify the nature of interaction as either quantitative or qualitative. A quantitative interaction between treatment and center indicates that the treatment differences are in the same direction across centers but the magnitude differs from center to center, while a qualitative interaction reveals that substantial treatment differences occur in different directions in different centers. More discussion regarding treatment-by-center interaction can be found in Chow and Shao (2002).

### 2.1.3 Remark

In clinical trials, a stratified randomization is usually employed with respect to some prognostic factors or covariates, which may have confounding and interaction effects on the evaluation of the test drug under investigation. Confounding or interaction effects may alter the conclusion of the evaluation of the test drug under investigation. Thus, a stratified randomization is desirable if the presence of the confounding and/or interaction effects of some factors is doubtful. In practice, although sample size calculation according to some stratification factors can be similarly performed within each combination of the stratification factors, it is not desirable to have too many stratification factors. Therefore, it is suggested that the possible confounding and/or interaction effects of the stratification factors should be carefully evaluated before a sample size calculation is performed and a stratified randomization is carried out.

## 2.2 One-Sided Test Versus Two-Sided Test

In clinical research, it has been a long discussion regarding whether a one-sided test or a two-sided test should be used for clinical evaluation of a test drug under investigation. Sample size calculations based on a one-sided test and a two-sided test are different at a fixed $\alpha$ level of significance. As it can be seen from (1.3.3), sample size for comparing the two means can be obtained as

$$n = \frac{(\sigma_1^2 + \sigma_2^2)(z_{\alpha/2} + z_\beta)^2}{\delta^2}.$$

When $\sigma_1^2 = \sigma_2^2 = \sigma^2$, the above formula reduces to

$$n = \frac{2\sigma^2(z_{\alpha/2} + z_\beta)^2}{\delta^2}.$$

If $\delta = c\sigma$, then the sample size formula can be rewritten as

$$n = \frac{2(z_{\alpha/2} + z_\beta)^2}{c^2}.$$

Table 2.2.1 provides a comparison for sample sizes obtained based on a one-sided test or a two-sided test at the $\alpha$ level of significance. The results indicate that sample size may be reduced by about 21% when switching from a two-sided test to a one-sided test for testing at the 5% level of significance with an 80% power for detection of a difference of 0.5 standard deviation.

The pharmaceutical industry prefers a one-sided test for demonstration of clinical superiority based on the argument that they will not run a study if the test drug would be worse. In practice, however, many drug products such as drug products in central nervous system may show a superior placebo effect as compared to the drug effect. This certainly argues against the use of a one-sided test. Besides, a one sided test allows more *bad* drug products to be approved because of chances as compared to a two-sided test.

As indicated earlier, the FDA requires that at least two adequate and well-controlled clinical studies be conducted to provide substantial evidence regarding the effectiveness and safety of a test drug under investigation. For each of the two adequate and well-controlled clinical trials, suppose the test drug is evaluated at the 5% level of significance. Table 2.2.2 provides a summary of comparison between one-sided test and two-sided test in clinical research. For the one-sided test procedure, the false positive rate is one out of 400 trials (i.e., 0.25%) for the two trials, while the false positive rate is one out of 1,600 trials (i.e., 0.0625%) for two trials when applying a two-sided test.

## 2.2. One-Sided Test Versus Two-Sided Test

Table 2.2.1: Sample Sizes Based on One-Sided Test and Two-Sided Test At $\alpha$-level of Significance

|  |  | One-sided Test | | Two-sided Test | |
| --- | --- | --- | --- | --- | --- |
| $\alpha$ | $\delta^*$ | 80% | 90% | 80% | 90% |
| 0.05 | $0.25\sigma$ | 198 | 275 | 252 | 337 |
|  | $0.50\sigma$ | 50 | 69 | 63 | 85 |
|  | $1.00\sigma$ | 13 | 18 | 16 | 22 |
| 0.01 | $0.25\sigma$ | 322 | 417 | 374 | 477 |
|  | $0.50\sigma$ | 81 | 105 | 94 | 120 |
|  | $1.00\sigma$ | 21 | 27 | 24 | 30 |

Some researchers from the academia and the pharmaceutical industry consider this false positive rate as acceptable and the evidence provided by the two clinical trials using the one-sided test procedure as rather substantial. Hence, the one-sided test procedure should be recommended. However, in practice a two-sided test may be preferred because placebo effect may be substantial in many drug products such as drug products regarding diseases in the central nervous system.

### 2.2.1 Remark

Dubey (1991) indicated that the FDA prefers a two-sided test over a one-sided test procedure in clinical research and development of drug products. In situations where (i) there is truly concern with outcomes in only one tail, and (ii) it is completely inconceivable that results could go in the opposite direction, one-sided test procedure may be appropriate (Dubey, 1991). Dubey (1991) provided situations where one-sided test procedure

Table 2.2.2: Comparison Between One-Sided Test and Two-Sided Test At $\alpha$-level of Significance

| Characteristic | One-sided Test | Two-sided Test |
| --- | --- | --- |
| Hypotheses | Non-inferiority | Equality |
|  | Superiority | Equivalence |
| One Trial | 1/20 | 1/40 |
| Two Trials | 1/400 | 1/1600 |

may be justified. These situations include (i) toxicity studies, (ii) safety evaluation, (iii) the analysis of occurrences of adverse drug reaction data, (iv) risk evaluation, and (v) laboratory data.

## 2.3 Crossover Design Versus Parallel Design

As indicated earlier, an adequate and well-controlled clinical trial requires that a valid study design be employed for a valid assessment of the effect of the test drug under investigation. As indicated in Chow and Liu (1998), commonly used study designs in clinical research include parallel design, crossover design, enrichment design, titration design, or a combination of these designs. Among these designs, crossover and parallel designs are probably the two most commonly employed study designs.

### 2.3.1 Inter-Subject and Intra-Subject Variabilities

Chow and Liu (1998) suggested that relative merits and disadvantages of candidate designs should be carefully evaluated before an appropriate design is chosen for the intended trial. The clarification of the intra-subject and inter-subject variabilities is essential for sample size calculation in clinical research when a crossover design or a parallel design is employed.

Intra-subject variability is the variability that could be observed by repeating experiments on the same subject under the same experiment condition. The source of intra-subject variability could be multifold. One important source is biological variability. Exactly the same results may not be obtained even if they are from the same subject under the same experiment condition. Another important source is measurement or calculation error. For example, in a bioequivalence study with healthy subjects, it could be (i) the error when measuring the blood or plasma concentration-time curve, (ii) the error when calculating AUC (area under the curve), and/or (iii) the error of rounding after log-transformation. Intra-subject variability could be eliminated if we could repeat the experiment infinitely many times (in practice, this just means a large number of times) on the same subject under the same experiment condition and then take the average. The reason is that intra-subject variability tends to cancel each other on average in a large scale. If we repeat the experiment on different subjects infinitely many times, it is possible that we may still see that the averages of the responses from different subjects are different from each other even if the experiments are carried out under the exactly the same conditions. Then, what causes this difference or variation? It is not due to intra-subject variability, which has been eliminated by averaging infinitely repeated experiments; it is not due to experiment conditions, which are exactly the

## 2.3. Crossover Design Versus Parallel Design

same for different subjects. Therefore, this difference or variation can only be due to the unexplained difference between the two subjects.

It should be pointed out that sometimes people may call the variation observed from different subjects under the same experiment condition inter-subject variability, which is different from the inter-subject variability defined here. The reason is that the variability observed from different subjects under the same experiment condition could be due to unexplained difference among subjects (pure inter-subject variability); it also could be due to the biological variability, or measurement error associated with different experiments on different subjects (intra-subject variability). Therefore, it is clear that the observed variability from different subjects incorporates two components. They are, namely, pure inter-subject variability and intra-subject variability. We refer to it as the total inter-subject variability. For simplicity, it is also called total variability, which is the variability one would observe from a parallel design.

In practice, no experiment can be carried out infinitely many times. It is also not always true the experiment can be repeatedly carried out on the same subject under the same experiment condition. But, we can still assess these two variability components (intra- and inter-) under certain statistical models, e.g., a mixed effects model.

### 2.3.2 Crossover Design

A crossover design is a modified randomized block design in which each block receives more than one treatment at different dosing periods. In a crossover design, subjects are randomly assigned to receive a sequence of treatments, which contains all the treatments in the study. For example, for a standard two-sequence, two-period $2 \times 2$ crossover design, subjects are randomly assigned to receive one of the two sequences of treatments (say, RT and TR), where T and R represent the test drug and the reference drug, respectively. For subjects who are randomly assigned to the sequence of RT, they receive the reference drug first and then crossover to receive the test drug after a sufficient length of washout. The major advantage of a crossover design is that it allows a within subject (or intra-subject) comparison between treatments (each subject serves as its own control) by removing the between subject (or inter-subject) variability from the comparison. Let $\mu_T$ and $\mu_R$ be the mean of the responses of the study endpoint of interest. Also, let $\sigma_S^2$ and $\sigma_e^2$ be the inter-subject variance and intra-subject variance, respectively. Define $\theta = (\mu_T - \mu_R)/\mu_R$ and assume that the equivalence limit is $\delta = 0.2\mu_R$. Then, under a two-sequence, two-period crossover design, the formula for sample size calculation is given by

(see, also Chow and Wang, 2001)

$$n \geq \frac{CV^2(t_{\alpha,2n-2} + t_{\beta/2,2n-2})^2}{(0.2 - |\theta|)^2},$$

where $CV = \sigma_e/\mu_R$.

### 2.3.3 Parallel Design

A parallel design is a complete randomized design in which each subject receives one and only one treatment in a random fashion. The parallel design does not provide independent estimates for the intra-subject variability for each treatment. As a result, the assessment of treatment effect is made based on the total variability, which includes the inter-subject variability and the intra-subject variability.

Under a parallel design, assuming that the equivalence limit $\delta = 0.2\mu_R$, the following formula is useful for sample size calculation (Chow and Wang, 2001):

$$n \geq \frac{2CV^2(t_{\alpha,2n-2} + t_{\beta/2,2n-2})^2}{(0.2 - |\theta|)^2},$$

where $CV = \sigma/\mu_R$ and $\sigma^2 = \sigma_S^2 + \sigma_e^2$.

### 2.3.4 Remark

In summary, in a parallel design, the comparison is made based on the inter-subject variation, while the comparison is made based on the intra-subject variation in a crossover design. As a result, sample size calculation under a parallel design or a crossover design is similar and yet different. Note that the above formulas for sample size calculation are obtained based on raw data. Sample size formulas based on log-transformation data under a parallel design or a crossover design can be similarly obtained (Chow and Wang, 2001). More discussion regarding data transformation such as a log-transformation is given in Section 2.5.

## 2.4 Subgroup/Interim Analyses

In clinical research, subgroup analyses are commonly performed in clinical trials. Subgroup analyses may be performed with respect to subject prognostic or confounding factors such as demographics or subject characteristics at baseline. The purpose of this type of subgroup analysis is to isolate the variability due to the prognostic or confounding factors for an

## 2.4. Subgroup/Interim Analyses

unbiased and reliable assessment of the efficacy and safety of the test drug under investigation. In addition, many clinical trial protocols may call for an interim analysis or a number of interim analyses during the conduct of the trials for the purpose of establishing early efficacy and/or safety monitoring. The rationale for interim analyses of accumulating data in clinical trials have been well established in the literature. See, for example, Armitage, et al. (1969), Haybittle (1971), Peto et al. (1976), Pocock (1977), O'Brien and Fleming (1979), Lan and DeMets (1983), PMA (1993), and DeMets and Lan (1994).

### 2.4.1 Group Sequential Boundaries

For interim analyses in clinical trials, it is suggested that the number of planned interim analyses should be specified in the study protocol. Let $N$ be the total planned sample size with equal allocation to the two treatments. Suppose that $K$ interim analyses is planned with equal increment of accumulating data. Then we can divide the duration of the clinical trial into $K$ intervals. Within each stage, the data of $n = N/K$ patients are accumulated. At the end of each interval, an interim analysis can be performed using the Z-statistic, denoted by $Z_i$, with the data accumulated up to that point. Two decisions will be made based on the result of each interim analysis. First, the trial will continue if

$$\mid Z_i \mid \leq z_i, \quad i = 1, ..., K-1, \qquad (2.4.1)$$

where the $z_i$ are some critical values that are known as the *group sequential boundaries*. We fail to reject the null hypothesis if

$$\mid Z_i \mid \leq z_i, \quad \text{for all } i = 1, ..., K. \qquad (2.4.2)$$

Note that we may terminate the trial if the null hypothesis is rejected at any of the $K$ interim analyses ($\mid Z_i \mid > z_i$, $i = 1, ..., K$). For example, at the end of the first interval, an interim analysis is carried out with data from $n$ subjects. If we fail to reject the null hypothesis, we continue the trial to the second planned interim analysis. Otherwise, we reject the null hypothesis and we may stop the trial. The trial may be terminated at the final analysis if we fail to reject the null hypothesis at the final analysis. Then we declare that the data from the trial provide sufficient evidence to doubt the validity of the null hypothesis. Otherwise, the null hypothesis is rejected and we conclude that there is statistically significant difference in change from baseline between the test drug and the control.

In contrast to the fixed sample where only one final analysis is performed, $K$ analyses are carried out for the $K$-stage group sequential procedure. Suppose that the nominal significance level for each of the $K$ interim analyses is still 5%. Then, because of repeated testing based on the accumulated data, the overall significance level is inflated. In other words, the probability of declaring at least one significance result increases due to $K$ interim analyses. Various methods have been proposed to maintain the overall significance level at the pre-specified nominal level. One of the early methods was proposed by Haybittle (1971) and Peto et al. (1976). They proposed to use 3.0 as group sequential boundaries for all interim analyses except for the final analysis for which they suggested 1.96. In other words,

$$z_i = \begin{cases} 3.0, & \text{if } i = 1, ..., K - 1, \\ 1.96, & \text{if } i = K. \end{cases}$$

Therefore, their method can be summarized as follows:

Step 1: At each of the $K$ interim analyses, compute $Z_i$, $i = 1, ..., K - 1$.
Step 2: If the absolute value of $Z_i$ crosses 3.0, then reject the null hypothesis and recommend a possible early termination of the trial; otherwise continue the trial to the next planned interim analysis and repeat steps 1 and 2.
Step 3: For the final analysis, use 1.96 for the boundary. Trial stops here regardless if the null hypothesis is rejected.

Haybittle and Peto's method is very simple. However, it is a procedure with ad hoc boundaries that are independent of the number of planned interim analyses and stage of interim analyses. Pocock (1977) proposed different group sequential boundaries which depend upon the number of planned interim analyses. However, his boundaries are constant at each stage of interim analyses. Since limited information is included in the early stages of interim analyses, O'Brien and Fleming (1979) suggested posing conservative boundaries for interim analyses scheduled to be carried out during an early phase of the trial. Their boundaries not only depend upon the number of interim analyses but also are a function of stages of interim analysis. As a result, the O'Brien-Fleming boundaries can be calculated as follows:

$$z_{ik} = \frac{c_k \sqrt{k}}{i}, \quad 1 \leq i \leq k \leq K, \qquad (2.4.3)$$

where $c_k$ is the critical value for a total of $k$ planned interim analyses. As an example, suppose that 5 planned interim analyses are scheduled. Then $c_5 = 2.04$ and boundaries for each stage of these 5 interim analyses are given as

$$z_{i5} = \frac{2.04\sqrt{5}}{i}, \quad 1 \leq i \leq 5.$$

## 2.4. Subgroup/Interim Analyses

Thus, O'Brien-Fleming boundary for the first interim analysis is equal to $(2.04)(\sqrt{5}) = 4.561$. The O'Brien-Fleming boundaries for the other 4 interim analyses can be similarly computed as 3.225, 2.633, 2.280, and 2.040, respectively. The O'Brien-Fleming boundaries are very conservative so that the early trial results must be extreme for any prudent and justified decision-making in recommendation of a possible early termination when very limited information is available. On the other hand, for the late phase of the trial when the accumulated information approaches the required maximum information, their boundaries also become quite close to the critical value when no interim analysis had been planned. As a result, the O'Brien-Fleming method does not require a significant increase in the sample size for what has already planned. Therefore, the O'Brien-Fleming group sequential boundaries have become one of the most popular procedures for the planned interim analyses of clinical trials.

### 2.4.2 Alpha Spending Function

The idea of the alpha spending function proposed by Lan and DeMets (1983) is to spend (i.e., distribute) the total probability of false positive risk as a continuous function of the information time. The implementation of the alpha spending function requires the selection and specification of the spending function in advance in the protocol. One cannot change and choose another spending function in the middle of trial. Geller (1994) suggested that the spending function should be convex and have the property that the same value of a test statistic is more compelling as the sample sizes increase. Since its flexibility and no requirement for total information and equal increment of information, there is a potential to abuse the alpha spending function by increasing the frequency of interim analyses as the results approach to the boundary. However, DeMets and Lan (1994) reported that alteration of the frequency of interim analyses has very little impact on the overall significance level if the O'Brien-Fleming-type or Pocock-type continuous spending function is used.

Pawitan and Hallstrom (1990) studied the alpha spending function with the use of the permutation test. The permutation test is conceptually simple and it provides an exact test for small sample sizes. In addition, it is valid for complicated stratified analysis in which the exact sampling distribution is in general unknown and large-sample approximation may not be adequate. Consider the one-sided alternative. For the $k$th interim analyses, under the assumption of no treatment effect, the null joint permutation distribution of test statistics $(Z_1, ..., Z_K)$ can be obtained by random permutation of treatment assignments on the actual data. Let $(Z^*_{1b}, ..., Z^*_{Kb}), b = 1, ..., B$, be the statistics computed from $B$ treatment assignments and $B$ be the total number of possible permutations. Given

$\alpha(s_1), \alpha(s_2) - \alpha(s_1),..., \alpha(s_k) - \alpha(s_{K-1})$, the probabilities of type I error allowed to spend at successive interim analyses, the one-sided boundaries $z_1,...z_K$ can be determined by

$$\frac{\# \text{ of } (Z_1^* > z_1)}{B} = \alpha(s_1),$$

and

$$\frac{\# \text{ of } (Z_1^* > z_1 \text{ or } Z_2^* > z_2, ..., \text{ or} Z_k^* > z_k)}{B} = \alpha(s_k) - \alpha(s_{k-1}),$$

$k = 1, ..., K$. If $B$ is very large, then the above method can be executed with a random sample with replacement of size $B$. The $\alpha$ spending function for an overall significance level of 2.5% for one-sided alternative is given by

$$\alpha(s) = \begin{cases} \frac{\alpha}{2}s, & \text{if } s < 1, \\ \alpha, & \text{if } s = 1. \end{cases}$$

In the interest of controlling the overall type I error rate at the $\alpha$ level of significance, sample size is necessarily adjusted according to the $\alpha$ spending function to account for the planned interim analyses. In some cases, sample size re-estimation without unblinding may be performed according to the procedure described in Section 1.3 of Chapter 1. More details can be found in Chapter 8.

## 2.5 Data Transformation

In clinical research, data transformation on clinical response of the primary study endpoint may be necessarily performed before statistical analysis for a more accurate and reliable assessment of the treatment effect. For example, for bioavailability and bioequivalence studies with healthy human subjects, the FDA requires that a log-transformation be performed before data analysis. Two drug products are claimed bioequivalent in terms of drug absorption if the 90% confidence interval of the ratio of means of the primary pharmacokinetic (PK) parameters, such as area under the blood or plasma concentration-time curve (AUC) and maximum concentration (Cmax), is entirely within the bioequivalence limits of (80%,125%). Let $\mu_T$ and $\mu_R$ be the population means of the test drug and the reference drug, respectively. Also, let $X$ and $Y$ be the PK responses for the test drug and the reference drug. After log-transformation, we assume that $\log X$ and $\log Y$ follow normal distributions with means $\mu_X^*$ and $\mu_Y^*$ and variance $\sigma^2$. Then

$$\mu_T = E(X) = e^{\mu_X^* + \frac{\sigma^2}{2}} \quad \text{and} \quad \mu_R = E(Y) = e^{\mu_Y^* + \frac{\sigma^2}{2}},$$

## 2.5. Data Transformation

which implies

$$\log\left(\frac{\mu_T}{\mu_R}\right) = \log(e^{\mu_X^* - \mu_Y^*}) = \mu_X^* - \mu_Y^*.$$

Under both the crossover and parallel design, an exact $(1-\alpha)100\%$ confidence interval for $\mu_X^* - \mu_Y^*$ can be obtained based on the log transformed data. Hence, an exact $(1-\alpha)100\%$ confidence interval for $\mu_T/\mu_R$ can be obtained after the back transformation.

Chow and Wang (2001) provided sample size formulas under a parallel design or a crossover design with and without log-transformation. These formulas are different but very similar. In practice, scientists often confuse them with one another. The following discussion may be helpful for clarification.

We note that the sample size derivation is based on normality assumption for the raw data and log-normality assumption for the transformed data. Thus, it is of interest to study the distribution of $\log X$ when $X$ is normally distributed with mean $\mu$ and variance $\sigma^2$. Note that

$$\text{Var}\left(\frac{X-\mu}{\mu}\right) = \frac{\sigma^2}{\mu^2} = CV^2.$$

If CV is sufficiently small, $(X-\mu)/\mu$ is close to 0. As a result, by Taylor's expansion,

$$\log X - \log \mu = \log\left(1 + \frac{X-\mu}{\mu}\right) \approx \frac{X-\mu}{\mu}.$$

Then,

$$\log X \approx \log \mu + \frac{X-\mu}{\mu} \sim N(\log \mu, CV^2).$$

This indicates that when $CV$ is small, $\log X$ is still approximately normally distributed, even if $X$ is from a normal population. Therefore, the procedure based on log-transformed data is robust in some sense. In addition, the $CV$ observed from the raw data is very similar to the variance obtained from the log-transformed data.

Traditionally, for the example regarding bioavailability and bioequivalence with raw data, BE can be established if the 90% confidence interval for $\mu_T - \mu_R$ is entirely within the interval of $(-0.2\mu_R, 0.2\mu_R)$ (Chow and Liu, 1992). This is the reason why 0.2 appears in the formula for raw data. However, both the 1992 FDA and the 2000 FDA guidances recommended that a log-transformation be performed before bioequivalence assessment is made. For log-transformed data, the BE can be established if the 90% confidence interval for $\mu_T/\mu_R$ is entirely located in the interval (80%,125%). That is why $\log 1.25$ appears in the formula for log-transformed data. It

Table 2.5.1: Posterior Power Evaluation Under a Crossover Design

| Data Type | Power |
|---|---|
| Raw Data | $1 - 2\Phi\left(\dfrac{0.2}{CV\sqrt{\frac{1}{n_1}+\frac{1}{n_2}}} - t_{\alpha, n_1+n_2-2}\right)$ |
| Log-transformed Data | $1 - 2\Phi\left(\dfrac{0.223}{\sigma_e\sqrt{\frac{1}{n_1}+\frac{1}{n_2}}} - t_{\alpha, n_1+n_2-2}\right)$ |

should be noted that $\log 1.25 = -\log 0.8 = 0.2231$. In other words, the BE limit for the raw data is symmetric about 0 (i.e., $\pm 0.2\mu_R$), while the BE limit for the log-transformed data is also symmetric about 0 after log transformation.

### 2.5.1 Remark

For the crossover design, since each subject serves as its own control, the inter-subject variation is removed from comparison. As a result, the formula for sample size calculation derived under a crossover design only involves the intra-subject variability. On the other hand, for the parallel design, formula for sample size calculation under a parallel design includes both the inter- and intra-subject variabilities. In practice, it is easy to get confused with the sample size calculation and/or evaluation of posterior power based on either raw data or log-transformed data under either a crossover design or a parallel design (Chow and Wang, 2001). As an example, posterior powers based on raw data and log-transformed data under a crossover design when the true mean difference is 0 are given in Table 2.5.1.

## 2.6 Practical Issues

### 2.6.1 Unequal Treatment Allocation

In a parallel design or a crossover design comparing two or more than two treatments, sample sizes in each treatment group (for parallel design) or in each sequence of treatments (for crossover design) may not be the same. For example, when conducting a placebo-control clinical trial with very ill patients or patients with severe or life-threatening diseases, it may

## 2.6. Practical Issues

not be ethical to put too many patients in the placebo arm. In this case, the investigator may prefer to put fewer patients in the placebo (if the placebo arm is considered necessary to demonstrate the effectiveness and safety of the drug under investigation). A typical ratio of patient allocation for situations of this kind is 1:2, i.e., each patient will have a one-third chance to be assigned to the placebo group and two-third chance to receive the active drug. For different ratios of patient allocation, the sample size formulae discussed can be directly applied with appropriate modification of the corresponding degrees of freedom in the formulas.

When there is unequal treatment allocation, say $\kappa$ to 1 ratio, sample size for comparing two means can be obtained as

$$n = \frac{(\sigma_1^2/\kappa + \sigma_2^2)(z_{\alpha/2} + z_\beta)^2}{\delta^2}.$$

When $\kappa = 1$, the above formula reduces to (1.3.3). When $\sigma_1^2 = \sigma_2^2 = \sigma^2$, we have

$$n = \frac{(\kappa+1)\sigma^2(z_{\alpha/2} + z_\beta)^2}{\kappa\delta^2}.$$

Note that unequal treatment allocation will have an impact on randomization in clinical trials, especially in multicenter trials. To maintain the integrity of blinding of an intended trial, a blocking size of 2 or 4 in randomization is usually employed. A blocking size of 2 guarantees that one of the subjects in the block will be randomly assigned to the treatment group and the other one will be randomly assigned to the control group. In a multicenter trial comparing two treatments, if we consider a 2 to 1 allocation, the size of each block has to be a mutiple of 3, i.e., 3, 6, or 9. In the treatment of having a minimum of two blocks in each center, each center is required to enroll a minimum of 6 subjects. As a result, this may have an impact on the selection of the number of centers. As indicated in Chow and Liu (1998), as a rule of thumb, it is not desirable to have the number of subjects in each center less than the number of centers. As a result, it is suggested that the use of a $\kappa$ to 1 treatment allocation in multicenter trials should take into consideration of blocking size in randomization and the number of centers selected.

### 2.6.2 Adjustment for Dropouts or Covariates

At the planning stage of a clinical study, sample size calculation provides the number of *evaluable* subjects required for achieving a desired statistical assurance (e.g., an 80% power). In practice, we may have to enroll more subjects to account for potential dropouts. For example, if the sample size required for an intended clinical trial is $n$ and the potential dropout rate is

$p$, then we need to enroll $n/(1-p)$ subjects in order to obtain $n$ evaluable subjects at the completion of the trial. It should also be noted that the investigator may have to screen more patients in order to obtain $n/(1-p)$ *qualified* subjects at the entry of the study based on inclusion/exclusion criteria of the trial.

Fleiss (1986) pointed out that a required sample size may be reduced if the response variable can be described by a covariate. Let $n$ be the required sample size per group when the design does not call for the experimental control of a prognostic factor. Also, let $n^*$ be the required sample size for the study with the factor controlled. The relative efficiency ($RE$) between the two designs is defined as

$$RE = \frac{n}{n^*}.$$

As indicated by Fleiss (1986), if the correlation between the prognostic factor (covariate) and the response variable is $r$, then $RE$ can be expressed as

$$RE = \frac{100}{1 - r^2}.$$

Hence, we have

$$n^* = n(1 - r^2).$$

As a result, the required sample size per group can be reduced if the correlation exists. For example, a correlation of $r = 0.32$ could result in a 10% reduction in the sample size.

## 2.6.3 Mixed-Up Randomization Schedules

*Randomization* plays an important role in the conduct of clinical trials. Randomization not only generates comparable groups of patients who constitute representative samples from the intended patient population, but also enables valid statistical tests for clinical evaluation of the study drug. Randomization in clinical trials involves random recruitment of the patients from the targeted patient population and random assignment of patients to the treatments. Under randomization, statistical inference can be drawn under some probability distribution assumption of the intended patient population. The probability distribution assumption depends on the method of randomization under a randomization model. A study without randomization results in the violation of the probability distribution assumption and consequently no accurate and reliable statistical inference on the evaluation of the safety and efficacy of the study drug can be drawn.

A problem commonly encountered during the conduct of a clinical trial is that a proportion of treatment codes are mixed-up in randomization

## 2.6. Practical Issues

schedules. Mixing up treatment codes can distort the statistical analysis based on the population or randomization model. Chow and Shao (2002) quantatively studied the effect of mixed-up treatment codes on the analysis based on the intention-to-treat (ITT) population, which are described below.

Consider a two-group parallel design for comparing a test drug and a control (placebo), where $n_1$ patients are randomly assigned to the treatment group and $n_2$ patients are randomly assigned to the control group. When randomization is properly applied, the population model holds and responses from patients are normally distributed. Consider first the simplest case where two patient populations (treatment and control) have the same variance $\sigma^2$ and $\sigma^2$ is known. Let $\mu_1$ and $\mu_2$ be the population means for the treatment and the control, respectively. The null hypothesis that $\mu_1 = \mu_2$ (i.e., there is no treatment effect) is rejected at the $\alpha$ level of significance if

$$\frac{|\bar{x}_1 - \bar{x}_2|}{\sigma\sqrt{\frac{1}{n_1} + \frac{1}{n_2}}} > z_{\alpha/2}, \quad (2.6.1)$$

where $\bar{x}_1$ is the sample mean of responses from patients in the treatment group, $\bar{x}_2$ is the sample mean of responses from patients in the control group, and $z_{\alpha/2}$ is the upper $(\alpha/2)$th percentile of the standard normal distribution. Intuitively, mixing up treatment codes does not affect the significance level of the test.

The power of the test, i.e., the probability of correctly detecting a treatment difference when $\mu_1 \neq \mu_2$, is

$$p(\theta) = P\left(\frac{|\bar{x}_1 - \bar{x}_2|}{\sigma\sqrt{\frac{1}{n_1} + \frac{1}{n_2}}} > z_{\alpha/2}\right) = \Phi(\theta - z_{\alpha/2}) + \Phi(-\theta - z_{\alpha/2}),$$

where $\Phi$ is the standard normal distribution function and

$$\theta = \frac{\mu_1 - \mu_2}{\sigma\sqrt{\frac{1}{n_1} + \frac{1}{n_2}}}. \quad (2.6.2)$$

This follows from the fact that under the randomization model, $\bar{x}_1 - \bar{x}_2$ has the normal distribution with mean $\mu_1 - \mu_2$ and variance $\sigma^2\left(\frac{1}{n_1} + \frac{1}{n_2}\right)$.

Suppose that there are $m$ patients whose treatment codes are randomly mixed-up. A straightforward calculation shows that $\bar{x}_1 - \bar{x}_2$ is still normally distributed with variance $\sigma^2\left(\frac{1}{n_1} + \frac{1}{n_2}\right)$, but the mean of $\bar{x}_1 - \bar{x}_2$ is equal to

$$\left[1 - m\left(\frac{1}{n_1} + \frac{1}{n_2}\right)\right](\mu_1 - \mu_2).$$

It turns out that the power for the test defined above is

$$p(\theta_m) = \Phi(\theta_m - z_{\alpha/2}) + \Phi(-\theta_m - z_{\alpha/2}),$$

where

$$\theta_m = \left[1 - m\left(\frac{1}{n_1} + \frac{1}{n_2}\right)\right] \frac{\mu_1 - \mu_2}{\sigma\sqrt{\frac{1}{n_1} + \frac{1}{n_2}}}. \qquad (2.6.3)$$

Note that $\theta_m = \theta$ if $m = 0$, i.e., there is no mix-up.

The effect of mixed-up treatment codes can be measured by comparing $p(\theta)$ with $p(\theta_m)$. Suppose that $n_1 = n_2$. Then $p(\theta_m)$ depends on $m/n_1$, the proportion of mixed-up treatment codes. For example, suppose that when there is no mix-up, $p(\theta) = 80\%$, which gives that $|\theta| = 2.81$. When 5% of treatment codes are mixed-up, i.e., $m/n_1 = 5\%$, $p(\theta_m) = 70.2\%$. When 10% of treatment codes are mixed-up, $p(\theta_m) = 61.4\%$. Hence, a small proportion of mixed-up treatment codes may seriously affect the probability of detecting treatment effect when such an effect exists. In this simple case we may plan ahead to ensure a desired power when the maximum proportion of mixed-up treatment codes is known. Assume that the maximum proportion of mixed-up treatment codes is $p$ and that the original sample size is $n_1 = n_2 = n_0$. Then

$$\theta_m = (1 - 2p)\theta = \frac{\mu_1 - \mu_2}{\sigma\sqrt{2}}\sqrt{(1 - 2p)^2 n_0}.$$

Thus, a new sample size $n_{\text{new}} = n_0/(1 - 2p)^2$ will maintain the desired power when the proportion of mixed-up treatment codes is no larger than $p$. For example, if $p = 5\%$, then $n_{\text{new}} = 1.23 n_0$, i.e., a 23% increase of the sample size will offset a 5% mix-up in randomization schedules.

The effect of mixed-up treatment codes is higher when the study design becomes more complicated. Consider the two-group parallel design with an unknown $\sigma^2$. The test statistic is necessarily modified by replacing $z_{\alpha/2}$ and $\sigma^2$ by $t_{\alpha/2;n_1+n_2-2}$ and

$$\hat{\sigma}^2 = \frac{(n_1 - 1)s_1^2 + (n_2 - 1)s_2^2}{n_1 + n_2 - 2},$$

where $s_1^2$ is the sample variance based on responses from patients in the treatment group, $s_2^2$ is the sample variance based on responses from patients in the control group, and $t_{\alpha/2;n_1+n_2-2}$ is the upper $(\alpha/2)$th percentile of the t-distribution with $n_1 + n_2 - 2$ degrees of freedom. When randomization is properly applied without mix-up, the two-sample t-test has the $\alpha$ level of significance and the power is given by

$$1 - \mathcal{T}_{n_1+n_2-2}(t_{\alpha/2;n_1+n_2-2}|\theta) + \mathcal{T}_{n_1+n_2-2}(-t_{\alpha/2;n_1+n_2-2}|\theta),$$

## 2.6. Practical Issues

where $\theta$ is defined by (2.6.2) and $\mathcal{T}_{n_1+n_2-2}(\cdot|\theta)$ is the non-central t-distribution function with $n_1 + n_2 - 2$ degrees of freedom and the non-centrality parameter $\theta$. When there are $m$ patients with mixed-up treatment codes and $\mu_1 \neq \mu_2$, the effect on the distribution of $\bar{x}_1 - \bar{x}_2$ is the same as that in the case of known $\sigma^2$. In addition, the distribution of $\hat{\sigma}^2$ is also changed. A direct calculation shows that the expectation of $\hat{\sigma}^2$ is

$$E(\hat{\sigma}^2) = \sigma^2 + \frac{2(\mu_1 - \mu_2)^2 m}{n_1 + n_2 - 2}\left[2 - m\left(\frac{1}{n_1} + \frac{1}{n_2}\right)\right].$$

Hence, the actual power of the two-sample t-test is less than

$$1 - \mathcal{T}_{n_1+n_2-2}(t_{0.975;n_1+n_2-2}|\theta_m) + \mathcal{T}_{n_1+n_2-2}(-t_{0.975;n_1+n_2-2}|\theta_m),$$

where $\theta_m$ is given by (2.6.3).

### 2.6.4 Treatment or Center Imbalance

In multicenter clinical trials, sample size calculation is usually performed under the assumption that there are equal numbers of subjects in each center. In practice, however, we may end up with an imbalance in sample sizes across centers. It is a concern (i) what the impact is of this imbalance on the power of the test and (ii) whether sample size calculation should be performed in a way to account for this imbalance. In this section, we examine this issue by studying the power with sample size imbalance across centers.

For a multicenter trial, the following model is usually considered:

$$y_{ijk} = \mu + T_i + C_j + (TC)_{ij} + \epsilon_{ijk},$$

where $i = 1, 2$ (treatment), $j = 1, ..., J$ (center), $k = 1, ..., n_{ij}$, $T_i$ is the $i$th treatment effect, $C_j$ is the effect due to the $j$th center, $(TC)_{ij}$ is the effect due to the interaction between the $i$th treatment in the $j$th center, and $\epsilon_{ijk}$ are random error which are normally distributed with mean 0 and variance $\sigma^2$. Under the above model, a test statistic for

$$\mu_1 - \mu_2 = (\mu + T_1) - (\mu + T_2) = T_1 - T_2$$

is given by

$$T^* = \frac{1}{J}\sum_{j=1}^{J}(\bar{y}_{1j} - \bar{y}_{2j})$$

with $E(T^*) = T_1 - T_2$ and

$$\text{Var}(T^*) = \frac{\sigma^2}{J^2}\sum_{j=1}^{J}\left(\frac{1}{n_{1j}} + \frac{1}{n_{2j}}\right).$$

If we assume that $n_{1j} = n_{2j} = n_j$ for all $j = 1, ..., J$, then

$$\mathrm{Var}(T^*) = \frac{\sigma^2}{J^2} \sum_{j=1}^{J} \frac{2}{n_j}.$$

In this case, the power of the test is given by

$$\text{Power} = 1 - \Phi\left(z_{\alpha/2} - \frac{\delta}{\frac{\sigma}{J}\sqrt{\sum_{j=1}^{J} 2/n_j}}\right).$$

When $n_j = n$ for all $j$,

$$\mathrm{Var}(T^*) = \frac{2\sigma^2}{Jn}$$

and the power of the test becomes

$$\text{Power} = 1 - \Phi\left(z_{\alpha/2} - \frac{\delta}{\sigma\sqrt{2/(Jn)}}\right).$$

As it can be seen that

$$1 - \Phi\left(z_{\alpha/2} - \frac{\delta}{\frac{\sigma}{J}\sqrt{\sum_{j=1}^{J} 2/n_j}}\right) \leq 1 - \Phi\left(z_{\alpha/2} - \frac{\delta}{\sigma\sqrt{2/(Jn)}}\right).$$

To achieve the same power, the only choice is to increase the sample size if we assume that the variance remains the same. In this situation, the total sample size $N = \sum_{j=1}^{J} n_j$ should satisfy

$$\frac{\delta}{\frac{\sigma}{J}\sqrt{\sum_{j=1}^{J} 2/n_j}} = \frac{\delta}{\sigma\sqrt{2/n}}.$$

The difficulty is that $n_j, j = 1, ..., J$, are not fixed and we are unable to predict how many subjects will be in each center at the end of the trial although we may start with the same number of subjects in each center. The loss in power due to treatment and/or center imbalance may be substantial in practice.

### 2.6.5 Multiplicity

In many clinical trials, multiple comparisons may be performed. In the interest of controlling the overall type I error rate at the $\alpha$ level, an adjustment for multiple comparisons such as the Bonferroni adjustment is necessary. The formulas for sample size calculation can still be applied by simply replacing the $\alpha$ level with an adjusted $\alpha$ level. In practice, it may be too conservative to adjust the $\alpha$ level when there are too many primary clinical endpoints or there are too many comparisons to be made. As a rule of thumb, Biswas, Chan and Ghosh (2000) suggested that a multiplicity adjustment to the significance level be made when at least one significant result (e.g., one of several primary clinical endpoints or several pairwise comparison) is required to draw conclusion. On the other hand, a multiplicity adjustment is not needed when (i) all results are required to be significant in order to draw conclusion or (ii) the testing problem is closed. A test procedure is said to be *closed* if the rejection region of a particular univariate null hypothesis at a given significance $\alpha$-level implies the rejection of all higher dimensional null hypotheses containing the univariate null hypothesis at the same significance $\alpha$-level (Marcus, Peritz, and Gabriel, 1976). When a multiplicity adjustment is required, it is recommended that either the method of Bonferroni or the procedures described in Hochberg and Tamhane (1987) be used.

### 2.6.6 Multiple-Stage Design for Early Stopping

In phase II cancer trials, it is undesirable to stop a study early when the treatment appears to be effective but desirable to terminate the trial when the treatment seems to be ineffective. For this purpose, a multiple-stage design is often employed to determine whether a test drug is promising enough to warrant further testing (Simon, 1989). The concept of a multiple-stage design is to permit early stopping when a moderately long sequence of initial failures occurs. For example, in Simon's two-stage optimal design, $n_1$ subjects are treated and the trial terminates if all $n_1$ are treatment failures. If there are one or more successes in stage 1, then stage 2 is implemented by including the other $n_2$ subjects. A decision is then made based on the response rate of the $n_1+n_2$ subjects. The drawback of Simon's design is that it does not allow early termination if there is a long run of failures at the start. To overcome this disadvantage, Ensign et al. (1994) proposed an optimal three-stage design which modifies the Simon's two-stage design. Let $p_0$ be the response rate that is not of interest for conducting further studies and $p_1$ be the response rate of definite interest ($p_1 > p_0$). The optimal three-stage design is implemented by testing the following hypotheses:

$$H_0 : p \leq p_0 \quad \text{versus} \quad H_a : p \geq p_1.$$

Rejection of $H_0$ indicates that further study of the test drug should be carried out. At stage 1, $n_1$ subjects are treated. We would reject $H_a$ (i.e., the test drug is not promising) and stop the trial if there is no response. If there are one or more responses, then proceed to stage 2 by including additional $n_2$ subjects. We would then reject $H_1$ and stop the trial if the total number of responses is less than a prespecified number of $r_2$; otherwise continue to stage 3. At stage 3, $n_3$ more subjects are treated. We reject $H_a$ if the total number of responses is less than a prespecified number of $r_3$. In this case, we conclude the test treatment is ineffective. Based on the three-stage design described above, Ensign et al. (1994) considered the following to determine the sample size. For each value of $n_2$ satisfying

$$(1-p_1)^{n_1} < \beta,$$

where

$$\beta = P(\text{reject } H_1 | p_1),$$

compute the values of $r_2, n_2, r_3$, and $n_3$ that minimize the null expected sample size $EN(p_0)$ subject to the error constraints $\alpha$ and $\beta$, where

$$EN(p) = n_1 + n_2\{1 - \beta_1(p)\} + n_3\{1 - \beta_1(p) - \beta_2(p)\},$$

and $\beta_i$ are the probability of making type II error evaluated stage $i$. Ensign et al. (1994) use the value of

$$\beta - (1-p_1)^{n_1}$$

as the type II error rate in the optimization along with type I error

$$\alpha = P(\text{reject } H_0 | p_0)$$

to obtain $r_2, n_2, r_3$, and $n_3$. Repeating this, $n_1$ can be chosen to minimize the overall $EN(p_0)$.

### 2.6.7 Rare Incidence Rate

In most clinical trials, although the primary objectives are usually for evaluation of the effectiveness and safety of the test drug under investigation, the assessment of drug safety has not received the same level of attention as the assessment of efficacy. Sample size calculations are usually performed based on a pre-study power analysis based on the primary efficacy variable. If sample size is determined based on the primary safety variable such as adverse event rate, a large sample size may be required especially when the incidence rate is extremely rare. For example, if the incidence rate is one per 10,000, then we will need to include 10,000 subjects in order to observe a single incidence. In this case, we may justify a selected sample size based on the concept of probability statement as described in Section 1.3.5. O'Neill (1988) indicated that the magnitude of rates that can be feasibly studied in most clinical trials is about 0.01 and higher. However,

## 2.6. Practical Issues

observational cohort studies usually can assess rates on the order of 0.001 and higher. O'Neill (1988) also indicated that it is informative to examine the sample sizes that would be needed to estimate a rate or to detect or estimate differences of specified amounts between rates for two different treatment groups.

# Chapter 3

# Comparing Means

In clinical research, clinical trials are usually conducted for evaluation of the efficacy and safety of a test drug as compared to a placebo control or an active control agent (e.g., a standard therapy) in terms of mean responses of some primary study endpoints. The objectives of the intended clinical trials usually include (i) the evaluation of the effect, (ii) the demonstration of therapeutic equivalence/non-inferiority, and (iii) the establishment of superiority. For evaluation of the effect within a given treatment, the null hypothesis of interest is to test whether there is a significant difference in mean response between pre- and post-treatment or mean change from baseline to endpoint. We refer to this testing problem as a one-sample problem. For establishment of the efficacy and safety of the test drug, a typical approach is to test whether there is a difference between the test drug and the placebo control and then evaluate the chance of correctly detecting a clinically meaningful difference if such a difference truly exists. Thus, it is of interest to first test the null hypothesis of equality and then evaluate the power under the alternative hypothesis to determine whether the evidence is substantial for regulatory approval. For demonstration of therapeutic equivalence/non-inferiority and/or superiority as compared to an active control or standard therapy, it is of interest to test hypotheses for equivalence/non-inferiority and/or superiority as described in Chapter 1. In this chapter, under a valid design (e.g., a parallel design or a crossover design), methods for sample size calculation are provided to achieve a desired power of statistical tests for appropriate hypotheses.

In Section 3.1, testing in one-sample problems is considered. Sections 3.2 and 3.3 summarize procedures for sample size calculation in two-sample problems under a parallel design and a crossover design, respectively. Sections 3.4 and 3.5 present procedures in multiple-sample problems under a parallel design (one-way analysis of variance) and a crossover design

(Williams design), respectively. Section 3.6 discusses some practical issues regarding sample size calculation for comparing means in clinical research, including sample size reduction when switching from a two-sided test to a one-sided test or from a parallel design to a crossover design, sensitivity analysis with respect to change in variability, and a brief discussion regarding Bayesian approach.

## 3.1 One-Sample Design

Let $x_i$ be the response from the $i$th sampled subject, $i = 1, ..., n$. In clinical research, $x_i$ could be the difference between matched pairs such as the pre-treatment and post-treatment responses or changes from baseline to endpoint within a treatment group. It is assumed that $x_i$'s are independent and identically distributed (i.i.d.) normal random variables with mean 0 and variance $\sigma^2$. Let

$$\bar{x} = \frac{1}{n} \sum_{i=1}^{n} x_i \quad \text{and} \quad s^2 = \frac{1}{n-1} \sum_{i=1}^{n} (x_i - \bar{x})^2 \qquad (3.1.1)$$

be the sample mean and sample variance of $x_i$'s, respectively. Also, let $\epsilon = \mu - \mu_0$ be the difference between the true mean response of a test drug ($\mu$) and a reference value ($\mu_0$). Without loss of generality, consider $\epsilon > 0$ ($\epsilon < 0$) an indication of *improvement* (*worsening*) of the test drug as compared to the reference value.

### 3.1.1 Test for Equality

To test whether there is a difference between the mean response of the test drug and the reference value, the following hypotheses are usually considered:

$$H_0 : \epsilon = 0 \quad \text{versus} \quad H_a : \epsilon \neq 0.$$

When $\sigma^2$ is known, we reject the null hypothesis at the $\alpha$ level of significance if

$$\left| \frac{\bar{x} - \mu_0}{\sigma/\sqrt{n}} \right| > z_{\alpha/2},$$

where $z_a$ is the upper $a$th quantile of the standard normal distribution. Under the alternative hypothesis that $\epsilon \neq 0$, the power of the above test is given by

$$\Phi\left( \frac{\sqrt{n}\epsilon}{\sigma} - z_{\alpha/2} \right) + \Phi\left( -\frac{\sqrt{n}\epsilon}{\sigma} - z_{\alpha/2} \right),$$

## 3.1. One-Sample Design

where $\Phi$ is the cumulative standard normal distribution function. By ignoring a small value $\leq \alpha/2$, the power is approximately

$$\Phi\left(\frac{\sqrt{n}|\epsilon|}{\sigma} - z_{\alpha/2}\right).$$

As a result, the sample size needed to achieve power $1 - \beta$ can be obtained by solving the following equation

$$\frac{\sqrt{n}|\epsilon|}{\sigma} - z_{\alpha/2} = z_\beta.$$

This leads to

$$n = \frac{(z_{\alpha/2} + z_\beta)^2 \sigma^2}{\epsilon^2} \qquad (3.1.2)$$

(if the solution of (3.1.2) is not an integer, then the smallest integer that is larger than the solution of (3.1.2) should be taken as the required sample size). An initial value of $\epsilon$ (or $\epsilon/\sigma$) is needed to calculate the sample size according to (3.1.2). A lower bound of $\epsilon/\sigma$, usually obtained from a pilot study or historical data, can be used as the initial value. A lower bound of $\epsilon/\sigma$ can also be defined as the clinically meaningful difference between the response means relative to the standard deviation $\sigma$.

When $\sigma^2$ is unknown, it can be replaced by the sample variance $s^2$ given in (3.1.1), which results in the usual one-sample t-test, i.e., we reject the null hypothesis $H_0$ if

$$\left|\frac{\bar{x} - \mu_0}{s/\sqrt{n}}\right| > t_{\alpha/2, n-1},$$

where $t_{a, n-1}$ is the upper $a$th quantile of a t-distribution with $n-1$ degrees of freedom. Under the alternative hypothesis that $\epsilon \neq 0$, the power of the one-sample t-test is given by

$$1 - \mathcal{T}_{n-1}\left(t_{\alpha/2, n-1} \middle| \frac{\sqrt{n}\epsilon}{\sigma}\right) + \mathcal{T}_{n-1}\left(-t_{\alpha/2, n-1} \middle| \frac{\sqrt{n}\epsilon}{\sigma}\right),$$

where $\mathcal{T}_{n-1}(\cdot|\theta)$ is the cumulative distribution function of a non-central t-distribution with $n-1$ degrees of freedom and the non-centrality parameter $\theta$. When an initial value of $\epsilon/\sigma$ is given, the sample size needed to achieve power $1 - \beta$ can be obtained by solving

$$\mathcal{T}_{n-1}\left(t_{\alpha/2, n-1} \middle| \frac{\sqrt{n}\epsilon}{\sigma}\right) - \mathcal{T}_{n-1}\left(-t_{\alpha/2, n-1} \middle| \frac{\sqrt{n}\epsilon}{\sigma}\right) = \beta. \qquad (3.1.3)$$

By ignoring a small value $\leq \alpha/2$, the power is approximately

$$1 - \mathcal{T}_{n-1}\left(t_{\alpha/2, n-1} \middle| \frac{\sqrt{n}|\epsilon|}{\sigma}\right).$$

Hence, the required sample size can also be obtained by solving

$$\mathcal{T}_{n-1}\left(t_{\alpha/2,n-1}\bigg|\frac{\sqrt{n}|\epsilon|}{\sigma}\right) = \beta. \tag{3.1.4}$$

Table 3.1.1 lists the solutions of this equation for some values of $\alpha$, $\beta$, and $\theta = |\epsilon|/\sigma$.

When $n$ is sufficiently large, $t_{\alpha/2,n-1} \approx z_{\alpha/2}$, $t_{\beta,n-1} \approx z_\beta$, and

$$\mathcal{T}_{n-1}\left(t_{\alpha/2,n-1}\bigg|\frac{\sqrt{n}\epsilon}{\sigma}\right) \approx \Phi\left(z_{\alpha/2} - \frac{\sqrt{n}\epsilon}{\sigma}\right). \tag{3.1.5}$$

Hence, formula (3.1.2) may still be used in the case of unknown $\sigma$.

## 3.1.2 Test for Non-Inferiority/Superiority

The problem of testing non-inferiority and superiority can be unified by the following hypotheses:

$$H_0 : \epsilon \leq \delta \quad \text{versus} \quad H_a : \epsilon > \delta,$$

where $\delta$ is the superiority or non-inferiority margin. When $\delta > 0$, the rejection of the null hypothesis indicates superiority over the reference value. When $\delta < 0$, the rejection of the null hypothesis implies non-inferiority against the reference value.

When $\sigma^2$ is known, we reject the null hypothesis $H_0$ at the $\alpha$ level of significance if

$$\frac{\bar{x} - \mu_0 - \delta}{\sigma/\sqrt{n}} > z_\alpha.$$

If $\epsilon > \delta$, the power of the above test is

$$\Phi\left(\frac{\sqrt{n}(\epsilon - \delta)}{\sigma} - z_\alpha\right).$$

As a result, the sample size needed to achieve power $1 - \beta$ can be obtained by solving

$$\frac{\sqrt{n}(\epsilon - \delta)}{\sigma} - z_\alpha = z_\beta,$$

which leads to

$$n = \frac{(z_\alpha + z_\beta)^2 \sigma^2}{(\epsilon - \delta)^2}. \tag{3.1.6}$$

When $\sigma^2$ is unknown, it can be replaced by $s^2$ given in (3.1.1). The null hypothesis $H_0$ is rejected at the $\alpha$ level of significance if

$$\frac{\bar{x} - \mu_0 - \delta}{s/\sqrt{n}} > t_{\alpha,n-1}.$$

## 3.1. One-Sample Design

Table 3.1.1: Smallest $n$ with $\mathcal{T}_{n-1}\left(t_{\alpha,n-1}|\sqrt{n}\theta\right) \leq \beta$

| | $\alpha = 2.5\%$ | | $\alpha = 5\%$ | | | $\alpha = 2.5\%$ | | $\alpha = 5\%$ | |
|---|---|---|---|---|---|---|---|---|---|
| | $1 - \beta =$ | | $1 - \beta =$ | | | $1 - \beta =$ | | $1 - \beta =$ | |
| $\theta$ | 80% | 90% | 80% | 90% | $\theta$ | 80% | 90% | 80% | 90% |
| 0.10 | 787 | 1053 | 620 | 858 | 0.54 | 29 | 39 | 23 | 31 |
| 0.11 | 651 | 871 | 513 | 710 | 0.56 | 28 | 36 | 22 | 29 |
| 0.12 | 547 | 732 | 431 | 597 | 0.58 | 26 | 34 | 20 | 27 |
| 0.13 | 467 | 624 | 368 | 509 | 0.60 | 24 | 32 | 19 | 26 |
| 0.14 | 403 | 539 | 317 | 439 | 0.62 | 23 | 30 | 18 | 24 |
| 0.15 | 351 | 469 | 277 | 382 | 0.64 | 22 | 28 | 17 | 23 |
| 0.16 | 309 | 413 | 243 | 336 | 0.66 | 21 | 27 | 16 | 22 |
| 0.17 | 274 | 366 | 216 | 298 | 0.68 | 19 | 25 | 15 | 20 |
| 0.18 | 245 | 327 | 193 | 266 | 0.70 | 19 | 24 | 15 | 19 |
| 0.19 | 220 | 293 | 173 | 239 | 0.72 | 18 | 23 | 14 | 18 |
| 0.20 | 199 | 265 | 156 | 216 | 0.74 | 17 | 22 | 13 | 18 |
| 0.21 | 180 | 241 | 142 | 196 | 0.76 | 16 | 21 | 13 | 17 |
| 0.22 | 165 | 220 | 130 | 179 | 0.78 | 15 | 20 | 12 | 16 |
| 0.23 | 151 | 201 | 119 | 164 | 0.80 | 15 | 19 | 12 | 15 |
| 0.24 | 139 | 185 | 109 | 151 | 0.82 | 14 | 18 | 11 | 15 |
| 0.25 | 128 | 171 | 101 | 139 | 0.84 | 14 | 17 | 11 | 14 |
| 0.26 | 119 | 158 | 93 | 129 | 0.86 | 13 | 17 | 10 | 14 |
| 0.27 | 110 | 147 | 87 | 119 | 0.88 | 13 | 16 | 10 | 13 |
| 0.28 | 103 | 136 | 81 | 111 | 0.90 | 12 | 16 | 10 | 13 |
| 0.29 | 96 | 127 | 75 | 104 | 0.92 | 12 | 15 | 9 | 12 |
| 0.30 | 90 | 119 | 71 | 97 | 0.94 | 11 | 14 | 9 | 12 |
| 0.32 | 79 | 105 | 62 | 86 | 0.96 | 11 | 14 | 9 | 11 |
| 0.34 | 70 | 93 | 55 | 76 | 0.98 | 11 | 14 | 8 | 11 |
| 0.36 | 63 | 84 | 50 | 68 | 1.00 | 10 | 13 | 8 | 11 |
| 0.38 | 57 | 75 | 45 | 61 | 1.04 | 10 | 12 | 8 | 10 |
| 0.40 | 52 | 68 | 41 | 55 | 1.08 | 9 | 12 | 7 | 9 |
| 0.42 | 47 | 62 | 37 | 50 | 1.12 | 9 | 11 | 7 | 9 |
| 0.44 | 43 | 57 | 34 | 46 | 1.16 | 8 | 10 | 7 | 8 |
| 0.46 | 40 | 52 | 31 | 42 | 1.20 | 8 | 10 | 6 | 8 |
| 0.48 | 37 | 48 | 29 | 39 | 1.30 | 7 | 9 | 6 | 7 |
| 0.50 | 34 | 44 | 27 | 36 | 1.40 | 7 | 8 | 5 | 7 |
| 0.52 | 32 | 41 | 25 | 34 | 1.50 | 6 | 7 | 5 | 6 |

The power of this test is given by

$$1 - \mathcal{T}_{n-1}\left(t_{\alpha,n-1}\left|\frac{\sqrt{n}(\epsilon - \delta)}{\sigma}\right|\right).$$

The sample size needed to achieve power $1 - \beta$ can be obtained by solving

$$\mathcal{T}_{n-1}\left(t_{\alpha,n-1}\left|\frac{\sqrt{n}(\epsilon - \delta)}{\sigma}\right|\right) = \beta.$$

By letting $\theta = (\epsilon - \delta)/\sigma$, Table 3.1.1 can be used to find the required sample size. From approximation (3.1.5), formula (3.1.6) can be used to calculate the required sample size when $n$ is sufficiently large.

### 3.1.3 Test for Equivalence

The objective is to test the following hypotheses

$$H_0 : |\epsilon| \geq \delta \quad \text{versus} \quad H_a : |\epsilon| < \delta.$$

The test drug is concluded to be equivalent to a gold standard on average if the null hypothesis is rejected at significance level $\alpha$.

When $\sigma^2$ is known, the null hypothesis $H_0$ is rejected at significance level $\alpha$ if

$$\frac{\sqrt{n}(\bar{x} - \mu_0 - \delta)}{\sigma} < -z_\alpha \quad \text{and} \quad \frac{\sqrt{n}(\bar{x} - \mu_0 + \delta)}{\sigma} > z_\alpha.$$

The power of this test is given by

$$\Phi\left(\frac{\sqrt{n}(\delta - \epsilon)}{\sigma} - z_\alpha\right) + \Phi\left(\frac{\sqrt{n}(\delta + \epsilon)}{\sigma} - z_\alpha\right) - 1. \quad (3.1.7)$$

Although the sample size $n$ can be obtained by setting the power in (3.1.7) to $1 - \beta$, it is more convenient to use the following method. Note that the power is larger than

$$2\Phi\left(\frac{\sqrt{n}(\delta - |\epsilon|)}{\sigma} - z_\alpha\right) - 1. \quad (3.1.8)$$

Hence, the sample size needed to achieve power $1 - \beta$ can be obtained by solving

$$\Phi\left(\frac{\sqrt{n}(\delta - |\epsilon|)}{\sigma} - z_\alpha\right) = 1 - \frac{\beta}{2}.$$

This leads to

$$n = \frac{(z_\alpha + z_{\beta/2})^2 \sigma^2}{(\delta - |\epsilon|)^2}. \quad (3.1.9)$$

## 3.1. One-Sample Design

Note that the quantity in (3.1.8) is a conservative approximation to the power. Hence, the sample size calculated according to (3.1.9) is conservative. A different approximation is given in Chow and Liu (1992, 2000), which leads to the following formula for sample size calculation:

$$n = \begin{cases} \frac{(z_\alpha + z_{\beta/2})^2 \sigma^2}{\delta^2} & \text{if } \epsilon = 0 \\ \frac{(z_\alpha + z_\beta)^2 \sigma^2}{(\delta - |\epsilon|)^2} & \text{if } \epsilon \neq 0. \end{cases}$$

When $\sigma^2$ is unknown, it can be estimated by $s^2$ given in (3.1.1). The null hypothesis $H_0$ is rejected at significance level $\alpha$ if

$$\frac{\sqrt{n}(\bar{x} - \mu_0 - \delta)}{s} < -t_{\alpha,n-1} \quad \text{and} \quad \frac{\sqrt{n}(\bar{x} - \mu_0 + \delta)}{s} > t_{\alpha,n-1}.$$

The power of this test can be estimated by

$$1 - \mathcal{T}_{n-1}\left(t_{\alpha,n-1} \left| \frac{\sqrt{n}(\delta - \epsilon)}{\sigma} \right. \right) - \mathcal{T}_{n-1}\left(t_{\alpha,n-1} \left| \frac{\sqrt{n}(\delta + \epsilon)}{\sigma} \right. \right).$$

Hence, the sample size needed to achieve power $1 - \beta$ can be obtained by setting the power to $1 - \beta$. Since the power is larger than

$$1 - 2\mathcal{T}_{n-1}\left(t_{\alpha,n-1} \left| \frac{\sqrt{n}(\delta - |\epsilon|)}{\sigma} \right. \right),$$

a conservative approximation to the sample size needed to achieve power $1 - \beta$ can be obtained by solving

$$\mathcal{T}_{n-1}\left(t_{\alpha,n-1} \left| \frac{\sqrt{n}(\delta - |\epsilon|)}{\sigma} \right. \right) = \frac{\beta}{2},$$

which can be done by using Table 3.1.1 with $\theta = (\delta - |\epsilon|)/\sigma$. From approximation (3.1.5), formula (3.1.9) can be used to calculate the required sample size when $n$ is sufficiently large.

### 3.1.4 An Example

To illustrate the use of sample size formulas derived above, we first consider an example concerning a study of osteoporosis in post-menopausal women. Osteoporosis and osteopenia (or decreased bone mass) most commonly develop in post-menopausal women. The consequences of osteoporosis are vertebral crush fractures and hip fractures. The diagnosis of osteoporosis is made when vertebral bone density is more than 10% below what is expected for sex, age, height, weight, and race. Usually, bone density is reported in terms of standard deviation (SD) from mean values. The World Health

Organization (WHO) defines osteopenia as bone density value greater than one SD below peak bone mass levels in young women and osteoporosis as a value of greater than 2.5 SD below the same measurement scale. In medical practice, most clinicians suggest therapeutic intervention should be begun in patients with osteopenia to prevent progression to osteoporosis.

**Test for Equality**

Suppose that the mean bone density before the treatment is 1.5 SD ($\mu_0 = 1.5$ SD) and after treatment is expected to be 2.0 SD (i.e., $\mu_1 = 2.0$ SD). We have $\epsilon = \mu_1 - \mu_0 = 2.0$ SD $-1.5$ SD $= 0.5$ SD. By (3.1.2), at $\alpha = 0.05$, the required sample size for having an 80% power (i.e., $\beta = 0.2$) for correctly detecting a difference of $\epsilon = 0.5$ SD change from pre-treatment to post-treatment can be obtained by normal approximation as

$$n = \frac{(z_{\alpha/2} + z_\beta)^2 \sigma^2}{\epsilon^2} = \frac{(1.96 + 0.84)^2}{(0.5)^2} \approx 32.$$

On the other hand, the sample size can also be obtained by solving equation (3.1.4). Note that

$$\theta = \frac{|\epsilon|}{\sigma} = 0.5.$$

By referring to the column under $\alpha = 2.5\%$ (two-sided test) at the row with $\theta = 0.5$ in Table 3.1.1, it can be found that the sample size needed is 34.

**Test for Non-Inferiority**

For prevention of progression from osteopenis to osteoporosis, we wish to show that the mean bone density post-treatment is no less than pre-treatment by a clinically meaningful difference $\delta = -0.5$ SD. As a result, by (3.1.6), at $\alpha=0.05$, the required sample size for having an 80% power (i.e., $\beta=0.20$) can be obtained by normal approximation as

$$n = \frac{(z_\alpha + z_\beta)^2 \sigma^2}{(\epsilon - \delta)^2} = \frac{(1.64 + 0.84)^2}{(0.5 + 0.5)^2} \approx 7.$$

On the other hand, the sample size can also be obtained by using Table 3.1.1. Note that

$$\theta = \frac{\epsilon - \delta}{\sigma} = 0.5 + 0.5 = 1.00.$$

By referring to the column under $\alpha = 5\%$ at the row with $\theta = 1.0$ in Table 3.1.1, it can be found that the sample size needed is 8.

## Test for Equivalence

To illustrate the use of the sample size formula for testing equivalence, we consider another example concerning the effect of a test drug on body weight change in terms of body mass index (BMI) before and after the treatment. Suppose clinicians consider that a less than 5% change in BMI from baseline (pre-treatment) to endpoint (post-treatment) is not a safety concern for the indication of the disease under study. Thus, we consider $\delta=5\%$ as the equivalence limit. The objective is then to demonstrate safety by testing equivalence in mean BMI between pre-treatment and post-treatment of the test drug. Assume the true BMI difference is 0 ($\epsilon = 0$) and the standard deviation is 10% ($\sigma = 0.1$), by (3.1.9) with $\alpha=0.05$, the sample size required for achieving an 80% power can be obtained by normal approximation as

$$n = \frac{(z_\alpha + z_{\beta/2})^2 \sigma^2}{\delta^2} = \frac{(1.64 + 1.28)^2 0.10^2}{0.05^2} \approx 35.$$

On the other hand, the sample size calculation can also be performed by using Table 3.1.1. Note that

$$\theta = \frac{\delta}{\sigma} = \frac{0.05}{0.10} = 0.50.$$

By referring to the column under $\alpha = 5\%$ and $1 - \beta = 90\%$ at the row with $\theta = 0.50$ in Table 3.1.1, it can be found the sample size needed is 36.

## 3.2 Two-Sample Parallel Design

Let $x_{ij}$ be the response observed from the $j$th subject in the $i$th treatment group, $j = 1, ..., n_i$, $i = 1, 2$. It is assumed that $x_{ij}$, $j = 1, ..., n_i$, $i = 1, 2$, are independent normal random variables with mean $\mu_i$ and variance $\sigma^2$. Let

$$\bar{x}_{i\cdot} = \frac{1}{n_i} \sum_{j=1}^{n_i} x_{ij} \quad \text{and} \quad s^2 = \frac{1}{n_1 + n_2 - 2} \sum_{i=1}^{2} \sum_{j=1}^{n_i} (x_{ij} - \bar{x}_{i\cdot})^2 \quad (3.2.1)$$

be the sample means for $i$th treatment group and the pooled sample variance, respectively. Also, let $\epsilon = \mu_2 - \mu_1$ be the true mean difference between a test drug ($\mu_2$) and a placebo control or an active control agent ($\mu_1$). Without loss of generality, consider $\epsilon > 0$ ($\epsilon < 0$) as an indication of *improvement (worsening)* of the test drug as compared to the placebo control or active control agent. In practice, it may be desirable to have an unequal treatment allocation, i.e., $n_1/n_2 = \kappa$ for some $\kappa$. Note that $\kappa = 2$ indicates a 2 to 1 test-control allocation, whereas $\kappa = 1/2$ indicates a 1 to 2 test-control allocation.

## 3.2.1 Test for Equality

The objective is to test whether there is a difference between the mean responses of the test drug and the placebo control or active control. Hence, the following hypotheses are considered:

$$H_0 : \epsilon = 0 \quad \text{versus} \quad H_a : \epsilon \neq 0.$$

When $\sigma^2$ is known, the null hypothesis $H_0$ is rejected at the significance level $\alpha$ if

$$\left| \frac{\bar{x}_{1\cdot} - \bar{x}_{2\cdot}}{\sigma \sqrt{\frac{1}{n_1} + \frac{1}{n_2}}} \right| > z_{\alpha/2}.$$

Under the alternative hypothesis that $\epsilon \neq 0$, the power of the above test is

$$\Phi\left( \frac{\epsilon}{\sigma \sqrt{\frac{1}{n_1} + \frac{1}{n_2}}} - z_{\alpha/2} \right) + \Phi\left( \frac{-\epsilon}{\sigma \sqrt{\frac{1}{n_1} + \frac{1}{n_2}}} - z_{\alpha/2} \right)$$

$$\approx \Phi\left( \frac{|\epsilon|}{\sigma \sqrt{\frac{1}{n_1} + \frac{1}{n_2}}} - z_{\alpha/2} \right),$$

after ignoring a small term of value $\leq \alpha/2$. As a result, the sample size needed to achieve power $1 - \beta$ can be obtained by solving the following equation

$$\frac{|\epsilon|}{\sigma \sqrt{\frac{1}{n_1} + \frac{1}{n_2}}} - z_{\alpha/2} = z_\beta.$$

This leads to

$$n_1 = \kappa n_2 \quad \text{and} \quad n_2 = \frac{(z_{\alpha/2} + z_\beta)^2 \sigma^2 (1 + 1/\kappa)}{\epsilon^2}. \tag{3.2.2}$$

When $\sigma^2$ is unknown, it can be replaced by $s^2$ given in (3.2.1). The null hypothesis $H_0$ is rejected if

$$\left| \frac{\bar{x}_{1\cdot} - \bar{x}_{2\cdot}}{s \sqrt{\frac{1}{n_1} + \frac{1}{n_2}}} \right| > t_{\alpha/2, n_1+n_2-2}.$$

Under the alternative hypothesis that $\epsilon \neq 0$, the power of this test is

$$1 - \mathcal{T}_{n_1+n_2-2}\left( t_{\alpha/2, n_1+n_2-2} \middle| \frac{\epsilon}{\sigma \sqrt{\frac{1}{n_1} + \frac{1}{n_2}}} \right)$$

## 3.2. Two-Sample Parallel Design

$$+ \mathcal{T}_{n_1+n_2-2}\left(-t_{\alpha/2,n_1+n_2-2}\left|\frac{\epsilon}{\sigma\sqrt{\frac{1}{n_1}+\frac{1}{n_2}}}\right.\right).$$

Thus, with $n_1 = \kappa n_2$, the sample size $n_2$ needed to achieve power $1 - \beta$ can be obtained by setting the power equal to $1 - \beta$.

After ignoring a small term of value $\leq \alpha/2$, the power is approximately

$$1 - \mathcal{T}_{n_1+n_2-2}\left(t_{\alpha/2,n_1+n_2-2}\left|\frac{|\epsilon|}{\sigma\sqrt{\frac{1}{n_1}+\frac{1}{n_2}}}\right.\right).$$

Hence, the required sample size $n_2$ can also be obtained by solving

$$\mathcal{T}_{(1+\kappa)n_2-2}\left(t_{\alpha/2,(1+\kappa)n_2-2}\left|\frac{\sqrt{n_2}|\epsilon|}{\sigma\sqrt{1+1/\kappa}}\right.\right) = \beta.$$

Table 3.2.1 can be used to obtain the solutions for $\kappa = 1, 2$, and some values of $\theta = |\epsilon|/\sigma$, $\alpha$, and $\beta$. When $\kappa = 1/2$, Table 3.2.1 can be used to find the required $n_1$ and $n_2 = 2n_1$.

From approximation (3.1.5), formula (3.2.2) can be used when both $n_1$ and $n_2$ are large.

### 3.2.2 Test for Non-Inferiority/Superiority

The problem of testing non-inferiority and superiority can be unified by the following hypotheses:

$$H_0 : \epsilon \leq \delta \quad \text{versus} \quad H_a : \epsilon > \delta,$$

where $\delta$ is the superiority or non-inferiority margin. When $\delta > 0$, the rejection of the null hypothesis indicates the superiority of the test drug over the control. When $\delta < 0$, the rejection of the null hypothesis indicates the non-inferiority of the test drug against the control.

When $\sigma^2$ is known, the null hypothesis $H_0$ is rejected at the $\alpha$ level of significance if

$$\frac{\bar{x}_1 - \bar{x}_2 - \delta}{\sigma\sqrt{\frac{1}{n_1}+\frac{1}{n_2}}} > z_\alpha.$$

Under the alternative hypothesis that $\epsilon > \delta$, the power of the above test is given by

$$\Phi\left(\frac{\epsilon - \delta}{\sigma\sqrt{\frac{1}{n_1}+\frac{1}{n_2}}} - z_\alpha\right).$$

Table 3.2.1: Smallest $n$ with $\mathcal{T}_{(1+\kappa)n-2}\left(t_{\alpha,(1+\kappa)n-2}|\sqrt{n}\theta/\sqrt{1+1/\kappa}\right) \leq \beta$

| | $\kappa = 1$ | | | | $\kappa = 2$ | | | |
| --- | --- | --- | --- | --- | --- | --- | --- | --- |
| | $\alpha = 2.5\%$ | | $\alpha = 5\%$ | | $\alpha = 2.5\%$ | | $\alpha = 5\%$ | |
| | $1 - \beta =$ | | $1 - \beta =$ | | $1 - \beta =$ | | $1 - \beta =$ | |
| $\theta$ | 80% | 90% | 80% | 90% | 80% | 90% | 80% | 90% |
| 0.30 | 176 | 235 | 139 | 191 | 132 | 176 | 104 | 144 |
| 0.32 | 155 | 207 | 122 | 168 | 116 | 155 | 92 | 126 |
| 0.34 | 137 | 183 | 108 | 149 | 103 | 137 | 81 | 112 |
| 0.36 | 123 | 164 | 97 | 133 | 92 | 123 | 73 | 100 |
| 0.38 | 110 | 147 | 87 | 120 | 83 | 110 | 65 | 90 |
| 0.40 | 100 | 133 | 78 | 108 | 75 | 100 | 59 | 81 |
| 0.42 | 90 | 121 | 71 | 98 | 68 | 90 | 54 | 74 |
| 0.44 | 83 | 110 | 65 | 90 | 62 | 83 | 49 | 67 |
| 0.46 | 76 | 101 | 60 | 82 | 57 | 76 | 45 | 62 |
| 0.48 | 70 | 93 | 55 | 76 | 52 | 70 | 41 | 57 |
| 0.50 | 64 | 86 | 51 | 70 | 48 | 64 | 38 | 52 |
| 0.52 | 60 | 79 | 47 | 65 | 45 | 59 | 35 | 48 |
| 0.54 | 55 | 74 | 44 | 60 | 42 | 55 | 33 | 45 |
| 0.56 | 52 | 68 | 41 | 56 | 39 | 51 | 31 | 42 |
| 0.58 | 48 | 64 | 38 | 52 | 36 | 48 | 29 | 39 |
| 0.60 | 45 | 60 | 36 | 49 | 34 | 45 | 27 | 37 |
| 0.65 | 39 | 51 | 30 | 42 | 29 | 38 | 23 | 31 |
| 0.70 | 34 | 44 | 26 | 36 | 25 | 33 | 20 | 27 |
| 0.75 | 29 | 39 | 23 | 32 | 22 | 29 | 17 | 24 |
| 0.80 | 26 | 34 | 21 | 28 | 20 | 26 | 15 | 21 |
| 0.85 | 23 | 31 | 18 | 25 | 17 | 23 | 14 | 19 |
| 0.90 | 21 | 27 | 16 | 22 | 16 | 21 | 12 | 17 |
| 0.95 | 19 | 25 | 15 | 20 | 14 | 19 | 11 | 15 |
| 1.00 | 17 | 23 | 14 | 18 | 13 | 17 | 10 | 14 |
| 1.05 | 16 | 21 | 12 | 17 | 12 | 15 | 9 | 13 |
| 1.10 | 15 | 19 | 11 | 15 | 11 | 14 | 9 | 12 |
| 1.15 | 13 | 17 | 11 | 14 | 10 | 13 | 8 | 11 |
| 1.20 | 12 | 16 | 10 | 13 | 9 | 12 | 7 | 10 |
| 1.25 | 12 | 15 | 9 | 12 | 9 | 11 | 7 | 9 |
| 1.30 | 11 | 14 | 9 | 11 | 8 | 11 | 6 | 9 |
| 1.35 | 10 | 13 | 8 | 11 | 8 | 10 | 6 | 8 |
| 1.40 | 10 | 12 | 8 | 10 | 7 | 9 | 6 | 8 |
| 1.45 | 9 | 12 | 7 | 9 | 7 | 9 | 5 | 7 |
| 1.50 | 9 | 11 | 7 | 9 | 6 | 8 | 5 | 7 |

## 3.2. Two-Sample Parallel Design

The sample size needed to achieve power $1 - \beta$ can be obtained by solving

$$\frac{\epsilon - \delta}{\sigma\sqrt{\frac{1}{n_1} + \frac{1}{n_2}}} - z_\alpha = z_\beta.$$

This leads to

$$n_1 = \kappa n_2 \quad \text{and} \quad n_2 = \frac{(z_\alpha + z_\beta)^2 \sigma^2 (1 + 1/\kappa)}{(\epsilon - \delta)^2}. \tag{3.2.3}$$

When $\sigma^2$ is unknown, it can be replaced by $s^2$ given in (3.2.1). The null hypothesis $H_0$ is rejected if

$$\frac{\bar{x}_1 - \bar{x}_2 - \delta}{s\sqrt{\frac{1}{n_1} + \frac{1}{n_2}}} > t_{\alpha, n_1 + n_2 - 2}.$$

Under the alternative hypothesis that $\epsilon > \delta$, the power of this test is given by

$$1 - \mathcal{T}_{n_1 + n_2 - 2}\left(t_{\alpha, n_1 + n_2 - 2} \middle| \frac{\epsilon - \delta}{\sigma\sqrt{\frac{1}{n_1} + \frac{1}{n_2}}}\right).$$

The sample size needed to achieve power $1 - \beta$ can be obtained by solving the following equation:

$$\mathcal{T}_{n_1 + n_2 - 2}\left(t_{\alpha, n_1 + n_2 - 2} \middle| \frac{\epsilon - \delta}{\sigma\sqrt{\frac{1}{n_1} + \frac{1}{n_2}}}\right) = \beta.$$

By letting $\theta = (\epsilon - \delta)/\sigma$, Table 3.2.1 can be used to find the required sample size.

From approximation (3.1.5), formula (3.2.3) can be used to calculate the required sample size when $n_1$ and $n_2$ are sufficiently large.

### 3.2.3 Test for Equivalence

The objective is to test the following hypotheses

$$H_0 : |\epsilon| \geq \delta \quad \text{versus} \quad H_a : |\epsilon| < \delta.$$

The test drug is concluded to be equivalent to the control in average if the null hypothesis is rejected at significance level $\alpha$.

When $\sigma^2$ is known, the null hypothesis $H_0$ is rejected at the $\alpha$ level of significance if

$$\frac{\bar{x}_1 - \bar{x}_2 - \delta}{\sigma\sqrt{\frac{1}{n_1} + \frac{1}{n_2}}} < -z_\alpha \quad \text{and} \quad \frac{\bar{x}_1 - \bar{x}_2 + \delta}{\sigma\sqrt{\frac{1}{n_1} + \frac{1}{n_2}}} > z_\alpha.$$

Under the alternative hypothesis that $|\epsilon| < \delta$, the power of this test is

$$\Phi\left(\frac{\delta - \epsilon}{\sigma\sqrt{\frac{1}{n_1} + \frac{1}{n_2}}} - z_\alpha\right) + \Phi\left(\frac{\delta + \epsilon}{\sigma\sqrt{\frac{1}{n_1} + \frac{1}{n_2}}} - z_\alpha\right) - 1$$

$$\approx 2\Phi\left(\frac{\delta - |\epsilon|}{\sigma\sqrt{\frac{1}{n_1} + \frac{1}{n_2}}} - z_\alpha\right) - 1.$$

As a result, the sample size needed to achieve power $1 - \beta$ can be obtained by solving the following equation

$$\frac{\delta - |\epsilon|}{\sigma\sqrt{\frac{1}{n_1} + \frac{1}{n_2}}} - z_\alpha = z_{\beta/2}.$$

This leads to

$$n_1 = \kappa n_2 \quad \text{and} \quad n_2 = \frac{(z_\alpha + z_{\beta/2})^2 \sigma^2 (1 + 1/\kappa)}{(\delta - |\epsilon|)^2}. \tag{3.2.4}$$

When $\sigma^2$ is unknown, it can be replaced by $s^2$ given in (3.2.1). The null hypothesis $H_0$ is rejected at the $\alpha$ level of significance if

$$\frac{\bar{x}_1 - \bar{x}_2 - \delta}{s\sqrt{\frac{1}{n_1} + \frac{1}{n_2}}} < -t_{\alpha, n_1 + n_2 - 2} \quad \text{and} \quad \frac{\bar{x}_1 - \bar{x}_2 + \delta}{s\sqrt{\frac{1}{n_1} + \frac{1}{n_2}}} > t_{\alpha, n_1 + n_2 - 2}.$$

Under the alternative hypothesis that $|\epsilon| < \delta$, the power of this test is

$$1 - \mathcal{T}_{n_1+n_2-2}\left(t_{\alpha, n_1+n_2-2} \left| \frac{\delta - \epsilon}{\sigma\sqrt{\frac{1}{n_1} + \frac{1}{n_2}}}\right.\right)$$

$$-\mathcal{T}_{n_1+n_2-2}\left(t_{\alpha, n_1+n_2-2} \left| \frac{\delta + \epsilon}{\sigma\sqrt{\frac{1}{n_1} + \frac{1}{n_2}}}\right.\right).$$

Hence, with $n_1 = \kappa n_2$, the sample size $n_2$ needed to achieve power $1 - \beta$ can be obtained by setting the power to $1 - \beta$. Since the power is larger than

$$1 - 2\mathcal{T}_{n_1+n_2-2}\left(t_{\alpha, n_1+n_2-2} \left| \frac{\delta - |\epsilon|}{\sigma\sqrt{\frac{1}{n_1} + \frac{1}{n_2}}}\right.\right),$$

## 3.2. Two-Sample Parallel Design

a conservative approximation to the sample size $n_2$ can be obtained by solving

$$\mathcal{T}_{(1+\kappa)n_2-2}\left(t_{\alpha,(1+\kappa)n_2-2}\left|\frac{\sqrt{n_2}(\delta-|\epsilon|)}{\sigma\sqrt{1+1/\kappa}}\right.\right) = \frac{\beta}{2}.$$

Table 3.2.1 can be used to calculate $n_1$ and $n_2$.

From approximation (3.1.5), formula (3.2.4) can be used to calculate the required sample size when $n_1$ and $n_2$ are sufficiently large.

### 3.2.4 An Example

Consider an example concerning a clinical trial for evaluation of the effect of a test drug on cholesterol in patients with coronary heart disease (CHD). Cholesterol is the main lipid associated with arteriosclerotic vascular disease. The purpose of cholesterol testing is to identify patients at risk for arteriosclerotic heart disease. The liver metabolizes the cholesterol to its free form which is transported in the bloodtream by lipoproteins. As indicated by Pagana and Pagana (1998), nearly 75% of the cholesterol is bound to low density lipoproteins (LDLs) and 25% is bound to high density lipoproteins (HDLs). Therefore, cholesterol is the main component of LDLs and only a minimal component of HDLs and very low density lipoproteins. LDL is the most directly associated with increased risk of CHD.

A pharmaceutical company is interested in conducting a clinical trial to compare two cholesterol lowering agents for treatment of patients with CHD through a parallel design. The primary efficacy parameter is the LDL. In what follows, we will consider the situations where the intended trial is for (i) testing equality of mean responses in LDL, (ii) testing non-inferiority or superiority of the test drug as compared to the active control agent, and (iii) testing for therapeutic equivalence. All sample size calculations in this section are performed for achieving an 80% power (i.e., $\beta = 0.20$) at the 5% level of significance (i.e., $\alpha = 0.05$).

**Test for Equality**

As discussed in Chapter 1, hypotheses for testing equality are point hypotheses. A typical approach for sample size calculation is to reject the null hypothesis of no treatment difference and conclude that there is a significant difference between treatment groups. Then, sample size can be chosen to achieve an 80% power for detecting a clinically meaningful difference (i.e., $\epsilon$). In this example, suppose a difference of 5% (i.e., $\epsilon = 5\%$) in percent change of LDL is considered of clinically meaningful difference. By (3.2.2), assuming that the standard deviation is 10% (i.e., $\sigma = 10\%$), the sample size by normal approximaton can be determined by

$$n_1 = n_2 = \frac{2(z_{\alpha/2} + z_\beta)^2 \sigma^2}{\epsilon^2} = \frac{2 \times (1.96 + 0.84)^2 \times 0.1^2}{0.05^2} \approx 63.$$

On the other hand, the sample size can also be obtained by using Table 3.2.1. Note that

$$\theta = \frac{\epsilon}{\sigma} = \frac{0.05}{0.10} = 0.50.$$

By referring to the column under $\alpha = 2.5\%$ at the row with $\theta = 0.50$ in Table 3.2.1, it can be found that the sample size needed is 64.

### Test for Non-Inferiority

Suppose that the pharmaceutical company is interested in establishing non-inferiority of the test drug as compared to the active control agent. Similarly, we assume that the non-inferiority margin is chosen to be 5% (i.e., $\delta = -0.05$). Also, suppose the true difference in mean LDL between treatment groups is 0% (i.e., $\epsilon = \mu_2$(test)$-\mu_1$(control)$= 0.00$). Then, by (3.2.3), the sample size by normal approximation can be determined by

$$n_1 = n_2 = \frac{2(z_\alpha + z_\beta)^2 \sigma^2}{(\epsilon - \delta)^2} = \frac{2 \times (1.64 + 0.84)^2 \times 0.1^2}{(-0.00 - (-0.05))^2} \approx 50.$$

On the other hand, the sample size can also be obtained by using Table 3.2.1. Note that

$$\theta = \frac{|\epsilon - \delta|}{\sigma} = \frac{0.05}{0.10} = 0.50.$$

By referring to the column under $\alpha = 5\%$ at the row with $\theta = 0.50$ in Table 3.2.1, it can be found that the sample size needed is 51.

### Test for Equivalence

For establishment of equivalence, suppose the true mean difference is 1% (i.e., $\epsilon = 0.01$) and the equivalence limit is 5% (i.e., $\delta = 0.05$). According to (3.2.4), the sample size by normal approximation can be determined by

$$n_1 = n_2 = \frac{2(z_\alpha + z_{\beta/2})^2 \sigma^2}{(\delta - |\epsilon|)^2} = \frac{2 \times (1.64 + 1.28)^2 \times 0.1^2}{(0.05 - 0.01)^2} \approx 107.$$

On the other hand, the sample size can also be obtained by using Table 3.2.1. Note that

$$\theta = \frac{\delta - |\epsilon|}{\sigma} = \frac{0.04}{0.10} = 0.40.$$

By referring to the column under $\alpha = 5\%$, $\beta = 0.10$ at the row with $\theta = 0.40$ in Table 3.2.1, it can be found that the sample size needed is 108.

## 3.2.5 Remarks

The assumption that $\sigma_1^2 = \sigma_2^2$ may not hold. When $\sigma_1^2 \neq \sigma_2^2$, statistical procedures are necessarily modified. If $\sigma_1^2$ and $\sigma_2^2$ are unknown, this becomes the well-known Behrens-Fisher problem. Extensive literature have been devoted to this topic in the past several decades. Miller (1997) gave a comprehensive review of research work done in this area.

In practice, it is suggested that superiority be established by testing non-inferiority first. Once the null hypothesis of inferiority is rejected, test for superiority is performed. This test procedure controls the overall type I error rate at the nominal level $\alpha$ because it is a closed test procedure. More details regarding closed testing procedures can be found in Marcus, Peritz and Gabriel (1976).

## 3.3 Two-Sample Crossover Design

In this section, we consider a $2 \times 2m$ replicated crossover design comparing mean responses of a test drug and a reference drug. Let $y_{ijkl}$ be the $l$th replicate or response ($l = 1, ..., m$) observed from the $j$th subject ($j = 1, ..., n$) in the $i$th sequence ($i = 1, 2$) under the $k$th treatment ($k = 1, 2$). The following model is considered:

$$y_{ijkl} = \mu_k + \gamma_{ik} + s_{ijk} + e_{ijkl}, \qquad (3.3.1)$$

where $\mu_k$ is the $k$th treatment effect, $\gamma_{ik}$ is the fixed effect of the $i$th sequence under treatment $k$, and $s_{ijk}$ is the random effect of the $j$th subject in the $i$th sequence under treatment $k$. $(s_{ij1}, s_{ij2}), i = 1, 2, j = 1, ..., n$, are assumed to be i.i.d. as bivariate normal random variables with mean 0 and covariance matrix

$$\Sigma = \begin{pmatrix} \sigma_{BT}^2 & \rho\sigma_{BT}\sigma_{BR} \\ \rho\sigma_{BT}\sigma_{BR} & \sigma_{BR}^2 \end{pmatrix}.$$

$e_{ij1l}$ and $e_{ij2l}$ are assumed to be independent normal random variables with mean 0 and variance $\sigma_{WT}^2$ or $\sigma_{WR}^2$ (depending on the treatment). Define

$$\sigma_D^2 = \sigma_{BT}^2 + \sigma_{BR}^2 - 2\rho\sigma_{BT}\sigma_{BR}.$$

$\sigma_D^2$ is the variability due to the effect of subject-by-treatment interaction, which reflects the heteroscedasticity of the subject random effect between the test drug and the reference drug.

Let $\epsilon = \mu_2 - \mu_1$ (test − reference),

$$\bar{y}_{ijk\cdot} = \frac{1}{m}(y_{ijk1} + \cdots + y_{ijkm}) \quad \text{and} \quad d_{ij} = \bar{y}_{ij1\cdot} - \bar{y}_{ij2\cdot}.$$

An unbiased estimate for $\epsilon$ is given by

$$\hat{\epsilon} = \frac{1}{2n} \sum_{i=1}^{2} \sum_{j=1}^{n} d_{ij}.$$

Under model (3.3.1), $\hat{\epsilon}$ follows a normal distribution with mean $\epsilon$ and variance $\sigma_m^2/(2n)$, where

$$\sigma_m^2 = \sigma_D^2 + \frac{1}{m}(\sigma_{WT}^2 + \sigma_{WR}^2). \quad (3.3.2)$$

An unbiased estimate for $\sigma_m^2$ can be obtained by

$$\hat{\sigma}_m^2 = \frac{1}{2(n-1)} \sum_{i=1}^{2} \sum_{j=1}^{n} (d_{ij} - \bar{d}_{i\cdot})^2,$$

where

$$\bar{d}_{i\cdot} = \frac{1}{n} \sum_{j=1}^{n} d_{ij}.$$

Without loss of of generality, consider $\epsilon > 0$ ($\epsilon < 0$) as an indication of *improvement* (*worsening*) of the test drug as compared to the reference drug. In practice, $\sigma_m$ is usually unknown.

### 3.3.1 Test for Equality

The objective is to test the following hypotheses

$$H_0: \epsilon = 0 \quad \text{versus} \quad H_a: \epsilon \neq 0.$$

The null hypothesis $H_0$ is rejected at $\alpha$ level of significance if

$$\left| \frac{\hat{\epsilon}}{\hat{\sigma}_m/\sqrt{2n}} \right| > t_{\alpha/2, 2n-2}.$$

Under the alternative hypothesis that $\epsilon \neq 0$, the power of this test is given by

$$1 - T_{2n-2}\left(t_{\alpha/2, 2n-2} \left| \frac{\sqrt{2n}\epsilon}{\sigma_m} \right.\right) + T_{2n-2}\left(-t_{\alpha/2, 2n-2} \left| \frac{\sqrt{2n}\epsilon}{\sigma_m} \right.\right).$$

As a result, the sample size needed to achieve power $1 - \beta$ can be obtained by setting the power to $1 - \beta$ or, after ignoring a small term $\leq \alpha/2$, by solving

$$T_{2n-2}\left(t_{\alpha/2, 2n-2} \left| \frac{\sqrt{2n}|\epsilon|}{\sigma_m} \right.\right) = \beta.$$

## 3.3. Two-Sample Crossover Design

Table 3.2.1 with $\kappa = 1$ and $\theta = 2|\epsilon|/\sigma_m$ can be used to obtain $n$. From approximation (3.1.5),

$$n = \frac{(z_{\alpha/2} + z_\beta)^2 \sigma_m^2}{2\epsilon^2} \qquad (3.3.3)$$

for sufficiently large $n$.

### 3.3.2 Test for Non-Inferiority/Superiority

Similar to test for non-inferiority/superiority under a parallel design, the problem can be unified by testing the following hypotheses:

$$H_0 : \epsilon \leq \delta \quad \text{versus} \quad H_a : \epsilon > \delta,$$

where $\delta$ is the non-inferiority or superiority margin. When $\delta > 0$, the rejection of the null hypothesis indicates the superiority of test drug against the control. When $\delta < 0$, the rejection of the null hypothesis indicates the non-inferiority of the test drug over the control. The null hypothesis $H_0$ is rejected at the $\alpha$ level of significance if

$$\frac{\hat{\epsilon} - \delta}{\hat{\sigma}_m/\sqrt{2n}} > t_{\alpha, 2n-2}.$$

Under the alternative hypothesis that $\epsilon > \delta$, the power of this test is given by

$$1 - \mathcal{T}_{2n-2}\left(t_{\alpha,2n-2} \left| \frac{\sqrt{2n}(\epsilon - \delta)}{\sigma_m} \right.\right).$$

As a result, the sample size needed to achieve power $1 - \beta$ can be obtained by solving

$$\mathcal{T}_{2n-2}\left(t_{\alpha,2n-2} \left| \frac{\sqrt{2n}(\epsilon - \delta)}{\sigma_m} \right.\right) = \beta,$$

which can be done by using Table 3.2.1 with $\kappa = 1$ and $\theta = 2(\epsilon - \delta)/\sigma_m$. When $n$ is sufficiently large, approximation (3.1.5) leads to

$$n = \frac{(z_\alpha + z_\beta)^2 \sigma_m^2}{2(\epsilon - \delta)^2}. \qquad (3.3.4)$$

### 3.3.3 Test for Equivalence

The objective is to test the following hypotheses

$$H_0 : |\epsilon| \geq \delta \quad \text{versus} \quad H_a : |\epsilon| < \delta.$$

The test drug is concluded equivalent to the control in average, i.e., the null hypothesis $H_0$ is rejected at significance level $\alpha$ when

$$\frac{\sqrt{2n}(\hat{\epsilon} - \delta)}{\hat{\sigma}_m} < -t_{\alpha, 2n-2} \quad \text{and} \quad \frac{\sqrt{2n}(\hat{\epsilon} + \delta)}{\hat{\sigma}_m} > t_{\alpha, 2n-2}.$$

Under the alternative hypothesis that $|\epsilon| < \delta$, the power of this test is

$$1 - \mathcal{T}_{2n-2}\left(t_{\alpha,2n-2}\left|\frac{\sqrt{2n}(\delta - \epsilon)}{\sigma_m}\right.\right)$$

$$-\mathcal{T}_{2n-2}\left(t_{\alpha,2n-2}\left|\frac{\sqrt{2n}(\delta + \epsilon)}{\sigma_m}\right.\right).$$

As a result, the sample size needed to achieve power $1 - \beta$ can be obtained by setting the power to $1 - \beta$. Since the power is larger than

$$1 - 2\mathcal{T}_{2n-2}\left(t_{\alpha,2n-2}\left|\frac{\sqrt{2n}(\delta - |\epsilon|)}{\sigma_m}\right.\right),$$

a conservative approximation of $n$ can be obtained by solving

$$\mathcal{T}_{2n-2}\left(t_{\alpha,2n-2}\left|\frac{\sqrt{2n}(\delta - |\epsilon|)}{\sigma_m}\right.\right) = \frac{\beta}{2},$$

which can be done by using Table 3.2.1 with $\kappa = 1$ and $\theta = 2(\delta - |\epsilon|)/\sigma_m$. When $n$ is large, approximation (3.1.5) leads to

$$n = \frac{(z_\alpha + z_{\beta/2})^2 \sigma_m^2}{2(\delta - |\epsilon|)^2}. \tag{3.3.5}$$

Note that an important application of testing for equivalence under crossover design is testing average bioequivalence (see Section 10.2). By applying a similar idea as introduced by Chow and Liu (2000), a different approximate sample size formula can be obtained as

$$n = \begin{cases} \frac{(z_\alpha + z_{\beta/2})^2 \sigma_m^2}{2\delta^2} & \text{if } \epsilon = 0 \\ \frac{(z_\alpha + z_\beta)^2 \sigma_m^2}{2(\delta - |\epsilon|)^2} & \text{if } \epsilon \neq 0 \end{cases}.$$

## 3.3.4 An Example

### Therapeutic Equivalence

Consider a standard two-sequence, two-period crossover design ($m = 1$) for trials whose objective is to establish therapeutic equivalence between a test drug and a standard therapy. The sponsor is interested in having an 80% ($1 - \beta = 0.8$) power for establishing therapeutic equivalence. Based on the results from previous studies, it is estimated that the variance is 20% ($\sigma_m = 0.20$). Suppose the true mean difference is $-10\%$ (i.e., $\epsilon = \mu_2(\text{test}) - \mu_1(\text{reference}) = -0.10$). Furthermore, we assume that the equivalence limit is 25% (i.e., $\delta = 0.25$). According to (3.3.5),

$$n = \frac{(z_\alpha + z_{\beta/2})^2 \sigma_m^2}{2(\delta - |\epsilon|)^2} = \frac{(1.64 + 1.28)^2 0.20^2}{2(0.25 - 0.10)^2} \approx 8.$$

On the other hand, the sample size calculation can also be performed by using Table 3.2.1. Note that

$$\theta = \frac{2(\delta - |\epsilon|)}{\sigma_m} = \frac{2(0.25 - |-0.10|)}{0.20} = 1.50.$$

By referring to the column under $\alpha = 5\%$, $1 - \beta = 90\%$ at the row with $\theta = 1.50$ in Table 3.2.1, it can be found that the sample size needed is 9.

### Non-Inferiority

Suppose that the sponsor is interested in showing non-inferiority of the test drug against the reference with a non-inferiority margin of $-20\%$ ($\delta = -20\%$). According to (3.3.4), the sample size needed is given by

$$n = \frac{(z_\alpha + z_\beta)^2 \sigma_m^2}{2(\epsilon - \delta)^2} = \frac{(1.64 + 0.84)^2 0.20^2}{2(-0.1 - (-0.2))^2} \approx 13.$$

On the other hand, the sample size calculation can also be performed by using Table 3.2.1. Note that

$$\theta = \frac{2(\epsilon - \delta)}{\sigma_m} = \frac{2(-0.10 - (-0.20))}{0.20} = 1.00.$$

By referring to the column under $\alpha = 5\%$, $1 - \beta = 80\%$ at the row with $\theta = 1.00$ in Table 3.2.1, it can be found that the sample size needed is 14.

## 3.3.5 Remarks

Sample size calculation for assessment of bioequivalence under higher-order crossover designs including Balaam's design, two-sequence dual design, and four-period optimal design with or without log-transformation can be found in Chen, Li, and Chow (1997). For assessment of bioequivalence, the FDA requires that a log-transformation of the pharmacokinetic (PK) responses be performed before analysis.

In this section, we focus on $2 \times 2m$ replicated crossover designs. When $m = 1$, it reduces to the standard two-sequence, two-period crossover design. The standard $2 \times 2$ crossover design suffers the following disadvantages: (i) it does not allow independent estimates of the intra-subject variabilities because each subject only receives each treatment once, (ii) the effects of sequence, period, and carry-over are confounded and cannot be separated under the study design. On the other hand, the $2 \times 2m$ ($m \geq 2$) replicated crossover design not only provides independent estimates of the intra-subject variabilities, but also allows separate tests of the sequence, period, and carry-over effects under appropriate statistical assumption.

## 3.4 Multiple-Sample One-Way ANOVA

Let $x_{ij}$ be the $j$th subject from the $i$th treatment group, $,i = 1,...,k$, $j = 1,...,n$. Consider the following one-way analysis of variance (ANOVA) model:

$$x_{ij} = \mu_i + \epsilon_{ij},$$

where $\mu_i$ is the fixed effect of the $i$th treatment and $\epsilon_{ij}$ is a random error in observing $x_{ij}$. It is assumed that $\epsilon_{ij}$ are i.i.d. normal random variables with mean 0 and variance $\sigma^2$. Let

$$\text{SSE} = \sum_{i=1}^{k} \sum_{j=1}^{n} (x_{ij} - \bar{x}_{i\cdot})^2$$

$$\text{SSA} = \sum_{i=1}^{k} (\bar{x}_{i\cdot} - \bar{x}_{\cdot\cdot})^2,$$

where

$$\bar{x}_{i\cdot} = \frac{1}{n} \sum_{j=1}^{n} x_{ij} \quad \text{and} \quad \bar{x}_{\cdot\cdot} = \frac{1}{k} \sum_{i=1}^{k} \bar{x}_{i\cdot}.$$

Then, $\sigma^2$ can be estimated by

$$\hat{\sigma}^2 = \frac{\text{SSE}}{k(n-1)}. \tag{3.4.1}$$

## 3.4.1 Pairwise Comparison

In practice, it is often of interest to compare means among treatments under study. Thus, the hypotheses of interest are

$$H_0 : \mu_i = \mu_j \quad \text{versus} \quad H_a : \mu_i \neq \mu_j$$

for some pairs $(i, j)$. Under the above hypotheses, there are $k(k-1)/2$ possible comparisons. For example, if there are four treatments in the study, then we can also a maximum of six pairwise comparisons. In practice, it is well recognized that multiple comparison will inflate the type I error. As a result, it is suggested that an adjustment be made for controlling the overall type I error rate at the desired significance level. Assume that there are $\tau$ comparisons of interest, where $\tau \leq k(k-1)/2$. We reject the null hypothesis $H_0$ at the $\alpha$ level of significance if

$$\left| \frac{\sqrt{n}(\bar{x}_{i\cdot} - \bar{x}_{j\cdot})}{\sqrt{2}\hat{\sigma}} \right| > t_{\alpha/(2\tau), k(n-1)}.$$

The power of this test is given by

$$1 - \mathcal{T}_{k(n-1)} \left( t_{\alpha/(2\tau), k(n-1)} \left| \frac{\sqrt{n}\epsilon_{ij}}{\sqrt{2}\sigma} \right. \right) + \mathcal{T}_{k(n-1)} \left( -t_{\alpha/(2\tau), k(n-1)} \left| \frac{\sqrt{n}\epsilon_{ij}}{\sqrt{2}\sigma} \right. \right)$$

$$\approx 1 - \mathcal{T}_{k(n-1)} \left( t_{\alpha/(2\tau), k(n-1)} \left| \frac{\sqrt{n}|\epsilon_{ij}|}{\sqrt{2}\sigma} \right. \right),$$

where $\epsilon_{ij} = \mu_i - \mu_j$. As a result, the sample size needed to achieve power $1 - \beta$ in for detecting a clinically meaningful difference between $\mu_i$ and $\mu_j$ is

$$n = \max\{n_{ij}, \text{ for all interested comparison}\}, \tag{3.4.2}$$

where $n_{ij}$ is obtained by solving

$$\mathcal{T}_{k(n_{ij}-1)} \left( t_{\alpha/(2\tau), k(n_{ij}-1)} \left| \frac{\sqrt{n_{ij}}|\epsilon_{ij}|}{\sqrt{2}\sigma} \right. \right) = \beta.$$

When the sample size is sufficiently large, approximately

$$n_{ij} = \frac{2(z_{\alpha/(2\tau)} + z_\beta)^2 \sigma^2}{\epsilon_{ij}^2}.$$

## 3.4.2 Simultaneous Comparison

The hypotheses of interest is

$$H_0 : \mu_1 = \mu_2 = \cdots = \mu_k$$
$$\text{versus} \quad H_a : \mu_i \neq \mu_j \text{ for some } 1 \leq i < j \leq k.$$

The null hypothesis $H_0$ is rejected at the $\alpha$ level of significance if

$$F_A = \frac{n\text{SSA}/(k-1)}{\text{SSE}/[k(n-1)]} > F_{\alpha, k-1, k(n-1)},$$

where $F_{\alpha, k-1, k(n-1)}$ is the $\alpha$ upper quantile of the F-distribution with $k-1$ and $k(n-1)$ degrees of freedom. Under the alternative hypothesis, the power of this test is given by

$$P(F_A > F_{\alpha, k-1, k(n-1)}) \approx P(n\text{SSA} > \sigma^2 \chi^2_{\alpha, k-1}),$$

where $\chi^2_{\alpha, k-1}$ is the $\alpha$th upper quantile for a $\chi^2$ distribution with $k-1$ degrees of freedom and the approximation follows from the fact that $\text{SSE}/[k(n-1)]$ is approximately $\sigma^2$ and $\chi^2_{\alpha, k-1} \approx (k-1)F_{\alpha, k-1, k(n-1)}$ when $k(n-1)$ is large. Under the alternative hypothesis, $n\text{SSA}/\sigma^2$ is distributed as a non-central $\chi^2$ distribution with degrees of freedom $k-1$ and non-centrality parameter $\lambda = n\Delta$, where

$$\Delta = \frac{1}{\sigma^2} \sum_{i=1}^{k}(\mu_i - \bar{\mu})^2, \qquad \bar{\mu} = \frac{1}{k}\sum_{j=1}^{k}\mu_j.$$

Hence, the sample size needed to achieve power $1-\beta$ can be obtained by solving

$$\chi^2_{k-1}\left(\chi^2_{\alpha, k-1}\big|\lambda\right) = \beta,$$

where $\chi^2_{k-1}(\cdot|\lambda)$ is the cumulative distribution function of the non-central $\chi^2$ distribution with degrees of freedom $k-1$ and non-centrality parameter $\lambda$. Some values of $\lambda$ needed to achieve different power (80% and 90%) with different significance level (1% and 5%) for different number of treatment groups are listed in Table 3.4.1. Once an initial value $\Delta$ is given and a $\lambda$ is obtained from Table 3.4.1, the required sample size is $n = \lambda/\Delta$.

### 3.4.3 An Example

To illustrate the use of Table 3.4.1 for sample size determination when comparing more than two treatments, consider the following example. Suppose that we are interested in conducting a four-arm ($k = 4$) parallel group, double-blind, randomized clinical trial to compare four treatments. The comparison will be made with a significance level of $\alpha = 0.05$. Assume that the standard deviation within each group is $\sigma = 3.5$ and that the true mean responses for the four treatment groups are given by

$$\mu_1 = 8.25, \ \mu_2 = 11.75, \ \mu_3 = 12.00, \text{ and } \mu_4 = 13.00.$$

Then, $\Delta^2 = 1.05$. From Table 3.4.1, for a four-group parallel design ($k = 4$), the non-centrality parameter $\lambda$ needed to achieve a power of 80% ($\beta =$

## 3.4. Multiple-Sample One-Way ANOVA

Table 3.4.1: $\lambda$ Values Satisfying $\chi^2_{k-1}(\chi^2_{\alpha,k-1}|\lambda) = \beta$

| k | $1-\beta = 0.80$ | | $1-\beta = 0.90$ | |
|---|---|---|---|---|
| | $\alpha = 0.01$ | $\alpha = 0.05$ | $\alpha = 0.01$ | $\alpha = 0.05$ |
| 2 | 11.68 | 7.85 | 14.88 | 10.51 |
| 3 | 13.89 | 9.64 | 17.43 | 12.66 |
| 4 | 15.46 | 10.91 | 19.25 | 14.18 |
| 5 | 16.75 | 11.94 | 20.74 | 15.41 |
| 6 | 17.87 | 12.83 | 22.03 | 16.47 |
| 7 | 18.88 | 13.63 | 23.19 | 17.42 |
| 8 | 19.79 | 14.36 | 24.24 | 18.29 |
| 9 | 20.64 | 15.03 | 25.22 | 19.09 |
| 10 | 21.43 | 15.65 | 26.13 | 19.83 |
| 11 | 22.18 | 16.25 | 26.99 | 20.54 |
| 12 | 22.89 | 16.81 | 27.80 | 21.20 |
| 13 | 23.57 | 17.34 | 28.58 | 21.84 |
| 14 | 24.22 | 17.85 | 29.32 | 22.44 |
| 15 | 24.84 | 18.34 | 30.04 | 23.03 |
| 16 | 25.44 | 18.82 | 30.73 | 23.59 |
| 17 | 26.02 | 19.27 | 31.39 | 24.13 |
| 18 | 26.58 | 19.71 | 32.04 | 24.65 |
| 19 | 27.12 | 20.14 | 32.66 | 25.16 |
| 20 | 27.65 | 20.56 | 33.27 | 25.66 |

0.20) at 5% level of significance is 10.91. As a result, the sample size per treatment group can be obtained as

$$n = \frac{10.91}{1.05} \approx 11.$$

### 3.4.4 Remarks

In practice, a question concerning when pairwise comparisons or a simultaneous comparison should be used often rises. To address this question, consider the following example. Suppose a sponsor is investigating a pharmaceutical compound for treatment of patients with cancer. The investigator is not only interested in showing efficacy of the test drug but also in establishing dose response curve. To achieve this study objective, a four-group parallel trial is designed with four treatments: P(Placebo), A(10 mg), B(20 mg), and C(30 mg). Let $\mu_p$, $\mu_A$, $\mu_B$, and $\mu_C$ represent the true mean of the clinical response under the four treatments, respectively. Since the primary objective of the trial is to demonstrate the efficacy of the test drug. The following hypotheses for pairwise comparison with the placebo are useful for demonstration of efficacy of the test drug.

$$H_0 : \mu_P = \mu_A \quad \text{versus} \quad H_a : \mu_P \neq \mu_A$$
$$H_0 : \mu_P = \mu_B \quad \text{versus} \quad H_a : \mu_P \neq \mu_B$$
$$H_0 : \mu_P = \mu_C \quad \text{versus} \quad H_a : \mu_P \neq \mu_C.$$

On the other hand, the following hypotheses for simultaneous comparison among doses is usually considered for studying dose response

$$H_0 : \mu_A = \mu_B = \mu_C \quad \text{versus} \quad H_a : \text{ not } H_0.$$

Note that in practice, it is often of interest to test the null hypothesis of no treatment difference against an ordered alternative hypothesis, e.g., $H_a : \mu_A < \mu_B < \mu_C$. In this case, some robust contrast-based trend tests can be used for sample size calculation.

## 3.5 Multiple-Sample Williams Design

In clinical research, crossover design is attractive because each subject serves as his/her control. In addition, it removes the inter-subject variability from comparison under appropriate statistical assumption. For example, the United States Food and Drug Administration (FDA) identifies crossover design as the design of choice for bioequivalence trials. As a result, a two-sequence, two-period crossover design comparing two treatments is often considered in clinical research. In practice, it is often of interest to compare more than two treatments under a crossover design. When there are more than two treatments, it is desirable to compare pairwise treatment effects with the same degrees of freedom. Hence, it is suggested that Williams design be considered. Under a Williams design, the following model is assumed:

$$y_{ijl} = P_{j'} + \gamma_i + \mu_l + e_{ijl}, \quad i, l = 1, ..., k, j = 1, ..., n,$$

where $y_{ijl}$ is the response from the $j$th subject in the $i$th sequence under the $l$th treatment, $P_{j'}$ is the fixed effect for the $j'$ period, $j'$ is the number of the period for the $i$th sequence's $l$th treatment, $\sum_{j=1}^{a} P_j = 0$, $\gamma_i$ is the fixed sequence effect, $\mu_j$ is the fixed treatment effect, and $e_{ijl}$ is a normal random variable with mean 0 and variance $\sigma_{il}^2$. For fixed $i$ and $l$, $e_{ijl}, j = 1, ..., n$ are independent and identically distributed. For fixed $i$ and $j$, $e_{ijl}, l = 1, ..., a$ are usually correlated because they all come from the same subject.

## 3.5. Multiple-Sample Williams Design

In bioequivalence trials, Williams designs comparing three treatments (a $6 \times 3$ crossover design) or four treatments (a $4 \times 4$ crossover design) are commonly employed. The construction of a Williams design can be found in Jones and Kenward (1989) and Chow and Liu (1992, 2000). Note that if $k$ is an odd integer, a Williams design results in a $2k \times k$ crossover design. On the other hand, if $k$ is an even integer, a Williams design reduces to a $k \times k$ crossover design.

It should be noted that the sequence-by-period interaction is not included in the above model. This is because that the responses from a given sequence's given treatment are all from the same period. Therefore, the fixed effect of the sequence-by-period interaction cannot be separated from the treatment effect without appropriate statistical assumption.

Without loss of generality, assume we want to compare treatments 1 and 2. Let

$$d_{ij} = y_{ij1} - y_{ij2}.$$

Then, the true mean difference between treatment 1 and 2 can be estimated by

$$\hat{\epsilon} = \frac{1}{kn} \sum_{i=1}^{k} \sum_{j=1}^{n} d_{ij},$$

which is normally distributed with mean $\epsilon = \mu_1 - \mu_2$ and variance $\sigma_d^2/(kn)$, where $\sigma_d^2$ is defined to be the variance of $d_{ij}$ and can be estimated by

$$\hat{\sigma}_d^2 = \frac{1}{k(n-1)} \sum_{i=1}^{k} \sum_{j=1}^{n} \left( d_{ij} - \frac{1}{n} \sum_{j'=1}^{n} d_{ij'} \right)^2.$$

### 3.5.1 Test for Equality

The objective is to test

$$H_0 : \epsilon = 0 \quad \text{versus} \quad H_a : \epsilon \neq 0.$$

The null hypothesis $H_0$ is rejected at $\alpha$ level of significance if

$$\left| \frac{\hat{\epsilon}}{\hat{\sigma}_d/\sqrt{kn}} \right| > t_{\alpha/2, k(n-1)}.$$

Under the alternative hypothesis that $\epsilon \neq 0$, the power of this test is approximately

$$1 - \mathcal{T}_{k(n-1)} \left( t_{\alpha/2, k(n-1)} \left| \frac{\sqrt{kn}\epsilon}{\sigma_d} \right| \right).$$

The sample size needed to achieve power $1-\beta$ can be obtained by setting the power to $1-\beta$. When $n$ is sufficiently large, approximation (3.1.5) leads to

$$n = \frac{(z_{\alpha/2} + z_\beta)^2 \sigma_d^2}{k\epsilon^2}. \tag{3.5.1}$$

## 3.5.2 Test for Non-Inferiority/Superiority

The problem of testing superiority and non-inferiority can be unified by the following hypotheses:

$$H_0 : \epsilon \leq \delta \quad \text{versus} \quad H_a : \epsilon > \delta,$$

where $\delta$ is the superiority or non-inferiority margin. When $\delta > 0$, the rejection of the null hypothesis indicates the superiority of test drug over the control. When $\delta < 0$, the rejection of the null hypothesis indicates the non-inferiority of the test drug against the control. The null hypothesis $H_0$ is rejected at $\alpha$ level of significance if

$$\frac{\hat{\epsilon} - \delta}{\hat{\sigma}_d/\sqrt{kn}} > t_{\alpha,k(n-1)}.$$

Under the alternative hypothesis that $\epsilon > \delta$, the power of this test is given by

$$1 - \mathcal{T}_{k(n-1)}\left(t_{\alpha,k(n-1)} \left| \frac{\epsilon - \delta}{\sigma_d/\sqrt{kn}} \right.\right).$$

As a result, the sample size needed to achieve power $1-\beta$ can be obtained by setting the power to $1-\beta$. When $n$ is sufficiently large, approximation (3.1.5) leads to

$$n = \frac{(z_\alpha + z_\beta)^2 \sigma_d^2}{k(\epsilon - \delta)^2}. \tag{3.5.2}$$

## 3.5.3 Test for Equivalence

The objective is to test the following hypotheses

$$H_0 : |\epsilon| \geq \delta \quad \text{versus} \quad H_a : |\epsilon| < \delta.$$

The test drug is concluded equivalent to the control in average if the null hypothesis $H_0$ is rejected at significance level $\alpha$, i.e.,

$$\frac{\sqrt{kn}(\hat{\epsilon} - \delta)}{\hat{\sigma}_d} < -t_{\alpha,k(n-1)} \quad \text{and} \quad \frac{\sqrt{kn}(\hat{\epsilon} + \delta)}{\hat{\sigma}_d} > t_{\alpha,k(n-1)}.$$

## 3.6. Practical Issues

Under the alternative hypothesis that $|\epsilon| < \delta$, the power of the above test is

$$1 - T_{k(n-1)}\left(t_{\alpha,k(n-1)} \left| \frac{\sqrt{kn}(\delta - \epsilon)}{\sigma_d} \right. \right) - T_{k(n-1)}\left(t_{\alpha,k(n-1)} \left| \frac{\sqrt{kn}(\delta + \epsilon)}{\sigma_d} \right. \right).$$

The sample size needed to achieve power $1 - \beta$ can be obtained by setting the power to $1 - \beta$. A conservative approximation to the required sample size can be obtained by solving

$$T_{k(n-1)}\left(t_{\alpha,k(n-1)} \left| \frac{\sqrt{kn}(\delta - |\epsilon|)}{\sigma_d} \right. \right) = \frac{\beta}{2}.$$

When $n$ is large, approximation (3.1.5) leads to

$$n = \frac{(z_\alpha + z_{\beta/2})^2 \sigma_d^2}{k(\delta - |\epsilon|)^2}.$$

### 3.5.4 An Example

Consider a randomized, placebo-controlled, double-blind, three-way (three-sequence, three-period) crossover trial, which is known as a Williams $6 \times 3$ ($k = 3$) crossover trial comparing cardiovascular safety of three different treatments (A, B, and C). Based on the results from the pilot study, it is estimated that the standard deviation is 0.10 (i.e. $\delta_d = 0.10$). Suppose the true mean for A, B, and C are given by 0.20, 0.15, 0.25, respectively. At the 5% level of significance, the sample size needed for achieving a power of 80% to reject

$$H_0: \mu_i = \mu_j \text{ vs. } H_a: \mu_i \neq \mu_j$$

can be obtained by

$$n_{AB} = \frac{(1.96 + 0.84)^2 0.10^2}{6(0.20 - 0.15)^2} \approx 6$$

$$n_{AC} = \frac{(1.96 + 0.84)^2 0.10^2}{6(0.20 - 0.25)^2} \approx 6$$

$$n_{BC} = \frac{(1.96 + 0.84)^2 0.10^2}{6(0.15 - 0.25)^2} \approx 2.$$

As a result, the sample size need per sequence is given by

$$n = \max\{6, 6, 2\} = 6.$$

It should be noted that the sample size can also be obtained by using the non-central t-distribution like before. However, since there are 6 sequences in this example, which alternates the degrees of freedom. Both Tables 3.1.1 and 3.2.1 cannot be used.

## 3.6 Practical Issues

At the planning stage of a clinical trial, sample size calculation is necessarily performed based on appropriate statistical test for the hypotheses that reflect the study objectives under a valid study design. In this section, some practical issues that are commonly encountered are discussed.

### 3.6.1 One-Sided Versus Two-Sided Test

In this chapter, statistical tests used for sample size calculation under either a parallel design or a crossover design can be classified into either a one-sided test (i.e., test for non-inferiority and test for superiority) or a two-sided test (i.e., test for equality and test for equivalence). In clinical research, test for non-inferiority or test for superiority are also known as one-sided equivalence test. As discussed in Chapter 1, it is very controversial to use a one-sided test or a two-sided test in clinical research. When switching from a two-sided test for therapeutic equivalence to a one-sided test for non-inferiority under a parallel design with 1 to 1 allocation, sample size could be reduced substantially at a fixed $\alpha$ level of significance. Suppose that the true mean difference between two treatments is $\epsilon = 0$. Based on (3.2.3) and (3.2.4), the ratio of the sample sizes needed for non-inferiority and therapeutic equivalence is given by

$$\frac{n_{\text{non-inferiority}}}{n_{\text{equivalence}}} = \frac{(z_\alpha + z_\beta)^2}{(z_\alpha + z_{\beta/2})^2}.$$

Table 3.6.1 summarizes possible sample size reduction when switching from testing equivalence to testing non-inferiority (one-sided equivalence). As it can be seen from Table 3.6.1, the sample size could be reduced by 27.8% when switching from testing equivalence to testing non-inferiority at the $\alpha = 0.05$ level of significance but still maintain the same power of 80%.

### 3.6.2 Parallel Design Versus Crossover Design

As indicated in the previous sections, sample size required for achieving a desired power under a crossover design may be less than that under a parallel design. Under a parallel design, treatment comparison is made based on both inter-subject and intra-subject variabilities, whereas treatment comparison is made based on the intra-subject variability under a crossover design under appropriate statistical assumption. If both designs are equally *efficient* regardless their relative merits and disadvantages, then the choice of the design should be based on an evaluation of the relative cost-effectiveness between the increase of an additional treatment period in

## 3.6. Practical Issues

Table 3.6.1: Sample Size Reduction from Testing Equivalence to Testing Non-Inferiority

| $\alpha$ | $\beta$ | Sample Size Reduction(%) |
|---|---|---|
| 0.10 | 0.1 | 23.3 |
|  | 0.2 | 31.4 |
| 0.05 | 0.1 | 20.9 |
|  | 0.2 | 27.8 |
| 0.01 | 0.1 | 17.5 |
|  | 0.2 | 22.9 |

a crossover design with respect to the increase of additional subjects in a parallel design.

Consider the sample size in testing equality or equivalence. The ratio of the sample size for a $2 \times 2$ crossover design ($m = 1$) over the sample size for a parallel deisgn is given by

$$\frac{n_{\text{crossover}}}{n_{\text{parallel}}} = \frac{\sigma_{WT}^2 + \sigma_{WR}^2 + \sigma_D^2}{\sigma_{WR}^2 + \sigma_{WT}^2 + \sigma_{BR}^2 + \sigma_{BT}^2}.$$

Table 3.6.2 summarizes possible sample size reduction when switching from a parallel design to a crossover design under the assumption that $\sigma_{WT} = \sigma_{WR} = \sigma_{BR} = \sigma_{BR} = 1$. As it can be seen, the sample size could be reduced by 30% by switching a parallel design to a crossover design when $\rho = 0.6$.

### 3.6.3 Sensitivity Analysis

Sample size calculation is usually performed by using initial values of the difference in mean responses between treatment groups (i.e., $\epsilon$), the standard deviation (i.e., $\sigma$), and the clinically meaningful difference or a pre-specified superiority/non-inferiority margin or equivalence limit (i.e., $\delta$). Any slight or moderate deviations from these initial values could result in a substantial change in the calculated sample sizes. Thus, it is suggested that a sensitivity analysis with respect to these initial values be performed. Sensitivity analysis provides useful information regarding what to expect if a deviation in any of the initial values shall occur. For example, consider a one-sample problem

$$H_0 : \mu = \mu_0 \quad \text{versus} \quad H_a : \mu \neq \mu_0.$$

Table 3.6.2: Sample Size Reduction from Parallel Design to Crossover Design

| $\rho$ | Sample Size Reduction(%) |
|---|---|
| 0.0 | 0.00 |
| 0.1 | 0.05 |
| 0.2 | 0.10 |
| 0.3 | 0.15 |
| 0.4 | 0.20 |
| 0.5 | 0.25 |
| 0.6 | 0.30 |
| 0.7 | 0.35 |
| 0.8 | 0.40 |
| 0.9 | 0.45 |
| 1.0 | 0.50 |

Table 3.6.3: Sample Size Reduction When Variability Decreases

| $c$ | Sample Size Reduction(%) |
|---|---|
| 1.0 | 0.00 |
| 0.9 | 0.19 |
| 0.8 | 0.36 |
| 0.7 | 0.51 |
| 0.6 | 0.64 |
| 0.5 | 0.75 |
| 0.4 | 0.84 |
| 0.3 | 0.91 |
| 0.2 | 0.96 |
| 0.1 | 0.99 |

## 3.6. Practical Issues

According to (3.1.2), if the standard deviation changes from $\sigma$ to $c\sigma$ for some $c > 0$, the ratio of the sample sizes needed before and after the change is given by

$$\frac{n_{c\sigma}}{n_\sigma} = c^2,$$

which is independent of the choice of $\alpha$ and $\beta$. Table 3.6.3 summarizes possible sample size reduction when the standard deviation changes from $\sigma$ to $c\sigma$. People in practice may want to see how much the sample size would increase when the variability increases, which is equivalent to study how much sample size would be saved if the variability decreases. As a result, without loss of generality, we would assume $c < 1$.

From Table 3.6.3, when the standard deviation decreases by 20% (i.e., $c = 0.8$), the sample size could be reduced by 36% when performing a test for equivalence at the $\alpha = 0.05$ level of significance but still maintain the same power of 80%.

# Chapter 4

# Large Sample Tests for Proportions

In clinical research, primary clinical endpoints for evaluation of the treatment effect of the compound under study could be discrete variables, for example, clinical response (e.g., complete response, partial response, and stable disease), survival in cancer trials, and the presence of adverse events in clinical trials. For evaluation of treatment effect based on discrete clinical endpoint, the proportions of events that have occurred between treatment groups are often compared. Under a given study design, statistical tests for specific hypotheses such as equality or equivalence/non-inferiority can be carried out based on the large sample theory in a similar manner as continuous responses discussed in Chapter 3. In this chapter, our primary focus will be placed on comparing proportions between treatment groups with binary responses.

The remaining sections of this chapter are organized as follows. In the next section, a general procedure of power analysis for sample size calculation for testing one-sample problem is given. Sections 4.2 and 4.3 summarize statistical procedures for sample size calculation for a two-sample problem under a parallel-group design and a crossover design, respectively. Sections 4.4 and 4.5 discuss statistical procedures for testing a multiple-sample problem under a parallel design and a crossover design (Williams design), respectively. Formulas for sample size calculation for comparing relative risks between treatment groups under a parallel design and a crossover design are given in Section 4.6 and 4.7, respectively. Section 4.8 provides some practical issues regarding sample size calculation for comparing proportions in clinical research.

## 4.1 One-Sample Design

Let $x_i, i = 1, ..., n$ be the binary response observed from the $i$th subject. In clinical research, $x_i$ could be the indicator for the response of tumor in cancer trials, i.e., $x_i = 1$ for responder (e.g., complete response plus partial response) or $x_i = 0$ for non-responder. It is assumed that $x_i$'s are i.i.d with $P(x_i = 1) = p$, where $p$ is the true response rate. Since $p$ is unknown, it is usually estimated by

$$\hat{p} = \frac{1}{n} \sum_{i=1}^{n} x_i.$$

Also, let $\epsilon = p - p_0$ be the difference between the true response rate of a test drug ($p$) and a reference value ($p_0$). Without loss of generality, consider $\epsilon > 0$ ($\epsilon < 0$) an indication of *improvement* (*worsening*) of the test drug as compared to the reference value. In practice, it is of interest to test for equality (i.e., $p = p_0$), non-inferiority (i.e., $p - p_0$ is greater than or equal to a pre-determined non-inferiority margin), superiority (i.e., $p - p_0$ is greater than a pre-determined superiority margin), and equivalence (i.e., the absolute difference between $p$ and $p_0$ is within a difference of clinical importance). In what follows, formulas for sample size calculation for testing equality, non-inferiority/superiority, and equivalence are derived. The formulas provide required sample sizes for achieving a desired power under the alternative hypothesis.

### 4.1.1 Test for Equality

To test whether there is a difference between the true response rate of the test drug and the reference value, the following hypotheses are usually considered:

$$H_0 : p = p_0 \text{ versus } H_a : p \neq p_0.$$

or

$$H_0 : \epsilon = 0 \text{ versus } H_a : \epsilon \neq 0.$$

Under the null hypothesis, the test statistic

$$\frac{\sqrt{n}\hat{\epsilon}}{\sqrt{\hat{p}(1-\hat{p})}}, \tag{4.1.1}$$

where $\hat{\epsilon} = \hat{p} - p_0$ approximately has a standard normal distribution for large $n$. Thus, we reject the null hypothesis at the $\alpha$ level of significance if

$$\left| \frac{\sqrt{n}\hat{\epsilon}}{\sqrt{\hat{p}(1-\hat{p})}} \right| > z_{\alpha/2}.$$

## 4.1. One-Sample Design

Under the alternative hypothesis that $p = p_0 + \epsilon$, where $\epsilon \neq 0$, the power of the above test is approximately

$$\Phi\left(\frac{\sqrt{n}|\epsilon|}{\sqrt{p(1-p)}} - z_{\alpha/2}\right).$$

As a result, the sample size needed for achieving a desired power of $1 - \beta$ can be obtained by solving the following equation

$$\frac{\sqrt{n}|\epsilon|}{\sqrt{p(1-p)}} - z_{\alpha/2} = z_\beta.$$

This leads to

$$n = \frac{(z_{\alpha/2} + z_\beta)^2 p(1-p)}{\epsilon^2}. \tag{4.1.2}$$

To use (4.1.2), information regarding $p$ is needed, which may be obtained through a pilot study or based on historical data. Note that $p(1-p)$ is a quadratic function symmetric about 0.5 on its domain $(0, 1)$. Thus, using (4.1.2) requires an upper bound on $p$ and a lower bound on $\epsilon^2$. For example, if we know that $p \leq \tilde{p}$, $1 - p \leq \tilde{p}$, and $\epsilon^2 \geq \tilde{\epsilon}^2$, where $\tilde{p}$ is a known value between 0 and 0.5 and $\tilde{\epsilon}^2$ is a known positive value, then $p(1-p) \leq \tilde{p}(1-\tilde{p})$ and a conservative $n$ can be obtained by using (4.1.2) with $\epsilon$ and $p$ replaced by $\tilde{\epsilon}$ and $\tilde{p}$, respectively.

### 4.1.2  Test for Non-Inferiority/Superiority

The problem of testing non-inferiority and superiority can be unified by the following hypotheses:

$$H_0 : p - p_0 \leq \delta \text{ versus } H_a : p - p_0 > \delta$$

or

$$H_0 : \epsilon \leq \delta \text{ versus } H_a : \epsilon > \delta,$$

where $\delta$ is the non-inferiority or superiority margin. When $\delta > 0$, the rejection of the null hypothesis indicates superiority over the reference value. When $\delta < 0$, the rejection of the null hypothesis implies non-inferiority against the reference value.

When $p - p_0 = \delta$, the test statistic

$$\frac{\sqrt{n}(\hat{\epsilon} - \delta)}{\sqrt{\hat{p}(1-\hat{p})}}$$

approximately has a standard normal distribution for large $n$. Thus, we reject the null hypothesis at the $\alpha$ level of significance if

$$\frac{\sqrt{n}(\hat{\epsilon} - \delta)}{\sqrt{\hat{p}(1-\hat{p})}} > z_\alpha.$$

If $\epsilon > \delta$, the power of the above test is given by

$$\Phi\left(\frac{\sqrt{n}(\epsilon - \delta)}{\sqrt{p(1-p)}} - z_\alpha\right).$$

As a result, the sample size needed for achieving a power of $1 - \beta$ can be obtained by solving the following equation

$$\frac{\sqrt{n}(\epsilon - \delta)}{\sqrt{p(1-p)}} - z_\alpha = z_\beta.$$

This leads to

$$n = \frac{(z_\alpha + z_\beta)^2 p(1-p)}{(\epsilon - \delta)^2}. \qquad (4.1.3)$$

### 4.1.3   Test for Equivalence

To establish equivalence, the following hypotheses are usually considered

$$H_0 : |p - p_0| \geq \delta \text{ versus } H_a : |p - p_0| < \delta$$

or

$$H_0 : |\epsilon| \geq \delta \text{ versus } H_a : |\epsilon| < \delta.$$

The proportion of the responses is concluded to be equivalent to the reference value of $p_0$ if the null hypothesis is rejected at a given significance level.

The above hypotheses can be tested using two one-sided test procedures as described in Chapter 3. The null hypothesis is rejected at approximately $\alpha$ level of significance if

$$\frac{\sqrt{n}(\hat\epsilon - \delta)}{\sqrt{\hat p(1-\hat p)}} < -z_\alpha \quad \text{and} \quad \frac{\sqrt{n}(\hat\epsilon + \delta)}{\sqrt{\hat p(1-\hat p)}} > z_\alpha.$$

When $n$ is large, the power of this test is approximately

$$\Phi\left(\frac{\sqrt{n}(\delta - \epsilon)}{\sqrt{p(1-p)}} - z_\alpha\right) + \Phi\left(\frac{\sqrt{n}(\delta + \epsilon)}{\sqrt{p(1-p)}} - z_\alpha\right) - 1$$

$$\geq 2\Phi\left(\frac{\sqrt{n}(\delta - |\epsilon|)}{\sqrt{p(1-p)}} - z_\alpha\right) - 1.$$

As a result, the sample size needed for achieving a power of $1 - \beta$ can be obtained by solving the following equations

$$\frac{\sqrt{n}(\delta - |\epsilon|)}{\sqrt{p(1-p)}} - z_\alpha = z_{\beta/2},$$

## 4.1. One-Sample Design

which leads to
$$n = \frac{(z_\alpha + z_{\beta/2})^2 p(1-p)}{(\delta - |\epsilon|)^2}. \qquad (4.1.4)$$

### 4.1.4 An Example

To illustrate the use of sample size formulas, consider the same example concerning a study of osteoporosis in post-menopausal women as described in Section 3.1.4. Suppose in addition to the study of the change in bone density post-treatment, it is also of interest to evaluate the treatment effect in terms of the response rate at the end of the study. Sample size calculation can then be carried out based on the response rate for achieving a desired power. The definition of a responder, however, should be given in the study protocol prospectively. For example, a subject may be defined as a responder if there is an improvement in bone density by more than one standard deviation (SD) or 30% of the measurements of bone density.

**Test for Equality**

Suppose that the response rate of the patient population under study after treatment is expected to be around 50% (i.e., $p = 0.50$). By (4.1.2), at $\alpha = 0.05$, the required sample size for having an 80% power (i.e., $\beta = 0.2$) for correctly detecting a difference between the post-treatment response rate and the reference value of 30% (i.e., $p_0 = 0.30$) is

$$n = \frac{(z_{\alpha/2} + z_\beta)^2 p(1-p)}{(p - p_0)^2} = \frac{(1.96 + 0.84)^2 0.5(1 - 0.5)}{(0.5 - 0.3)^2} = 49.$$

**Test for Non-Inferiority**

For prevention of progression from osteopenia to osteoporosis, we wish to show that the majority of patients whose change in bone density after treatment is at least as good as the reference value (30%) ($p_0 = 30\%$). Also assume that a difference of 10% in responder rate is considered of no clinical significance ($\delta = -10\%$). Assume the true response rate is 50% ($p = 50\%$). According to (4.1.3), at $\alpha=0.05$, the required sample size for having an 80% power (i.e., $\beta=0.2$) is

$$n = \frac{(z_\alpha + z_\beta)^2 p(1-p)}{(p - p_0 - \delta)^2} = \frac{(1.64 + 0.84)^2 0.5(1 - 0.5)}{(0.5 - 0.3 + 0.1)^2} \approx 18.$$

**Test for Equivalence**

Assume that one brand name drug for osteoporosis on the market has a responder rate of 60% (i.e., $p_0 = 0.60$). It is believed that a 20% difference in responder rate is of no clinical significance (i.e., $\delta = 0.2$). Hence, the investigator wants to show the study drug is equivalent to the market drug in terms of responder rate. By (4.1.4), at $\alpha = 0.05$, assuming that the true response rate is 60% (i.e., $p = 0.60$), the sample size required for achieving an 80% power is

$$n = \frac{(z_\alpha + z_{\beta/2})^2 p(1-p)}{(\delta - |p - p_0|)^2} = \frac{(1.64 + 1.28)^2 \times 0.6(1-0.6)}{(0.2 - |0.6 - 0.6|)^2} \approx 52.$$

### 4.1.5 Remarks

For one-sample test for equality, there exists another approach, which is very similar to (4.1.1) but not exactly the same. This approach will reject the null hypothesis that $\epsilon = 0$ if

$$\left| \frac{\sqrt{n}\hat{\epsilon}}{\sqrt{p_0(1-p_0)}} \right| > z_{\alpha/2}. \tag{4.1.5}$$

Since (4.1.1) estimates the variance of $\sqrt{n}\hat{\epsilon}$ without any constraints, we refer to (4.1.1) as the unconditional method. On the other hand, since (4.1.5) estimates the variance of $\sqrt{n}\hat{\epsilon}$ conditional on the null hypothesis, we refer to (4.1.5) as the conditional method. Note that both (4.1.1) and (4.1.5) have asymptotic size $\alpha$ when $n$ is sufficiently large. Then, which one should be used is always a dilemma because one is not necessarily more powerful than the other. For the purpose of completeness, the sample size calculation formula based on (4.1.5) is given below. The same idea can be applied to the testing problems of non-inferiority/superiority.

Under the alternative hypothesis ($\epsilon \neq 0$), the power of the test defined by (4.1.5) is approximately

$$\Phi\left( \frac{\sqrt{n}|\epsilon| - z_{\alpha/2}\sqrt{p_0(1-p_0)}}{\sqrt{p(1-p)}} \right).$$

As a result, the sample size needed for achieving a desired power of $1 - \beta$ can be obtained by solving the following equation:

$$\frac{\sqrt{n}|\epsilon| - z_{\alpha/2}\sqrt{p_0(1-p_0)}}{\sqrt{p(1-p)}} = z_\beta.$$

This leads to

$$n = \frac{[z_{\alpha/2}\sqrt{p_0(1-p_0)} + z_\beta \sqrt{p(1-p)}]^2}{\epsilon^2}.$$

## 4.2  Two-Sample Parallel Design

Let $x_{ij}$ be a binary response from the $j$th subject in the $i$th treatment group, $j = 1, ..., n_i$, $i = 1, 2$. For a fixed $i$, it is assumed that $x_{ij}$'s are i.i.d. with $P(x_{ij} = 1) = p_i$. In practice, $p_i$ is usually estimated by the observed proportion in the $i$th treatment group:

$$\hat{p}_i = \frac{1}{n_i} \sum_{j=1}^{n_i} x_{ij}.$$

Let $\epsilon = p_1 - p_2$ be the difference between the true mean response rates of a test drug ($p_1$) and a control ($p_2$). Without loss of generality, consider $\epsilon > 0$ ($\epsilon < 0$) an indication of *improvement* (*worsening*) of the test drug as compared to the control value. In what follows, formulas for sample size calculation to achieve a desired power under the alternative hypothesis are derived for testing equality, non-inferiority/superiority, and equivalence.

### 4.2.1  Test for Equality

To test whether there is a difference between the mean response rates of the test drug and the reference drug, the following hypotheses are usually considered:

$$H_0 : \epsilon = 0 \quad \text{versus} \quad H_a : \epsilon \neq 0.$$

We reject the null hypothesis at the $\alpha$ level of significance if

$$\left| \frac{\hat{p}_1 - \hat{p}_2}{\sqrt{\hat{p}_1(1-\hat{p}_1)/n_1 + \hat{p}_2(1-\hat{p}_2)/n_2}} \right| > z_{\alpha/2}. \tag{4.2.1}$$

Under the alternative hypothesis that $\epsilon \neq 0$, the power of the above test is approximately

$$\Phi\left( \frac{|\epsilon|}{\sqrt{p_1(1-p_1)/n_1 + p_2(1-p_2)/n_2}} - z_{\alpha/2} \right).$$

As a result, the sample size needed for achieving a power of $1 - \beta$ can be obtained by the following equation:

$$\frac{|\epsilon|}{\sqrt{p_1(1-p_1)/n_1 + p_2(1-p_2)/n_2}} - z_{\alpha/2} = z_\beta.$$

This leads to

$$n_1 = \kappa n_2$$
$$n_2 = \frac{(z_{\alpha/2}+z_\beta)^2}{\epsilon^2} \left[ \frac{p_1(1-p_1)}{\kappa} + p_2(1-p_2) \right]. \tag{4.2.2}$$

## 4.2.2 Test for Non-Inferiority/Superiority

The problem of testing non-inferiority and superiority can be unified by the following hypotheses:

$$H_0: \epsilon \leq \delta \quad \text{versus} \quad H_a: \epsilon > \delta,$$

where $\delta$ is the superiority or non-inferiority margin. When $\delta > 0$, the rejection of the null hypothesis indicates the superiority of the test drug over the control. When $\delta < 0$, the rejection of the null hypothesis indicates the non-inferiority of the test drug against the control.

We reject the null hypothesis at the $\alpha$ level of significance if

$$\frac{\hat{p}_1 - \hat{p}_2 - \delta}{\sqrt{\hat{p}_1(1-\hat{p}_1)/n_1 + \hat{p}_2(1-\hat{p}_2)/n_2}} > z_\alpha.$$

Under the alternative hypothesis that $\epsilon > \delta$, the power of the above test is approximately

$$\Phi\left(\frac{\epsilon - \delta}{\sqrt{p_1(1-p_1)/n_1 + p_2(1-p_2)/n_2}} - z_\alpha\right).$$

As a result, the sample size needed for achieving a power of $1 - \beta$ can be obtained by solving

$$\frac{\epsilon - \delta}{\sqrt{p_1(1-p_1)/n_1 + p_2(1-p_2)/n_2}} - z_\alpha = z_\beta,$$

which leads to

$$n_1 = \kappa n_2$$
$$n_2 = \frac{(z_\alpha + z_\beta)^2}{(\epsilon - \delta)^2}\left[\frac{p_1(1-p_1)}{\kappa} + p_2(1-p_2)\right]. \tag{4.2.3}$$

## 4.2.3 Test for Equivalence

The objective is to test the following hypotheses:

$$H_0: |\epsilon| \geq \delta \quad \text{versus} \quad H_a: |\epsilon| < \delta.$$

The null hypothesis is rejected and the test drug is concluded to be equivalent to the control if

$$\frac{\hat{p}_1 - \hat{p}_2 - \delta}{\sqrt{\hat{p}_1(1-\hat{p}_1)/n_1 + \hat{p}_2(1-\hat{p}_2)/n_2}} < -z_\alpha$$

## 4.2. Two-Sample Parallel Design

and

$$\frac{\hat{p}_1 - \hat{p}_2 + \delta}{\sqrt{\hat{p}_1(1-\hat{p}_1)/n_1 + \hat{p}_2(1-\hat{p}_2)/n_2}} > z_\alpha.$$

Under the alternative hypothesis that $|\epsilon| < \delta$, the power of the above test is approximately

$$2\Phi\left(\frac{\delta - |\epsilon|}{\sqrt{p_1(1-p_1)/n_1 + p_2(1-p_2)/n_2}} - z_\alpha\right) - 1.$$

As a result, the sample size needed for achieving a power of $1 - \beta$ can be obtained by solving the following equation:

$$\frac{\delta - |\epsilon|}{\sqrt{p_1(1-p_1)/n_1 + p_2(1-p_2)/n_2}} - z_\alpha = z_{\beta/2},$$

which leads to

$$n_1 = \kappa n_2$$
$$n_2 = \frac{(z_\alpha + z_{\beta/2})^2}{(\delta - |\epsilon|)^2}\left[\frac{p_1(1-p_1)}{\kappa} + p_2(1-p_2)\right]. \quad (4.2.4)$$

### 4.2.4 An Example

Consider the following example concerning the evaluation of anti-infective agents in the treatment of patients with skin and skin structure infections. As it is well known, gram-positive and gram-negative pathogens are commonly associated with skin and skin structure infections such as streptococci, staphylococci, and various strains of enterobacteriaceae. For the evaluation of the effectiveness of a test antibiotic agent, clinical assessments and cultures are usually done at a post-treatment visits (e.g., between 4 and 8 days) after treatment has been completed but prior to treatment with another anti-microbial agent. If the culture is positive, the pathogen(s) is usually identified and susceptibility testing is performed. The effectiveness of therapy is usually assessed based on clinical and bacteriological responses at post-treatment visit. For example, clinical responses may include cure (e.g., no signs of skin infection at post-treatment visits), improvment (e.g., the skin infection has resolved to the extent that no further systemic antibiotic therapy is needed based on the best judgment of the investigator), failure (e.g., lack of significant improvement in the signs and symptoms of the skin infection at or before post-treatment visits such that a change in antibiotic treatment is required). On the other hand, bacteriological responses may include cure (e.g., all pathogens eradicated at post-treatment day 4-8 or material suitable for culturing has diminished to a degree that proper cultures cannot be obtained), colonization (e.g., isolation of pathogen(s) from the original site of infection in the absence of local or systemic signs of infection at post-treatment visits), and failure (e.g., any pathogen(s) isolated at post-treatment visits coupled with the investigator's decision to prescribe alternate antibiotic therapy).

Suppose that a pharmaceutical company is interested in conducting a clinical trial to compare the efficacy, safety, and tolerability of two anti-microbial agents when administered orally once daily in the treatment of patients with skin and skin structure infections. In what follows, we will consider the situations where the intended trial is for (i) testing equality of mean cure rates, (ii) testing non-inferiority or superiority of the test drug as compared to the active control agent, and (iii) testing for therapeutic equivalence. For this purpose, the following assumptions are made. First, sample size calculation will be performed for achieving an 80% power (i.e., $\beta = 0.2$) at the 5% level of significance (i.e., $\alpha = 0.05$).

**Test for Equality**

In this example, suppose that a difference of $\epsilon = 20\%$ in clinical response of cure is considered of clinically meaningful difference between the two anti-microbial agents. By (4.2.2), assuming that the true cure rate for the active control agent is 65% ($p_1 = 0.80$ and $p_2 = p_1 + \epsilon = 0.85$), respectively, the sample size with $\kappa = 1$ (equal allocation) can be determined by

$$n_1 = n_2 = \frac{(z_{\alpha/2} + z_\beta)^2 (p_1(1-p_1) + p_2(1-p_2))}{\epsilon^2}$$

$$= \frac{(1.96 + 0.84)^2 (0.65(1-0.65) + 0.85(1-0.85))}{0.2^2}$$

$$\approx 70.$$

**Test for Non-Inferiority**

Now, suppose it is of interest to establish non-inferiority of the test drug as compared to the active control agent. Similarly, we consider the difference less than 10% is of no clinical importance. Thus, the non-inferiority margin is chosen to be 10% (i.e., $\delta = -0.10$). Also, suppose the true mean cure rates of the treatment agents and the active control are 85% and 65%, respectively. Then, by (4.2.3), the sample size with $\kappa = 1$ (equal allocation) can be determined by

$$n_1 = n_2 = \frac{(z_\alpha + z_\beta)^2 (p_1(1-p_1) + p_2(1-p_2))}{(\epsilon - \delta)^2}$$

$$= \frac{(1.64 + 0.84)^2 (0.65(1-0.65) + 0.85(1-0.85))}{(0.20 + 0.10)^2}$$

$$\approx 25.$$

## 4.2. Two-Sample Parallel Design

**Test for Superiority**

On the other hand, the pharmaceutical company may want to show superiority of the test drug over the active control agent. Assume the superiority margin is 5% ($\delta = 0.05$). According to (4.2.3), the sample size with $\kappa = 1$ (equal allocation) can be determined by

$$n_1 = n_2 = \frac{(z_\alpha + z_\beta)^2 (p_1(1-p_1) + p_2(1-p_2))}{(\epsilon - \delta)^2}$$

$$= \frac{(1.64 + 0.84)^2 (0.65(1-0.65) + 0.85(1-0.85))}{(0.20 - 0.05)^2}$$

$$\approx 98.$$

As it can be seen, testing superiority usually requires larger sample size than testing non-inferiority and equalty.

**Test for Equivalence**

For establishment of equivalence, suppose the true cure rate for the two agents are 75% ($p_1 = 0.75$) and 80% ($p_2 = 0.80$) and the equivalence limit is 20% (i.e., $\delta = 0.20$). According to (4.2.4), the sample size with $\kappa = 1$ (equal allocation) can be determined by

$$n_1 = n_2 = \frac{(z_\alpha + z_{\beta/2})^2 (p_1(1-p_1) + p_2(1-p_2))}{(\delta - |\epsilon|)^2}$$

$$= \frac{(1.64 + 1.28)^2 (0.75(1-0.75) + 0.80(1-0.80))}{(0.20 - 0.05)^2}$$

$$\approx 132.$$

### 4.2.5 Remarks

For two-sample test for equality there exists another approach, which is very similar to (4.2.1) but not exactly the same. This approach will reject the null hypothesis that $\epsilon = 0$ if

$$\frac{\hat{p}_1 - \hat{p}_2}{\sqrt{(\frac{1}{n_1} + \frac{1}{n_2})\hat{p}(1-\hat{p})}}, \tag{4.2.5}$$

where

$$\hat{p} = \frac{n_1 \hat{p}_1 + n_2 \hat{p}_2}{n_1 + n_2}.$$

Note that the difference between (4.2.1) and (4.2.5) is the following. In (4.2.1) the variance of $\hat{p}_1 - \hat{p}_2$ is estimated by maximum likelihood estimate

(MLE) without any constraint, which is given by $\hat{p}_1(1-\hat{p}_1)/n_1 + \hat{p}_2(1-\hat{p}_2)/n_2$. On the other side, in (4.2.5) the same quantity is estimated by MLE under the null hypothesis ($p_1 = p_2$), which gives $(1/n_1 + 1/n_2)\hat{p}(1-\hat{p})$. We will refer to (4.2.1) as unconditional approach and (4.2.5) as conditional approach. Which test (conditional/unconditional) should be used is always a problem because one is not necessarily always more powerful than the other. However, a drawback of the conditional approach is that it is difficult to be generalized to other testing problems, e.g., superiority, non-inferiority/equivalence. Let

$$p = \frac{n_1 p_1 + n_2 p_2}{n_1 + n_2}.$$

When $n = n_1 = n_2$, which is a very important special case, it can be shown that

$$\left(\frac{1}{n_1} + \frac{1}{n_2}\right)\hat{p}(1-\hat{p}) \approx \left(\frac{1}{n_1} + \frac{1}{n_2}\right)p(1-p)$$
$$\geq \frac{p_1(1-p_1)}{n_1} + \frac{p_2(1-p_2)}{n_2}$$
$$\approx \frac{\hat{p}_1(1-\hat{p}_1)}{n_1} + \frac{\hat{p}_2(1-\hat{p}_2)}{n_2},$$

which implies that under the alternative hypothesis, the unconditional approach has more power than the conditional method. As a result, in this section and also the following section, we will focus on the unconditional method because it provides a unified approach for all the testing problems mentioned above.

Nevertheless, for the purpose of completeness, the conditional approach for a two-sample test of equality is also presented below. Under the alternative hypothesis that $\epsilon \neq 0$ and $n_1 = \kappa n_2$, the power of (4.2.5) is approximately

$$\Phi\left(\frac{|\epsilon|}{\sqrt{p_1(1-p_1)/n_1 + p_2(1-p_2)/n_2}} - z_{\alpha/2}\frac{\sqrt{(1/n_1 + 1/n_2)p(1-p)}}{\sqrt{p_1(1-p_1)/n_1 + p_2(1-p_2)/n_2}}\right),$$

where $p = (p_1 + \kappa p_2)/(1 + \kappa)$. As a result, the sample size needed for achieving a power of $1-\beta$ can be obtained by solving the following equation

$$\frac{|\epsilon|}{\sqrt{p_1(1-p_1)/n_1 + p_2(1-p_2)/n_2}} - z_{\alpha/2}\frac{\sqrt{(1/n_1 + 1/n_2)p(1-p)}}{\sqrt{p_1(1-p_1)/n_1 + p_2(1-p_2)/n_2}} = z_\beta.$$

This leads to

$$n_1 = \kappa n_2$$
$$n_2 = \tfrac{1}{\epsilon^2}[z_{\alpha/2}\sqrt{(1+1/\kappa)p(1-p)} + z_\beta\sqrt{p_1(1-p_1)/\kappa + p_2(1-p_2)}]^2.$$

## 4.3  Two-Sample Crossover Design

In this section, we consider a $2 \times 2m$ replicated crossover design comparing mean response rates of a test drug and a reference drug. Let $x_{ijkl}$ be the $l$th replicate of a binary response ($l = 1, ..., m$) observed from the $j$th subject ($j = 1, ..., n$) in the $i$th sequence ($i = 1, 2$) under the $k$th treatment ($k = 1, 2$). Assume that $(x_{ij11}, ..., x_{ij1m}, ..., x_{ijk1}, ..., x_{ijkm}), i = 1, 2, j = 1, ..., n$ are i.i.d. random vectors with each component's marginal distribution specified by $P(x_{ijkl} = 1) = p_k$. Note that the observations from the same subject can be correlated with each other. By specifying that $P(x_{ijkl} = 1) = p_k$, it implies that there are no sequence, period, and crossover effects. The statistical model incorporates those effects are more complicated for binary data compared with continuous data. Its detailed discussion is beyond the scope of this book.

Let $\epsilon = p_2(\text{test}) - p_1(\text{reference})$,

$$\bar{x}_{ijk\cdot} = \frac{1}{m}(x_{ijk1} + \cdots + x_{ijkm}) \quad \text{and} \quad d_{ij} = \bar{x}_{ij1\cdot} - \bar{x}_{ij2\cdot}.$$

An unbiased estimator of $\epsilon$ is given by

$$\hat{\epsilon} = \frac{1}{2n}\sum_{i=1}^{a}\sum_{j=1}^{n} d_{ij}.$$

According to the central limit theorem, $\hat{\epsilon}$ is asymptotically normally distributed as $N(0, \sigma_d^2)$, where $\sigma_d^2 = \text{var}(d_{ij})$ and can be estimated by

$$\hat{\sigma}_d^2 = \frac{1}{2(n-1)}\sum_{i=1}^{a}\sum_{j=1}^{n}(d_{ij} - \bar{d}_{i\cdot})^2,$$

where

$$\bar{d}_{i\cdot} = \frac{1}{n}\sum_{j=1}^{n} d_{ij}.$$

Without loss of of generality, consider $\epsilon > 0$ ($\epsilon < 0$) as an indication of *improvement* (*worsening*) of the test drug as compared to the reference drug.

## 4.3.1 Test for Equality

The objective is to test the following hypotheses

$$H_0 : \epsilon = 0 \quad \text{versus} \quad H_a : \epsilon \neq 0.$$

Then, the null hypothesis will be rejected at $\alpha$ level of significance if

$$\left| \frac{\hat{\epsilon}}{\hat{\sigma}_d/\sqrt{2n}} \right| > z_{\alpha/2}.$$

Under the alternative hypothesis that $\epsilon \neq 0$, the power of the above test is approximately

$$\Phi\left( \frac{\sqrt{2n}\epsilon}{\sigma_d} - z_{\alpha/2} \right).$$

As a result, the sample size needed for achieving a power of $1 - \beta$ can be obtained by solving

$$\frac{\sqrt{2n}|\epsilon|}{\sigma_d} - z_{\alpha/2} = t_\beta.$$

This leads to

$$n = \frac{(z_{\alpha/2} + z_\beta)^2 \sigma_d^2}{2\epsilon^2}. \tag{4.3.1}$$

## 4.3.2 Test for Non-Inferiority/Superiority

Similar to test for non-inferiority/superiority under a parallel design, the problem can be unified by testing the following hypotheses:

$$H_0 : \epsilon \leq \delta \quad \text{versus} \quad H_a : \epsilon > \delta,$$

where $\delta$ is the non-inferiority or superiority margin. When $\delta > 0$, the rejection of the null hypothesis indicates the superiority of test drug against the control. When $\delta < 0$, the rejection of the null hypothesis indicates the non-inferiority of the test drug over the control. The null hypothesis will be rejected at the $\alpha$ level of significance if

$$\frac{\hat{\epsilon} - \delta}{\hat{\sigma}_d/\sqrt{2n}} > z_\alpha.$$

Under the alternative hypothesis that $\epsilon > \delta$, the power of the above test is approximately

$$\Phi\left( \frac{\epsilon - \delta}{\sigma_d/\sqrt{2n}} - z_{\alpha/2} \right).$$

## 4.3. Two-Sample Crossover Design

As a result, the sample size needed for achieving a power of $1 - \beta$ can be obtained by solving

$$\frac{\epsilon - \delta}{\sigma_d/\sqrt{2n}} - z_{\alpha/2} \geq z_\beta.$$

This leads to

$$n = \frac{(z_\alpha + z_\beta)^2 \sigma_d^2}{2(\epsilon - \delta)^2}. \tag{4.3.2}$$

### 4.3.3 Test for Equivalence

The objective is to test the following hypotheses

$$H_0 : |\epsilon| \geq \delta \quad \text{versus} \quad H_a : |\epsilon| < \delta.$$

The test drug will be concluded equivalent to the control on average if the null hypothesis is rejected at a given significance level. At the significance level of $\alpha$, the null hypothesis will be rejected if

$$\frac{\sqrt{2n}(\hat{\epsilon} - \delta)}{\hat{\sigma}_d} < -z_\alpha \quad \text{and} \quad \frac{\sqrt{2n}(\hat{\epsilon} + \delta)}{\hat{\sigma}_d} > z_\alpha.$$

Under the alternative hypothesis that $|\epsilon| < \delta$, the power of the above test is approximately

$$2\Phi\left(\frac{\sqrt{2n}(\delta - |\epsilon|)}{\sigma_d} - z_\alpha\right) - 1.$$

As a result, the sample size needed for achieving a power of $1 - \beta$ can be obtained by solving

$$\frac{\sqrt{2n}(\delta - |\epsilon|)}{\sigma_d} - z_\alpha \geq z_{\beta/2}.$$

This leads to

$$n \geq \frac{(z_\alpha + z_{\beta/2})^2 \sigma_d^2}{2(\delta - |\epsilon|)^2}. \tag{4.3.3}$$

### 4.3.4 An Example

Suppose a sponsor is interested in conducting an open label randomized crossover trial to compare an inhaled insulin formulation manufactured for commercial usage for patients with type I diabetes to the inhaled insulin formulation utilized in phase III clinical trials. Unlike subcutaneous injection, the efficiency and reproducibility of pulmonary insulin delivery is a concern. As a result, a replicated crossover consisting of two sequences of ABAB and BABA is recommended ($a = 2, m = 2$), where A is the inhaled insulin formulation for commercial usage and B is the inhaled insulin formulation utilized in phase III clinical trials. Qualified subjects are to be randomly assigned to receive one of the two sequences. In each sequence, subjects will receive single doses with a replicate of treatments A and B as specified in the sequence on days 1, 3, 5, and 7. In this trial, in addition to the comparison of pharmacokinetic parameters such as area under the blood concentration time curve and peak concentration (Cmax), it is also of interest to compare the safety profiles between the two formulations in terms of the incidence rate of adverse events.

**Test for Equality**

Assuming $\sigma_d = 50\%$, according to (4.3.1), the sample size needed in order to achieve a 80% ($\beta = 0.2$) power in detecting 20% ($\epsilon = 0.20$) difference in adverse events rate is given by

$$n = \frac{(z_{\alpha/2} + z_\beta)^2 \sigma_d^2}{2\epsilon^2} = \frac{(1.96 + 0.84)^2 \times 0.5^2}{2 \times 0.2^2} = 24.5 \approx 25.$$

**Test for Non-Inferiority**

Assume $\sigma_d = 50\%$, no difference in the mean adverse event rates between the two treatments ($\epsilon = 0$), and a non-inferiority margin is $\delta = -20\%$. According to (4.3.2), the sample size needed in order to achieve 80% ($\beta = 0.2$) power is given by

$$n = \frac{(z_\alpha + z_\beta)^2 \sigma_d^2}{2(\epsilon - \delta)^2} = \frac{(1.64 + 0.84)^2 \times 0.5^2}{2 \times (0 - (-0.2))^2} = 19.2 \approx 20.$$

**Test for Equivalence**

Assume $\sigma_d = 50\%$, no difference in the mean adverse event rate between the two treatments ($\epsilon = 0$), and the equivalence limit is 20% ($\delta = 0.2$). According to (4.3.3), the sample size needed in order to achieve 80% ($\beta = 0.2$) is given by

$$n = \frac{(z_\alpha + z_{\beta/2})^2 \sigma_d^2}{2\delta^2} = \frac{(1.64 + 1.28)^2 0.5^2}{0.2^2} = 26.6 \approx 27.$$

### 4.3.5 Remarks

For a crossover design, two ways exist to increase the power. One is to increase the number of subjects, i.e., increase $n$. An other way is to increase the number of the replicates from each subject, i.e., increase $m$. In practice, usually increasing $m$ is more cost-effective compared to increasing $n$. The power of the test is mainly determined by the variability of $\hat{\epsilon}$ under the alternative assumption. Heuristically, the variability of $\hat{\epsilon}$ can be considered to consist of two parts, i.e., inter- and intra-subject variability components. From a statistical point of view, increasing $n$ can decrease both inter- and intra-subject components of $\hat{\epsilon}$. As a result, as long as $n$ is sufficiently large, the power can be arbitrarily close to 1. However, increasing the number of replicates ($m$) can only decrease the intra-subject variability component of $\hat{\epsilon}$. When $m \to \infty$, the intra-subject variability will go to 0, but the inter-subject variability still remains. Consequently, the power cannot be increased arbitrarily by increasing $m$.

In practice, if the intra-subject variability is relatively small compared with the inter-subject variability, simply increasing the number of replicates may not provide sufficient power. In such a situation, the number of subjects should be sufficiently large to acheive the desired statistical power. On the other side, if the intra-subject variability is relatively large compared with the inter-subject variability, it may be preferable to increase the number of repilcates to achieve the desired power and retain a relatively low cost.

## 4.4 One-Way Analysis of Variance

Let $x_{ij}$ be a binary response from the $j$th subject in the $i$th treatment group, $i = 1, ..., a$, $j = 1, \cdots, n$. Assume that $P(x_{ij} = 1) = p_i$. Define

$$\hat{p}_{i\cdot} = \frac{1}{n} \sum_{j=1}^{n} x_{ij}.$$

### 4.4.1 Pairwise Comparison

In practice, it is often of interest to compare proportions among treatments under study. Thus, the hypotheses of interest are

$$H_0 : \mu_i = \mu_j \quad \text{versus} \quad H_a : \mu_i \neq \mu_j, \text{ for some } i \neq j.$$

Under the above hypotheses, there are $a(a-1)/2$ possible comparisons. For example, if there are four treatments in the study, then we can have a maximum of six pairwise comparisons. In practice, it is well recognized that multiple comparison will inflate the type I error. As a result, it is suggested that an adjustment be made for controlling the overall type I error rate at the desired significance level. Assume that there are $\tau$ comparisons of interest, where $\tau \leq a(a-1)/2$. We reject the null hypothesis $H_0$ at the $\alpha$

level of significance if

$$\left| \frac{\sqrt{n}(\bar{p}_i - \bar{p}_j)}{\sqrt{\hat{p}_i(1-\hat{p}_i) + \hat{p}_j(1-\hat{p}_j)}} \right| > z_{\alpha/(2\tau)}.$$

The power of this test is approximately

$$\Phi\left( \frac{\sqrt{n}|\epsilon_{ij}|}{\sqrt{p_i(1-p_i) + p_j(1-p_j)}} - z_{\alpha/(2\tau)} \right),$$

where $\epsilon_{ij} = p_i - p_j$. As a result, the sample size needed for detecting a clinically meaningful difference between $p_i$ and $p_j$ can be obtained by solving

$$\frac{\sqrt{n}|\epsilon_{ij}|}{\sqrt{p_i(1-p_i) + p_j(1-p_j)}} - z_{\alpha/(2\tau)} = z_\beta.$$

This leads to

$$n_{ij} = \frac{(z_{\alpha/(2\tau)} + z_\beta)^2 [p_1(1-p_1) + p_2(1-p_2)]}{\epsilon_{ij}^2}. \qquad (4.4.1)$$

The final sample size needed can be estimated by

$$n = \max\{n_{ij}, \text{ all interested pairs } (i,j)\}. \qquad (4.4.2)$$

### 4.4.2 An Example

Suppose an investigator is interested in conducting a parallel-group clinical trial comparing two active doses of a test compound against a standard therapy in patients with a specific carcinoma. Suppose the standard therapy, which is referred to as treatment 0, has a 20% response rate. For illustration purpose, the two active doses of the test compound are referred to as treatment 1 and treatment 2, respectively. Suppose the investigator would like to determine whether test treatments 1 and 2 will achieve the response rates of 40% and 50%, respectively. As a result, statistical comparisons of interest include the comparison between the standard therapy (treatment 0) vs. treatment 1 and between the standard therapy (treatment 0) vs. treatment 2. In this case, $\tau = 2$. According to (4.4.1), we have

$$n_{01} = \frac{(z_{0.05/(2\times 2)} + z_{0.2})^2 [0.2(1-0.2) + 0.4(1-0.4)]}{(0.2 - 0.4)^2} \approx 95$$

and

$$n_{02} = \frac{(2.24 + 0.84)^2 [0.2(1-0.2) + 0.5(1-0.5)]}{0.09} \approx 44.$$

By (4.4.2), the sample size needed in order to achieve an 80% power is given by $n = \max\{95, 44\} = 95$.

### 4.4.3 Remarks

It should be noted that the maximum approach described in this section is somewhat conservative in two aspects. First, the $\alpha$ adjustment based on the method of Bonferrouni is conservative. Other less conservative methods for $\alpha$ adjustment may be used. Second, the formula is designed to detect statistically significant differences for all comparisons of interest. In practice, the comparisons of interest may not be equally important to the investigator. Hence, one of the comparisons is usually considered as the primary comparison and sample size calculation is performed based on the primary comparison. Once the sample size is determined, it can be justified under appropriate statistical assumption for other comparisons (secondary comparison) of interest.

## 4.5 Williams Design

We consider the Williams design described in Section 3.5. Let $x_{ijl}$ be a binary response from the $j$th ($j = 1, ..., n$) subject in the $i$th ($i = 1, ..., a$) sequence under the $l$th ($l = 1, ..., b$) treatment. It is assumed that $(x_{ij1}, ..., x_{ijb}), i = 1, ..., a, j = 1, ..., n$ are i.i.d. random vectors with $P(x_{ijl} = 1) = p_l$. The observations from the same subject can be correlated with each other. By specifying that $P(x_{ijl} = 1) = p_l, l = 1, ..., m$, it implies that there is no sequence, period, or crossover effects. The statistical model incorporates those effects that are more complicated for binary data compared with continuous data. Its detailed discussion is beyond the scope of this book.

Without loss of generality, assume that we want to compare treatment 1 and treatment 2. Let

$$d_{ij} = y_{ij1} - y_{ij2}.$$

The true mean difference between treatment 1 and treatment 2 can be estimated by

$$\hat{\epsilon} = \frac{1}{an} \sum_{i=1}^{a} \sum_{j=1}^{n} d_{ij},$$

which is asymptotically normally distributed with mean $\epsilon = p_1 - p_2$ and variance $\sigma_d^2/an$, where $\sigma_d^2$ is defined to be the variance of $d_{ij}$ and can be estimated by

$$\hat{\sigma}_d^2 = \frac{1}{a(n-1)} \sum_{i=1}^{a} \sum_{j=1}^{n} (d_{ij} - \frac{1}{n} \sum_{j'=1}^{n} d_{ij'})^2.$$

### 4.5.1 Test for Equality

Let $\epsilon = \mu_1 - \mu_2$ be the true mean difference. The objective is to test the following hypotheses:

$$H_0 : \epsilon = 0 \quad \text{versus} \quad H_a : \epsilon \neq 0.$$

Then, the null hypothesis will be rejected at $\alpha$ level of significance if

$$\left| \frac{\hat{\epsilon}}{\hat{\sigma}_d/\sqrt{an}} \right| > z_{\alpha/2}.$$

Under the alternative hypothesis that $\epsilon \neq 0$, the power of this test is approximately

$$\Phi\left( \frac{\sqrt{an}\epsilon}{\sigma_d} - z_{\alpha/2} \right).$$

As a result, the sample size needed for achieving a power of $1 - \beta$ can be obtained as

$$n = \frac{(z_{\alpha/2} + z_\beta)^2 \sigma_d^2}{a\epsilon^2}. \tag{4.5.1}$$

### 4.5.2 Test for Non-Inferiority/Superiority

The problem of testing superiority and non-inferiority can be unified by the following hypothesis:

$$H_0 : \epsilon \leq \delta \quad \text{versus} \quad H_a : \epsilon > \delta,$$

where $\delta$ is the superiority or non-inferiority margin. When $\delta > 0$, the rejection of the null hypothesis indicates the superiority of the test drug over the control. When $\delta < 0$, the rejection of the null hypothesis indicates the non-inferiority of the test drug against the control. The null hypothesis will be rejected at $\alpha$ level of significance if

$$\frac{\hat{\epsilon} - \delta}{\hat{\sigma}_d/\sqrt{an}} > z_\alpha.$$

Under the alternative hypothesis that $\epsilon > \delta$, the power of the above test is approximately

$$\Phi\left( \frac{\epsilon - \delta}{\sigma_d/\sqrt{an}} - z_\alpha \right).$$

As a result, the sample size needed for achieving a power of $1 - \beta$ can be obtained by solving

$$\frac{\epsilon - \delta}{\sigma_d/\sqrt{an}} - z_\alpha = z_\beta.$$

This leads to

$$n = \frac{(z_\alpha + z_\beta)^2 \sigma_d^2}{a(\epsilon - \delta)^2}. \tag{4.5.2}$$

## 4.5.3 Test for Equivalence

The objective is to test the following hypotheses:

$$H_0 : |\epsilon| \geq \delta \quad \text{versus} \quad H_a : |\epsilon| < \delta.$$

The test drug will be concluded equivalent to the control on average if the null hypothesis is rejected at a given significance level. For example, at the significance level of $\alpha$, the null hypothesis will be rejected if

$$\frac{\sqrt{an}(\hat{\epsilon} - \delta)}{\hat{\sigma}_d} < -z_\alpha$$

and

$$\frac{\sqrt{an}(\hat{\epsilon} + \delta)}{\hat{\sigma}_d} > z_\alpha.$$

Under the alternative hypothesis that $|\epsilon| < \delta$, the power of the above test is approximately

$$2\Phi\left(\frac{\sqrt{an}(\delta - |\epsilon|)}{\sigma_d} - z_\alpha\right) - 1.$$

As a result, the sample size needed for achieving a power of $1 - \beta$ can be obtained by solving

$$\frac{\sqrt{an}(\delta - |\epsilon|)}{\sigma_d} - z_\alpha = z_{\beta/2}.$$

This leads to

$$n = \frac{(z_\alpha + z_{\beta/2})^2 \sigma_d^2}{a(\delta - |\epsilon|)^2}. \quad (4.5.3)$$

## 4.5.4 An Example

Suppose that a sponsor is interested in conducting a $6 \times 3$ (Williams design) crossover experiment (i.e., $a = 6$) to compare two active doses (i.e., morning dose and evening dose) of a test compound against a placebo in patients with sleep disorder. Similarly, we will refer to the placebo and the two active doses as treatment 0, treatment 1, and treatment 2, respectively. Qualified subjects will be randomly assigned to receive one of the six sequences of treatments. The trial consists of three visits. Each visit consists of two nights and three days with subjects in attendance at a designated Sleep Laboratory. On day two of each visit, the subject will receive one of the three treatments. Polysomnography will be applied to examine the treatment effect on sleep quality. Suppose the sponsor is interested in examining the existence of awakeness after the onset of sleep. As a result, sample size calculation is performed based on the proportion of subjects experiencing wakeness after the onset of sleep. Based on a pilot study, about

50%, 30%, and 35% of subjects receiving treatment 0, 1, and 2, respectively, experienced awakeness after the onset of sleep. As a result, for performing sample size calculation, we assume that the response rates for subjects receiving treatment 0, 1, and 2 are 50%, 30%, and 35%, respectively. Since the comparisons of interest include the comparison between treatment 1 and the placebo and between treatment 2 and the placebo, without loss of generality and for simplicity without adjusting type I error, we will focus on sample size calculation based on the comparison between treatment 1 and the placebo.

According to the information given above, it follows that the difference in proportion of subjects experiencing awakeness between treatment 1 and the placebo is given by 20% ($\epsilon = 20\%$). From the pilot study, it is estimated that $\sigma_d = 75\%$. The significance level is fixed to be $\alpha = 5\%$.

**Test for Equality**

Since this is a $6 \times 3$ crossover design, the number of sequence is $a = 6$. According to (4.5.1), the sample size needed in order to achieve 80% power ($\beta = 0.2$) is given by

$$n = \frac{(z_{\alpha/2} + z_\beta)^2 \sigma_d^2}{a\epsilon^2} = \frac{(1.96 + 0.84)^2 0.75^2}{6 \times 0.2^2} \approx 19.$$

**Test for Superiority**

Assuming the superiority margin is 5% ($\delta = 0.05$), the sample size needed in order to achieve 80% power ($\beta = 0.2$) is given by

$$n = \frac{(z_\alpha + z_\beta)^2 \sigma_d^2}{a(\epsilon - \delta)^2} = \frac{(1.64 + 0.84)^2 0.75^2}{6 \times (0.2 - 0.05)^2} \approx 27.$$

**Test for Equivalence**

Assuming the equivalence margin is 30% ($\delta = 0.30$), the sample size needed is given by

$$n = \frac{(z_\alpha + z_{\beta/2})^2 \sigma_d^2}{a(\delta - |\epsilon|)^2} = \frac{(1.64 + 1.28)^2 0.75^2}{6 \times (0.3 - 0.2)^2} \approx 80.$$

## 4.6 Relative Risk—Parallel Design

In clinical trials, it is often of interest to investigate the relative effect (e.g., risk or benefit) of the treatments for the disease under study. Odds ratio has

## 4.6. Relative Risk—Parallel Design

been frequently used to assess the association between a binary exposure variable and a binary disease outcome since it was introduced by Cornfield (1956). Let $p_T$ be the probability of observing an outcome of interest for a patient treatment by a test treatment and $p_C$ for a patient treated by a control. For a patient receiving the test treatment, the odds that he/she will have an outcome of interest over that he/she will not have an outcome are given by

$$O_T = \frac{p_T}{1 - p_T}.$$

Similarly, for a patient receiving the control, the odds are given by

$$O_C = \frac{p_C}{1 - p_C}.$$

As a result, the odds ratio between the test treatment and the control is defined as

$$OR = \frac{O_T}{O_C} = \frac{p_T(1 - p_C)}{p_C(1 - p_T)}.$$

The odds ratio is always positive and usually has a range from 0 to 4. $OR = 1$ (i.e., $p_T = p_C$) implies that there is no difference between the two treatments in terms of the outcome of interest. When $1 < OR < 4$, patients in the treatment group are more likely to have outcomes of interest than those in the control group. Note that $1 - OR$ is usually referred to as relative odds reduction in the literature. Intuitively, $OR$ can be estimated by

$$\widehat{OR} = \frac{\hat{p}_T(1 - \hat{p}_C)}{\hat{p}_C(1 - \hat{p}_T)},$$

where $\hat{p}_T$ and $\hat{p}_C$ are the maximum likelihood estimators of $p_T$ and $p_C$, respectively, given by

$$\hat{p}_T = \frac{x_T}{n_T} \quad \text{and} \quad \hat{p}_C = \frac{x_C}{n_C}, \quad (4.6.1)$$

and $x_T$ and $x_C$ are the observed numbers of patients in the respective treatment and control groups who have the outcome of interest. The asymptotic variance for $\log(\widehat{OR})$ can be obtained as

$$\text{var}[\log(\widehat{OR})] = \frac{1}{n_T p_T(1 - p_T)} + \frac{1}{n_C p_C(1 - p_C)},$$

which can be estimated by simply replacing $p_T$ and $p_C$ with their maximum likelihood estimator $\hat{p}_T$ and $\hat{p}_C$.

### 4.6.1 Test for Equality

The hypotheses of interest are given by

$$H_0 : OR = 1 \quad \text{versus} \quad H_a : OR \neq 1.$$

The test statistic is given by

$$T = \log(\widehat{OR}) \left[ \frac{1}{n_T \hat{p}_T (1 - \hat{p}_T)} + \frac{1}{n_C \hat{p}_C (1 - \hat{p}_C)} \right]^{-1/2},$$

which approximately follows a standard normal distribution when $n_T$ and $n_C$ are sufficiently large. Thus, we reject the null hypothesis that $OR = 1$ if $|T| > z_{\alpha/2}$. Under the alternative hypothesis that $OR \neq 1$, the power of the above test can be approximated by

$$\Phi \left( |\log(OR)| \left[ \frac{1}{n_T p_T (1 - p_T)} + \frac{1}{n_C p_C (1 - p_C)} \right]^{-1/2} - z_{\alpha/2} \right).$$

As a result, the sample size needed for achieving a desired power of $1 - \beta$ can be obtained by solving

$$|\log(OR)| \left[ \frac{1}{n_T p_T (1 - p_T)} + \frac{1}{n_C p_C (1 - p_C)} \right]^{-1/2} - z_{\alpha/2} = z_\beta.$$

Under the assumption that $n_T/n_C = \kappa$ (a known ratio), we have

$$n_C = \frac{(z_{\alpha/2} + z_\beta)^2}{\log^2(OR)} \left( \frac{1}{\kappa p_T (1 - p_T)} + \frac{1}{p_C (1 - p_C)} \right). \qquad (4.6.2)$$

### 4.6.2 Test for Non-Inferiority/Superiority

The problem of testing non-inferiority and superiority can be unified by the following hypotheses:

$$H_0 : OR \leq \delta' \quad \text{versus} \quad H_a : OR > \delta',$$

where $\delta'$ is the non-inferiority or superiority margin in raw scale. The above hypotheses are the same as

$$H_0 : \log(OR) \leq \delta \quad \text{versus} \quad H_a : \log(OR) > \delta,$$

where $\delta$ is the non-inferiority or superiority margin in log-scale. When $\delta > 0$, the rejection of the null hypothesis indicates superiority over the reference value. When $\delta < 0$, the rejection of the null hypothesis implies non-inferiority against the reference value.

## 4.6. Relative Risk—Parallel Design

Let

$$T = (\log(\widehat{OR}) - \delta) \left[ \frac{1}{n_T \hat{p}_T(1-\hat{p}_T)} + \frac{1}{n_C \hat{p}_C(1-\hat{p}_C)} \right]^{-1/2}.$$

We reject the null hypothesis at the $\alpha$ level of significance if $T > z_\alpha$. Under the alternative hypothesis that $\log(OR) > \delta$, the power of the above test is approximately

$$\Phi \left( (\log(OR) - \delta) \left[ \frac{1}{n_T p_T(1-p_T)} + \frac{1}{n_C p_C(1-p_C)} \right]^{-1/2} - z_\alpha \right).$$

As a result, the sample size needed for achieving a desired power of $1 - \beta$ can be obtained by solving

$$|\log(OR) - \delta| \left[ \frac{1}{n_T p_T(1-p_T)} + \frac{1}{n_C p_C(1-p_C)} \right]^{-1/2} - z_{\alpha/2} = z_\beta.$$

Under the assumption that $n_T/n_C = \kappa$, we have

$$n_C = \frac{(z_\alpha + z_\beta)^2}{(\log(OR) - \delta)^2} \left( \frac{1}{\kappa p_T(1-p_T)} + \frac{1}{p_C(1-p_C)} \right). \quad (4.6.3)$$

### 4.6.3 Test for Equivalence

To establish equivalence, the following hypotheses are usually considered

$$H_0 : |\log(OR)| \geq \delta \quad \text{versus} \quad H_a : |\log(OR)| < \delta.$$

The above hypotheses can be tested using the two one-sided tests procedure as described in previous sections. We reject the null hypothesis at $\alpha$ level of significance if

$$(\log(\widehat{OR}) - \delta) \left[ \frac{1}{n_T \hat{p}_T(1-\hat{p}_T)} + \frac{1}{n_C \hat{p}_C(1-\hat{p}_C)} \right]^{-1/2} < -z_\alpha$$

and

$$(\log(\widehat{OR}) + \delta) \left[ \frac{1}{n_T \hat{p}_T(1-\hat{p}_T)} + \frac{1}{n_C \hat{p}_C(1-\hat{p}_C)} \right]^{-1/2} > z_\alpha.$$

When $|\log(OR)| < \delta$, the power of this test is approximately

$$2\Phi \left( (\delta - |\log(OR)|) \left[ \frac{1}{n_T p_T(1-p_T)} + \frac{1}{n_C p_C(1-p_C)} \right]^{-1} - z_{\alpha/2} \right) - 1.$$

Under the assumption that $n_T/n_C = \kappa$, the sample size needed for achieving a desired power of $1 - \beta$ is given by

$$n_C = \frac{(z_\alpha + z_{\beta/2})^2}{(\delta - |\log(OR)|)^2} \left( \frac{1}{\kappa p_T(1-p_T)} + \frac{1}{p_C(1-p_C)} \right). \quad (4.6.4)$$

### 4.6.4 An Example

Suppose that a sponsor is interested in conducting a clinical trial to study the relative risk between a test compound and a standard therapy for prevention of relapse in subjects with schizophrenia and schizoaffective disorders. Based on the results from a previous study with 365 subjects (i.e., 177 subjects received the test compound and 188 received the standard therapy), about 25% (45/177) and 40% (75/188) of subjects receiving the test compound and the standard therapy experienced relapse after the treatment. Subjects who experienced first relapse may withdraw from the study or continue on. Among the subjects who experienced the first relapse and stayed on the study, about 26.7% (8/30) and 32.0% (16/50) experienced the second relapse. the sponsor is interested in studying the odds ratio of the test compound as compared to the standard therapy for prevention of experiencing the first relapse. In addition, it also of interest to examine the odds ratio for prevention of experiencing the second relapse.

**Test for Equality**

Assume the responder rate in control group is 25% and the rate in test is 40%, which produces a relative risk

$$OR = \frac{0.40(1 - 0.25)}{(1 - 0.4)0.25} = 2.$$

According to (4.6.2) and $n = n_T = n_C$ ($k = 1$), the sample size needed in order to achieve 80% ($\beta = 0.2$) at 0.05 ($\alpha = 0.05$) level of significance is given by

$$n = \frac{(1.96 + 0.84)^2}{\log^2(2)} \left[ \frac{1}{0.4(1 - 0.4)} + \frac{1}{0.25(1 - 0.25)} \right] \approx 156.$$

**Test for Superiority**

Assume that 20% ($\delta = 0.2$) is considered as a clinically important superiority margin for log-scale relative risk. According to (4.6.3) the sample size needed to achieve 80% power ($\beta = 0.2$) is given by

$$n = \frac{(1.64 + 0.84)^2}{(\log(2) - 0.2)^2} \left[ \frac{1}{0.4(1 - 0.4)} + \frac{1}{0.25(1 - 0.25)} \right] \approx 241.$$

**Test for Equivalence**

Assume that the relapse rate of the study drug (25%) is approximately equal to a market drug ($\log(OR) = 0$) and that the equivalence margin in log-scale relative risk is 50% ($\delta = 0.50$). According to (4.6.4) the sample size needed to achieve 80% ($\beta = 0.2$) power to establish equivalence is given by

$$n = \frac{(z_{0.05} + z_{0.2/2})^2}{0.5^2} \left[ \frac{1}{0.25(1-0.25)} + \frac{1}{0.25(1-0.25)} \right] \approx 364.$$

## 4.7 Relative Risk—Crossover Design

Consider a $1 \times 2$ crossover design with no period effects. Without loss of generality, we assume that every subject will receive test first and then be crossed over to control. Let $x_{ij}$ be a binary response from the $j$th subject in the $i$th period, $j = 1, ..., n$. The number of outcomes of interest under treatment is given by $x_T = \sum_{j=1}^{n} x_{1j}$. The number of outcomes of interest under control, $x_C$, is similarly defined. Then the true response rates under treatment and control can still be estimated according to (4.6.1). According to Taylor's expansion, it can be shown that

$$\sqrt{n}(\log(\widehat{OR}) - \log(OR))$$
$$= \sqrt{n} \left[ \frac{1}{p_T(1-p_T)}(\hat{p}_T - p_T) - \frac{1}{p_C} p_C(1-p_C)(\hat{p}_C - p_C) \right] + o_p(1)$$
$$= \frac{1}{\sqrt{n}} \sum_{j=1}^{n} \left[ \frac{x_{1j} - p_T}{p_T(1-p_T)} - \frac{x_{2j} - p_C}{p_C(1-p_C)} \right] + o_p(1)$$
$$\to_d N(0, \sigma_d^2),$$

where

$$\sigma_d^2 = \text{var}\left( \frac{x_{1j} - p_T}{p_T(1-p_T)} - \frac{x_{2j} - p_C}{p_C(1-p_C)} \right).$$

Let

$$d_j = \left( \frac{x_{1j}}{\hat{p}_T(1-\hat{p}_T)} - \frac{x_{2j}}{\hat{p}_C(1-\hat{p}_C)} \right).$$

Then, $\sigma_d^2$ can be estimated by $\hat{\sigma}_d^2$, the sample variance based on $d_j, j = 1, ..., n$.

### 4.7.1 Test for Equality

The hypotheses of interest are given by

$$H_0 : \log(OR) = 0 \quad \text{versus} \quad H_a : \log(OR) \neq 0.$$

Under the null hypothesis, the test statistic

$$T = \frac{\sqrt{n}\log(\widehat{OR})}{\hat{\sigma}_d}$$

approximately follows a standard normal distribution when $n_T$ and $n_C$ are sufficiently large. Thus, we reject the null hypothesis that $OR = 1$ if $|T| > z_{\alpha/2}$. Under the alternative hypothesis that $OR \neq 1$, the power of the above test can be approximated by

$$\Phi\left(\frac{\sqrt{n}|\log(OR)|}{\sigma_d} - z_{\alpha/2}\right).$$

As a result, the sample size needed for achieving a desired power of $1 - \beta$ can be obtained by solving

$$\frac{\sqrt{n}|\log(OR)|}{\sigma_d} - z_{\alpha/2} = z_\beta.$$

This leads to

$$n = \frac{(z_{\alpha/2} + z_\beta)^2 \sigma_d^2}{\log^2(OR)}. \tag{4.7.1}$$

## 4.7.2 Test for Non-Inferiority/Superiority

The problem of testing non-inferiority and superiority can be unified by the following hypotheses:

$$H_0 : \log(OR) \leq \delta \quad \text{versus} \quad H_a : \log(OR) > \delta,$$

where $\delta$ is the non-inferiority or superiority margin in log-scale. When $\delta > 0$, the rejection of the null hypothesis indicates superiority over the reference value. When $\delta < 0$, the rejection of the null hypothesis implies non-inferiority against the reference value.

When $\log(OR) = \delta$, the test statistic

$$T = \frac{\sqrt{n}(\log(\widehat{OR}) - \delta)}{\hat{\sigma}_d}$$

approximately follows the standard normal distribution when $n_T$ and $n_C$ are sufficiently large. Thus, we reject the null hypothesis at the $\alpha$ level of significance if $T > z_\alpha$. Under the alternative hypothesis that $\log(OR) > \delta$, the power of the above test is approximately

$$\Phi\left(\frac{\log(OR) - \delta}{\sigma_d} - z_\alpha\right).$$

As a result, the sample size needed for achieving a desired power of $1 - \beta$ can be obtained by solving

$$\frac{\log(OR) - \delta}{\sigma_d} - z_\alpha = z_\beta.$$

It leads to

$$n = \frac{(z_\alpha + z_\beta)^2 \sigma_d^2}{[\log(OR) - \delta]^2}. \tag{4.7.2}$$

### 4.7.3 Test for Equivalence

To establish equivalence, the following hypotheses are usually considered:

$$H_0 : |\log(OR)| \geq \delta \quad \text{versus} \quad H_a : |\log(OR)| < \delta.$$

The above hypotheses can be tested using the two one-sided tests procedure (see, e.g., Chow and Liu, 1998). We reject the null hypothesis at the $\alpha$ level of significance if

$$\frac{\sqrt{n}(\log(\widehat{OR}) - \delta)}{\hat{\sigma}_d} < -z_\alpha$$

and

$$\frac{\sqrt{n}(\log(\widehat{OR}) + \delta)}{\hat{\sigma}_d} > z_\alpha.$$

When $|\log(OR)| < \delta$, the power of the above test is approximately

$$2\Phi\left(\frac{(\delta - |\log(OR)|)}{\sigma_d} - z_\alpha\right) - 1.$$

Then, the sample size needed for achieving a desired power of $1 - \beta$ can be obtained by

$$n = \frac{(z_\alpha + z_{\beta/2})^2 \sigma_d^2}{(\delta - |\log(OR)|)^2}. \tag{4.7.3}$$

## 4.8 Practical Issues

### 4.8.1 Exact and Asymptotic Tests

It should be noted that all of the formulas for sample size calculation given in this chapter are derived based on asymptotic theory. In other words, the formulas are valid when the sample size is sufficiently large. However, "how large is considered sufficiently large" is always a question to researchers who are trying to determine the sample size at the planning stage of an intended study. Unfortunately, there is no simple rule which can be used to evaluate whether the sample size is sufficiently large. As an alternative, some exact tests may be useful when the expected sample size of the intended study is small (due to budget constraint and/or slow enrollment). Details of various commonly used exact tests, such as binomial test, Fisher's exact test, and mutiple-stage optimal design will be discussed in the next chapter.

### 4.8.2 Variance Estimates

For testing equality, non-inferiority/superiority, and equivalence, the following test statistic is always considered:

$$Z = \frac{\hat{p}_1 - \hat{p}_2 + \epsilon}{\hat{\sigma}},$$

where $\hat{p}_1$ and $\hat{p}_2$ are observed response rates from treatment 1 and treatment 2, respectively, and $\hat{\sigma}$ is an estimate of the standard error $\sigma$, which is given by

$$\sigma = \sqrt{\frac{p_1(1-p_1)}{n_1} + \frac{p_2(1-p_2)}{n_2}}.$$

Under the null hypothesis, $Z$ is asymptotically normally distributed with mean 0 and standard deviation 1. As an example, for testing non-inferiority between an active treatment (treatment 1) and an active control (treatment 2), large $Z$ values (i.e., treatment is better than control) favor the alternative hypothesis. Blackwelder (1982) recommended $\sigma^2$ be estimated by the observed variance, which is given by

$$\hat{\sigma}^2 = \frac{\hat{p}_1(1-\hat{p}_1)}{n_1} + \frac{\hat{p}_2(1-\hat{p}_2)}{n_2}.$$

In practice, however, $\sigma^2$ can be estimated by different methods. For example, Dunnett and Gent (1977) proposed to estimate variance from fixed marginal totals. The idea is to estimate $p_1$ and $p_2$ under the null hypothesis restriction $p_1 - p_2 = \epsilon$, subject to the marginal totals remaining equal to those observed. This approach leads to the estimates

$$\tilde{p}_1 = \left[\hat{p}_1 + \left(\frac{n_2}{n_1}\right)(\hat{p}_2 + \epsilon)\right] \bigg/ \left(1 + \frac{n_2}{n_1}\right),$$

$$\tilde{p}_2 = \left[\hat{p}_1 + \left(\frac{n_2}{n_1}\right)(\hat{p}_2 - \epsilon)\right] \bigg/ \left(1 + \frac{n_2}{n_1}\right).$$

As a result, an estimate of $\sigma$ can then be obtained based on $\tilde{p}_1$ and $\tilde{p}_2$. Tu (1997) suggested $\sigma^2$ be estimated by the unbiased observed variance

$$\hat{\sigma}_U^2 = \frac{\hat{p}_1(1-\hat{p}_1)}{n_1 - 1} + \frac{\hat{p}_2(1-\hat{p}_2)}{n_2 - 1}.$$

In addition, Miettinen and Nurminen (1985) and Farrington and Manning (1990) considered estimating $\sigma^2$ using the constrained maximum likelihood estimate (MLE) as follows

$$\tilde{\sigma}^2_{MLE} = \frac{\tilde{p}_1(1-\tilde{p}_1)}{n_1} + \frac{\tilde{p}_2(1-\tilde{p}_2)}{n_2},$$

where $\tilde{p}_1$ and $\tilde{p}_2$ are the constrained MLE of $p_1$ and $p_2$ under the null hypothesis. As indicated in Farrington and Manning (1990), $\tilde{p}_1$ can be obtained as the unique solution of the following maximum likelihood equation:

$$ax^3 + bx^2 + cx + d = 0,$$

where

$$a = 1 + \frac{n_2}{n_1},$$

$$b = -\left[1 + \frac{n_2}{n_1} + \hat{p}_1 + \left(\frac{n_2}{n_1}\right)\hat{p}_2 + \epsilon\left(\frac{n_2}{n_1} + 2\right)\right],$$

$$c = \epsilon^2 + \epsilon\left(2\hat{p}_1 + \frac{n_2}{n_1} + 1\right) + \hat{p}_1 + \left(\frac{n_2}{n_1}\right)\hat{p}_2,$$

$$d = -\hat{p}_1\epsilon(1+\epsilon).$$

The solution is given by

$$\tilde{p}_1 = 2u\cos(w) - b/3a \quad \text{and} \quad \tilde{p}_2 = \tilde{p}_1 - \epsilon,$$

where

$$w = \frac{1}{3}\left[\pi + \cos^{-1}(v/u^3)\right],$$
$$v = b^3/(3a)^3 - bc/(6a^2) + d/(2a),$$
$$u = \text{sign}(v)[b^2/(3a)^2 - c/(3a)]^{1/2}.$$

Biswas, Chan, and Ghosh (2000) showed that the method of the constrained MLE performs better than methods by Blackwelder (1982) and Dunnett and Gent (1977) in terms of controlling type I error rate, power and confidence interval coverage through a simulation study. The power function (sample size calculation) is sensitive to the difference between true response rates. A small difference (i.e., $\epsilon \neq 0$) will drop the power rapidly. Consequently, a large sample size is required for achieving a desired power.

### 4.8.3 Stratified Analysis

In clinical research, stratified randomization is often employed to isolate the possible confounding or interaction effects that may be caused by prognostic factors (e.g., age, weight, disease status, and medical history) and/or non-prognostic factors (e.g., study center). Responses in these strata are expected to be similar and yet they may be systematically different or subject to random fluctuation across strata. In the interest of a fair and reliable assessment of the treatment difference, it is suggested that the stratified analysis be performed. The purpose of the stratified analysis is to obtain an unbiased estimate of treatment difference with a desired precision.

Stratified analysis can be performed based on Blackwelder's approach or the method proposed by Miettinen and Nurminen (1985) and Farrington and Manning (1990) by adapting different weights in each strata. In practice, several weights are commonly considered. These weights include (i) equal weights, (ii) sample size, (iii) Cochran-Mantel-Haenszel, (iv) inverse of variance, and (v) minimum risk. Suppose there are $K$ strata. Let $n_{ik}$ be the sample size of the $k$th stratum in the $i$th treatment group and $w_k$ be the weight assigned to the $k$th stratum, where $k = 1, ..., K$. Basically, equal weights, i.e., $w_k = w$ for all $k$ imply that no weights are considered. Intuitively, one may consider using the weight based on sample size, i.e.,

$$w_k \propto (n_{1k} + n_{2k}).$$

In other words, larger strata will carry more weights as compared to smaller strata. Alternatively, we may consider the weight suggested by Cochran-Mantel-Haenszel as follows:

$$w_k \propto \frac{n_{1k} n_{2k}}{n_{1k} + n_{2k}}.$$

These weights, however, do not take into consideration of the heterogeneity of variability across strata. To overcome this problem, the weight based on the inverse of variance for the $k$th stratum is useful, i.e.,

$$w_k \propto \sigma_k^{-1},$$

where $\sigma_k^2$ is the variance of the $k$th stratum. The weight of minimum risk is referred to as the weight that minimizes the mean squared error (Mehrotra and Railkar, 2000).

Biswas, Chan, and Ghosh (2000) conducted a simulation study to compare the relative performances of Blackwelder's approach and Miettinen and Nurminen's method with different weights for stratified analysis. The results indicate that Cochran-Mantel-Haenszel weight for Miettinen and Nurminen's method and minimum risk weight for Blackwelder's approach perform very well even in the case of extreme proportions and/or the presence of interactions. Inverse variance weight is biased which leads to liberal confidence interval coverage probability.

## 4.8.4 Equivalence Test for More Than Two Proportions

In clinical trials, it may be of interest to demonstrate therapeutic equivalence among a group of drug products for treatment of certain disease under study. In this case, a typical approach is to perform a pairwise equivalence testing with or without adjusting the $\alpha$ level for multiple comparisons. Suppose a clinical trial was conducted to establish therapeutic equivalence among three drug products (A, B and C) for treatment of women with advanced breast cancer. For a given equivalence limit, equivalence test can be performed for testing (i) drug A versus drug B, (ii) drug A versus drug C, and (iii) drug B versus drug C. It is very likely that we may conclude that drug A is equivalent to drug B and drug B is equivalent to drug C but drug A is not equivalent drug C based on pairwise comparison. In this case, equivalence among the three drug products can not be established. As an alternative approach, Wiens, Heyse, and Matthews (1996) consider the following hypotheses for testing equivalence among a group of treatments:

$$H_0 : \max_{1 \leq i \leq j \leq K} |p_i - p_j| \geq \delta \quad \text{versus} \quad H_a : \max_{1 \leq i \leq j \leq K} |p_i - p_j| < \delta .$$

Testing the above hypotheses is equivalent to testing the following hypotheses:

$$H_0 : \max_{1 \leq i \leq K} p_i - \max_{1 \leq j \leq K} p_j \geq \delta \quad \text{versus} \quad H_a : \max_{1 \leq i \leq K} p_i - \max_{1 \leq j \leq K} p_j < \delta .$$

Under the above hypotheses, formulas for sample size calculation can be similarly derived.

# Chapter 5

# Exact Tests for Proportions

In the previous chapter, formulas for sample size calculation for comparing proportions were derived based on asymptotic approximations. In practice, sample sizes for some clinical trials such as phase II cancer trials are usually small and, hence, the formulas given in the previous chapter may not be useful. In this chapter, our primary focus is placed on procedures for sample size calculation based on exact tests for small samples. Unlike the tests based on asymptotic distribution, the power functions of the exact tests usually do not have explicit forms. Hence, exact formulas for sample size calculation cannot be obtained. However, the sample size can be obtained numerically by greedy search over the sample space.

In the next two sections, procedures for obtaining sample sizes based on exact tests for comparing proportions such as the binomial test and Fisher's exact test are discussed. In Section 5.3, procedures for sample size calculation under various optimal multiple-stage designs such as an optimal two-stage design, an optimal three-stage design and a flexible optimal design for single-arm phase II cancer trials are given. Section 5.4 provides procedures for sample size calculation under a flexible design for multiple armed clinical trials. Some practical issues are presented in the last section.

## 5.1 Binomial Test

In this section, we describe the binomial test, which is probably the most commonly used exact test for one-sample testing problem with binary response in clinical research, and the related sample size calculation formula.

## 5.1.1 The Procedure

The test for equality and non-inferiority/superiority can all be unified by the following hypotheses:

$$H_0 : p = p_0^* + \delta \quad \text{versus} \quad H_a : p = p_1, \tag{5.1.1}$$

where $p_0^*$ is a predefined reference value and $p_1 > p_0 + \delta$ is an unknown proportion. When $\delta = 0$, (5.1.1) becomes the (one-sided) test for equality. When $\delta < 0$ ($\delta > 0$), it becomes the test for non-inferiority (superiority). Let $n$ be the sample size of a single arm clinical study and $m$ be the number of observed outcome of interest. When $p = p_0 = p_0^* + \delta$, $m$ is distributed as a binomial random variable with parameters $(p_0, n)$. If the number of the observed responses is greater than or equal to $m$, then it is considered at least as favorable as the observed outcome of $H_a$. The probability of observing these responses is defined as the exact p-value for the observed outcome. In other words,

$$\text{exact p-value} = \sum_{i=m}^{n} \frac{n!}{m!(n-m)!} p_0^i (1-p_0)^{n-i}.$$

For a given significance level $\alpha$, there exists a nonnegative integer $r$ (called the critical value) such that

$$\sum_{i=r}^{n} \frac{n!}{i!(n-i)!} p_0^i (1-p_0)^{n-i} \leq \alpha$$

and

$$\sum_{i=r-1}^{n} \frac{n!}{i!(n-i)!} p_0^i (1-p_0)^{n-i} > \alpha.$$

We then reject the null hypothesis at the $\alpha$ level of significance if $m \geq r$. Under the alternative hypothesis that $p = p_1 > p_0$, the power of this test can be evaluated as

$$P(m \geq r | H_a) = \sum_{i=r}^{n} \frac{n!}{i!(n-i)!} p_1^i (1-p_1)^{n-i}.$$

For a given power, the sample size required for achieving a desired power of $1 - \beta$ can be obtained by solving $P(m \geq r | H_a) \geq 1 - \beta$.

Tables 5.1.1 and 5.1.2 provide sample sizes required for achieving a desired power (80% or 90%) for $p_1 - p_0 = 0.15$ and $p_1 - p_0 = 0.20$, respectively. As an example, a sample size of 40 subjects is required for detection of a 15% difference (i.e., $p_1 - p_0 = 0.15$) with a 90% power assuming that $p_0 = 0.10$. Note that with the selected sample size, we would reject the null hypothesis that $p_0 = 0.10$ at the $\alpha$ level of significance if there are 7 (out of 40) responses.

## 5.1. Binomial Test

Table 5.1.1: Sample Size $n$ and Critical Value $r$ for Binomial Test $(p_1 - p_0 = 0.15)$

| $\alpha$ | $p_0$ | $p_1$ | $1-\beta=80\%$ $r$ | $n$ | $1-\beta=90\%$ $r$ | $n$ |
|---|---|---|---|---|---|---|
| 0.05 | 0.05 | 0.20 | 3 | 27 | 4 | 38 |
|  | 0.10 | 0.25 | 7 | 40 | 9 | 55 |
|  | 0.15 | 0.30 | 11 | 48 | 14 | 64 |
|  | 0.20 | 0.35 | 16 | 56 | 21 | 77 |
|  | 0.25 | 0.40 | 21 | 62 | 27 | 83 |
|  | 0.30 | 0.45 | 26 | 67 | 35 | 93 |
|  | 0.35 | 0.50 | 30 | 68 | 41 | 96 |
|  | 0.40 | 0.55 | 35 | 71 | 45 | 94 |
|  | 0.45 | 0.60 | 38 | 70 | 52 | 98 |
|  | 0.50 | 0.65 | 41 | 69 | 54 | 93 |
|  | 0.55 | 0.70 | 45 | 70 | 58 | 92 |
|  | 0.60 | 0.75 | 43 | 62 | 58 | 85 |
|  | 0.65 | 0.80 | 41 | 55 | 55 | 75 |
|  | 0.70 | 0.85 | 39 | 49 | 54 | 69 |
|  | 0.75 | 0.90 | 38 | 45 | 46 | 55 |
|  | 0.80 | 0.95 | 27 | 30 | 39 | 44 |
| 0.10 | 0.05 | 0.20 | 2 | 21 | 3 | 32 |
|  | 0.10 | 0.25 | 5 | 31 | 6 | 40 |
|  | 0.15 | 0.30 | 8 | 37 | 11 | 53 |
|  | 0.20 | 0.35 | 12 | 44 | 16 | 61 |
|  | 0.25 | 0.40 | 15 | 46 | 20 | 64 |
|  | 0.30 | 0.45 | 19 | 50 | 26 | 71 |
|  | 0.35 | 0.50 | 21 | 49 | 30 | 72 |
|  | 0.40 | 0.55 | 24 | 50 | 35 | 75 |
|  | 0.45 | 0.60 | 28 | 53 | 39 | 75 |
|  | 0.50 | 0.65 | 31 | 53 | 41 | 72 |
|  | 0.55 | 0.70 | 31 | 49 | 44 | 71 |
|  | 0.60 | 0.75 | 32 | 47 | 43 | 64 |
|  | 0.65 | 0.80 | 33 | 45 | 44 | 61 |
|  | 0.70 | 0.85 | 29 | 37 | 41 | 53 |
|  | 0.75 | 0.90 | 25 | 30 | 33 | 40 |
|  | 0.80 | 0.95 | 22 | 25 | 28 | 32 |

Table 5.1.2: Sample Size $n$ and Critical Value $r$ for Binomial Test $(p_1 - p_0 = 0.20)$

|  |  |  | $1-\beta = 80\%$ | | $1-\beta = 90\%$ | |
|---|---|---|---|---|---|---|
| $\alpha$ | $p_0$ | $p_1$ | $r$ | $N$ | $r$ | $N$ |
| 0.05 | 0.05 | 0.25 | 2 | 16 | 3 | 25 |
|  | 0.10 | 0.30 | 5 | 25 | 6 | 33 |
|  | 0.15 | 0.35 | 7 | 28 | 9 | 38 |
|  | 0.20 | 0.40 | 11 | 35 | 14 | 47 |
|  | 0.25 | 0.45 | 13 | 36 | 17 | 49 |
|  | 0.30 | 0.50 | 16 | 39 | 21 | 53 |
|  | 0.35 | 0.55 | 19 | 41 | 24 | 53 |
|  | 0.40 | 0.60 | 22 | 42 | 28 | 56 |
|  | 0.45 | 0.65 | 24 | 42 | 30 | 54 |
|  | 0.50 | 0.70 | 23 | 37 | 32 | 53 |
|  | 0.55 | 0.75 | 25 | 37 | 33 | 50 |
|  | 0.60 | 0.80 | 26 | 36 | 32 | 45 |
|  | 0.65 | 0.85 | 24 | 31 | 32 | 42 |
|  | 0.70 | 0.90 | 23 | 28 | 30 | 37 |
|  | 0.75 | 0.95 | 20 | 23 | 25 | 29 |
|  | 0.80 | 1.00 | 13 | 14 | 13 | 14 |
| 0.10 | 0.05 | 0.25 | 2 | 16 | 2 | 20 |
|  | 0.10 | 0.30 | 3 | 18 | 4 | 25 |
|  | 0.15 | 0.35 | 5 | 22 | 7 | 32 |
|  | 0.20 | 0.40 | 7 | 24 | 10 | 36 |
|  | 0.25 | 0.45 | 9 | 26 | 13 | 39 |
|  | 0.30 | 0.50 | 12 | 30 | 15 | 39 |
|  | 0.35 | 0.55 | 13 | 29 | 19 | 44 |
|  | 0.40 | 0.60 | 15 | 30 | 20 | 41 |
|  | 0.45 | 0.65 | 16 | 29 | 24 | 44 |
|  | 0.50 | 0.70 | 17 | 28 | 23 | 39 |
|  | 0.55 | 0.75 | 19 | 29 | 25 | 39 |
|  | 0.60 | 0.80 | 17 | 24 | 25 | 36 |
|  | 0.65 | 0.85 | 16 | 21 | 24 | 32 |
|  | 0.70 | 0.90 | 17 | 21 | 20 | 25 |
|  | 0.75 | 0.95 | 13 | 15 | 17 | 20 |
|  | 0.80 | 1.00 | 10 | 11 | 10 | 11 |

### 5.1.2 Remarks

The exact p-value is well defined only if the sample distribution is completely specified under the null hypothesis. On the other hand, the test for equivalence usually involves interval hypothesis, which means that, under the null hypothesis, we only know the parameter of interest is located within certain interval but are unaware of its exact value. As a result, the distribution under the null hypothesis cannot be completely specified and, hence, exact test is not well defined in such a situation.

### 5.1.3 An Example

Suppose the investigator is interested in conducting a trial to study the treatment effect of a test compound in curing patients with certain types of cancer. The responder is defined to be the subject who is completely cured by the study treatment. According to literature, the standard therapy available on the market can produce a cure rate of 10% ($p_0 = 10\%$). A pilot study of the test compound shows that the test compound may produce a cure rate of 30% ($p_1 = 30\%$). The objective of the planning trial is to confirm such a difference truly exists. It is desirable to have a sample size, which can produce 80% power at 5% level of significance. According to Table 5.1.1, the total sample size needed is given by 25. The null hypothesis should be rejected if there are at least 5 subjects who are classified as responders.

## 5.2 Fisher's Exact Test

For comparing proportions between two treatment groups, the hypotheses of interest are given by

$$H_0 : p_1 = p_2 \quad \text{versus} \quad H_a : p_1 \neq p_2,$$

where $p_1$ and $p_2$ are the true proportions of treatment 1 and treatment 2, respectively. Unlike the one-sample binomial test, under the null hypothesis that $p_1 = p_2$, the exact values of $p_1$ and $p_2$ are unknown. Hence, it is impossible to track the marginal distribution of the events observed from different treatment groups. In this case, a conditional test such as Fisher's exact test is usually considered. In this section, we describe Fisher's exact test and the related sample size calculation formula.

## 5.2.1 The Procedure

Let $m_i$ be the number of responses observed in the $i$th treatment group. Then, the total number of observed responses is $m = m_1 + m_2$. Under the null hypothesis that $p_1 = p_2$ and conditional on $m$, it can be shown that $m_1$ follows a hypergeometric distribution with parameters $(m, n_1, n_2)$, i.e.,

$$P(m_1 = i | m, n_1, n_2) = \frac{\binom{n_1}{i} \binom{n_2}{m-i}}{\binom{n_1+n_2}{m}}.$$

Any outcomes with the same $m$ but larger than $m_1$ would be considered at least as favorable to $H_a$ as the observed outcome. Then, the probability of observing these outcomes, which is at least as observed, is defined as the exact p-value. In other words,

$$\text{exact p-value} = \sum_{i=m_1}^{m} \frac{\binom{n_1}{i} \binom{n_2}{m-i}}{\binom{n_1+n_2}{m}}.$$

We reject the null hypothesis at the $\alpha$ level of significance when the exact p-value is less than $\alpha$. Under the alternative hypothesis that $p_1 \neq p_2$ and for a fixed $n$, the power of Fisher's exact test can be obtained by summing the probabilities of all the outcomes such that the exact p-value is less than $\alpha$. However, it should be noted that no closed form exists for the power of Fisher's exact test. As a result, sample size required for achieving a desired power can only be obtained numerically such as by greedy search for all possible outcomes.

Table 5.2.1 provides sample sizes required for achieving the desired power (80% or 90%) under various parameters (i.e., $p_2 - p_1$ ranging from 0.10 to 0.35) when testing the null hypothesis that $p_1 = p_2$. As an example, a sample size of 34 subjects is required for detection of a 25% difference in proportion between treatment groups (i.e., $p_2 - p_1 = 0.25$) with an 80% power assuming that $p_1 = 0.15$.

## 5.2.2 Remarks

For Fisher's exact test, the exact p-value is well defined only if the conditional sample distribution is completely specified under the null hypothesis. On the other side, the test for non-inferiority/superiority and equivalence

Table 5.2.1: Sample Size for Fisher's Exact Test

|             |       |       | $\alpha = 0.10$ |               | $\alpha = 0.05$ |               |
| ----------- | ----- | ----- | ------------- | ------------- | ------------- | ------------- |
| $p_2 - p_1$ | $p_1$ | $p_2$ | $\beta = 0.20$ | $\beta = 0.10$ | $\beta = 0.20$ | $\beta = 0.10$ |
| 0.25 | 0.05 | 0.30 | 25 | 33 | 34 | 42 |
|      | 0.10 | 0.35 | 31 | 41 | 39 | 52 |
|      | 0.15 | 0.40 | 34 | 48 | 46 | 60 |
|      | 0.20 | 0.45 | 39 | 52 | 49 | 65 |
|      | 0.25 | 0.50 | 40 | 56 | 54 | 71 |
|      | 0.30 | 0.55 | 41 | 57 | 55 | 72 |
|      | 0.35 | 0.60 | 41 | 57 | 56 | 77 |
|      | 0.40 | 0.65 | 41 | 57 | 56 | 77 |
|      | 0.45 | 0.70 | 41 | 57 | 55 | 72 |
|      | 0.50 | 0.75 | 40 | 56 | 54 | 71 |
|      | 0.55 | 0.80 | 39 | 52 | 49 | 65 |
|      | 0.60 | 0.85 | 34 | 48 | 46 | 60 |
|      | 0.65 | 0.90 | 31 | 41 | 39 | 52 |
|      | 0.70 | 0.95 | 25 | 33 | 34 | 42 |
| 0.30 | 0.05 | 0.35 | 20 | 26 | 25 | 33 |
|      | 0.10 | 0.40 | 23 | 32 | 30 | 39 |
|      | 0.15 | 0.45 | 26 | 35 | 34 | 45 |
|      | 0.20 | 0.50 | 28 | 39 | 36 | 47 |
|      | 0.25 | 0.55 | 29 | 40 | 37 | 51 |
|      | 0.30 | 0.60 | 29 | 40 | 41 | 53 |
|      | 0.35 | 0.65 | 33 | 40 | 41 | 53 |
|      | 0.40 | 0.70 | 29 | 40 | 41 | 53 |
|      | 0.45 | 0.75 | 29 | 40 | 37 | 51 |
|      | 0.50 | 0.80 | 28 | 39 | 36 | 47 |
|      | 0.55 | 0.85 | 26 | 35 | 34 | 45 |
|      | 0.60 | 0.90 | 23 | 32 | 30 | 39 |
| 0.35 | 0.05 | 0.40 | 16 | 21 | 20 | 25 |
|      | 0.10 | 0.45 | 19 | 24 | 24 | 31 |
|      | 0.15 | 0.50 | 20 | 28 | 26 | 34 |
|      | 0.20 | 0.55 | 23 | 29 | 27 | 36 |
|      | 0.25 | 0.60 | 24 | 29 | 30 | 36 |
|      | 0.30 | 0.65 | 24 | 33 | 31 | 40 |
|      | 0.35 | 0.70 | 24 | 33 | 31 | 40 |
|      | 0.40 | 0.75 | 24 | 29 | 30 | 36 |
|      | 0.45 | 0.80 | 23 | 29 | 27 | 36 |
|      | 0.50 | 0.85 | 20 | 28 | 26 | 34 |
|      | 0.55 | 0.90 | 19 | 24 | 24 | 31 |
|      | 0.60 | 0.95 | 16 | 21 | 20 | 25 |

usually involves interval hypothesis, which means under the null hypothesis, we only know the parameter of interest is located within certain interval but unaware of its exact value. As a result, the distribution under the null hypothesis can not be completely specified and, hence, Fisher's exact test is not well defined in such a situation.

### 5.2.3 An Example

Suppose the investigator is interested in conducting a two-arm trial to study the treatment effect of a test compound in preventing the relapse rate in EAE score. The active control involved in the trial is a standard therapy aleady available on market. It is assumed that the responder rates for the test compound and the control are given by 10% ($p_1 = 20\%$) and 35% ($p_2 = 35\%$), respectively. The objective of the planning trial is to confirm such a difference truly exists. It is desirable to have a sample size, which can produce 80% power at 5% level of significance. According to Table 5.2.1, the sample size needed per arm is given by 39.

## 5.3 Optimal Multiple-Stage Designs for Single Arm Trials

In phase II cancer trials, it is undesirable to stop a study early when the test drug is promising. On the other hand, it is desirable to terminate the study as early as possible when the treatment is not effective. For this purpose, an optimal multiple-stage design is often employed to determine whether a study drug holds sufficient promise to warrant further testing. In what follows, procedures for sample size calculation under various optimal multiple-stage designs are introduced.

### 5.3.1 Optimal Two-Stage Designs

The concept of an optimal two-stage design is to permit early stopping when a moderately long sequence of initial failures occurs. Denote the number of subjects studied in the first and second stage by $n_1$ and $n_2$, respectively. Under a two-stage design, $n_1$ patients are treated at the first stage. If there are less than $r_1$ responses, then stop the trial. Otherwise, stage 2 is implemented by including the other $n_2$ patients. A decision regarding whether the test drug is a promising compound is then made based on the response rate of the $N = n_1 + n_2$ subjects. Let $p_0$ be the undesirable response rate and $p_1$ be the desirable response rate ($p_1 > p_0$). If the response rate of a test drug is at the undesirable level, one wishes to reject it as an

## 5.3. Optimal Multiple-Stage Designs for Single Arm Trials

ineffective compound with a high probability (or the false positive rate is low), and if its response rate is at the desirable level, not to reject it as a promising compound with a high probability (or the false negative rate is low). As a result, it is of interest to test the following hypotheses:

$$H_0 : p \leq p_0 \quad \text{versus} \quad H_a : p \geq p_1.$$

Rejection of $H_0$ (or $H_a$) means that further (or no further) study of the test drug should be carried out. Note that under the above hypotheses, the usual type I error is the false positive rate in accepting an ineffective drug and the type II error is the false negative rate in rejecting a promising compound.

To select among possible two-stage designs with specific type I and type II errors, Simon (1989) proposed to use the optimal design that achieves the minimum expected sample size when the response rate is $p_0$. Let $EN$ be the expected sample size. Then, $EN$ can be obtained as

$$EN = n_1 + (1 - PET)n_2,$$

where $PET$ is the probability of early termination after the first stage, which depends upon the true probability of response $p$. At the end of the first stage, we would terminate the trial early and reject the test drug if $r_1$ or fewer responses are observed. As a result, $PET$ is given by

$$PET = B(r_1; p, n_1),$$

where $B(\cdot; p, n_1)$ denotes the cumulative binomial distribution with parameter $(p, n_1)$. We would reject the test drug at the end of the second stage if $r$ or fewer responses are observed. Hence, the probability of rejecting the test drug with success probability $p$ is given by

$$B(r_1; p, n_1) + \sum_{x=r_1+1}^{\min(n_1, r)} b(x; p, n_1) B(r - x; p, n_2),$$

where $b(\cdot; p, n_1)$ denotes the binomial probability function with parameter $(p, n_1)$. For specified values of $p_0$, $p_1$, $\alpha$, and $\beta$, Simon's optimal two-stage design can be obtained as the two-stage design that satisfies the error constraints and minimizes the expected sample size when the response probability is $p_0$. As an alternative design, Simon (1989) also proposed to seek the minimum total sample size first and then achieve the minimum expected sample size for the fixed total sample size when the response rate is $p_0$. This design is referred to as the minimax design.

Tables 5.3.1 and 5.3.2 provide sample sizes for optimal two-stage designs and minimax designs for a variety of design parameters, respectively. The

Table 5.3.1: Sample Sizes and Critical Values for Two-Stage Designs $(p_1 - p_0 = 0.15)$

|       |       |          |         | Optimal Design | | Minimax Design | |
|-------|-------|----------|---------|--------|--------|--------|--------|
| $p_0$ | $p_1$ | $\alpha$ | $\beta$ | $r_1/n_1$ | $r/N$ | $r_1/n_1$ | $r/N$ |
| 0.05  | 0.20  | 0.10     | 0.10    | 0/12   | 3/37   | 0/13   | 3/32   |
|       |       | 0.05     | 0.20    | 0/10   | 3/29   | 0/13   | 3/27   |
|       |       | 0.05     | 0.10    | 1/21   | 4/41   | 1/29   | 4/38   |
| 0.10  | 0.25  | 0.10     | 0.10    | 2/21   | 7/50   | 2/27   | 6/40   |
|       |       | 0.05     | 0.20    | 2/18   | 7/43   | 2/22   | 7/40   |
|       |       | 0.05     | 0.10    | 2/21   | 10/66  | 3/31   | 9/55   |
| 0.20  | 0.35  | 0.10     | 0.10    | 5/27   | 16/63  | 6/33   | 15/58  |
|       |       | 0.05     | 0.20    | 5/22   | 19/72  | 6/31   | 15/53  |
|       |       | 0.05     | 0.10    | 8/37   | 22/83  | 8/42   | 21/77  |
| 0.30  | 0.45  | 0.10     | 0.10    | 9/30   | 29/82  | 16/50  | 25/69  |
|       |       | 0.05     | 0.20    | 9/27   | 30/81  | 16/46  | 25/65  |
|       |       | 0.05     | 0.10    | 13/40  | 40/110 | 27/77  | 33/88  |
| 0.40  | 0.55  | 0.10     | 0.10    | 16/38  | 40/88  | 18/45  | 34/73  |
|       |       | 0.05     | 0.20    | 11/26  | 40/84  | 28/59  | 34/70  |
|       |       | 0.05     | 0.10    | 19/45  | 49/104 | 24/62  | 45/94  |
| 0.50  | 0.65  | 0.10     | 0.10    | 18/35  | 47/84  | 19/40  | 41/72  |
|       |       | 0.05     | 0.20    | 15/28  | 48/83  | 39/66  | 40/68  |
|       |       | 0.05     | 0.10    | 22/42  | 60/105 | 28/57  | 54/93  |
| 0.60  | 0.75  | 0.10     | 0.10    | 21/34  | 47/71  | 25/43  | 43/64  |
|       |       | 0.05     | 0.20    | 17/27  | 46/67  | 18/30  | 43/62  |
|       |       | 0.05     | 0.10    | 21/34  | 64/95  | 48/72  | 57/84  |
| 0.70  | 0.85  | 0.10     | 0.10    | 14/20  | 45/59  | 15/22  | 40/52  |
|       |       | 0.05     | 0.20    | 14/19  | 46/59  | 16/23  | 39/49  |
|       |       | 0.05     | 0.10    | 18/25  | 61/79  | 33/44  | 53/68  |
| 0.80  | 0.95  | 0.10     | 0.10    | 5/7    | 27/31  | 5/7    | 27/31  |
|       |       | 0.05     | 0.20    | 7/9    | 26/29  | 7/9    | 26/29  |
|       |       | 0.05     | 0.10    | 16/19  | 37/42  | 31/35  | 35/40  |

## 5.3. Optimal Multiple-Stage Designs for Single Arm Trials

Table 5.3.2: Sample Sizes and Critical Values for Two-Stage Designs
$(p_1 - p_0 = 0.20)$

|       |       |       |       | Optimal Design | | Minimax Design | |
|-------|-------|-------|-------|---------|-------|---------|-------|
| $p_0$ | $p_1$ | $\alpha$ | $\beta$ | $r_1/n_1$ | $r/n$ | $r_1/n_1$ | $r/n$ |
| 0.05  | 0.25  | 0.10  | 0.10  | 0/9   | 2/24  | 0/13  | 2/20  |
|       |       | 0.05  | 0.20  | 0/9   | 2/17  | 0/12  | 2/16  |
|       |       | 0.05  | 0.10  | 0/9   | 3/30  | 0/15  | 3/25  |
| 0.10  | 0.30  | 0.10  | 0.10  | 1/12  | 5/35  | 1/16  | 4/25  |
|       |       | 0.05  | 0.20  | 1/10  | 5/29  | 1/15  | 5/25  |
|       |       | 0.05  | 0.10  | 2/18  | 6/35  | 2/22  | 6/33  |
| 0.20  | 0.40  | 0.10  | 0.10  | 3/17  | 10/37 | 3/19  | 10/36 |
|       |       | 0.05  | 0.20  | 3/13  | 12/43 | 4/18  | 10/33 |
|       |       | 0.05  | 0.10  | 4/19  | 15/54 | 5/24  | 13/45 |
| 0.30  | 0.50  | 0.10  | 0.10  | 7/22  | 17/46 | 7/28  | 15/39 |
|       |       | 0.05  | 0.20  | 5/15  | 18/46 | 6/19  | 16/39 |
|       |       | 0.05  | 0.10  | 8/24  | 24/63 | 7/24  | 21/53 |
| 0.40  | 0.60  | 0.10  | 0.10  | 7/18  | 22/46 | 11/28 | 20/41 |
|       |       | 0.05  | 0.20  | 7/16  | 23/46 | 17/34 | 20/39 |
|       |       | 0.05  | 0.10  | 11/25 | 32/66 | 12/29 | 27/54 |
| 0.50  | 0.70  | 0.10  | 0.10  | 11/21 | 26/45 | 11/23 | 23/39 |
|       |       | 0.05  | 0.20  | 8/15  | 26/43 | 12/23 | 23/37 |
|       |       | 0.05  | 0.10  | 13/24 | 35/61 | 14/27 | 32/53 |
| 0.60  | 0.80  | 0.10  | 0.10  | 6/11  | 26/38 | 18/27 | 14/35 |
|       |       | 0.05  | 0.20  | 7/11  | 30/43 | 8/13  | 25/35 |
|       |       | 0.05  | 0.10  | 12/19 | 37/53 | 15/26 | 32/45 |
| 0.70  | 0.90  | 0.10  | 0.10  | 6/9   | 22/28 | 11/16 | 20/25 |
|       |       | 0.05  | 0.20  | 4/6   | 22/27 | 19/23 | 21/26 |
|       |       | 0.05  | 0.10  | 11/15 | 29/36 | 13/18 | 26/32 |

tabulated results include the optimal sample size $n_1$ for the first stage, the maximum sample size $n$, the critical value $r_1$ at the end of the first stage, and the critical value $r$ at the end of the trial. For example, the first line in Table 5.3.2 corresponds to a design with $p_0 = 0.20$ and $p_1 = 0.40$. The optimal two-stage design gives $(r_1/n_1, r/n) = (3/13, 12/43)$ for achieving an 80% power at the 5% level of significance, i.e., $(\alpha, \beta) = (0.05, 0.20)$. In other words, at the first stage, thirteen subjects are tested. If no more than 3 subjects respond, then terminate the trial. Otherwise, accrual continues to a total of 43 subjects. We would conclude that the test drug is effective if there are more than 12 (out of 43 subjects) responses.

## 5.3.2 Flexible Two-Stage Designs

Chen and Ng (1998) proposed optimal multiple-stage flexible designs for phase II trials by simply assuming that the sample sizes are uniformly distributed on a set of $k$ consecutive possible values. As an example, the procedure for obtaining an optimal two-stage flexible design is outlined below.

Let $r_i$ and $n_i$ be the critical value and the sample size for the first stage and $R_j$ and $N_j$ be the critical value and sample size for the second stage. Thus, for a given combination of $(n_i, N_j)$, the expected sample size is given by

$$EN = n_i + (1 - PET)(N_j - n_i),$$

where

$$PET = B(r_i; p, n_i) = \sum_{x \leq r_i} b(x; p, n_i).$$

The probability of rejecting the test drug is then given by

$$B(r_i; p, n_i) + \sum_{x=r_i+1}^{\min(n_i, R_j)} b(x; p, n_i) B(R_j - x; p, N_j - n_i).$$

The average probability of an early termination ($APET$) is the average of $PET$ for all possible $n_i$. The average total probability of rejecting the test drug ($ATPRT$) is the average of the above probability for all possible combinations of $(n_i, N_j)$. The average expected sample size ($AEN$) is the average of $EN$. Chen and Ng (1998) considered the following criteria for obtaining an optimal flexible design. If the true response rate is $p_0$, we reject the test drug with a very high probability (i.e., $ATPRT \geq 1-\alpha$). If the true response rate is $p_1$, we reject the test drug with a very low probability (i.e., $ATPRT \leq \beta$). There are many solutions of $(r_i, n_i, R_j, N_j)'s$ that satisfy the $\alpha$ and $\beta$ requirements for the specific $p_0$ and $p_1$. The optimal design is the one that has minimum $AEN$ when $p = p_0$. The minimax design is the one that has the minimum $N_k$ and the minimum $AEN$ within this fixed $N_k$ when $p = p_0$.

Tables 5.3.3-5.3.4 and Tables 5.3.5-5.3.6 provide sample sizes for flexible two-stage designs and minimax designs for a variety of design parameters, respectively. The tabulated results include the optimal sample size $n_i$ and the critical value $r_i$ for the first stage and the total sample size $N_j$ and critical value $R_j$ at the end of the second stage. For example, the second line in Table 5.3.3 corresponds to a design with $p_0 = 0.10$ and $p_1 = 0.30$. The flexible two-stage design gives 1/11-17, 2/18 for the first stage and 3/24, 4/25-28, 5/29-31 for the second stage for achieving a 90% power at the 10% level of significance. The optimal flexible two-stage design allows the first stage sample size to range from 11 ($n_1$) to 18 ($n_8$). The critical value $r_i$ is 1 if $n_i$ ranges from 11 to 17, and 2 if $n_i$ is 18. If the observed responses are greater than $r_i$, we accrue $27 - n_i$ additional subjects at the second stage. The flexible optimal two-stage design allows the total sample size to range from 24 ($N_1$) to 31 ($N_8$). The rejection boundary $R_j$ is 3 if $N_j$ is 24, 4 if $N_j$ ranges from 25 to 28, and 5 if $N_j$ ranges from 29 to 31.

### 5.3.3 Optimal Three-Stage Designs

The advantage of a two-stage design is that it does not allow early termination if there is a long run of failures at the start. To overcome this disadvantage, Ensign et al. (1994) proposed an optimal three-stage design, which modifies the optimal two-stage design. The optimal three-stage design is implemented by testing the following similar hypotheses:

$$H_0 : p \leq p_0 \quad \text{versus} \quad H_a : p \geq p_1.$$

Rejection of $H_0$ (or $H_a$) means that further (or not further) study of the test drug should be carried out. At stage 1, $n_1$ patients are treated. We would reject $H_a$ (i.e., the test treatment is not responding) and stop the trial if there is no response. If there are one or more responses, then proceed to stage 2 by including additional $n_2$ patients. We would reject $H_a$ and stop the trial if the total number of responses is less than or equal to a pre-specified number of $r_2$; otherwise continue to stage 3. At stage 3, $n_3$ more patients are treated. We would reject $H_a$ if the total responses for the three stages combined is less than or equal to $r_3$. In this case, we conclude the test drug is ineffective. On the other hand, if there are more than $r_3$ responses, we reject $H_0$ and conclude the test drug is effective. Based on the concept of the above three-stage design, Ensign et al. (1994) considered the following to determine the sample size. For each value of $n_1$ satisfying

$$(1 - p_1)^{n_1} < \beta,$$

Table 5.3.3: Sample Sizes and Critical Values for Optimal Flexible Two-Stage Designs ($p_1 - p_0 = 0.15$)

| $p_0$ | $p_1$ | $\alpha$ | $\beta$ | $r_i/n_i$ | $R_j/N_j$ |
|---|---|---|---|---|---|
| 0.05 | 0.20 | 0.10 | 0.10 | 0/15-16,1/17-22 | 2/30-31,3/32-37 |
|  |  | 0.05 | 0.20 | 0/10-12,1/13-17 | 3/27-34 |
|  |  | 0.05 | 0.10 | 1/17-24 | 4/41-46,5/47-48 |
| 0.10 | 0.25 | 0.10 | 0.10 | 2/19-25,3/26 | 6/44-45,7/46-51 |
|  |  | 0.05 | 0.20 | 1/13-15,2/16-20 | 6/40,7/41-45,8/46-47 |
|  |  | 0.05 | 0.10 | 2/21-24,3/25-28 | 9/57-61,10/62-64 |
| 0.20 | 0.35 | 0.10 | 0.10 | 6/28-31,7/32-35 | 15/62,16/63-65, 17/66-68,18/69 |
|  |  | 0.05 | 0.20 | 4/18-21,5/22-24,6/25 | 17/62-64,18/65-69, |
|  |  | 0.05 | 0.20 | 6/31,7/32-34,8/35-38 | 22/82-85,23/86-89 |
| 0.30 | 0.45 | 0.10 | 0.10 | 9/31,10/32-33 11/34-37,12/38 | 27/75-77,28/78-80 29/81-82 |
|  |  | 0.05 | 0.20 | 7/23,8/24-25, 9/26-29,10/30 | 27/73,28/74-76, 29/77-78,30/79-80 |
|  |  | 0.05 | 0.20 | 11/35-36,12/37-39, 13/40-42 | 36/98-99,37/100-102, 38/103-104,39/105 |
| 0.40 | 0.55 | 0.10 | 0.10 | 12/30-31,13/32-33, 14/34-35,15/36-37 | 37/80-81,38/82-84, 39/85-86,40/87 |
|  |  | 0.05 | 0.20 | 11/25-26,12/27-29, 13/30-31,14/32 | 37/78,38/79-80, 39/81-82,40/83-85 |
|  |  | 0.05 | 0.10 | 16/38-39,17/40-41, 18/42-44,19/45 | 49/104-105,50/106-107, 51/108-109,52/110-111 |
| 0.50 | 0.65 | 0.10 | 0.10 | 15/30,16/31-32,17/33-34, 18/35-36,19/37 | 44/78-79,45/80-81, 46/82-83,47/84,48/85 |
|  |  | 0.05 | 0.20 | 12/23,13/24-25,14/26-27, 15/28-29,16/30 | 45/77-78,46/79-80, 47/81-82,48/83,49/84 |
|  |  | 0.05 | 0.10 | 21/40,22/41-42,23/43-44, 24/45-46,25/47 | 59/103-104,60/105-106, 61/107,62/108-109,63/110 |
| 0.60 | 0.75 | 0.10 | 0.10 | 16/27,17/28,18/29-30, 19/31-32,20/33,21/34 | 44/67,45/68,46/69-70, 47/71,48/72,49/73-74 |
|  |  | 0.05 | 0.20 | 14/22-23,15/24,16/25 | 46/68,47/69,48/70-71 |
|  |  | 0.05 | 0.10 | 20/32-33,21/34,22/36-36, 23/37/24/38-39 | 61/90-91,62/92,63/93-94, 64/95,65/96-97 |
| 0.70 | 0.85 | 0.10 | 0.10 | 13/19,14/20,15/21, 16/22-23,17/24,18/25-26 | 40/53,41/54,42/55,43/56, 44/57-58,45/59,46/60 |
|  |  | 0.05 | 0.20 | 9/13,10/14,11/15,12/16-17, 13/18,14/19,15/20 | 44/56-57,45/58,46/59, 47/60,48/61-62,49/63 |
|  |  | 0.05 | 0.10 | 17/24,18/26,19/26, 20/27-28,21/29,22/30, 23/31 | 57/73-74,58/75,59/76-77, 60/78,61/79,62/80 |
| 0.80 | 0.95 | 0.10 | 0.10 | 8/10,9/11,10/12-13, 11/14,12/15,13/16,14/17 | 24/28,25/29,26/30,27/31, 28/32,29/33,30/34-35 |
|  |  | 0.05 | 0.20 | 7/9,8/10,9/11,10/12, 11/13,12/14,13/15,14/16 | 25/28,26/29,27/30, 28/31-32,29/33,30/34, 31/35 |
|  |  | 0.05 | 0.10 | 10/12,11/13-14,12/15, 13/16,14/17,15/18,16/19 | 35/40,36/41,37/42,38/43, 39/44,40/45-46,41/47 |

Table 5.3.4: Sample Sizes and Critical Values for Optimal Flexible Two-Stage Designs ($p_1 - p_0 = 0.20$)

| $p_0$ | $p_1$ | $\alpha$ | $\beta$ | $r_i/n_i$ | $R_j/N_j$ |
|---|---|---|---|---|---|
| 0.05 | 0.25 | 0.10 | 0.10 | 0/8-13,1/14-15 | 1/18,2/19-25 |
|      |      | 0.05 | 0.20 | 0/5-10,1/11-12 | 2/17-22,3/23-24 |
|      |      | 0.05 | 0.10 | 0/8-13,1/14-15 | 2/24,3/25-31 |
| 0.10 | 0.30 | 0.10 | 0.10 | 1/11-17,2/18 | 3/24,4/25-28,5/29-31 |
|      |      | 0.05 | 0.20 | 1/8-12,2/13-15 | 4/26,5/27-32,6/33 |
|      |      | 0.05 | 0.10 | 1/12-14,2/15-19 | 6/36-39,7/40-43 |
| 0.20 | 0.40 | 0.10 | 0.10 | 2/14,3/15-17,4/18-21 | 9/35-36,10/37-38,11/39-42 |
|      |      | 0.05 | 0.20 | 2/10-12,3/13-15,4/16-17 | 10/33-35,11/36-40 |
|      |      | 0.05 | 0.10 | 4/18-20,5/21-24,6/25 | 13/48,14/49-51,15/52-55 |
| 0.30 | 0.50 | 0.10 | 0.10 | 4/14-16,5/17-19, 6/20-21 | 15/40-41,16/42-44, 17/45-46,18/47 |
|      |      | 0.05 | 0.20 | 3/11,4/12-14, 5/15-16/6/17-18 | 16/40-41,16/42-44, 18/45-46,18/47 |
|      |      | 0.05 | 0.10 | 6/19-20,7/21-23, 8/24-26 | 21/55,22/56-58, 23/59-60,24/61-62 |
| 0.40 | 0.60 | 0.10 | 0.10 | 6/15-16,7/17-19, 8/20,9/21-22 | 21/44-45,22/46-47, 23/48-49,24/50-51 |
|      |      | 0.05 | 0.20 | 5/12-13,6/14, 7/15-16,8/17-19 | 22/44-45,23/46-47,24/48-49, 25/50,26/51 |
|      |      | 0.05 | 0.10 | 8/20,9/21-22,10/23-24, 11/25-26,12/27 | 28/58,29/59-60,30/61-62, 31/63,32/64-65 |
| 0.50 | 0.70 | 0.10 | 0.10 | 7/15,8/16-17,9/18, 10/19-20,11/21,12/22 | 24/41-42,25/43/44, 26/45,27/46-47,28/48 |
|      |      | 0.05 | 0.20 | 5/10,6/11-12, 7/13-14,8/15,9/16-17 | 25/42,26/43-44,27-45, 28/46-47,29/48,30/49 |
|      |      | 0.05 | 0.10 | 10/19-20,11/21, 12/22-23,13/24-25,14/26 | 33/55-56,34/57-58, 35/59,36/60-61,37/62 |
| 0.60 | 0.80 | 0.10 | 0.10 | 7/12,8/13-14,9/15, 10/16-17,11/18,12/19 | 24/35-36,25/37,26/38 27/39-40,28/41,29/42 |
|      |      | 0.05 | 0.20 | 5/8-9,6/10,7/11, 8/12-13,9/14-15 | 25/35-36,26/37,27/38, 28/39-40,29/41,30/42 |
|      |      | 0.05 | 0.10 | 11/17-18,12/19,13/20-21, 14/22,15/23,16/24 | 34/48-49,35/50-51, 36/52,37/53-54,38/55 |
| 0.70 | 0.90 | 0.10 | 0.10 | 6/9,7/10,8/11,9/12-13, 10/14,11/15-16 | 18/23,19/24,20/25-26, 21/27,22/28,23/29,24/30 |
|      |      | 0.05 | 0.20 | 4/6,5/7,6/8,7/9, 8/10-11,9/12,10/13 | 22/27,23/28-29,24/30, 25/31,26/32-33,27/34 |
|      |      | 0.05 | 0.10 | 7/10,8/11,9/12-13, 10/14,11/15,12/16,13/17 | 27/34/28/35,29/36,30/37-38, 31/39,32/40,33/41 |

Table 5.3.5: Sample Sizes and Critical Values for Minimax Flexible Two-Stage Designs ($p_1 - p_0 = 0.15$)

| $p_0$ | $p_1$ | $\alpha$ | $\beta$ | $r_i/n_i$ | $R_j/N_j$ |
|---|---|---|---|---|---|
| 0.05 | 0.20 | 0.10 | 0.10 | 0/16-22,1/23 | 2/26-28,3/29-33 |
|  |  | 0.05 | 0.20 | 0/10-17 | 2/23,2/24-30 |
|  |  | 0.05 | 0.10 | 0/22-27,1/28-29 | 3/33-34,4/35-40 |
| 0.10 | 0.25 | 0.10 | 0.10 | 1/25-27,2/28-32 | 5/37,6/38-42,7/43-44 |
|  |  | 0.05 | 0.20 | 1/22-24,2/25-29 | 6/33-37,7/38-40 |
|  |  | 0.05 | 0.10 | 2/25-29,3/30-32 | 8/49-52,9/53-56 |
| 0.20 | 0.35 | 0.10 | 0.10 | 6/37-39,7/40-42,8/43-440 | 14/54-55,15/56-59,16/60-61 |
|  |  | 0.05 | 0.20 | 6/28,6/29-31,7/32-35 | 14/50-51,15/52-54,16/55-57 |
|  |  | 0.05 | 0.10 | 8/41-45,9/46-48 | 19/71-72,20/73-74,21/75-78 |
| 0.30 | 0.45 | 0.10 | 0.10 | 11/43,12/44-46 13/47-48,14/49-50 | 23/64,24/65-67, 25/68-69,26/70-71 |
|  |  | 0.05 | 0.20 | 10/36,11/37, 12/38-39,13/40-43 | 23/60,24/61-63, 25/64-65,26/66-67 |
|  |  | 0.05 | 0.10 | 15/50-52,16/53-55, 17/56-57 | 32/85-86,33/87-89, 34/90-91,35/92 |
| 0.40 | 0.55 | 0.10 | 0.10 | 16/43-44,17/45-46, 18/47,19/48-49,20/50 | 32/69-70,33/71, 34/72-73,35/74-75,36/76 |
|  |  | 0.05 | 0.20 | 13/34-35,14/36, 15/37-39,16/40-41 | 32/65-66,33/67-68, 34/69-70,35/71,36/72 |
|  |  | 0.05 | 0.10 | 23/60-61,24/62-63, 25/64-65,26/66-67 | 43/91,44/92-93, 45/94,46/95-96,47/97-98 |
| 0.50 | 0.65 | 0.10 | 0.10 | 19/41,20/42-43, 21/44-45,22/57-57,23/48 | 38/67,39/68-69,40/70-71, 41/72,42/73-74 |
|  |  | 0.05 | 0.20 | 16/33,17/34-35, 18/36-37,19/38-39,20/40 | 38/64-65,39/66, 40/67-68,41/69,42/70-71 |
|  |  | 0.05 | 0.10 | 26/53,27/54-55,28/56, 29/57,30/58-59,31/60 | 52/89-90,53/91-92, 54/93-94,55/95,56/96 |
| 0.60 | 0.75 | 0.10 | 0.10 | 22/38-39,23/40,24/41-42, 25/43,26/44-45 | 40/60,41/61,42/62-63, 43/64,44/65-66,45/67 |
|  |  | 0.05 | 0.20 | 18/31,19/32,20/33-34, 21/35,22/36-37,23/38 | 40/57-58,41/59, 42/60-61,43/62,44/63-64 |
|  |  | 0.05 | 0.10 | 23/39,24/40-41,25/42-43, 26/44,27/45,28/46 | 54/80,55/81,56/82, 57/83-84,58/85,59/86-87 |
| 0.70 | 0.85 | 0.10 | 0.10 | 19/28-29,20/30,21/31, 22/32,23/33-34,24/35 | 36/46-47,37/48,38/49, 39/50-51,40/52,41/53 |
|  |  | 0.05 | 0.20 | 18/25,19/26,20/27-28, 21/29,22/30,23/31,24/32 | 36/45,37/46-47,38/48, 39/49,40/50-51,41/52 |
|  |  | 0.05 | 0.10 | 26/38,27/39,28/40,29/41, 30/42-43,31/44/32/45 | 48/62,49/63,50/64,51/65, 52/66,53/67,54/68-69 |
| 0.80 | 0.95 | 0.10 | 0.10 | 9/12,10/13,11/14,12/15, 13/16,14/17,15/18,16/19 | 23/26,24/27-28,25/29, 26/30,27/31,28/32,29/33 |
|  |  | 0.05 | 0.20 | 6/8,7/9,8/10,9/11, 10/12-13,11/14,12/15 | 23/26,24/27,25/28,26/29, 27/30,28/31,29/32,30/33 |
|  |  | 0.05 | 0.10 | 22/26,23/27,24/28,25/29, 26/30,27/31,28/32,29/33 | 31/35,32/36,33/37,34/38, 35/39-40,36/41,37/42 |

Table 5.3.6: Sample Sizes and Critical Values for Minimax Flexible Two-Stage Designs ($p_1 - p_0 = 0.20$)

| $p_0$ | $p_1$ | $\alpha$ | $\beta$ | $r_i/n_i$ | $R_j/N_j$ |
|---|---|---|---|---|---|
| 0.05 | 0.25 | 0.10 | 0.10 | 0/8-15 | 1/17,2/18-24 |
|  |  | 0.05 | 0.20 | 0/6-12,1/13 | 2/14-21 |
|  |  | 0.05 | 0.10 | 0/10-16,1/17 | 2/21-22,3/23-28 |
| 0.10 | 0.30 | 0.10 | 0.10 | 0/11-13,1/14-18 | 3/22-23,4/24-26,5/27-29 |
|  |  | 0.05 | 0.20 | 0/11-14,1/15-18 | 3/19,4/20-22,5/23-26 |
|  |  | 0.05 | 0.10 | 1/17-20,2/21-23,3/24 | 5/28-30,6/31-35 |
| 0.20 | 0.40 | 0.10 | 0.10 | 3/22-23,4/24, 5/25-27,6/28-29 | 8/30-31,9/32/33, 10/34-37 |
|  |  | 0.05 | 0.20 | 2/14,3/15-18,4/19-21 | 9/28-31,10/32-34,11/35 |
|  |  | 0.05 | 0.10 | 5/27-29,11/40,12/41-42, 6/30-32,7/33-34 | 13/43-45,14/46-47 |
| 0.30 | 0.50 | 0.10 | 0.10 | 6/24-25,7/26-29, 8/30,9/31 | 13/35,14/36-37, 15/38-40,16/41-42 |
|  |  | 0.05 | 0.20 | 5/18-19,6/20-22,14/33-35, 15/36-37,7/23-24,8/25 | 16/38-39,17/40 |
|  |  | 0.05 | 0.10 | 7/27,8/28-29,19/47-49, 20/50-51,9/30-31,10/32-34 | 21/52-53,22/54 |
| 0.40 | 0.60 | 0.10 | 0.10 | 8/23-24,9/25-26, 10/27,11/28-29,12/30 | 18/37-38,19/39-40, 20/41,21/42-43,22/44 |
|  |  | 0.05 | 0.20 | 6/18,7/19-20,8/21-22, 9/23,10/24-25 | 18/35-36,19/37, 20/38-39,21/40,22/41-42 |
|  |  | 0.05 | 0.10 | 10/26-27,11/28, 12/29-31,13/32-33 | 25/50-51,26/52, 27/53-54,28/55-56,29/57 |
| 0.50 | 0.70 | 0.10 | 0.10 | 8/18,9/19-20,10/21, 11/22-23,12/24,13/25 | 21/36,22/37-38,23/39, 24/40-41,25/42-43 |
|  |  | 0.05 | 0.20 | 7/15,8/16-17,9/18-19, 10/20,11/21,12/22 | 21/34,22/35-36,23/37-38, 24/39,25/40,26/41 |
|  |  | 0.05 | 0.10 | 14/30-31,15/32,16/33-34, 17/35,18/36,19/37 | 18/47,29/48,30/49-50, 31/51,32/52-53,33/54 |
| 0.60 | 0.80 | 0.10 | 0.10 | 9/17-18,10/19,11/20, 12/21,13/22-23,14/24 | 21/30-31,22/32,23/33, 24/34-35,25/36,26/37 |
|  |  | 0.05 | 0.20 | 6/11,7/12-13,8/14, 9/15-16,10/17,11/18 | 21/29,22/30-31,23/32, 24/33,25/34-35,26/36 |
|  |  | 0.05 | 0.10 | 11/19,12/20-21, 13/22,14/23,15/24-26 | 29/41,30/42-43,31/44, 32/45,33/46-47,34/48 |
| 0.70 | 0.90 | 0.10 | 0.10 | 5/8,6/9,7/10-11,8/12, 9/13,10/14-15 | 17/22,18/23,19/24,20/25, 21/26,22/27-28,23/29 |
|  |  | 0.05 | 0.20 | 5/8,6/9,7/10,8/11, 9/12-13,10/14,11/15 | 17/21,18/22,19/23,20/24, 21/25,22/26-27,23/28 |
|  |  | 0.05 | 0.10 | 8/12,9/13,10/14,11/15, 12/16-17,13/18,14/19 | 24/30,35/31,26/32,27/33, 28/34-35,29/36,30/37 |

where
$$\beta = P(\text{reject } H_a \mid p_1),$$
computing the values of $r_2, n_2, r_3$, and $n_3$ that minimize the null expected sample size $EN(p_0)$ subject to the error constraints $\alpha$ and $\beta$, where
$$EN(p) = n_1 + n_2\{1 - \beta_1(p)\} + n_3\{1 - \beta_1(p) - \beta_2(p)\},$$
and $\beta_i$ are the probability of making type II error evaluated at stage $i$. Ensign et al. (1994) use the value of
$$\beta - (1 - p_1)^{n_1}$$
as the type II error rate in the optimization along with type I error
$$\alpha = P(\text{reject } H_0 \mid p_0)$$
to obtain $r_2, n_2, r_3$, and $n_3$. Repeating this, $n_i$ can then be chosen to minimize the overall $EN(p_0)$.

Tables 5.3.7 and 5.3.8 provide sample sizes for optimal three-stage designs based on the method proposed by Ensign et al. (1994) for a variety of design parameters. The tabulated results include the optimal size $n_i$ and the critical value $r_i$ of the $i$th stage. For example, the result in Table 5.3.7 corresponding to a design with $p_0 = 0.25$ and $p_1 = 0.40$ gives $0/6, 7/26, 24/75$ for achieving an 80% power at the 5% level of significance. In other words, at the first stage, six subjects are treated. If there is no response, then the trial is terminated. Otherwise, accrual continues to a total of 26 subjects at the second stage. If there are no more than 7 subjects respond, then stop the trial. Otherwise, proceed to the third stage by recruiting 49 additional subjects. We would conclude that the test drug is effective if there are more than 24 responses for the subjects in the three stages combined.

Note that the optimal three-stage designs proposed by Ensign et al. (1994) restrict the rejection region in the first stage to be zero response, and the sample size to at least 5. As an alternative, Chen (1997b) also extended Simon's two-stage to a three-stage design without these restrictions. As a result, sample sizes can be obtained by computing the values of $r_1, n_1, r_2, n_2, r_3$, and $n_3$ that minimize the expected sample size

$$EN = n_1 + (1 - PET_1)n_2 + (1 - PET_{all})n_3$$
$$PET_1 = B(r_1; n_1, p) = \sum_{x \leq r_1} b(x; n_1, p)$$
$$PET_{all} = PET_1 + \sum_{x=r_1+1}^{\min(n_1, r_2)} b(d; n, p) B(r_2 - x; n_2, p).$$

Table 5.3.7: Sample Sizes $n_i$ and Critical Values $r_i$ for Optimal Three-Stage Designs - Ensign et al. (1994) ($p_1 - p_0 = 0.15$)

| $p_0$ | $p_1$ | $\alpha$ | $\beta$ | Stage 1 $r_1/n_1$ | Stage 2 $r_2/(n_1+n_2)$ | Stage 3 $r_3/(n_1+n_2+n_3)$ |
|---|---|---|---|---|---|---|
| 0.05 | 0.20 | 0.10 | 0.10 | 0/12 | 1/25 | 3/38 |
|      |      | 0.05 | 0.20 | 0/10 | 2/24 | 3/31 |
|      |      | 0.05 | 0.10 | 0/14 | 2/29 | 4/43 |
| 0.10 | 0.25 | 0.10 | 0.10 | 0/11 | 3/29 | 7/50 |
|      |      | 0.05 | 0.20 | 0/9  | 3/25 | 7/43 |
|      |      | 0.05 | 0.10 | 0/13 | 3/27 | 10/66 |
| 0.15 | 0.30 | 0.10 | 0.10 | 0/12 | 4/28 | 11/55 |
|      |      | 0.05 | 0.20 | 0/9  | 5/27 | 12/56 |
|      |      | 0.05 | 0.10 | 0/13 | 6/35 | 16/77 |
| 0.20 | 0.35 | 0.10 | 0.10 | 0/11 | 7/34 | 16/63 |
|      |      | 0.05 | 0.20 | 0/6  | 6/28 | 18/67 |
|      |      | 0.05 | 0.10 | 0/9  | 10/44 | 23/88 |
| 0.25 | 0.40 | 0.10 | 0.10 | 0/8  | 8/32 | 23/76 |
|      |      | 0.05 | 0.20 | 0/6  | 7/26 | 24/75 |
|      |      | 0.05 | 0.10 | 0/9  | 11/41 | 30/95 |
| 0.30 | 0.45 | 0.10 | 0.10 | 0/7  | 13/41 | 28/79 |
|      |      | 0.05 | 0.20 | 0/7  | 9/27 | 31/84 |
|      |      | 0.05 | 0.10 | 0/9  | 14/43 | 38/104 |
| 0.35 | 0.50 | 0.10 | 0.10 | 0/9  | 12/34 | 33/81 |
|      |      | 0.05 | 0.20 | 0/5  | 12/31 | 37/88 |
|      |      | 0.05 | 0.10 | 0/8  | 17/45 | 45/108 |
| 0.40 | 0.55 | 0.10 | 0.10 | 0/11 | 16/38 | 40/88 |
|      |      | 0.05 | 0.20 | 0/5  | 14/32 | 40/84 |
|      |      | 0.05 | 0.10 | 0/10 | 19/45 | 49/104 |
| 0.45 | 0.60 | 0.10 | 0.10 | 0/6  | 15/34 | 40/78 |
|      |      | 0.05 | 0.20 | 0/5  | 12/25 | 47/90 |
|      |      | 0.05 | 0.10 | 0/6  | 20/42 | 59/114 |
| 0.50 | 0.65 | 0.10 | 0.10 | 0/5  | 16/32 | 46.84 |
|      |      | 0.05 | 0.20 | 0/5  | 12/25 | 47/90 |
|      |      | 0.05 | 0.10 | 0/6  | 20/42 | 59/114 |
| 0.55 | 0.70 | 0.10 | 0.10 | 0/7  | 19/34 | 46/75 |
|      |      | 0.05 | 0.20 | 0/5  | 15/26 | 48/76 |
|      |      | 0.05 | 0.10 | 0/5  | 23/40 | 64/96 |
| 0.60 | 0.75 | 0.10 | 0.10 | 0/5  | 21/34 | 47/71 |
|      |      | 0.05 | 0.20 | 0/5  | 13/21 | 49/72 |
|      |      | 0.05 | 0.10 | 0/5  | 14/23 | 90/98 |
| 0.65 | 0.80 | 0.10 | 0.10 | 0/5  | 17/26 | 47/66 |
|      |      | 0.05 | 0.20 | 0/5  | 12/18 | 49/67 |
|      |      | 0.05 | 0.20 | 0/5  | 8/13  | 74/78 |
| 0.70 | 0.85 | 0.10 | 0.10 | 0/5  | 14/20 | 45/59 |
|      |      | 0.05 | 0.20 | 0/5  | 14/19 | 46/59 |
|      |      | 0.05 | 0.10 | 0/5  | 12/17 | 68/72 |
| 0.75 | 0.90 | 0.10 | 0.10 | 0/5  | 16/21 | 36/44 |
|      |      | 0.05 | 0.20 | 0/5  | 10/13 | 40/48 |
|      |      | 0.05 | 0.10 | 0/5  | 8/11  | 55/57 |
| 0.80 | 0.95 | 0.10 | 0.10 | 0/5  | 5/7   | 27/31 |
|      |      | 0.05 | 0.20 | 0/5  | 7/9   | 26/29 |
|      |      | 0.05 | 0.10 | 0/5  | 8/10  | 44/45 |

Table 5.3.8: Sample Sizes $n_i$ and Critical Values $r_i$ for Optimal Three-Stage Designs - Ensign et al. (1994) ($p_1 - p_0 = 0.20$)

| | | | | Stage 1 | Stage 2 | Stage 3 |
|---|---|---|---|---|---|---|
| $p_0$ | $p_1$ | $\alpha$ | $\beta$ | $r_1/n_1$ | $r_2/(n_1+n_2)$ | $r_3/(n_1+n_2+n_3)$ |
| 0.05 | 0.25 | 0.10 | 0.10 | 0/9 | 1/19 | 2/25 |
| | | 0.05 | 0.20 | 0/7 | 1/15 | 3/26 |
| | | 0.05 | 0.10 | 0/9 | 1/22 | 3/30 |
| 0.10 | 0.30 | 0.10 | 0.10 | 0/10 | 2/19 | 4/26 |
| | | 0.05 | 0.20 | 0/6 | 2/17 | 5/29 |
| | | 0.05 | 0.10 | 0/9 | 3/22 | 7/45 |
| 0.15 | 0.35 | 0.10 | 0.10 | 0/9 | 2/16 | 7/33 |
| | | 0.05 | 0.20 | 0/5 | 3/17 | 9/41 |
| | | 0.05 | 0.10 | 0/9 | 4/23 | 10/44 |
| 0.20 | 0.40 | 0.10 | 0.10 | 0/8 | 3/16 | 11/42 |
| | | 0.05 | 0.20 | 0/5 | 4/17 | 12/43 |
| | | 0.05 | 0.10 | 0/9 | 4/23 | 15/54 |
| 0.25 | 0.45 | 0.10 | 0.10 | 0/6 | 6/23 | 14/44 |
| | | 0.05 | 0.20 | 0/5 | 5/17 | 16/48 |
| | | 0.05 | 0.10 | 0/7 | 6/22 | 20/61 |
| 0.30 | 0.50 | 0.10 | 0.10 | 0/6 | 6/20 | 17/46 |
| | | 0.05 | 0.20 | 0/5 | 5/15 | 19/49 |
| | | 0.05 | 0.10 | 0/8 | 8/24 | 24/63 |
| 0.35 | 0.55 | 0.10 | 0.10 | 0/6 | 7/20 | 20/47 |
| | | 0.05 | 0.20 | 0/6 | 8/20 | 19/42 |
| | | 0.05 | 0.10 | 0/5 | 10/26 | 29/67 |
| 0.40 | 0.60 | 0.10 | 0.10 | 0/5 | 8/20 | 22/46 |
| | | 0.05 | 0.20 | 0/5 | 7/16 | 24/48 |
| | | 0.05 | 0.10 | 0/5 | 9/22 | 30/61 |
| 0.45 | 0.65 | 0.10 | 0.10 | 0/5 | 10/21 | 26/50 |
| | | 0.05 | 0.20 | 0/5 | 7/15 | 24/43 |
| | | 0.05 | 0.10 | 0/5 | 15/30 | 32/59 |
| 0.50 | 0.70 | 0.10 | 0.10 | 0/5 | 11/21 | 26/45 |
| | | 0.05 | 0.20 | 0/5 | 8/15 | 26/43 |
| | | 0.05 | 0.10 | 0/5 | 12/23 | 34/57 |
| 0.55 | 0.75 | 0.10 | 0.10 | 0/5 | 10/18 | 26/41 |
| | | 0.05 | 0.20 | 0/5 | 9/15 | 28/43 |
| | | 0.05 | 0.10 | 0/5 | 10/18 | 35/54 |
| 0.60 | 0.80 | 0.10 | 0.10 | 0/5 | 6/11 | 26/38 |
| | | 0.05 | 0.20 | 0/5 | 7/11 | 30/43 |
| | | 0.05 | 0.10 | 0/5 | 12/19 | 37/53 |
| 0.65 | 0.85 | 0.10 | 0.10 | 0/5 | 10/15 | 25/34 |
| | | 0.05 | 0.20 | 0/5 | 10/14 | 25/33 |
| | | 0.05 | 0.20 | 0/5 | 10/15 | 33/44 |
| 0.70 | 0.90 | 0.10 | 0.10 | 0/5 | 6/9 | 22/28 |
| | | 0.05 | 0.20 | 0/5 | 4/6 | 22/27 |
| | | 0.05 | 0.10 | 0/5 | 11/15 | 29/36 |
| 0.75 | 0.95 | 0.10 | 0.10 | 0/5 | 6/8 | 16/19 |
| | | 0.05 | 0.20 | 0/5 | 9/11 | 19/22 |
| | | 0.05 | 0.10 | 0/5 | 7/9 | 24/28 |

5.3. Optimal Multiple-Stage Designs for Single Arm Trials 137

Table 5.3.9: Sample Sizes $n_i$ and Critical Values $r_i$ for Optimal Three-Stage Designs - Chen (1997b) ($p_1 - p_0 = 0.15$)

| $p_0$ | $p_1$ | $\alpha$ | $\beta$ | Stage 1 $r_1/n_1$ | Stage 2 $r_2/(n_1+n_2)$ | Stage 3 $r_3/(n_1+n_2+n_3)$ |
|---|---|---|---|---|---|---|
| 0.05 | 0.20 | 0.10 | 0.10 | 0/13 | 1/22 | 3/37 |
|  |  | 0.05 | 0.20 | 0/10 | 1/19 | 3/30 |
|  |  | 0.05 | 0.10 | 0/14 | 2/29 | 4/43 |
| 0.10 | 0.25 | 0.10 | 0.10 | 1/17 | 3/29 | 7/50 |
|  |  | 0.05 | 0.20 | 1/13 | 3/24 | 8/53 |
|  |  | 0.05 | 0.10 | 1/17 | 4/34 | 10/66 |
| 0.15 | 0.30 | 0.10 | 0.10 | 2/20 | 5/33 | 11/55 |
|  |  | 0.05 | 0.20 | 2/15 | 6/33 | 13/62 |
|  |  | 0.05 | 0.10 | 3/23 | 8/46 | 16/77 |
| 0.20 | 0.35 | 0.10 | 0.10 | 3/21 | 8/37 | 17/68 |
|  |  | 0.05 | 0.20 | 3/17 | 9/37 | 18/68 |
|  |  | 0.05 | 0.10 | 5/27 | 11/49 | 23/88 |
| 0.25 | 0.40 | 0.10 | 0.10 | 4/20 | 10/39 | 24/80 |
|  |  | 0.05 | 0.20 | 4/17 | 12/42 | 25/79 |
|  |  | 0.05 | 0.10 | 6/26 | 15/54 | 32/103 |
| 0.30 | 0.45 | 0.10 | 0.10 | 6/24 | 14/44 | 28/79 |
|  |  | 0.05 | 0.20 | 5/18 | 14/41 | 31/84 |
|  |  | 0.05 | 0.10 | 8/29 | 19/57 | 38/104 |
| 0.35 | 0.50 | 0.10 | 0.10 | 7/23 | 18/49 | 34/84 |
|  |  | 0.05 | 0.20 | 6/19 | 17/43 | 34/80 |
|  |  | 0.05 | 0.10 | 9/28 | 23/60 | 45/108 |
| 0.40 | 0.55 | 0.10 | 0.10 | 7/21 | 19/46 | 38/83 |
|  |  | 0.05 | 0.20 | 7/19 | 19/43 | 39/82 |
|  |  | 0.05 | 0.10 | 12/31 | 28/64 | 54/116 |
| 0.45 | 0.60 | 0.10 | 0.10 | 12/28 | 27/56 | 43/85 |
|  |  | 0.05 | 0.20 | 8/19 | 21/42 | 45/86 |
|  |  | 0.05 | 0.10 | 13/30 | 29/60 | 58/112 |
| 0.50 | 0.65 | 0.10 | 0.10 | 10/22 | 25/48 | 48/86 |
|  |  | 0.05 | 0.20 | 8/17 | 21/39 | 49/85 |
|  |  | 0.05 | 0.10 | 14/29 | 34/63 | 62/109 |
| 0.55 | 0.70 | 0.10 | 0.10 | 13/25 | 25/44 | 47/77 |
|  |  | 0.05 | 0.20 | 7/14 | 23/39 | 49/78 |
|  |  | 0.05 | 0.10 | 15/28 | 36/61 | 65/105 |
| 0.60 | 0.75 | 0.10 | 0.10 | 11/20 | 26/42 | 57/71 |
|  |  | 0.05 | 0.20 | 8/14 | 23/36 | 52/77 |
|  |  | 0.05 | 0.10 | 14/24 | 36/56 | 70/105 |
| 0.65 | 0.80 | 0.10 | 0.10 | 11/18 | 27/40 | 49/69 |
|  |  | 0.05 | 0.20 | 8/13 | 27/38 | 52/72 |
|  |  | 0.05 | 0.20 | 16/25 | 35/50 | 66/92 |
| 0.70 | 0.85 | 0.10 | 0.10 | 14/20 | 18/37 | 45/59 |
|  |  | 0.05 | 0.20 | 4/7 | 11/16 | 44/56 |
|  |  | 0.05 | 0.10 | 12/18 | 28/38 | 58/75 |
| 0.75 | 0.90 | 0.10 | 0.10 | 10/14 | 23/29 | 38/47 |
|  |  | 0.05 | 0.20 | 9/12 | 21/26 | 39/47 |
|  |  | 0.05 | 0.10 | 10/14 | 23/29 | 55/67 |
| 0.80 | 0.95 | 0.10 | 0.10 | 5/7 | 16/19 | 30/35 |
|  |  | 0.05 | 0.20 | 2/3 | 16/19 | 35/40 |
|  |  | 0.05 | 0.10 | 6/8 | 24/28 | 41/47 |

Table 5.3.10: Sample Sizes $n_i$ and Critical Values $r_i$ for Optimal Three-Stage Designs - Chen (1997b) ($p_1 - p_0 = 0.20$)

| $p_0$ | $p_1$ | $\alpha$ | $\beta$ | Stage 1 $r_1/n_1$ | Stage 2 $r_2/(n_1+n_2)$ | Stage 3 $r_3/(n_1+n_2+n_3)$ |
|---|---|---|---|---|---|---|
| 0.05 | 0.25 | 0.10 | 0.10 | 0/9 | 1/18 | 2/26 |
|  |  | 0.05 | 0.20 | 0/8 | 1/13 | 2/19 |
|  |  | 0.05 | 0.10 | 0/10 | 1/17 | 3/30 |
| 0.10 | 0.30 | 0.10 | 0.10 | 0/10 | 2/19 | 4/26 |
|  |  | 0.05 | 0.20 | 0/6 | 2/17 | 5/29 |
|  |  | 0.05 | 0.10 | 1/13 | 3/23 | 7/45 |
| 0.15 | 0.35 | 0.10 | 0.10 | 1/12 | 3/21 | 7/33 |
|  |  | 0.05 | 0.20 | 1/9 | 4/21 | 8/35 |
|  |  | 0.05 | 0.10 | 2/15 | 5/27 | 11/51 |
| 0.20 | 0.40 | 0.10 | 0.10 | 1/10 | 6/26 | 11/43 |
|  |  | 0.05 | 0.20 | 1/8 | 5/22 | 11/38 |
|  |  | 0.05 | 0.10 | 3/17 | 7/30 | 14/50 |
| 0.25 | 0.45 | 0.10 | 0.10 | 3/16 | 7/25 | 13/41 |
|  |  | 0.05 | 0.20 | 2/10 | 6/20 | 16/48 |
|  |  | 0.05 | 0.10 | 4/18 | 10/33 | 19/58 |
| 0.30 | 0.50 | 0.10 | 0.10 | 3/13 | 9/28 | 17/46 |
|  |  | 0.05 | 0.20 | 3/11 | 7/21 | 18/46 |
|  |  | 0.05 | 0.10 | 4/16 | 11/32 | 23/60 |
| 0.35 | 0.55 | 0.10 | 0.10 | 6/18 | 13/33 | 20/48 |
|  |  | 0.05 | 0.20 | 3/10 | 9/23 | 21/47 |
|  |  | 0.05 | 0.10 | 6/18 | 15/38 | 27/62 |
| 0.40 | 0.60 | 0.10 | 0.10 | 7/18 | 9/26 | 22/46 |
|  |  | 0.05 | 0.20 | 3/9 | 10/23 | 23/46 |
|  |  | 0.05 | 0.10 | 6/16 | 17/38 | 32/66 |
| 0.45 | 0.65 | 0.10 | 0.10 | 5/13 | 13/27 | 26/50 |
|  |  | 0.05 | 0.20 | 3/8 | 10/20 | 29/54 |
|  |  | 0.05 | 0.10 | 6/15 | 17/34 | 34/63 |
| 0.50 | 0.70 | 0.10 | 0.10 | 4/10 | 12/24 | 26/45 |
|  |  | 0.05 | 0.20 | 4/9 | 13/23 | 29/49 |
|  |  | 0.05 | 0.10 | 7/15 | 19/34 | 38/65 |
| 0.55 | 0.75 | 0.10 | 0.10 | 5/11 | 12/21 | 27/43 |
|  |  | 0.05 | 0.20 | 6/11 | 14/23 | 28/43 |
|  |  | 0.05 | 0.10 | 7/14 | 16/27 | 36/56 |
| 0.60 | 0.80 | 0.10 | 0.10 | 6/11 | 14/22 | 29/43 |
|  |  | 0.05 | 0.20 | 5/9 | 12/48 | 28/40 |
|  |  | 0.05 | 0.10 | 6/11 | 19/29 | 38/55 |
| 0.65 | 0.85 | 0.10 | 0.10 | 5/9 | 13/19 | 25/34 |
|  |  | 0.05 | 0.20 | 5/8 | 13/18 | 27/36 |
|  |  | 0.05 | 0.20 | 6/10 | 16/23 | 35/47 |
| 0.70 | 0.90 | 0.10 | 0.10 | 5/8 | 11/15 | 22/28 |
|  |  | 0.05 | 0.20 | 3/5 | 10/13 | 25/31 |
|  |  | 0.05 | 0.10 | 6/9 | 16/21 | 31/39 |
| 0.75 | 0.95 | 0.10 | 0.10 | 3/5 | 6/8 | 16/19 |
|  |  | 0.05 | 0.20 | 1/2 | 9/11 | 19/22 |
|  |  | 0.05 | 0.10 | 6/8 | 13/16 | 24/28 |

## 5.3. Optimal Multiple-Stage Designs for Single Arm Trials

Table 5.3.11: Sample Sizes $n_i$ and Critical Values $r_i$ for Minimax Three-Stage Designs - Chen (1997b) ($p_1 - p_0 = 0.15$)

| $p_0$ | $p_1$ | $\alpha$ | $\beta$ | Stage 1 $r_1/n_1$ | Stage 2 $r_2/(n_1+n_2)$ | Stage 3 $r_3/(n_1+n_2+n_3)$ |
|---|---|---|---|---|---|---|
| 0.05 | 0.20 | 0.10 | 0.10 | 0/18 | 1/26 | 3/32 |
|  |  | 0.05 | 0.20 | 0/14 | 1/20 | 3/27 |
|  |  | 0.05 | 0.10 | 0/23 | 1/30 | 4/38 |
| 0.10 | 0.25 | 0.10 | 0.10 | 1/23 | 3/33 | 6/40 |
|  |  | 0.05 | 0.20 | 1/17 | 3/30 | 7/40 |
|  |  | 0.05 | 0.10 | 1/21 | 4/39 | 9/55 |
| 0.15 | 0.30 | 0.10 | 0.10 | 2/23 | 5/36 | 11/53 |
|  |  | 0.05 | 0.20 | 2/19 | 6/36 | 11/48 |
|  |  | 0.05 | 0.10 | 4/35 | 8/51 | 14/64 |
| 0.20 | 0.35 | 0.10 | 0.10 | 5/30 | 9/45 | 15/58 |
|  |  | 0.05 | 0.20 | 3/22 | 7/35 | 15/53 |
|  |  | 0.05 | 0.10 | 16/65 | 19/72 | 20/74 |
| 0.25 | 0.40 | 0.10 | 0.10 | 6/31 | 11/46 | 20/64 |
|  |  | 0.05 | 0.20 | 7/30 | 12/42 | 20/60 |
|  |  | 0.05 | 0.10 | 9/47 | 17/67 | 27/83 |
| 0.30 | 0.45 | 0.10 | 0.10 | 7/29 | 16/51 | 25/69 |
|  |  | 0.05 | 0.20 | 8/29 | 14/42 | 25/65 |
|  |  | 0.05 | 0.10 | 12/46 | 25/73 | 33/88 |
| 0.35 | 0.50 | 0.10 | 0.10 | 12/39 | 20/57 | 30/72 |
|  |  | 0.05 | 0.20 | 10/33 | 18/48 | 29/66 |
|  |  | 0.05 | 0.10 | 11/36 | 22/60 | 40/94 |
| 0.40 | 0.55 | 0.10 | 0.10 | 10/30 | 19/48 | 34/73 |
|  |  | 0.05 | 0.20 | 13/33 | 30/63 | 34/70 |
|  |  | 0.05 | 0.10 | 20/55 | 32/77 | 45/94 |
| 0.45 | 0.60 | 0.10 | 0.10 | 18/41 | 35/69 | 38/74 |
|  |  | 0.05 | 0.20 | 13/32 | 25/53 | 38/70 |
|  |  | 0.05 | 0.10 | 26/58 | 47/90 | 50/95 |
| 0.50 | 0.65 | 0.10 | 0.10 | 19/40 | 24/64 | 41/72 |
|  |  | 0.05 | 0.20 | 18/36 | 36/62 | 40/68 |
|  |  | 0.05 | 0.10 | 19/43 | 34/67 | 54/93 |
| 0.55 | 0.70 | 0.10 | 0.10 | 23/43 | 36/60 | 42/68 |
|  |  | 0.05 | 0.20 | 18/33 | 41/64 | 42/66 |
|  |  | 0.05 | 0.10 | 23/43 | 42/84 | 45/89 |
| 0.60 | 0.75 | 0.10 | 0.10 | 19/35 | 30/50 | 43/64 |
|  |  | 0.05 | 0.20 | 19/32 | 40/58 | 42/61 |
|  |  | 0.05 | 0.10 | 18/46 | 50/75 | 57/84 |
| 0.65 | 0.80 | 0.10 | 0.10 | 22/33 | 26/41 | 43/60 |
|  |  | 0.05 | 0.20 | 16/26 | 27/40 | 41/55 |
|  |  | 0.05 | 0.20 | 25/41 | 37/56 | 55/75 |
| 0.70 | 0.85 | 0.10 | 0.10 | 15/22 | 18/37 | 40/52 |
|  |  | 0.05 | 0.20 | 11/17 | 16/24 | 39/49 |
|  |  | 0.05 | 0.10 | 13/20 | 31/42 | 43/68 |
| 0.75 | 0.90 | 0.10 | 0.10 | 11/17 | 22/29 | 33/40 |
|  |  | 0.05 | 0.20 | 8/12 | 16/21 | 33/39 |
|  |  | 0.05 | 0.10 | 12/17 | 23/30 | 45/54 |
| 0.80 | 0.95 | 0.10 | 0.10 | 1/3 | 17/20 | 26/30 |
|  |  | 0.05 | 0.20 | 7/9 | 16/19 | 26/29 |
|  |  | 0.05 | 0.10 | 16/20 | 31/35 | 35/40 |

Table 5.3.12: Sample Sizes $n_i$ and Critical Values $r_i$ for Minimax Three-Stage Designs - Chen (1997b) ($p_1 - p_0 = 0.20$)

|       |       |          |         | Stage 1     | Stage 2           | Stage 3                 |
|-------|-------|----------|---------|-------------|-------------------|-------------------------|
| $p_0$ | $p_1$ | $\alpha$ | $\beta$ | $r_1/n_1$   | $r_2/(n_1+n_2)$   | $r_3/(n_1+n_2+n_3)$     |
| 0.05  | 0.25  | 0.10     | 0.10    | 0/13        | 1/18              | 2/20                    |
|       |       | 0.05     | 0.20    | 0/12        | 1/15              | 2/16                    |
|       |       | 0.05     | 0.10    | 0/15        | 1/21              | 3/25                    |
| 0.10  | 0.30  | 0.10     | 0.10    | 0/12        | 1/16              | 4/25                    |
|       |       | 0.05     | 0.20    | 0/11        | 2/19              | 5/25                    |
|       |       | 0.05     | 0.10    | 0/14        | 2/22              | 6/33                    |
| 0.15  | 0.35  | 0.10     | 0.10    | 1/13        | 3/22              | 7/32                    |
|       |       | 0.05     | 0.20    | 1/12        | 3/19              | 7/28                    |
|       |       | 0.05     | 0.10    | 1/16        | 4/28              | 9/38                    |
| 0.20  | 0.40  | 0.10     | 0.10    | 2/16        | 5/26              | 10/36                   |
|       |       | 0.05     | 0.20    | 2/13        | 5/22              | 10/33                   |
|       |       | 0.05     | 0.10    | 2/16        | 6/28              | 13/45                   |
| 0.25  | 0.45  | 0.10     | 0.10    | 3/18        | 8/31              | 13/39                   |
|       |       | 0.05     | 0.20    | 3/15        | 6/23              | 13/36                   |
|       |       | 0.05     | 0.10    | 4/21        | 9/35              | 17/45                   |
| 0.30  | 0.50  | 0.10     | 0.10    | 6/26        | 11/35             | 15/39                   |
|       |       | 0.05     | 0.20    | 3/13        | 8/24              | 16/39                   |
|       |       | 0.05     | 0.10    | 5/20        | 12/36             | 21/53                   |
| 0.35  | 0.55  | 0.10     | 0.10    | 2/11        | 10/27             | 18/42                   |
|       |       | 0.05     | 0.20    | 4/14        | 9/24              | 18/39                   |
|       |       | 0.05     | 0.10    | 10/34       | 17/45             | 24/53                   |
| 0.40  | 0.60  | 0.10     | 0.10    | 5/17        | 9/26              | 20/41                   |
|       |       | 0.05     | 0.20    | 4/12        | 11/25             | 21/41                   |
|       |       | 0.05     | 0.10    | 7/20        | 17/39             | 27/54                   |
| 0.45  | 0.65  | 0.10     | 0.10    | 6/16        | 13/29             | 22/41                   |
|       |       | 0.05     | 0.20    | 6/15        | 12/24             | 22/39                   |
|       |       | 0.05     | 0.10    | 15/32       | 28/51             | 29/53                   |
| 0.50  | 0.70  | 0.10     | 0.10    | 7/17        | 14/28             | 23/39                   |
|       |       | 0.05     | 0.20    | 7/16        | 13/25             | 23/37                   |
|       |       | 0.05     | 0.10    | 8/18        | 18/34             | 32/53                   |
| 0.55  | 0.75  | 0.10     | 0.10    | 13/23       | 22/35             | 24/38                   |
|       |       | 0.05     | 0.20    | 8/15        | 14/23             | 24/36                   |
|       |       | 0.05     | 0.10    | 12/22       | 21/35             | 32/49                   |
| 0.60  | 0.80  | 0.10     | 0.10    | 8/15        | 14/22             | 24/35                   |
|       |       | 0.05     | 0.20    | 9/15        | 23/32             | 24/34                   |
|       |       | 0.05     | 0.10    | 15/26       | 24/37             | 32/45                   |
| 0.65  | 0.85  | 0.10     | 0.10    | 4/8         | 11/17             | 23/31                   |
|       |       | 0.05     | 0.20    | 6/10        | 13/18             | 23/30                   |
|       |       | 0.05     | 0.20    | 16/24       | 28/37             | 30/40                   |
| 0.70  | 0.90  | 0.10     | 0.10    | 5/9         | 13/18             | 20/25                   |
|       |       | 0.05     | 0.20    | 4/7         | 19/23             | 20/25                   |
|       |       | 0.05     | 0.10    | 5/9         | 12/17             | 26/32                   |
| 0.75  | 0.95  | 0.10     | 0.10    | 3/5         | 6/8               | 16/19                   |
|       |       | 0.05     | 0.20    | 6/8         | 14/16             | 17/20                   |
|       |       | 0.05     | 0.10    | 9/12        | 19/22             | 22/26                   |

## 5.4. Flexible Designs for Multiple-Arm Trials

Tables 5.3.9-5.3.10 and 5.3.11-5.3.12 provide sample sizes for optimal three-stage designs and minimax designs based on the method proposed by Chen (1997b) for a variety of design parameters. For example, the result in Table 5.3.9 corresponding to a design with $p_0 = 0.25$ and $p_1 = 0.40$ gives $4/17, 12/42, 25/79$ for achieving an 80% power at the 5% level of significance. In other words, at the first stage, seventeen subjects are treated. If no more than four responses are obtained, then the trial is terminated. Otherwise, accrual continues to a total of 42 subjects at the second stage. If there are no more than 12 subjects respond, then stop the trial. Otherwise, proceed to the third stage by recruiting 37 additional subjects. We would conclude that the test drug is effective if there are more than 25 responses for the subjects in the three stages combined.

## 5.4 Flexible Designs for Multiple-Arm Trials

In the previous section, we introduced procedures for sample size calculation under (flexible) optimal multiple-stage designs for single arm phase II cancer trials. Sargent and Goldberg (2001) proposed a flexible optimal design considering a phase II trial that allows clinical scientists to select the treatment to proceed for further testing for a phase III trial based on other factors when the difference in the observed responses rates between two treatments falls into the interval $[-\delta, \delta]$, where $\delta$ is a pre-specified quantity. The proposed rule is that if the observed difference in the response rates of the treatments is larger than $\delta$, then the treatment with the highest observed response rate is selected. On the other hand, if the observed difference is less than or equal to $\delta$, other factors may be considered in the selection. In this framework, it is not essential that the very best treatment is definitely selected, rather it is important that a substantially inferior treatment is not selected when a superior treatment exists.

To illustrate the concept proposed by Sargent and Golberg (2001), for simplicity, consider a two-arm trial. Let $p_1$ and $p_2$ denote the true response rates for the poor treatment and the better treatment, respectively. Without loss of generality, assume that $p_2 > p_1$.

Let $\hat{p}_1$ and $\hat{p}_2$ denote the corresponding observed response rates for treatment 1 and treatment 2, respectively. Sargent and Glodberg (2001) considered the probability of correctly choosing the better treatment, i.e.,

$$P_{Corr} = P\{\hat{p}_1 > \hat{p}_1 + \delta | p_1, p_2\}$$

and the probability of the difference between the two observed response rates falling into the ambiguous range of $[-\delta, \delta]$, i.e.,

$$P_{Amb} = P\{-\delta \leq \hat{p}_2 - \hat{p}_1 \leq \delta | p_1, p_2\}.$$

Assuming that each treatment arm has the same number of subjects (i.e., $n_1 = n_2 = n$). The above two probabilities are given by

$$P_{Corr} = \sum_{x=0}^{n}\sum_{y=0}^{n} I_{\{(x-y)/n > \delta\}} \binom{n}{x}\binom{n}{y} p_2^x(1-p_2)^{n-x} p_1^y(1-p_1)^{n-y}$$

and

$$P_{Arm} = \sum_{x=0}^{n}\sum_{y=0}^{n} I_{\{-\delta \leq (x-y)/n \leq \delta\}} \binom{n}{x}\binom{n}{y} p_2^x(1-p_2)^{n-x} p_1^y(1-p_1)^{n-y},$$

where $I_A$ is the indicator function of event $A$, i.e., $I_A = 1$ if event $A$ occurs and $I_A = 0$ otherwise. Sargent and Goldberg (2001) suggested that $n$ be selected such that $P_{corr} + \rho P_{Amb} > \gamma$, a pre-specified threshold. Table 5.4.1 provides results for $\rho = 0$ and $\rho = 0.5$ for different sample sizes for $p_2 = 0.35$ and $\delta = 0.05$.

Liu (2001) indicated that by the central limit theorem, we have

$$P_{Corr} \approx 1 - \Phi\left(\frac{\delta - \epsilon}{\sigma}\right)$$

and

$$P_{Amb} \approx \Phi\left(\frac{\delta - \epsilon}{\sigma}\right) - \Phi\left(\frac{-\delta - \epsilon}{\sigma}\right),$$

where $\Phi$ is the standard normal cumulative distribution function, $\epsilon = p_2 - p_1$ and

$$\sigma^2 = \frac{p_1(1-p_1) + p_2(1-p_2)}{n}.$$

As indicated in Chapter 4, the power of the test for the following hypotheses

$$H_0: p_1 = p_2 \quad \text{versus} \quad H_a: p_1 \neq p_2$$

Table 5.4.1: Probability of Various Outcomes for Different Sample Sizes ($\delta = 0.05$)

| $n$ | $p_1$ | $p_2$ | $P_{Corr}$ | $P_{Amb}$ | $P_{Corr} + 0.5 P_{Amb}$ |
|---|---|---|---|---|---|
| 50 | 0.25 | 0.35 | 0.71 | 0.24 | 0.83 |
| 50 | 0.20 | 0.35 | 0.87 | 0.12 | 0.93 |
| 75 | 0.25 | 0.35 | 0.76 | 0.21 | 0.87 |
| 75 | 0.20 | 0.35 | 0.92 | 0.07 | 0.96 |
| 100 | 0.25 | 0.35 | 0.76 | 0.23 | 0.87 |
| 100 | 0.20 | 0.35 | 0.94 | 0.06 | 0.97 |

## 5.4. Flexible Designs for Multiple-Arm Trials

Table 5.4.2: Sample Sizes Per Arm for Various $\lambda$ Assuming $\delta = 0.05$ and $\rho = 0$ or $\rho = 0.5$

| $p_1$ | $p_2$ | $\rho = 0$ | | $\rho = 0.5$ |
|---|---|---|---|---|
| | | $\lambda = 0.90$ | $\lambda = 0.80$ | $\lambda = 0.90$ |
| 0.05 | 0.20 | 32 | 13 | 16 |
| 0.10 | 0.25 | 38 | 15 | 27 |
| 0.15 | 0.30 | 0.53 | 17 | 31 |
| 0.20 | 0.35 | 57 | 19 | 34 |
| 0.25 | 0.40 | 71 | 31 | 36 |
| 0.30 | 0.45 | 73 | 32 | 38 |
| 0.35 | 0.50 | 75 | 32 | 46 |
| 0.40 | 0.55 | 76 | 33 | 47 |

is given by

$$1 - \beta = 1 - \Phi\left(z_{\alpha/2} - \frac{\epsilon}{\delta}\right) + \Phi\left(-z_{\alpha/2} - \frac{\epsilon}{\delta}\right).$$

Let $\lambda = P_{Corr} + P_{Amb}$. Then

$$\lambda = 1 - \Phi\left(z_{\alpha/2} - \frac{\epsilon}{\delta}\right) + \rho\beta.$$

As a result, sample size per arm required for a given $\lambda$ can be obtained. Table 5.4.2 gives sample sizes per arm for $\delta = 0.05$ and $\lambda = 0.80$ or $0.90$ assuming $\rho = 0$ or $\rho = 0.5$ based on exact binomial probabilities.

Note that the method proposed by Sargent and Goldberg (2001) can be extended to the case where there are three or more treatments. The selection of the best treatment, however, may be based on pairwise comparison or a global test. Table 5.4.3 provides sample sizes per arm with three or four arms assuming $\delta = 0.05$ and $\lambda = 0.80$ or $0.90$.

## 5.5 Remarks

Chen and Ng (1998) indicated that the optimal two-stage design described above is similar to the Pocock sequence design for randomized controlled clinical trials where the probability of early termination is high, the total possible sample size is larger, and the expected size under the alternative hypothesis is smaller (see also Pocock, 1977). The minimax design, on the other hand, is similar to the O'Brien-Fleming design where the probability

Table 5.4.3: Sample Size Per Arm for Trials with Three or Four Arms for $\epsilon = 0.15$, $\delta = 0.05$, and $\lambda = 0.80$ or $0.90$

|  | $n(\rho = 0)$ | | $n(\rho = 0.5)$ | |
| --- | --- | --- | --- | --- |
| $\epsilon$ | $r = 3$ | $r = 4$ | $r = 3$ | $r = 4$ |
| $\lambda = 0.80$ | | | | |
| 0.2 | 18 | 31 | 13 | 16 |
| 0.3 | 38 | 54 | 26 | 32 |
| 0.4 | 54 | 73 | 31 | 39 |
| 0.5 | 58 | 78 | 34 | 50 |
| $\lambda = 0.90$ | | | | |
| 0.2 | 39 | 53 | 30 | 34 |
| 0.3 | 77 | 95 | 51 | 59 |
| 0.4 | 98 | 119 | 68 | 78 |
| 0.5 | 115 | 147 | 73 | 93 |

of early termination is low, the total possible size is smaller, but the expected size under the alternative hypothesis is larger (O'Brien and Fleming, 1979). The minimum design is useful when the patient source is limited, such as a rare cancer or a single-site study.

Recently, multiple-stage designs have been proposed to monitor response and toxicity variables simultaneously. See, for example, Bryant and Day (1995), Conaway and Petroni (1996), Thall, Simon, and Estey (1995, 1996). In these designs, the multivariate outcomes are modeled and family-wise errors are controlled. It is suggested that this form of design should be frequently used in cancer clinical trials since delayed toxicity could be a problem in phase II trials. Chen (1997b) also pointed out that one can use optimal three-stage design for toxicity monitoring (not simultaneous with the response). The role of *response* with that of *no toxicity* can be exchanged and the designs are similarly optimal and minimax.

In practice, the actual size at each stage of the multiple-stage design may deviate slightly from the exact design. Green and Dahlberg (1992) reviewed various phase II designs and modified each design to have variable sample sizes at each stage. They compared various flexible designs and concluded that flexible designs work well across a variety of $p'_0s$, $p'_1s$, and powers.

# Chapter 6

# Tests for Goodness-of-Fit and Contingency Tables

In clinical research, the range of a categorical response variable often contains more than two values. Also, the dimension of a categorical variable can often be multivariate. The focus of this chapter is on categorical variables that are non-binary and on the association among the components of a multivariate categorical variable. A contingency table is usually employed to summarize results from multivariate categorical responses. In practice, hypotheses testing for goodness-of-fit, independence (or association), and categorical shift are usually conducted for evaluation of clinical efficacy and safety of a test compound under investigation. For example, a sponsor may be interested in determining whether the test treatment has any influence on the performance of some primary study endpoints, e.g., the presence/absence of a certain event such as disease progression, adverse event, or response (complete/partial) of a cancer tumor. It is then of interest to test the null hypothesis of independence or no association between the test treatment (e.g., before and after treatment) and the change in the study endpoint. In this chapter, formulas for sample size calculation for testing goodness-of-fit and independence (or association) under an $r \times c$ contingency table is derived based on various chi-square type test statistics such as Pearson's chi-square and likelihood ratio test statistics. In addition, procedures for sample size calculation for testing categorical shift using McNemar's test and/or Stuart-Maxwell test is also derived.

In the next section, a sample size calculation formula for goodness-of-fit based on Pearson's test is derived. Sample size calculation formulas for testing independence (or association) with single stratum and multiple strata are introduced based on various chi-square test statistics, respectively, in Sections 6.2 and 6.3. Test statistics and the corresponding sample size calculation for categorical shift is discussed in Sections 6.4. Section 6.5 considers testing for carry-over effect in a 2 × 2 crossover design. Some practical issues are presented in Section 6.6.

## 6.1 Tests for Goodness-of-Fit

In practice, it is often of interest to study the distribution of the primary study endpoint under the study drug with some reference distribution, which may be obtained from historical (control) data or literature review. If the primary study endpoint is a categorical response that is non-binary, Pearson's chi-square test is usually applied.

### 6.1.1 Pearson's Test

For the $i$th subject, let $X_i$ be the response taking values from $\{x_1, ..., x_r\}$, $i = 1, ..., n$. Assume that $X_i$'s are i.i.d. Let

$$p_k = P(X_i = x_k),$$

where $k = 1, ..., r$. $p_k$ can be estimated by $\hat{p}_k = n_k/n$, where $n_k$ is the frequency count of the subjects with response value $k$. For testing goodness-of-fit, the following hypotheses are usually considered:

$$H_0 : p_k = p_{k,0} \text{ for all } k \quad \text{vs.} \quad p_k \neq p_{k,0} \text{ for some } k,$$

where $p_{k,0}$ is a reference value (e.g., historical control), $k = 1, ..., r$. Pearson's chi-square statistic for testing goodness-of-fit is given by

$$T_G = \sum_{k=1}^{r} \frac{n(\hat{p}_k - p_{k,0})^2}{p_{k,0}}.$$

Under the null hypothesis $H_0$, $T_G$ is asymptotically distributed as a central chi-square random variable with $r - 1$ degrees of freedom. Hence, we reject the null hypothesis with approximate $\alpha$ level of significance if

$$T_G > \chi^2_{\alpha, r-1},$$

where $\chi^2_{\alpha, r-1}$ denotes the $\alpha$th upper quantile of a central chi-square random variable with $r - 1$ degrees of freedom. The power of Pearson's chi-square test can be evaluated under some local alternatives. (A local alternative typically means that the difference between treatment effects in terms of

## 6.1. Tests for Goodness-of-Fit

the parameters of interest decreases to 0 at the rate of $1/\sqrt{n}$ when the sample size $n$ increases to infinity.) More specifically, if

$$\lim_{n\to\infty} \sum_{k=1}^{r} \frac{n(p_k - p_{k,0})^2}{p_{k,0}} = \delta,$$

then $T_G$ is asymptotically distributed as a non-central chi-square random variable with $r - 1$ degrees of freedom and the non-centrality parameter $\delta$. For a given degrees of freedom $r - 1$ and a desired power $1 - \beta$, $\delta$ can be obtained by solving for

$$\chi^2_{r-1}(\chi^2_{\alpha,r-1}|\delta) = \beta, \tag{6.1.1}$$

where $\chi^2_{r-1}(\cdot|\delta)$ denotes the non-central chi-square distribution with $r - 1$ degrees of freedom and the non-centrality parameter $\delta$. Note that $\chi^2_{r-1}(t|\delta)$ is descreasing in $\delta$ for any fixed $t$. Hence, (6.1.1) has a unique solution. Let $\delta_{\alpha,\beta}$ be the solution of (6.1.1) for given $\alpha$ and $\beta$. The sample size needed in order to achieve the desired power of $1 - \beta$ is then given by

$$n = \delta_{\alpha,\beta} \left[ \sum_{k=1}^{r} \frac{(p_k - p_{k,0})^2}{p_{k,0}} \right]^{-1},$$

where $p_k$ should be replaced by an initial value.

### 6.1.2 An Example

Suppose a sponsor is interested in conducting a pilot study to evaluate clinical efficacy of a test compound on subjects with hypertension. The objective of the intended pilot study is to compare the distribution of the proportions of subjects whose blood pressures are below, within and above some pre-specified reference (normal) range with that from historical control. Suppose that it is expected that the proportions of subjects after treatments are 20% (below the reference range), 60% (within the reference range), and 20% (above the reference range), respectively. Thus, we have $r = 3$ and

$$(p_1, p_2, p_3) = (0.20, 0.60, 0.20)$$

Furthermore, suppose based on historical data or literature review, the proportions of subjects whose blood pressures are below, within, and above the reference range are given by 25%, 45%, and 30%, respectively. This is,

$$(p_{10}, p_{20}, p_{30}) = (0.25, 0.45, 0.30).$$

The sponsor would like to choose a sample size such that the trial will have an 80% ($\beta = 0.20$) power for detecting such a difference at the 5% ($\alpha = 0.05$) level of significance.

First, we need to find $\delta$ under the given parameters according to (6.1.1):

$$\chi_2^2(\chi_{0.05,3-1}^2|\delta) = 0.2.$$

This leads to $\delta_{0.05,0.2} = 9.634$. As a result, the sample size needed in order to achieve an 80% power is given by

$$n = 9.634 \left[\frac{(0.20-0.25)^2}{0.25} + \frac{(0.60-0.45)^2}{0.45} + \frac{(0.20-0.30)^2}{0.30}\right]^{-1} \approx 104.$$

## 6.2 Test for Independence—Single Stratum

A $r \times c$ (two-way) contingency table is defined as a two-way table representing the cross-tabulation of observed frequencies of two categorical response variables. Let $x_i$, $i = 1, ..., r$ and $y_j$, $j = 1, ..., c$ denote the categories (or levels) of variables $X$ and $Y$, respectively. Also, let $n_{ij}$ be the cell frequency of $X = x_i$ and $Y = y_j$. Then, we have the following $r \times c$ contingency table:

|       | $y_1$    | $y_2$    | $\cdots$ | $y_c$    |          |
|-------|----------|----------|----------|----------|----------|
| $x_1$ | $n_{11}$ | $n_{12}$ | $\cdots$ | $n_{1c}$ | $n_{1.}$ |
| $x_2$ | $n_{21}$ | $n_{22}$ | $\cdots$ | $n_{2c}$ | $n_{2.}$ |
| $\cdots$ | $\cdots$ | $\cdots$ | $\cdots$ | $\cdots$ | $\cdots$ |
| $x_r$ | $n_{r1}$ | $n_{r2}$ | $\cdots$ | $n_{rc}$ | $n_{r.}$ |
|       | $n_{.1}$ | $n_{.2}$ | $\cdots$ | $n_{.c}$ |          |

where

$$\begin{aligned} n_{.j} &= \sum_{i=1}^{r} n_{ij} & \text{(the } j\text{th column total)}, \\ n_{i.} &= \sum_{j=1}^{c} n_{ij} & \text{(the } i\text{th row total)}, \\ n &= \sum_{i=1}^{r} \sum_{j=1}^{c} n_{ij} & \text{(the overall total)}. \end{aligned}$$

In practice, the null hypothesis of interest is that there is no association between the row variable and the column variable, i.e., $X$ is independent of $Y$. When $r = c = 2$, Fisher's exact test introduced in the previous chapter can be applied. In the following we consider some popular tests for general cases.

### 6.2.1 Pearson's Test

The following Pearson's chi-square test statistic is probably the most commonly employed test statistic for independence: by

$$T_I = \sum_{i=1}^{r} \sum_{j=1}^{c} \frac{(n_{ij} - m_{ij})^2}{m_{ij}},$$

## 6.2. Test for Independence—Single Stratum

where
$$m_{ij} = \frac{n_{i\cdot} n_{\cdot j}}{n}.$$

Define $\hat{p}_{ij} = n_{ij}/n$, $\hat{p}_{i\cdot} = n_{i\cdot}/n$, and $\hat{p}_{\cdot j} = n_{\cdot j}/n$. Then $T_I$ can also be written as
$$T_I = \sum_{i=1}^{r} \sum_{j=1}^{c} \frac{n(\hat{p}_{ij} - \hat{p}_{i\cdot}\hat{p}_{\cdot j})^2}{\hat{p}_{i\cdot}\hat{p}_{\cdot j}}.$$

Under the null hypothesis that $X$ and $Y$ are independent, $T_I$ is asymptotically distributed as a central chi-square random variable with $(r-1)(c-1)$ degrees of freedom. Under the local-alternative with

$$\lim_{n \to \infty} \sum_{i=1}^{r} \sum_{j=1}^{c} \frac{n(p_{ij} - p_{i\cdot}p_{\cdot j})^2}{p_{i\cdot}p_{\cdot j}} = \delta, \quad (6.2.1)$$

where $p_{ij} = P(X = x_i, Y = y_j)$, $p_{i\cdot} = P(X = x_i)$, and $p_{\cdot j} = P(Y = y_j)$, $T_I$ is asymptotically distributed as a non-central chi-square random variable with $(r-1)(c-1)$ degrees of freedom and the non-centrality parameter $\delta$.

For given $\alpha$ and a desired power $1 - \beta$, $\delta$ can be obtained by solving

$$\chi^2_{(r-1)(c-1)}(\chi_{\alpha,(r-1)(c-1)}|\delta) = \beta. \quad (6.2.2)$$

Let the solution be $\delta_{\alpha,\beta}$. The sample size needed in order to achieve power $1 - \beta$ is then given by

$$n = \delta_{\alpha,\beta} \left[ \sum_{i=1}^{r} \sum_{j=1}^{c} \frac{(p_{ij} - p_{i\cdot}p_{\cdot j})^2}{p_{i\cdot}p_{\cdot j}} \right]^{-1}.$$

### 6.2.2 Likelihood Ratio Test

Another commonly used test for independence is the likelihood ratio test. More specifically, the likelihood function for a two-way contingency table is given by

$$L = \prod_{i=1}^{r} \prod_{j=1}^{c} p_{ij}^{n_{ij}}.$$

Without any constraint, the above likelihood function is maximized at $p_{ij} = n_{ij}/n$, which leads to

$$\max_{p_{ij}} \log L = \sum_{i=1}^{r} \sum_{j=1}^{c} n_{ij} \log \frac{n_{ij}}{n}.$$

Under the null hypothesis that $p_{ij} = p_{i.} p_{.j}$, the likelihood function can be re-written as

$$L = \prod_{i=1}^{r} p_{i.}^{n_{i.}} \prod_{j=1}^{c} p_{.j}^{n_{.j}}.$$

It is maximized at $p_{i.} = n_{i.}/n$ and $p_{.j} = n_{.j}/n$, which leads to

$$\max_{p_{ij}=p_{i.}p_{.j}} \log L = \sum_{i=1}^{r}\sum_{j=1}^{c} n_{ij} \log \frac{n_{i.}n_{.j}}{n^2}.$$

Hence, the likelihood ratio test statistic can be obtained as

$$T_L = 2\left(\max_{p_{ij}} \log L - \max_{p_{ij}=p_{i.}p_{.j}} \log L\right) = \sum_{i=1}^{r}\sum_{j=1}^{c} n_{ij} \log \frac{n_{ij}}{m_{ij}},$$

where $m_{ij} = n_{i.}n_{.j}/n$. Under the null hypothesis, $T_L$ is asymptotically distributed as a central chi-square random variable with $(r-1)(c-1)$ degrees of freedom. Thus, we reject the null hypothesis at approximate $\alpha$ level of significance if

$$T_L > \chi^2_{\alpha,(r-1)(c-1)}.$$

Note that the likelihood ratio test is asymptotically equivalent to Pearson's test for independence. Under the local alternative (6.2.1), it can be shown that $T_L$ is still asymptotically equivalent to Pearson's test for testing independence in terms of the power. Hence, the sample size formula derived based on Pearson's statistic can be used for obtaining sample size for the likelihood ratio test.

### 6.2.3 An Example

A small scaled pilot study was conducted to compare two treatment (treatment and control) in terms of the categorized hypotension. The results are summarized in the following $2 \times 3$ ($r = 2$ and $c = 3$) contingency table:

|           | Hypotension |        |       |    |
|-----------|:-----:|:------:|:-----:|:--:|
|           | below | normal | above |    |
| treatment | 2     | 7      | 1     | 10 |
| control   | 2     | 5      | 3     | 10 |
|           | 4     | 12     | 4     | 20 |

It can be seen that the treatment is better than the control in terms of lowering blood pressure. In order to confirm that such a difference truly exists, the investigator is planning a larger trial to confirm the finding by applying Pearson's chi-square test for independence. It is of interest to select a sample size such that there is an 80% ($\beta = 0.2$) power for detecting such a difference observed in the pilot study at the 5% ($\alpha = 0.05$) level of significance.

We first identify $\delta$ under the given parameters according to (6.2.2) by solving
$$\chi^2_{(2-1)(3-1)}(\chi^2_{0.05}|\delta) = 0.2.$$
This leads to $\delta_{0.05,0.2} = 9.634$. As a result, the sample size required for achieving an 80% power is given by

$$n = \delta_{0.05,0.2} \left[ \sum_{i=1}^{r} \sum_{j=1}^{c} \frac{(p_{ij} - p_{i\cdot} p_{\cdot j})^2}{p_{i\cdot} p_{\cdot j}} \right]^{-1} = \frac{9.634}{0.0667} \approx 145.$$

## 6.3 Test for Independence—Multiple Strata

In clinical trials, multiple study sites (or centers) are usually considered not only to make sure clinical results are reproducible but also to expedite patient recruitment so that the intended trials can be done within the desired time frame. In a multi-center trial, it is a concern whether the sample size within each center (or stratum) is sufficient for providing an accurate and reliable assessment of the treatment effect (and consequently for achieving the desired power) when there is significant treatment-by-center interaction. In practice, a typical approach is to pool data across all centers for an overall assessment of the treatment effect. However, how to control for center effect has become another issue in data analysis. When the data is binary, the Cochran-Mantel-Haenszel (CMH) test is probably the most commonly used test procedure, and can adjust for differences among centers.

### 6.3.1 Cochran-Mantel-Haenszel Test

To introduce the CMH method, consider summarizing data from a multi-center trial in the following series of $2 \times 2$ contingency tables:

| Treatment | Binary Reponse 0 | 1 | Total |
|---|---|---|---|
| Treatment 1 | $n_{h,10}$ | $n_{h,11}$ | $n_{h,1\cdot}$ |
| Treatment 2 | $n_{h,20}$ | $n_{h,21}$ | $n_{h,2\cdot}$ |
| Total | $n_{h,\cdot 0}$ | $n_{h,\cdot 1}$ | $n_{h,\cdot\cdot}$ |

where $h = 1, ..., H$, $n_{h,ij}$ is the number of patients in the $h$th center (stratum) under the $i$th treatment with response $j$. Let $p_{h,ij}$ be the probability that a patient in the $h$th stratum under the $i$th treatment has response $j$. The hypotheses of interest are given by

$$H_0 : p_{h,1j} = p_{h,2j} \text{ for all } h,j \quad \text{versus} \quad H_a : p_{h,1j} \neq p_{h,2j} \text{ for some } h,j.$$

The CMH test for the above hypotheses is defined as

$$T_{CMH} = \frac{[\sum_{h=1}^{H}(n_{h,11} - m_{h,11})]^2}{\sum_{h=1}^{H} v_h},$$

where

$$m_{h,11} = \frac{n_{h,1\cdot} n_{h,\cdot 1}}{n_h} \quad \text{and} \quad v_h = \frac{n_{h,1\cdot} n_{h,2\cdot} n_{h,\cdot 0} y_{h,\cdot 1}}{n_h^2(n_h-1)}, h = 1,...,H.$$

Under the null hypothesis $H_0$, $T_{CMH}$ is asymptotically distributed as a chi-square random variable with one degree of freedom. Hence, we reject the null hypothesis at approximate $\alpha$ level of significance if

$$T_{CMH} > \chi_{\alpha,1}^2.$$

In order to evaluate the power of this test under the alternative hypothesis, we assume that $n_h \to \infty$ and $n_h/n \to \pi_h$, where $n = \sum_{h=1}^{H} n_h$. Then, under the local alternative

$$\lim \left| \frac{\sum_{h=1}^{H} \pi_h(p_{h,11} - p_{h,1\cdot} p_{h,\cdot 1})}{\sqrt{\sum_{h=1}^{H} \pi_h p_{h,1\cdot} p_{h,2\cdot} p_{h,\cdot 0} p_{h,\cdot 1}}} \right| = \delta, \qquad (6.3.1)$$

where $p_{h,i\cdot} = p_{h,i0} + p_{h,i1}$ and $p_{h,\cdot j} = p_{h,1j} + p_{h,2j}$. $T_{CMH}$ is asymptotically distributed as a chi-square random variable with 1 degree of freedom and the non-centrality parameter $\delta^2$. In such a situation, it can be noted that $T_{CMH} > \chi_{\alpha,1}$ is equivalent to $N(\delta, 1) > z_{\alpha/2}$. Hence, the sample size required for achieving a desired power of $1 - \beta$ at the $\alpha$ level of significance is given by

$$n = \frac{(z_{\alpha/2} + z_\beta)^2}{\delta^2}.$$

### 6.3.2 An Example

Consider a multi-national, multi-center clinical trial conducted in four different countries (the United States of America, the United Kingdom, France, and Japan) for evaluation of clinical efficacy and safety of a test compound. Suppose the objective of this trial is to compare the test compound with a placebo in terms of the proportions of patients who experience certain types of adverse events. Let 0 and 1 denote the absence and presence of the adverse event. It is expected that the sample size will be approximately evenly distributed across the four centers (i.e., $\pi_h = 25\%, h = 1, 2, 3, 4$). Suppose based on a pilot study, the values of $p_{h,ij}$'s within each country are estimated as follows:

| center | Treatment | Binary Response 0 | Binary Response 1 | Total |
|---|---|---|---|---|
| 1 | Study Drug | 0.35 | 0.15 | 0.50 |
|   | Placebo | 0.25 | 0.25 | 0.50 |
|   | Total | 0.60 | 0.40 | 1.00 |
| 2 | Study Drug | 0.30 | 0.20 | 0.50 |
|   | Placebo | 0.20 | 0.30 | 0.50 |
|   | Total | 0.50 | 0.50 | 1.00 |
| 3 | Study Drug | 0.40 | 0.10 | 0.50 |
|   | Placebo | 0.20 | 0.30 | 0.50 |
|   | Total | 0.60 | 0.40 | 1.00 |
| 4 | Study Drug | 0.35 | 0.15 | 0.50 |
|   | Placebo | 0.15 | 0.35 | 0.50 |
|   | Total | 0.50 | 0.50 | 1.00 |

By (6.3.1), $\delta$ is given by 0.3030. Hence the sample size needed in order to achieve an 80% ($\beta = 0.20$) power at the 5% ($\alpha = 0.05$) level of significance is given by

$$n = \frac{(z_{\alpha/2} + z_\beta)^2}{\delta^2} = \frac{(1.96 + 0.84)^2}{0.3030^2} \approx 86.$$

## 6.4 Test for Categorical Shift

In clinical trials, it is often of interest to examine any change in laboratory values before and after the application of the treatment. When the response variable is categorical, this type of change is called a categorical shift. In this section, we consider testing for categorical shift.

### 6.4.1 McNemar's Test

For a given laboratory test, test results are usually summarized as either normal (i.e., the test result is within the normal range of the test) or abnormal (i.e., the test result is outside the normal range of the test). Let $x_{ij}$ be the binary response ($x_{ij} = 0$: normal and $x_{ij} = 1$: abnormal) from the $i$th ($i = 1, ..., n$) subject in the $j$th ($j = 1$: pre-treatment and $j = 2$: post treatment) treatment. The test results can be summarized in the following

$2 \times 2$ table:

|  | Post-Treatment | | |
|---|---|---|---|
| Pre-Treatment | Normal | Abnormal | |
| Normal | $n_{00}$ | $n_{01}$ | $n_{0\cdot}$ |
| Abnormal | $n_{10}$ | $n_{11}$ | $n_{1\cdot}$ |
| | $n_{\cdot 0}$ | $n_{\cdot 1}$ | $n_{\cdot\cdot}$ |

where

$$n_{00} = \sum_{i=1}^{n}(1-x_{i1})(1-x_{i2})$$

$$n_{01} = \sum_{i=1}^{n}(1-x_{i1})x_{i2}$$

$$n_{10} = \sum_{i=1}^{n}x_{i1}(1-x_{i2})$$

$$n_{11} = \sum_{i=1}^{n}x_{i1}x_{i2}.$$

Define

$$p_{00} = P(x_{i1}=0, x_{i2}=0)$$
$$p_{01} = P(x_{i1}=0, x_{i2}=1)$$
$$p_{10} = P(x_{i1}=1, x_{i2}=0)$$
$$p_{11} = P(x_{i1}=1, x_{i2}=1)$$
$$p_{1+} = P(x_{i1}=1) = p_{10} + p_{11}$$
$$p_{+1} = P(x_{i2}=1) = p_{01} + p_{11}.$$

It is then of interest to test whether there is a categorical shift after treatment. A categorical shift is defined as either a shift from 0 (normal) in pre-treatment to 1 (abnormal) in post-treatment or a shift from 1 (abnormal) in pre-treatment to 0 (normal) in post-treatment. Consider

$$H_0 : p_{1+} = p_{+1} \quad \text{versus} \quad H_a : p_{1+} \neq p_{+1},$$

which is equivalent to

$$H_0 : p_{10} = p_{01} \quad \text{versus} \quad H_a : p_{10} \neq p_{01}.$$

The most commonly used test procedure to serve the purpose is McNemar's test, whose test statistic is given by

$$T_{MN} = \frac{n_{10} - n_{01}}{\sqrt{n_{10} + n_{01}}}.$$

## 6.4. Test for Categorical Shift

Under the null hypothesis $H_0$, $T_{MN}$ is asymptotically distributed as a standard normal random variable. Hence, we reject the null hypothesis at approximate $\alpha$ level of significance if

$$|T_{MN}| > z_{\alpha/2}.$$

Under the alternative hypothesis that $p_{01} \neq p_{10}$, it follows that

$$T_{MN} = \frac{n_{01} - n_{10}}{\sqrt{n_{01} + n_{10}}}$$
$$= \sqrt{\frac{n}{n_{01} + n_{10}}} \sqrt{n} \left( \frac{n_{10}}{n} - \frac{n_{01}}{n} \right)$$
$$= \frac{1}{\sqrt{p_{10} + p_{01}}} \frac{1}{\sqrt{n}} \sum_{i=1}^{n} d_i,$$

where $d_i = x_{i1} - x_{i2}$. Note that $d_i$'s are independent and identically distributed random variables with mean $(p_{01} - p_{10})$ and variance $p_{01} + p_{10} - (p_{01} - p_{10})^2$. As a result, by the Central Limit Theorem, the power of McNemar's test can be approximated by

$$\Phi \left( \frac{\sqrt{n}(p_{01} - p_{10}) - z_{\alpha/2}\sqrt{p_{01} + p_{10}}}{\sqrt{p_{01} + p_{10} - (p_{01} - p_{10})^2}} \right).$$

In order to achieve a power of $1 - \beta$, the sample size needed can be obtained by solving

$$\frac{\sqrt{n}(p_{01} - p_{10}) - z_{\alpha/2}\sqrt{p_{01} + p_{10}}}{\sqrt{p_{01} + p_{10} - (p_{01} - p_{10})^2}} = -z_\beta.$$

which leads to

$$n = \frac{[z_{\alpha/2}\sqrt{p_{01} + p_{10}} + z_\beta \sqrt{p_{10} + p_{01} - (p_{01} - p_{10})^2}]^2}{(p_{10} - p_{01})^2}. \quad (6.4.1)$$

Define $\psi = p_{01}/p_{10}$ and $\pi_{\text{Discordant}} = p_{01} + p_{10}$. Then

$$n = \frac{[z_{\alpha/2}(\psi + 1) + z_\beta \sqrt{(\psi + 1)^2 - (\psi - 1)^2 \pi_{\text{Discordant}}}]^2}{(\psi - 1)^2 \pi_{\text{Discordant}}}.$$

### 6.4.2 Stuart-Maxwell Test

McNemar's test can be applied only to the case in which there are two possible categories for the outcome. In practice, however, it is possible that the outcomes are classified into more than two (multiple) categories. For example, instead of classifying the laboratory values into normal and abnormal (two categories), it is often to classify them into three categories (i.e., below, within, and above the normal range). Let $x_{ij} \in \{1,...,r\}$ be the categorical observation from the $i$th subject under the $j$th treatment ($j = 1$: pre-treatment and $j = 2$: post-treatment). In practice, the data are usually summarized by the following $r \times r$ contingency table:

|               | Post-Treatment |          |         |          |          |
|---------------|----------------|----------|---------|----------|----------|
| Pre-Treatment | 1              | 2        | $\cdots$ | $r$      |          |
| 1             | $n_{11}$       | $n_{12}$ | $\cdots$ | $n_{1r}$ | $n_{1.}$ |
| 2             | $n_{21}$       | $n_{22}$ | $\cdots$ | $n_{2r}$ | $n_{2.}$ |
| $\cdots$      | $\cdots$       | $\cdots$ | $\cdots$ | $\cdots$ |          |
| $r$           | $n_{r1}$       | $n_{r2}$ | $\cdots$ | $n_{rr}$ | $n_{r.}$ |
|               | $n_{.1}$       | $n_{.2}$ | $\cdots$ | $n_{.r}$ | $n_{..}$ |

Let
$$p_{ij} = P(x_{k1} = i, x_{k2} = j),$$
which is the probability that the subject will shift from $i$ pre-treatment to $j$ post-treatment. If there is no treatment effect, one may expect that $p_{ij} = p_{ji}$ for all $1 \leq i, j, \leq r$. Hence, it is of interest to test the hypotheses

$$H_0 : p_{ij} = p_{ij} \text{ for all } i \neq j \quad \text{versus} \quad H_a : p_{ij} \neq p_{ij} \text{ for some } i \neq j.$$

In order to test the above hypotheses, the test statistic proposed by Stuart and Maxwell is useful (see, e.g., Stuart, 1955). We refer to the test statistic as Stuart-Maxwell test, which is given by

$$T_{SM} = \sum_{i<j} \frac{(n_{ij} - n_{ji})^2}{n_{ij} + n_{ji}}.$$

Under the null hypothesis $H_0$, $T_{SM}$ follows a standard chi-square distribution with $r(r-1)/2$ degrees of freedom. Hence, for a given significance level of $\alpha$, the null hypothesis should be rejected if $T_{SM} > \chi^2_{\alpha, r(r-1)/2}$.

Under the local alternative given by

$$\lim_{n \to \infty} n \sum_{i<j} \frac{(p_{ij} - p_{ji})^2}{p_{ij} + p_{ji}} = \delta,$$

$T_{SM}$ is asymptotically distributed as a non-central chi-square random variable with $r(r-1)/2$ degrees of freedom and the non-centrality parameter $\delta$. For a given degrees of freedom ($r(r-1)/2$) and a desired power $(1-\beta)$, $\delta$ can be obtained by solving

$$\chi^2_{r(r-1)/2}(\chi_{\alpha, r(r-1)/2}|\delta) = \beta, \quad (6.4.2)$$

## 6.4. Test for Categorical Shift

where $\chi_a^2(\cdot|\delta)$ is the cumulative distribution function of the non-central chi-square distribution with degrees freedom $a$ and non-centraliity parameter $\delta$. Let $\delta_{\alpha,\beta}$ be the solution. Then, the sample size needed in order to achieve a power of $1-\beta$ is given by

$$n = \delta_{\alpha,\beta} \left[ \sum_{i<j} \frac{(p_{ij} - p_{ji})^2}{p_{ij} + p_{ji}} \right]^{-1}. \qquad (6.4.3)$$

### 6.4.3 Examples

**McNemar's Test**

Suppose that an investigator is planning to conduct a trial to study a test compound under investigation in terms of the proportions of the patients with nocturnal hypoglycaemia, which is defined to be the patients with the overnight glucose value $\leq 3.5$ mgL on two consecutive visits (15 minutes/per visit). At the first visit (pre-treatment), patients' overnight glucose levels will be measured every 15 minutes. Whether or not the patient experience nocturnal hypoglycaemia will be recorded. At the second visit, patients will receive the study compound and the overnight glucose levels will be obtained in a similar manner. Patients' experience on nocturnal hypoglycaemia will also be recorded. According to some pilot studies, it is expected that about 50% ($p_{10} = 0.50$) of patients will shift from 1 (nocturnal hypoglycaemia pre-treatment) to 0 (normal post-treatment) and 20% ($p_{01} = 0.20$) of patients will shift from 0 (normal pre-treatment) to 1 (nocturnal hypoglycaemia post-treatment). The investigator would like to select a sample size such that there is an 80% ($\beta = 0.20$) power for detecting such a difference if it truly exists at the 5% ($\alpha = 0.05$) level of significance. According to (6.4.1), the required sample size can be obtained as follows:

$$n = \frac{[z_{\alpha/2}\sqrt{p_{01} + p_{10}} + z_{\beta}\sqrt{p_{10} + p_{01} - (p_{01} - p_{10})^2}]^2}{(p_{10} - p_{01})^2}$$

$$= \frac{[1.96\sqrt{0.20 + 0.50} + 0.84\sqrt{0.20 + 0.50 - (0.20 - 0.50)^2}]^2}{(0.20 - 0.50)^2}$$

$$\approx 59.$$

**Stuart-Maxwell Test**

A pilot study was conducted to study the treatment effect of a test compound based on the number of monocytes in the blood. The primary study endpoint is the number of monocytes (i.e., below, within, and above normal range) in the blood (i.e., $r = 3$). The results were summarized in the following contingency table:

|  | Post-Treatment | | | |
| Pre-Treatment | below | normal | above | |
| --- | --- | --- | --- | --- |
| below | 3 | 4 | 4 | 11 |
| normal | 2 | 3 | 3 | 8 |
| above | 1 | 2 | 3 | 6 |
| | 6 | 9 | 10 | 25 |

From this pilot study, the results suggest that the test compound can increase the number of monocytes in the blood because the upper off diagonal elements are always larger than those in the lower off diagonal.

To confirm whether such a trend truly exists, a larger trial is planned to have an 80% ($\beta = 0.20$) power at the 5% ($\alpha = 0.05$) level of significance. For this purpose, we need to first estimate $\delta$ under the given parameters according to (6.4.2).

$$\chi^2_{3(3-1)/2}(\chi^2_{0.05,3(3-1)/2}|\delta) = 0.20,$$

which leads to $\delta_{\alpha,\beta} = 10.903$. As a result, the sample size needed for achieving an 80% power is given by

$$n = \delta_{\alpha,\beta} \left[ \sum_{i<j} \frac{(p_{ij} - p_{ji})^2}{p_{ij} + p_{ji}} \right]^{-1} = \frac{10.903}{0.107} \approx 102.$$

## 6.5 Carry-Over Effect Test

As discussed earlier, a standard $2 \times 2$ crossover design is commonly used in clinical research for evaluation of clinical efficacy and safety of a test compound of interest. When the response is binary, under the assumption of no period and treatment-by-period interaction (carry-over effect), McNemar's test can be applied to test for the treatment effect. In some cases, the investigator may be interested in testing the treatment-by-period interaction. In this section, statistical procedure for testing the treatment-by-period interaction, based on the model by Becker and Balagtas (1993), is introduced. The corresponding procedure for sample size calculation is derived.

### 6.5.1 Test Procedure

Consider a standard two-sequence, two-period crossover design, i.e., (AB, BA). Let $x_{ijk}$ be the binary response from the $k$th ($k = 1, ..., n_i$) subject

## 6.5. Carry-Over Effect Test

in the $i$th sequence at the $j$th dosing period. Let $p_{ij} = P(x_{ijk} = 1)$. In order to separate the treatment, period, and carryover effects, Becker and Balagtas (1993) considered the following logistic regression model

$$\log \frac{p_{11}}{1 - p_{11}} = \alpha + \tau_1 + \rho_1,$$

$$\log \frac{p_{12}}{1 - p_{12}} = \alpha + \tau_2 + \rho_2 + \gamma_1,$$

$$\log \frac{p_{21}}{1 - p_{21}} = \alpha + \tau_2 + \rho_1,$$

$$\log \frac{p_{22}}{1 - p_{22}} = \alpha + \tau_1 + \rho_2 + \gamma_2,$$

where $\tau_i$ is the $i$th treatment effect, $\rho_j$ is the $j$th period effect, and $\gamma_k$ is the carry-over effect from the first period in the $k$th sequence. It is assumed that

$$\tau_1 + \tau_2 = 0$$
$$\rho_1 + \rho_2 = 0$$
$$\gamma_1 + \gamma_2 = 0.$$

Let

$$\gamma = \gamma_1 - \gamma_2$$
$$= \log \frac{p_{11}}{1 - p_{11}} + \log \frac{p_{12}}{1 - p_{12}} - \log \frac{p_{21}}{1 - p_{21}} - \log \frac{p_{22}}{1 - p_{22}}.$$

The hypotheses of interest are given by

$$H_0 : \gamma = 0 \quad \text{versus} \quad H_a : \gamma \neq 0.$$

Let $\hat{p}_{ij} = n^{-1} \sum_k x_{ijk}$. Then, $\gamma$ can be estimated by

$$\hat{\gamma} = \log \frac{\hat{p}_{11}}{1 - \hat{p}_{11}} + \log \frac{\hat{p}_{12}}{1 - \hat{p}_{12}} - \log \frac{\hat{p}_{21}}{1 - \hat{p}_{21}} - \log \frac{\hat{p}_{22}}{1 - \hat{p}_{22}}.$$

It can be shown that $\hat{\gamma}$ is asymptotically distributed as a normal random variable with mean $\gamma$ and variance $\sigma_1^2 n_1^{-1} + \sigma_2^2 n_2^{-1}$, where

$$\sigma_i^2 = \text{var} \left( \frac{x_{i1k}}{p_{i1}(1 - p_{i1})} + \frac{x_{i2k}}{p_{i2}(1 - p_{i2})} \right),$$

which can be estimated by $\hat{\sigma}_i^2$, the sample variance of

$$\frac{x_{i1k}}{\hat{p}_{i1}(1 - \hat{p}_{i1})} + \frac{x_{i2k}}{\hat{p}_{i2}(1 - \hat{p}_{i2})}, \quad k = 1, ..., n_i.$$

Hence, the test statistic is given by

$$T = \hat{\gamma}\left(\frac{\hat{\sigma}_1^2}{n_1} + \frac{\hat{\sigma}_2^2}{n_2}\right)^{-1/2}.$$

Under the null hypothesis $H_0$, $T$ is asymptotically distributed as a standard normal random variable. We reject the null hypothesis at approximate $\alpha$ level of significance if

$$|T| > z_{\alpha/2}$$

Under the alternative hypothesis that $\gamma \neq 0$, the power of the this test procedure can be approximated by

$$\Phi\left(\gamma\left[\frac{\sigma_1^2}{n_1} + \frac{\sigma_2^2}{n_2}\right]^{-1/2} - z_{\alpha/2}\right).$$

For a given power of $1 - \beta$ and assuming that $n = n_1 = n_2$, the sample size needed can be obtained by solving

$$\gamma\left[\frac{\sigma_1^2}{n} + \frac{\sigma_2^2}{n}\right]^{-1/2} - z_{\alpha/2} = z_\beta,$$

which leads to

$$n = \frac{(z_{\alpha/2} + z_\beta)^2(\sigma_1^2 + \sigma_2^2)}{\gamma^2}.$$

## 6.5.2 An Example

Consider a single-center, open, randomized, active-controlled, two-sequence, two-period crossover design with the primary efficacy endpoint of nocturnal hypoglycaemia. The objective of the study is to compare the study drug with a standard therapy on the marketplace in terms of the proportion of the patients who will experience nocturnal hypoglycaemia. As a result, the investigator is interested in conducting a larger trial to confirm whether such an effect truly exists. However, based on the results of a small-scale pilot study, no evidence of statistical significance in the possible carry-over effect was detected. According to the pilot study, the following parameters were estimated: $\gamma = 0.89$, $\sigma_1 = 2.3$, and $\sigma_2 = 2.4$. The sample size needed in order to achieve an 80% ($\beta = 0.2$) power at the 5% ($\alpha = 0.05$) level of significance is given by

$$n = \frac{(z_{\alpha/2} + z_\beta)^2(\sigma_1^2 + \sigma_2^2)}{\gamma^2} = \frac{(1.96 + 0.84)^2(2.3^2 + 2.4^2)}{0.89^2} \approx 110.$$

Hence, a total of 110 subjects are required in order to have the desired power for the study.

## 6.6 Practical Issues

### 6.6.1 Local Alternative Versus Fixed Alternative

In this chapter, we introduced various chi-square type test statistics for contingency tables. When the chi-square test has only one degree of freedom, it is equivalent to a Z-test (i.e., a test based on standard normal distribution). Hence, the formula for sample size calculation can be derived under the ordinary fixed alternative. When the degrees of freedom of the chi-square test is larger than one (e.g., Pearson's test for goodness-of-fit and independence), it can be verified that the chi-square test statistic is distributed as a weighted non-central chi-square distribution under the fixed alternative hypothesis. In order words, it has the same distribution as the random variable $\sum_{i=1}^{k} \lambda_i \chi^2(\delta_i)$ for some $k$, $\lambda_i$ and $\delta_i$, where $\chi^2(\delta_i)$ denotes a chi-square random variable with one degree of freedom and the non-centrality parameter $\delta_i$. The power function based on a weighted non-central chi-square random variable could be very complicated and no standard table/software is available. As a result, all the sample size formulas for the chi-square tests with more than one degree of freedom are derived under the local alternative. Under the concept of local alternative, one assumes that the difference in the parameters of interest between the null hypothesis and the alternative hypothesis shrinks to 0 at a speed of $1/\sqrt{n}$. In practice, however, it is more appealing to consider the alternative as fixed. In other words, the alternative hypothesis does not change as the sample size changes. Further research in sample size estimation based on a fixed alternative is needed.

### 6.6.2 Random Versus Fixed Marginal Total

In randomized, controlled parallel clinical trials, the numbers of subjects assigned to each treatment group are usually fixed. Consequently, when the data are reported by a two-way contingency table (treatment and response), one of the margins (treatment) is fixed. However, it is not uncommon (e.g., in an observational study) that the number of subjects assigned to each treatment is also random. In this situation, Pearson's test for independence between treatment and response is still valid. Thus, Pearson's test is commonly used in the situation where the marginal distribution of the numbers of the subjects for each treatment is unknown. When the marginal distribution of the numbers of the subjects for each treatment is known or can be approximated by some distribution such as Poisson, Pearson's test may not be efficient. Alternatively, the likelihood ratio test may be useful (see, e.g., Shao and Chow, 1990).

### 6.6.3 $r \times c$ Versus $p \times r \times c$

In this chapter, we focus on procedures for sample size calculation for testing goodness-of-fit, independence (or association), and categorical shift under an $r \times c$ contingency table. In practice, we may encounter the situation which involves a $p \times r \times c$ contingency table when a third variable (e.g., sex, race, or age). In practice, how to handle this type of three-way contingency table is always a challenge. One simple solution is combining the third variable with the treatment variable and applying the standard procedure designed for a two-way contingency table. Further research regarding how to handle three-way contingency tables is necessary.

# Chapter 7

# Comparing Time-to-Event Data

In clinical research, in addition to continuous and discrete study endpoints described in the previous two chapters, the investigator may also be interested in the occurrence of certain *events* such as adverse experience, disease progression, relapse, or death. In most clinical trials, the occurrence of such an event is usually undesirable. Hence, one of the primary objectives of the intended clinical trials may be to evaluate the effect of the test drug on the prevention or delay of such events. The time to the occurrence of an event is usually referred to as the time-to-event. In practice, time-to-event has become a natural measure of the extent to which the event occurrence is delayed. When the event is the death, the time-to-event of a patient is the patient's survival time. Hence, the analysis of time-to-event is sometimes referred to as *survival analysis*.

In practice, statistical methods for analysis of time-to-event data are very different from those commonly used for continuous variables (e.g., analysis of variance) due to the following reasons. First, time-to-event is usually subject to censoring, e.g., right (left) or interval censoring, at which its exact value is unknown but we know that it is larger or smaller than an observed censoring time or within an interval. Second, time-to-event data are usually highly skewed, which violates the normality assumption of standard statistical methods such as the analysis of variance. In this chapter, for simplicity, we focus on sample size calculation based only on the most typical censor type (i.e., right censoring) and the most commonly used testing procedures such as the exponential model, Cox's proportional hazards model, and the weighted log-rank test.

The remainder of this chapter is organized as follows. In the next section, basic concepts regarding survival and hazard functions in the analysis of time-to-event data are provided. In Section 7.2, formulas for sample size calculation for testing equality, non-inferioirty/superiority, and equivalence in two-sample problems are derived under the commonly used exponential model. In Section 7.3, formulas for sample size calculation under Cox's proportional hazards model is presented. In Section 7.4, formulas for sample size estimation based on the weighted log-rank test are derived. Some practical issues are discussed in Section 7.5.

## 7.1 Basic Concepts

In this section, we introduce some basic concepts regarding survival and hazard functions, which are commonly used in the analysis of time-to-event data. In practice, hypotheses of clinical interest are often involved in comparing median survival times, surival functions, and hazard rates. Under a given set of hypotheses, appropriate statistical tests are then constructed based on consistent estimators of these parameters.

### 7.1.1 Survival Function

In the analysis of time-to-event data, the *survival function* is usually used to characterize the distribution of the time-to-event data. Let $X$ be the variable of time-to-event and $S(x)$ be the corresponding survival function. Then, $S(x)$ is defined as

$$S(x) = P(X > x).$$

Thus, $S(x)$ is the probability that the event will occur after time $x$. When the event is death, $S(x)$ is the probability of a patient who will survive until $x$. Theoretically, $X$ could be a continuous variable, a discrete response, or a combination of both. In this chapter, however, we consider only the case where $X$ is a continuous random variable with a density function $f(x)$. The relationship between $S(x)$ and $f(x)$ is given by

$$f(x) = \frac{dS(x)}{dx}.$$

A commonly used nonparametric estimator for $S(x)$ is the Kaplan-Meier estimator, which is given by

$$\hat{S}(t) = \prod_i \left(1 - \frac{d_i}{n_i}\right), \qquad (7.1.1)$$

where the product is over all event times, $d_i$ is the number of events observed at the $i$th event time, and $n_i$ is the number of subjects at risk just prior the $i$th event time.

## 7.1. Basic Concepts

### 7.1.2 Median Survival Time

In a clinical study, it is of interest to compare the median surival time, which is defined to be the 50% quantile of the surival distribution. In other words, if $m_{1/2}$ is the median survival time, then it should satisfy

$$P(X > m_{1/2}) = 0.5.$$

A commonly used nonparametric estimator for $m_{1/2}$ is given by $\hat{m}_{1/2} = \hat{S}^{-1}(0.5)$, where $\hat{S}$ is the Kaplan-Meier estimator. When the time-to-event is exponentially distributed with hazard rate $\lambda$, it can be shown that the median survival time is given by $\log 2/\lambda$.

### 7.1.3 Hazard Function

Another important concept in the analysis of time-to-event data is the so-called *hazard function*, which is defined as

$$h(x) = \lim_{\Delta x \to 0} \frac{P(x \leq X < x + \Delta x | X \geq x)}{\Delta x}.$$

As it can be seen, $h(x)$ can also be written as

$$h(x) = \frac{f(x)}{S(x)},$$

which implies that

$$S(x) = \exp\left\{-\int_0^x h(t)da\right\}.$$

If we assume a constant hazard rate (i.e., $h(t) = \lambda$ for some $\lambda$), $S(x)$ becomes

$$S(x) = \exp\{-\lambda x\}.$$

In this case, time-to-event $X$ is distributed as an exponential variable with hazard rate $\lambda$.

### 7.1.4 An Example

A clinical trial was conducted to study a test treatment on patients with small cell lung cancer. The trial lasted for 1 year with 10 patients entered in the study simultaneously. The data is given in Table 7.1.1 with "+" indicating censored observations.

The Kaplan-Meier estimator can be obtained based on (7.1.1) with median 0.310. The obtained Kaplan-Meier estimator is plotted in Figure 7.1.1.

Table 7.1.1: Survival Data

| Subject Number | Survival Time |
|---|---|
| 1 | 0.29 |
| 2 | 0.25 |
| 3 | 0.12 |
| 4 | 0.69 |
| 5 | 1.00+ |
| 6 | 0.33 |
| 7 | 0.19 |
| 8 | 1.00+ |
| 9 | 0.23 |
| 10 | 0.93 |

It can be seen from the Kaplan-Meier plot that approximately 80% patients in the patient population will live beyond 0.2 years. If we assume constant hazard rate over time, the estimated hazard rate according to (7.2.1) in the next section is 1.59.

## 7.2 Exponential Model

In what follows, formulas for sample size calculation based on hazard rates for median survival times and survival functions between treatment groups will be derived under an exponential model, which is the simplest parametric statistical model for time-to-event data. Under the exponential model, it is assumed that the time-to-event is exponentially distributed with a constant hazard rate. For survival analysis in clinical trials comparing two treatments, the hypothesis of interest could be either comparing the hazard rates or the median survival times. However, since the time-to-event is assumed to be exponentially distributed, the median survival time is determined by the hazard rate. As a result, comparing median survival times is equivalent to comparing hazard rates. Without loss of generality, we focus on comparing hazard rates between treatment groups. In this section, we will introduce the method by Lachin and Foulkes (1986).

Consider a two-arm parallel survival trial with accrural time period $T_0$ and the follow-up $T - T_0$. Let $a_{ij}$ denote the entry time of the $j$th patient of the $i$th treatment group. It is assumed that $a_{ij}$ follows a continuous

## 7.2. Exponential Model

Figure 7.1.1: Kaplan-Meier Estimator for $S(x)$

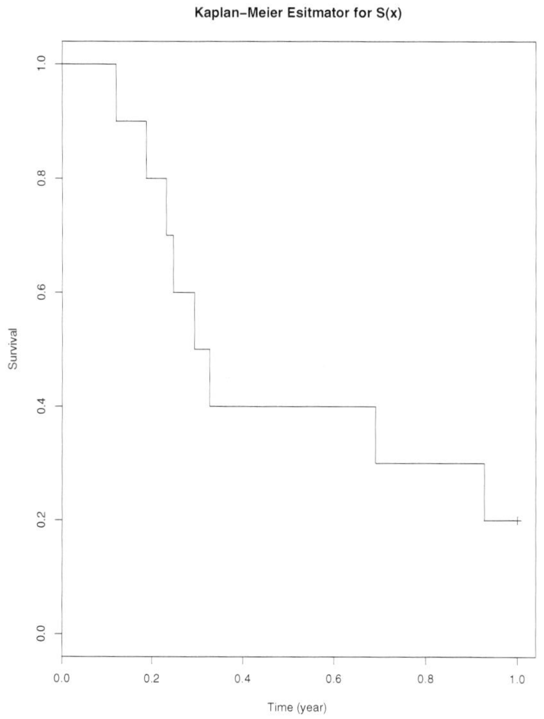

distribution with the density function given by

$$g(z) = \frac{\gamma e^{-\gamma z}}{1 - e^{-\gamma T_0}}, \quad 0 \leq z \leq T_0.$$

When $\gamma > 0$, the entry distribution is convex, which implies fast patient entry at beginning. When $\gamma < 0$, the entry distribution is concave, which implies lagging patient entry. For convenience, we define $g(z) = 1/T_0$ when $\gamma = 0$, which implies uniform patient entry. Let $t_{ij}$ be the time-to-event (i.e., the time from the patient entry to the time observing event) for the $j$th subject in the $i$th treatment group, $i = 1, 2, j = 1, ..., n_i$. It is assumed that $t_{ij}$ follows an exponential distribution with hazard rate $\lambda_i$. The information observed from the sample is $(x_{ij}, \delta_{ij}) = (\min(t_{ij}, T - a_{ij}), I\{t_{ij} \leq T - a_{ij}\})$.

168                     Chapter 7. Comparing Time-to-Event Data

For a fixed $i$, the joint likelihood for $x_{ij}, j = 1, ..., n_i$ can be written as

$$L(\lambda_i) = \frac{\gamma^n e^{-\gamma \sum_{j=1}^{n_i} a_{ij}}}{(1 - e^{-\gamma T_0})^n} \lambda_i^{\sum_{j=1}^{n_i} \delta_{ij}} e^{-\lambda_i \sum_{j=1}^{n_i} x_{ij}}.$$

It can be shown that the MLE for $\lambda_i$ is given by

$$\hat{\lambda}_i = \frac{\sum_{j=1}^{n_i} \delta_{ij}}{\sum_{j=1}^{n_i} x_{ij}}. \tag{7.2.1}$$

According to the Central Limit Theorem,

$$\sqrt{n_i}(\hat{\lambda}_i - \lambda_i) = \sqrt{n_i} \frac{\sum_{j=1}^{n_i} (\delta_{ij} - \lambda_i x_{ij})}{\sum_{j=1}^{n_i} x_{ij}}$$

$$= \frac{1}{E(x_{ij})} \frac{1}{\sqrt{n_i}} \sum_{j=1}^{n_i} (\delta_{ij} - \lambda_i x_{ij}) + o_p(1)$$

$$\to_d N(0, \sigma^2(\lambda_i)),$$

where

$$\sigma^2(\lambda_i) = \frac{1}{E^2(x_{ij})} \text{var}(\delta_{ij} - \lambda_i x_{ij})$$

and $\to_d$ denotes convergence in distribution. Note that

$$E(\delta_{ij}) = E(\delta_{ij}^2)$$

$$= 1 - \int_0^{T_0} g(a) e^{-\lambda_i (T-a)} da$$

$$= 1 - \int_0^{T_0} \frac{\gamma e^{-\gamma a}}{1 - e^{-\gamma T_0}} e^{-\lambda_i (T-a)} da$$

$$= 1 + \frac{\gamma e^{-\lambda_i T} \left(1 - e^{(\lambda_i - \gamma) T_0}\right)}{(\lambda_i - \gamma)(1 - e^{-\gamma T_0})},$$

$$E(x_{ij}) = \int_0^{T_0} g(a) da \int_0^{T-a} \lambda_i x e^{-\lambda_i x} dx + (T-a) e^{-\lambda_i (T-a)}$$

$$= \int_0^{T_0} g(a) \frac{1 - e^{-\lambda_i (T-a)}}{\lambda_i} da$$

$$= \frac{1}{\lambda_i} E(\delta_{ij}),$$

$$E(\delta_{ij} x_{ij}) = \int_0^{T_0} g(a) da \int_0^{T-a} \lambda_i x e^{-\lambda_i x} dx,$$

## 7.2. Exponential Model

and

$$E(x_{ij}^2) = \int_0^{T_0} g(a)da \int_0^{T-a} \lambda_i x^2 e^{-\lambda_i x} dx + (T-a)^2 e^{-\lambda_i(T-a)}$$

$$= \int_0^{T_0} g(a)da \int_0^{T-a} 2x e^{-\lambda_i x} dx$$

$$= \frac{2E(\delta_{ij} x_{ij})}{\lambda_i}.$$

Hence

$$\operatorname{var}(\delta_{ij} - \lambda_i x_{ij}) = E(\delta_{ij}^2) - 2\lambda_i E(\delta_{ij} x_{ij}) + \lambda_i^2 E(x_{ij}^2)$$

$$= E(\delta_{ij}^2) - 2\lambda_i E(\delta_{ij} x_{ij}) + 2\lambda_i E(\delta_{ij} x_{ij})$$

$$= E(\delta_{ij}^2) = E(\delta_{ij}).$$

That is,

$$\sigma^2(\lambda_i) = \frac{\lambda_i^2}{E(\delta_{ij})} = \lambda_i^2 \left[ 1 + \frac{\gamma e^{-\lambda_i T} \left(1 - e^{(\lambda_i - \gamma)T_0}\right)}{(\lambda_i - \gamma)(1 - e^{-\gamma T_0})} \right]^{-1}. \quad (7.2.2)$$

### 7.2.1 Test for Equality

Let $\epsilon = \lambda_1 - \lambda_2$ be the difference between the hazard rates of a control and a test drug. To test whether there is a difference between the hazard rates of the test drug and the reference drug, the following hypotheses are usually considered:

$$H_0 : \epsilon = 0 \quad \text{versus} \quad H_a : \epsilon \neq 0.$$

Under the null hypothesis, test statistic

$$T = (\hat{\lambda}_1 - \hat{\lambda}_2) \left[ \frac{\sigma^2(\hat{\lambda}_1)}{n_1} + \frac{\sigma^2(\hat{\lambda}_2)}{n_2} \right]^{-1/2}$$

approximately follows a standard normal distribution for large $n_1$ and $n_2$. We then reject the null hypothesis at approximate $\alpha$ level of significance if

$$\left| (\hat{\lambda}_1 - \hat{\lambda}_2) \left[ \frac{\sigma^2(\hat{\lambda}_1)}{n_1} + \frac{\sigma^2(\hat{\lambda}_2)}{n_2} \right]^{-1/2} \right| > z_{\alpha/2}. \quad (7.2.3)$$

Under the alternative hypothesis that $\lambda_1 - \lambda_2 \neq 0$, the power of the above test is approximately

$$\Phi \left( |\lambda_1 - \lambda_2| \left[ \frac{\sigma^2(\lambda_1)}{n_1} + \frac{\sigma^2(\lambda_2)}{n_2} \right]^{-1/2} - z_{\alpha/2} \right).$$

As a result, the sample size needed in order to achieve a desired power of $1 - \beta$ can be obtained by solving

$$|\lambda_1 - \lambda_2| \left[ \frac{\sigma^2(\lambda_1)}{n_1} + \frac{\sigma^2(\lambda_2)}{n_2} \right]^{-1/2} - z_{\alpha/2} = z_\beta.$$

Under the assumption that $n_1 = \kappa n_2$, we obtain that

$$n_2 = \frac{(z_{\alpha/2} + z_\beta)^2}{(\lambda_1 - \lambda_2)^2} \left[ \frac{\sigma^2(\lambda_1)}{k} + \sigma^2(\lambda_2) \right]. \quad (7.2.4)$$

## 7.2.2 Test for Non-Inferiority/Superiority

Since $\epsilon = \lambda_1 - \lambda_2$, where $\lambda_1$ and $\lambda_2$ are the hazard rates of the control and test drug, respectively, in practice, a smaller hazard rate is considered a favor of the test drug. In other words, a negative value of $\epsilon$ implies a better performance of the test drug than the control. Hence, the problem of testing non-inferiority and superiority can be unified by the following hypotheses:

$$H_0 : \epsilon \leq \delta \quad \text{versus} \quad H_a : \epsilon > \delta,$$

where $\delta$ is the superiority or non-inferiority margin. When $\delta > 0$, the rejection of the null hypothesis indicates the superiority of the test drug over the control. When $\delta < 0$, the rejection of the null hypothesis indicates the non-inferiority of the test drug against the control. Similarly, under the null hypothesis, test statistic

$$T = (\hat{\lambda}_1 - \hat{\lambda}_2 - \delta) \left[ \frac{\sigma^2(\hat{\lambda}_1)}{n_1} + \frac{\sigma^2(\hat{\lambda}_2)}{n_2} \right]^{-1/2}$$

is asymptotically distributed as a standard normal random variable. Thus, we reject the null hypothesis at approximate $\alpha$ level of significance if

$$(\hat{\lambda}_1 - \hat{\lambda}_2 - \delta) \left[ \frac{\sigma^2(\hat{\lambda}_1)}{n_1} + \frac{\sigma^2(\hat{\lambda}_2)}{n_2} \right]^{-1/2} > z_\alpha.$$

Under the alternative hypothesis that $\epsilon > \delta$, the power of the above test is approximately

$$\Phi \left( (\epsilon - \delta) \left[ \frac{\sigma^2(\lambda_1)}{n_1} + \frac{\sigma^2(\lambda_2)}{n_2} \right]^{-1/2} - z_\alpha \right).$$

As a result, the sample size needed in order to achieve a desired power of $1 - \beta$ can be obtained by solving

$$(\epsilon - \delta) \left[ \frac{\sigma^2(\lambda_1)}{n_1} + \frac{\sigma^2(\lambda_2)}{n_2} \right]^{-1/2} - z_\alpha = z_\beta.$$

## 7.2. Exponential Model

Under the assumption that $n_1 = \kappa n_2$, we have

$$n_2 = \frac{(z_\alpha + z_\beta)^2}{(\epsilon - \delta)^2}\left[\frac{\sigma^2(\lambda_1)}{k} + \sigma^2(\lambda_2)\right]. \tag{7.2.5}$$

### 7.2.3 Test for Equivalence

The objective is to test the following hypotheses:

$$H_0 : |\epsilon| \geq \delta \quad \text{versus} \quad H_a : |\epsilon| < \delta.$$

The null hypothesis is rejected and the test drug is concluded to be equivalent to the control on average if

$$(\hat\lambda_1 - \hat\lambda_2 - \delta)\left[\frac{\sigma^2(\hat\lambda_1)}{n_1} + \frac{\sigma^2(\hat\lambda_2)}{n_2}\right]^{-1/2} < -z_\alpha$$

and

$$(\hat\lambda_1 - \hat\lambda_2 + \delta)\left[\frac{\sigma^2(\hat\lambda_1)}{n_1} + \frac{\sigma^2(\hat\lambda_2)}{n_2}\right]^{-1/2} > z_\alpha.$$

Under the alternative hypothesis ($|\epsilon| < \delta$), the power of the above testing procedure is approximately

$$2\Phi\left((\delta - |\epsilon|)\left[\frac{\sigma^2(\lambda_1)}{n_1} + \frac{\sigma^2(\lambda_2)}{n_2}\right]^{-1/2} - z_\alpha\right) - 1.$$

As a result, the sample size needed for achieving a power of $1 - \beta$ can be obtained by solving the following equation

$$(\delta - |\epsilon|)\left[\frac{\sigma^2(\lambda_1)}{n_1} + \frac{\sigma^2(\lambda_2)}{n_2}\right]^{-1/2} - z_\alpha = z_{\beta/2}.$$

As a result, the sample size needed for achieving a power of $1 - \beta$ is given by $n_1 = kn_2$ and

$$n_2 = \frac{(z_\alpha + z_{\beta/2})^2}{(\delta - |\epsilon|)^2}\left(\frac{\sigma^2(\lambda_1)}{k} + \sigma^2(\lambda_2)\right). \tag{7.2.6}$$

### 7.2.4 An Example

Suppose that the sponsor is planning a trial among the patients with either Hodgkin's disease (HOD) or non-Hodgkin's lymphoma (NHL). The patients will be given either an allogeneic (allo) transplant from an HLA-matched sibling donor or an autologous (auto) transplant where their own marrow has been cleansed and returned to them after high dose of chemotherapy. The primary objective is to compare the patients with allo or auto transplant in terms of time to leukemia. The trial is planned to last for 3 ($T = 3$) years with 1 year accrual ($T_0 = 1$). Uniform patient entry for both allo and auto transplant groups is assumed ($\gamma = 0$). It is also assumed that the leukemia-free hazard rates for allo and auto transplant are given by 1 ($\lambda_1 = 1$) and 2 ($\lambda_2 = 2$), respectively. According to (7.2.2), the variance function is given by

$$\sigma^2(\lambda_i) = \lambda_i^2 \left(1 + \frac{e^{-\lambda_i T} - e^{-\lambda_i(T-T_0)}}{\lambda_i T_0}\right)^{-1}.$$

**Test for Equality**

Assume that $n = n_1 = n_2$. According to (7.2.4), the sample size needed in order to achieve a 80% ($\beta = 0.2$) power at 0.05 level of significance is

$$n = \frac{(z_{\alpha/2} + z_\beta)^2}{(\lambda_2 - \lambda_1)^2} \left(\frac{\sigma^2(\lambda_1)}{k} + \sigma^2(\lambda_2)\right)$$

$$= \frac{(1.96 + 0.84)^2}{(2-1)^2}(0.97 + 3.94)$$

$$\approx 39.$$

**Test for Superiority**

Assume that $n = n_1 = n_2$ and the superiority margin $\delta = 0.2$. According to (7.2.5), the sample size needed in order to achieve a 80% ($\beta = 0.2$) power at 0.05 level of significance is

$$n = \frac{(z_\alpha + z_\beta)^2}{(\lambda_2 - \lambda_1 - \delta)^2} \left(\frac{\sigma^2(\lambda_1)}{k} + \sigma^2(\lambda_2)\right)$$

$$= \frac{(1.64 + 0.84)^2}{(2 - 1 - 0.2)^2}(0.97 + 3.94)$$

$$\approx 48.$$

**Test for Equivalence**

Assume that $n = n_1 = n_2$, $\lambda_1 = \lambda_2 = 1$, and the equivalence margin is 0.5 ($\delta = 0.5$). According to (7.2.6), the sample size needed in order to achieve

## 7.2. Exponential Model

a 80% ($\beta = 0.2$) power at 0.05 level of significance is

$$n = \frac{(z_\alpha + z_{\beta/2})^2}{\delta^2} \left( \frac{\sigma^2(\lambda_1)}{k} + \sigma^2(\lambda_2) \right)$$
$$= \frac{(1.64 + 1.28)^2}{(0.5 - 0)^2}(0.97 + 0.97)$$
$$\approx 67.$$

### 7.2.5 Remarks

**Unconditional Versus Conditional**

According to Lachin (1981), for testing equality of hazard rates based on exponential model, there exists another way to construct the test statistic other than (7.2.3). More specifically, the testing procedure can be modified to reject the null hypothesis if

$$\left| (\hat{\lambda}_1 - \hat{\lambda}_2) \left[ \sigma^2(\hat{\bar{\lambda}}) \left( \frac{1}{n_1} + \frac{1}{n_2} \right) \right]^{-1/2} \right| > z_{\alpha/2}, \quad (7.2.7)$$

where

$$\hat{\bar{\lambda}} = \frac{n_1 \hat{\lambda}_1 + n_2 \hat{\lambda}_2}{n_1 + n_2}.$$

As it can be seen, (7.2.7) is very similar to (7.2.3) except using a different estimate for the variance of $\hat{\lambda}_1 - \hat{\lambda}_2$. The difference is that the variance estimate used in (7.2.3) is the MLE without constraint while the variance estimate used in (7.2.7) is a pooled estimate of $\hat{\lambda}_1 - \hat{\lambda}_2$, which is consistent conditional on $H_0$. We refer to (7.2.3) as the unconditional method and (7.2.7) conditional method. In practice, which method (unconditional/conditional) should be used to test equality is always a dilemma because one is not necessarily always more powerful than the other under the alternative hypothesis. However, it is difficult to generalize the conditional method to test non-inferiority/superiority and equivalence because the MLE under $H_0$ is difficult to find. Although both unconditional and conditional methods have asymptotic size $\alpha$ under the null hypothesis, the powers under the alternative hypothesis are not equal to each other. Hence, the sample size formula for (7.2.7) is different from the sample size formula for (7.2.3). For the purpose of completeness, it is derived below.

Under the alternative hypothesis ($\epsilon \neq 0$), the power of (7.2.7) is approximately

$$\Phi \left( \left[ |\epsilon| - \left[ \sigma^2(\bar{\lambda})(\frac{1}{n_1} + \frac{1}{n_2}) \right] z_{\alpha/2} \right] \left[ \frac{\sigma^2(\lambda_1)}{n_1} + \frac{\sigma^2(\lambda_2)}{n_2} \right]^{-1/2} \right),$$

where
$$\bar{\lambda} = \frac{n_1\lambda_1 + n_2\lambda_2}{n_1 + n_2}.$$

Hence the sample size needed in order to achieve a power of $1 - \beta$ can be achieved by solving

$$\left[|\epsilon| - \left[\sigma^2(\bar{\lambda})(\frac{1}{n_1} + \frac{1}{n_2})\right]z_{\alpha/2}\right]\left[\frac{\sigma^2(\lambda_1)}{n_1} + \frac{\sigma^2(\lambda_2)}{n_2}\right]^{-1/2} = z_\beta.$$

Under the assumption that $n_1 = \kappa n_2$, it implies that

$$n_2 = \frac{1}{\epsilon^2}\left[z_{\alpha/2}\sigma^2(\bar{\lambda})(\frac{1}{k} + 1) + z_\beta\left(\frac{\sigma(\lambda_1)}{k} + \sigma^2(\lambda_2)\right)^{1/2}\right]^2, \quad (7.2.8)$$

where
$$\bar{\lambda} = \frac{k\lambda_1 + \lambda_2}{k+1}.$$

**Losses to Follow-up, Dropout, and Noncompliance**

If we further assume that the losses are exponentially distributed with loss hazard rate $\eta_i$ in the $i$th treatment group, it has been shown by Lachin and Foulkes (1986) that variance of $\hat{\lambda}_i$ is given by

$$\sigma^2(\lambda_i, \eta_i, \gamma_i) = \lambda_i^2\left(\frac{\lambda_i}{\lambda_i + \eta_i} + \frac{\lambda_i\gamma_i e^{-(\lambda_i+\eta_i)T}\left[1 - e^{(\lambda_i+\eta_i-\gamma_i)T_0}\right]}{(1 - e^{-\gamma_i T_0})(\lambda_i + \eta_i)(\lambda_i + \eta_i - \gamma_i)}\right)^{-1}.$$

In such a situation, an appropriate test statistic can be constructed by replacing $\sigma(\hat{\lambda}_i)$ and $\sigma(\hat{\bar{\lambda}})$ by $\sigma(\hat{\lambda}_i, \hat{\eta}_i, \hat{\gamma}_i)$ and $\sigma(\hat{\bar{\lambda}}_i, \hat{\bar{\eta}}_i, \hat{\bar{\gamma}}_i)$, respectively, where $\hat{\eta}_i$ and $\hat{\gamma}_i$ are the MLE of $\eta_i$ and $\gamma_i$, respectively, and

$$\hat{\bar{\eta}}_i = \frac{n_1\hat{\eta}_1 + n_2\hat{\eta}_2}{n_1 + n_2} \text{ and } \hat{\bar{\gamma}}_i = \frac{n_1\hat{\gamma}_1 + n_2\hat{\gamma}_2}{n_1 + n_2}.$$

Hence, appropriate sample size calculation formulas can be obtained by replaing $\sigma(\lambda_i)$, $\sigma(\bar{\lambda})$ by $\sigma(\lambda_i, \eta_i, \gamma_i)$ and $\sigma(\bar{\lambda}, \bar{\eta}, \bar{\gamma})$, respectively, where

$$\bar{\eta}_i = \frac{n_1\eta_1 + n_2\eta_2}{n_1 + n_2} \text{ and } \bar{\gamma}_i = \frac{n_1\gamma_1 + n_2\gamma_2}{n_1 + n_2}.$$

## 7.3 Cox's Proportional Hazards Model

The most commonly used regression model in survival analysis is Cox's proportional hazards model. Let $t_i$ be the time-to-event for the $i$th subject

## 7.3. Cox's Proportional Hazards Model

and $C_i$ be the corresponding censoring time. Besides $t_i$ and $C_i$, each subject also provides a $p$-dimension column vector of covariates denoted by $z_i$. The most commonly encountered covariates include treatment indicator, demographical information, medical history, etc. Let $h(t|z)$ be the hazard rate at time $t$ for an individual with covariate vector $z$. Cox's proportional hazard model assumes

$$h(t|z) = h(t|0)e^{b'z},$$

where $b$, the coefficient vector with the same dimension as $z$, can be estimated by maximing the following partial likelihood function

$$L(b) = \prod_{i=1}^{d} \frac{e^{b'z_{(i)}}}{\sum_{j \in R_i} e^{b'z_j}},$$

the product is over all the observed deaths, $z_{(i)}$ is the covariate vector associated with the $i$th observed death, and $R_i$ is the set of individuals at risk just prior the $i$th observed death. Maximizing $L$ is equivalent to solving $U(b) = 0$, where

$$U(b) = \sum_{i=1}^{d} z_{(i)} - \sum_{i=1}^{d} \frac{\sum_{j \in R_i} z_j e^{b'z_j}}{\sum_{j \in R_i} e^{b'z_j}}. \tag{7.3.1}$$

The corresponding information matrix is given by $I(b)$ with the $(a,b)$th element given by

$$I(b) = \sum_{i=1}^{d} \frac{\sum_{j \in R_i} z_j z_j' e^{b'z_j}}{\sum_{j \in R_i} e^{b'z_j}}$$

$$- \sum_{i=1}^{d} \left( \frac{\sum_{j \in R_i} Z_j e^{b'z_j}}{\sum_{j \in R_i} e^{b'z_j}} \right) \left( \frac{\sum_{j \in R_i} Z_j e^{b'z_j}}{\sum_{j \in R_i} e^{b'z_j}} \right)'. \tag{7.3.2}$$

### 7.3.1 Test for Equality

In practice, it is of interest to test the following hypotheses:

$$H_0 : b = b_0 \quad \text{versus} \quad H_a : b \neq b_0.$$

To test $b = b_0$, the following score statistic proposed by Schoenfeld (1981) is used:

$$\chi^2_{SC} = U(b_0)' I^{-1}(b_0) U(b_0).$$

Under the null hypothesis of $b = b_0$, $\chi^2_{SC}$ is asymptotically distributed as a chi-square random variable with $p$ degrees of freedom. The null hypothesis is rejected if $\chi^2_{SC} > \chi^2_{\alpha,p}$, where $\chi^2_{\alpha,p}$ is the $\alpha$th upper quantile of a chi-square random variable with $p$ degrees of freedom.

The most typical situation in practice is to compare two treatments without adjusting for other covariates. As a result, we consider the indicator as the only covariate ($z_i = 0$: treatment 1; $z_i = 1$: treatment 2). Then, according to (7.3.3) and (7.3.4), it follows that

$$U(b) = d_1 - \sum_{i=1}^{d} \frac{Y_{2i} e^b}{Y_{1i} + Y_{2i} e^b}, \qquad (7.3.3)$$

and

$$I(b) = \sum_{i=1}^{d} \left[ \frac{Y_i e^b}{Y_{1i} + Y_{2i} e^b} - \frac{Y_{2i}^2 e^{2b}}{(Y_{1i} + Y_{2i} e^b)^2} \right] = \sum_{i=1}^{d} \frac{Y_{1i} Y_{2i} e^b}{(Y_{1i} + Y_{2i} e^b)^2}, \qquad (7.3.4)$$

where $Y_{ij}$ denotes the number of subjects at risk just prior the $i$th observed event and $i = 1, 2$. In order to test for equality of two survival curves, the following hypotheses are usually considered:

$$H_0 : b = 0 \quad \text{versus} \quad H_a : b \neq 0.$$

Under the null hypothesis, we have

$$U(b) = d_1 - \sum_{i=1}^{d} \frac{Y_{2i}}{Y_{1i} + Y_{2i}},$$

and

$$I(b) = \sum_{i=1}^{d} \left[ \frac{Y_{2i}}{Y_{1i} + Y_{2i}} - \frac{Y_{2i}^2}{(Y_{1i} + Y_{2i})^2} \right] = \sum_{i=1}^{d} \frac{Y_{2i} Y_{1i}}{(Y_{1i} + Y_{2i})^2}.$$

Note that the score test statistic $\chi^2_{SC} = U(0)^2 / I(0)$ reduces to the following log-rank test statistic for two-sample problem:

$$L = \frac{\sum_{k=1}^{d} \left( I_k - \frac{Y_{1i}}{Y_{1i} + Y_{2i}} \right)}{\left[ \sum_{k=1}^{d} \left( \frac{Y_{1i} Y_{2i}}{(Y_{1i} + Y_{2i})^2} \right) \right]^{-1/2}},$$

where $I_k$ is a binary variable indicating whether the $k$th event is from the first treatment group or not. Thus, we reject the null hypothesis at approximate $\alpha$ level of significance if $L > z_{\alpha/2}$. The formula for sample size calculation introduced below can be viewed as a special case of log-rank test under the assumption of proportional hazard.

Let $p_i$ be the proportion of patients in the $i$th treatment group, $H_i(t)$ be the distribution function of censoring, and $\lambda_i(t)$, $f_i(t)$, and $F_i(t)$ be the hazard, density, and distribution function of survival in group $i$, respectively. Define the functions

$$V(t) = p_1 f_0(t)(1 - H_1(t)) + p_2 f_1(t)(1 - H_2(t)),$$

## 7.3. Cox's Proportional Hazards Model

and
$$\pi(t) = \frac{p_2(1-F_1(t))(1-H_2(t))}{p_1(1-F_0(t))(1-H_1(t)) + p_2(1-F_1(t))(1-H_2(t))}.$$

Then $L$ is asymptotically distributed as a normal random variable with variance 1 and mean given by

$$\frac{n^{1/2} \int_0^\infty \log(\lambda_2(t)/\lambda_1(t))\pi(t)(1-\pi(t))V(t)dt}{\left[\int_0^\infty \pi(t)(1-\pi(t))V(t)dt\right]^{1/2}}. \quad (7.3.5)$$

Under the assumption of proportional hazard, $\log(\lambda_2(t)/\lambda_1(t)) = b$ is a constant. Assume that $H_2(t) = H_1(t)$. Let $d = \int_0^\infty V(t)dt$, which is the probability of observing an event. In practice, mostly commonly $F_1(t) \approx F_0(t)$. In such a situation, it can be noted that $\pi(t) \approx p_2$, then the (7.3.5) becomes

$$b(np_1p_2d)^{1/2}.$$

Therefore, the two-sided sample size formula with significance level $\alpha$ and power $1-\beta$ is given by

$$n = \frac{(z_{\alpha/2} + z_\beta)^2}{b^2 p_1 p_2 d}. \quad (7.3.6)$$

### 7.3.2 Test for Non-Inferiority/Superiority

We still assume that $z_i = 0$ for treatment 1 and $z_i = 1$ for treatment 2. The problem of testing non-inferiority and superiority can be unified by the following hypotheses:

$$H_0 : b \leq \delta \quad \text{versus} \quad H_a : b > \delta,$$

where $\delta$ is the superiority or non-inferiority margin. When $\delta > 0$, the rejection of the null hypothesis indicates superiority over the reference value. When $\delta < 0$, the rejection of the null hypothesis implies non-inferiority against the reference value. When $b = \delta$, the test statistic

$$L = \frac{\sum_{k=1}^d \left(I_k - \frac{Y_{1i}e^\delta}{Y_{1i}e^\delta + Y_{2i}}\right)}{\left[\sum_{k=1}^d \left(\frac{Y_{1i}Y_{2i}e^\delta}{(Y_{1i}e^\delta + Y_{2i})^2}\right)\right]^{-1/2}}$$

follows a standard normal distribution when the sample size is sufficiently large. Hence, the null hypothesis should be rejected if $L > z_\alpha$. Under the alternative hypothesis, $L$ is asymptotically distributed as a normal random variable with variance 1 and mean given by

$$\frac{n^{1/2} \int_0^\infty (\log(\lambda_2(t)/\lambda_1(t)) - \delta)\pi(t)(1-\pi(t))V(t)dt}{\left[\int_0^\infty \pi(t)(1-\pi(t))V(t)dt\right]^{1/2}}. \quad (7.3.7)$$

Under the assumption of proportional hazard, $\log(\lambda_2(t)/\lambda_1(t)) = b > \delta$ is a constant. Assume that $H_2(t) = H_1(t)$. Let $d = \int_0^\infty V(t)dt$, which is the probability of observing an event. In practice, mostly commonly $F_1(t) \approx F_0(t)$. In such a situation, it can be noted that $\pi(t) \approx p_2$, then the (7.3.7) becomes
$$(b-\delta)(np_1p_2d)^{1/2}.$$
Therefore, the sample size formula with significance level $\alpha$ and power $1-\beta$ is given by
$$n = \frac{(z_{\alpha/2} + z_\beta)^2}{(b-\delta)^2 p_1 p_2 d}. \quad (7.3.8)$$

### 7.3.3 Test for Equivalence

Assume that $z_i = 0$ for treatment 1 and $z_i = 1$ for treatment 2. To establish equivalence, the following hypotheses are usually considered
$$H_0: |b| \geq \delta \quad \text{versus} \quad H_a: |b| < \delta.$$
The above hypotheses can be tested using two one-sided test procedures. More specifically, the null hypothesis should be rejected if
$$\frac{\sum_{k=1}^d \left( I_k - \frac{Y_{1i} e^\delta}{Y_{1i} e^\delta + Y_{2i}} \right)}{\left[ \sum_{k=1}^d \left( \frac{Y_{1i} Y_{2i} e^\delta}{(Y_{1i} e^\delta + Y_{2i})^2} \right) \right]^{-1/2}} < -z_\alpha$$
and
$$\frac{\sum_{k=1}^d \left( I_k - \frac{Y_{1i} e^{-\delta}}{Y_{1i} e^{-\delta} + Y_{2i}} \right)}{\left[ \sum_{k=1}^d \left( \frac{Y_{1i} Y_{2i} e^{-\delta}}{(Y_{1i} e^{-\delta} + Y_{2i})^2} \right) \right]^{-1/2}} > z_\alpha.$$
The power of the above procedure is approximately
$$2\Phi((\delta - |b|)\sqrt{np_1p_2d} - z_\alpha) - 1.$$
Hence, the sample size needed in order to achieve a power of $1-\beta$ at $\alpha$ level of significance is given by
$$n = \frac{(z_\alpha + z_{\beta/2})^2}{(\delta - |b|)^2 p_1 p_2 d}. \quad (7.3.9)$$

### 7.3.4 An Example

Infection of a burn wound is a common complication resulting in extended hospital stays and in the death of severely burned patients. One of the important components of burn management is to prevent or delay the infection. Suppose an investigator is interested in conducting a trial to compare a new therapy with a routine bathing care method in terms of the time-to-infection. Assume that a hazard ratio of 2 (routine bathing care/test therapy) is considered of clinical importance ($b = \log(2)$). It is further assumed that about 80% of patients' infection may be observed during the trial period. Let $n = n_1 = n_2$ ($p_1 = p_2 = 0.5$).

**Test for Equality**

According to (7.3.6), the sample size per treatment group needed to achieve a power of 80% ($\beta = 0.2$) at the 5% level of significance ($\alpha = 0.05$) is given by

$$n = \frac{(z_{\alpha/2} + z_\beta)^2}{b^2 p_1 p_2 d} = \frac{(1.96 + 0.84)^2}{\log^2(2) \times 0.5 \times 0.5 \times 0.8} \approx 82.$$

**Test for Superiority**

Assume that the superiority margin is 0.3 ($\delta = 0.3$). By (7.3.8), the sample size per treatment group needed for achieving an 80% ($\beta = 0.2$) power at the 5% level of significance ($\alpha = 0.05$) is given by

$$n = \frac{(z_\alpha + z_\beta)^2}{(b-\delta)^2 p_1 p_2 d} = \frac{(1.64 + 0.84)^2}{(\log(2) - 0.3)^2 \times 0.5 \times 0.5 \times 0.8} \approx 200.$$

**Test for Equivalence**

Assume that the equivalence limit is 0.5 (i.e., $\delta = 0.5$) and $b = 0$. Then, by (7.3.9), the sample size per treatment group required in order to achieve an 80% power ($\beta = 0.2$) at the 5% level of significance ($\alpha = 0.05$) is given by

$$n = \frac{(z_\alpha + z_{\beta/2})^2}{(\delta - |b|)^2 p_1 p_2 d} = \frac{(1.64 + 1.28)^2}{(0.5 - 0.0)^2 \times 0.5 \times 0.5 \times 0.8} \approx 171.$$

## 7.4 Weighted Log-Rank Test

When the time-to-event is not exponentially distributed and the assumption of proportional hazard does not hold, the treatment effects are usually evaluated by comparing survival curves ($S_i(t)$). To test whether there is a difference between the true survival curves, the following hypotheses are usually considered:

$$H_0 : S_1(t) = S_2(t) \quad \text{versus} \quad H_a : S_1(t) \neq S_2(t).$$

In such a situation, testing non-inferiority/superiority or equivalence is usually difficult to be carried out, because $S_i(t)$ is an infinite dimensional parameter and, hence, how to define noninferiority/superiority and equivalence is not clear. As a result, we provide sample size calculation formula for testing equality only in this section.

## 7.4.1 Tarone-Ware Test

In order to compare two survival curves, weighted log tests are usually considered. The test statistic of weighted log-rank test (the Tarone-Ware statistic) is given by

$$L = \frac{\sum_{i=1}^{d} w_i \left( I_i - \frac{Y_{1i}}{Y_{1i}+Y_{2i}} \right)}{\left[ \sum_{i=1}^{d} w_i^2 \left( \frac{Y_{1i}Y_{2i}}{(Y_{1i}+Y_{2i})^2} \right) \right]^{1/2}},$$

where the sum is over all deaths, $I_i$ is the indicator of the first group, $w_i$ is the $i$th weight, and $Y_{ij}$ is number of subjects at risk just before the $j$th death in the $i$th group. When $w_i = 1$, $L$ becomes the commonly used log-rank statistic. Under the null hypothesis of $H_0 : S_1 = S_2$, $L$ is asymptotically distributed as a standard normal random variable. Hence, we would reject the null hypothesis at approximate $\alpha$ level of siginicance if $|L| > z_{\alpha/2}$.

The sample size calculation formula we are going to introduce in this section was developed by Lakatos (1986, 1988). According to Lakatos' method, the trial period should be first partioned into $N$ equally spaced intervals. Let $d_i$ denote the number of deaths within the $i$th interval. Define $\phi_{i_k}$ to be the ratio of patients in the two treatment groups at risk just prior to the $k$th death in the $i$th interval. The expectation of $L$ under a fixed local alternative can be approximated by

$$E = \frac{\sum_{i=1}^{N} \sum_{k=1}^{d_i} w_{i_k} \left[ \frac{\phi_{i_k}\theta_{i_k}}{1+\phi_{i_k}\theta_{i_k}} - \frac{\phi_{i_k}}{1+\phi_{i_k}} \right]}{\left[ \sum_{i=1}^{N} \sum_{k=1}^{d_i} \frac{w_{i_k}^2 \phi_{i_k}}{(1+\phi_{i_k})^2} \right]^{1/2}}, \qquad (7.4.1)$$

where the right summation of the each double summation is over the $d_i$ deaths in the $i$th interval, and the left summation is over the $N$ intervals that partition the trial period. Treating this statistic as $N(E, 1)$, the sample size needed in order to achieve a power of $1 - \beta$ can be obtained by solving

$$E = z_{\alpha/2} + z_\beta.$$

When $N$ is sufficiently large, we can assume that $\phi_{i_k} = \phi_i$ and $w_{i_k} = w_i$ for all $k$ in the $i$th interval. Let $\rho_i = d_i/d$, where $d = \sum d_i$. Then, $E$ can be written as

$$E = e(D)\sqrt{d},$$

## 7.4. Weighted Log-Rank Test

where

$$e(D) = \frac{\sum_{i=1}^{N} w_i \rho_i \gamma_i}{\left(\sum_{i=1}^{N} w_i^2 \rho_i \eta_i\right)^{1/2}},$$

$$\gamma_i = \frac{\phi_i \theta_i}{1 + \phi_i \theta_i} - \frac{\phi_i}{1 + \phi_i}, \quad (7.4.2)$$

and

$$\eta_i = \frac{\phi_i}{(1 + \phi_i)^2}. \quad (7.4.3)$$

It follows that

$$d = \frac{(z_{\alpha/2} + z_\beta)^2 \left(\sum_{i=1}^{N} w_i^2 \rho_i \eta_i\right)}{\left(\sum_{i=1}^{N} w_i \rho_i \gamma_i\right)^2}. \quad (7.4.4)$$

Let $n_i$ denote the sample size in the $i$th treatment group. Under the assumption that $n = n_1 = n_2$, the sample sized needed to achieve a power of $1 - \beta$ is given by

$$n = \frac{2d}{p_1 + p_2},$$

where $p_i$ is the cumulative event rates for the $i$th treatment group.

### 7.4.2 An Example

To illustrate the method described above, the example given in Lakatos (1988) is considered. In order to carry out Lakatos' method, we need to first partition the trial period into $N$ equal length intervals. Then, parameters like $\gamma_i$, $\eta_i$, $\rho_i$, $\theta_i$, and $\phi_i$ need to be specified. There are two ways we can specify them. One is directly specify them for each interval or estimate them from a pilot study. Then the whole procedure becomes relatively easy. However, some times only yearly rates are given for the necessary parameters. Then we need to calculate all those parameters by ourselves.

For example, consider a two-year cardiovascular trial. It is assumed that the yearly hazard rates in treatment group ($i = 1$) and control group ($i = 2$) are given by 1 and 0.5, respectively. Hence, the yearly event rates in the two treatment groups are given by $1 - e^{-1} = 63.2\%$ and $1 - e^{-0.5} = 39.3\%$, respectively. It is also assumed that the yearly loss to follow-up and non-compliance rates are 3% and 4%, respectively. The rate at which patients assigned to control begin taking a medication with an efficacy similar to the experimental treatment is called "drop-in." In cardiovascular trials, drop-ins often occur when the private physician of a patient assigned to control detects the condition of interest, such as hypertension, and prescribes treatment. In this example, it is assumed that the yearly drop-in rate is 5%. Assume that the patient's status follows a Markov chain with four possible states, i.e., lost to follow-up, event, active in treatment, and active in control, which are denoted by $L$, $E$, $A_E$ and $A_C$, respectively. Then, the yearly transition matrix of this Markov chain is given by

$$T = \begin{bmatrix} 1 & 0 & 0.03 & 0.03 \\ 0 & 1 & 0.3935 & 0.6321 \\ 0 & 0 & 1-\Sigma & 0.05 \\ 0 & 0 & 0.04 & 1-\Sigma \end{bmatrix}.$$

Entries denoted by $1 - \Sigma$ represent 1 minus the sum of the remainder of the column. Assume, however, we want to partition the 2-year period into 20 equal length intervals. Then we need the transition matrix within each interval. It can be obtained by replacing each off-diagonal entry $x$ in $T$ by $1 - (1-x)^{1/K}$. The resulting transition matrix is given by

$$T_{1/20} = \begin{bmatrix} 1.0000 & 0.0000 & 0.0030 & 0.0030 \\ 0.0000 & 1.0000 & 0.0951 & 0.0488 \\ 0.0000 & 0.0000 & 0.8978 & 0.0051 \\ 0.0000 & 0.0000 & 0.0041 & 0.9431 \end{bmatrix}.$$

Then, the patient distribution at the end of the $i/10$th year is given by $T_{1/20}^i x$, where $x$ is a four-dimension vector indicating the initial distribution of patients. So, for treatment group, $x = (0,0,1,0)'$ indicating that at the begining of the trial all patients active in treatment. Similarly, for control, $x = (0,0,0,1)$. For illustration purpose, consider at the time point 0.3 year, the patient distribution for the treatment group is given by

$$\begin{bmatrix} 1.0000 & 0.0000 & 0.0030 & 0.0030 \\ 0.0000 & 1.0000 & 0.0951 & 0.0488 \\ 0.0000 & 0.0000 & 0.8978 & 0.0051 \\ 0.0000 & 0.0000 & 0.0041 & 0.9431 \end{bmatrix}^3 \begin{pmatrix} 0 \\ 0 \\ 1 \\ 0 \end{pmatrix} = \begin{pmatrix} 0.0081 \\ 0.2577 \\ 0.7237 \\ 0.0104 \end{pmatrix}.$$

This indicates by the time of 0.3 year, we may expect 0.81% of patients were lossed to follow-up, 25.77% experienced events, 72.37% were still active in treatment, and 1.04% switched to some other medication with similar effects as control (noncompliance). Hence, this vector becomes the third row and first four columns of Table 7.4.1. Similary, we can produce all the rows for the first eight columns in Table 7.4.1.

Assuming equal allocation of patients across treatment groups, we have $\phi = 1$ when $t_i = 0.1$, which means just before time point $t_i = 0.1$, the ratio of patients at risk between treatment groups is 1. When $t_i = 0.2$, the patients at risk just prior to $t_i = 0.2$ in control groups are the patients still

## 7.4. Weighted Log-Rank Test

Table 7.4.1: Sample Size Calculation by Lakatos' Method

| $t_i$ | $\gamma$ | $\eta$ | $\rho$ | $\theta$ | $\phi$ | | $L$ | $E$ | $A_C$ | $A_E$ |
|---|---|---|---|---|---|---|---|---|---|---|
| 0.1 | 0.167 | 0.250 | 0.098 | 2.000 | 1.000 | $C$ | 0.003 | 0.095 | 0.897 | 0.005 |
| | | | | | | $E$ | 0.003 | 0.049 | 0.944 | 0.004 |
| 0.2 | 0.166 | 0.250 | 0.090 | 1.986 | 0.951 | $C$ | 0.006 | 0.181 | 0.804 | 0.009 |
| | | | | | | $E$ | 0.006 | 0.095 | 0.891 | 0.007 |
| 0.3 | 0.166 | 0.249 | 0.083 | 1.972 | 0.905 | $C$ | 0.008 | 0.258 | 0.721 | 0.013 |
| | | | | | | $E$ | 0.009 | 0.139 | 0.842 | 0.010 |
| 0.4 | 0.165 | 0.249 | 0.076 | 1.959 | 0.862 | $C$ | 0.010 | 0.327 | 0.647 | 0.016 |
| | | | | | | $E$ | 0.011 | 0.181 | 0.795 | 0.013 |
| 0.5 | 0.164 | 0.248 | 0.070 | 1.945 | 0.821 | $C$ | 0.013 | 0.389 | 0.580 | 0.018 |
| | | | | | | $E$ | 0.014 | 0.221 | 0.750 | 0.015 |
| 0.6 | 0.163 | 0.246 | 0.064 | 1.932 | 0.782 | $C$ | 0.014 | 0.445 | 0.520 | 0.020 |
| | | | | | | $E$ | 0.016 | 0.259 | 0.708 | 0.016 |
| 0.7 | 0.162 | 0.245 | 0.059 | 1.920 | 0.746 | $C$ | 0.016 | 0.496 | 0.466 | 0.022 |
| | | | | | | $E$ | 0.018 | 0.295 | 0.669 | 0.017 |
| 0.8 | 0.160 | 0.243 | 0.054 | 1.907 | 0.711 | $C$ | 0.017 | 0.541 | 0.418 | 0.023 |
| | | | | | | $E$ | 0.020 | 0.330 | 0.632 | 0.018 |
| 0.9 | 0.158 | 0.241 | 0.050 | 1.894 | 0.679 | $C$ | 0.019 | 0.582 | 0.375 | 0.024 |
| | | | | | | $E$ | 0.022 | 0.362 | 0.596 | 0.019 |
| 1.0 | 0.156 | 0.239 | 0.046 | 1.882 | 0.648 | $C$ | 0.020 | 0.619 | 0.336 | 0.024 |
| | | | | | | $E$ | 0.024 | 0.393 | 0.563 | 0.019 |
| 1.1 | 0.154 | 0.236 | 0.043 | 1.870 | 0.619 | $C$ | 0.021 | 0.652 | 0.302 | 0.025 |
| | | | | | | $E$ | 0.026 | 0.423 | 0.532 | 0.020 |
| 1.2 | 0.152 | 0.234 | 0.039 | 1.857 | 0.592 | $C$ | 0.022 | 0.682 | 0.271 | 0.025 |
| | | | | | | $E$ | 0.028 | 0.450 | 0.502 | 0.020 |
| 1.3 | 0.149 | 0.231 | 0.036 | 1.845 | 0.566 | $C$ | 0.023 | 0.709 | 0.243 | 0.025 |
| | | | | | | $E$ | 0.029 | 0.477 | 0.474 | 0.020 |
| 1.4 | 0.147 | 0.228 | 0.034 | 1.833 | 0.542 | $C$ | 0.024 | 0.734 | 0.218 | 0.025 |
| | | | | | | $E$ | 0.031 | 0.502 | 0.448 | 0.020 |
| 1.5 | 0.144 | 0.225 | 0.031 | 1.820 | 0.519 | $C$ | 0.025 | 0.755 | 0.195 | 0.025 |
| | | | | | | $E$ | 0.032 | 0.525 | 0.423 | 0.020 |
| 1.6 | 0.141 | 0.222 | 0.029 | 1.808 | 0.497 | $C$ | 0.025 | 0.775 | 0.175 | 0.024 |
| | | | | | | $E$ | 0.033 | 0.548 | 0.399 | 0.019 |
| 1.7 | 0.138 | 0.219 | 0.027 | 1.796 | 0.477 | $C$ | 0.026 | 0.793 | 0.157 | 0.024 |
| | | | | | | $E$ | 0.035 | 0.569 | 0.377 | 0.019 |
| 1.8 | 0.135 | 0.215 | 0.025 | 1.783 | 0.457 | $C$ | 0.026 | 0.809 | 0.141 | 0.023 |
| | | | | | | $E$ | 0.036 | 0.589 | 0.356 | 0.018 |
| 1.9 | 0.132 | 0.212 | 0.023 | 1.771 | 0.439 | $C$ | 0.027 | 0.824 | 0.127 | 0.023 |
| | | | | | | $E$ | 0.037 | 0.609 | 0.336 | 0.018 |
| 2.0 | 0.129 | 0.209 | 0.021 | 1.758 | 0.421 | $C$ | 0.027 | 0.837 | 0.114 | 0.022 |
| | | | | | | $E$ | 0.038 | 0.627 | 0.318 | 0.018 |

$C$ : Control
$E$ : Experimental

active $(A_C + A_E)$ in control group, which is given by $0.897 + 0.005 = 0.902$. Similarly, the patients at risk in experimental group just prior to $t = 0.1$ is given by $0.944 + 0.004 = 0.948$. Hence, at $t_i = 0.2$, the value of $\phi$ can be determined by $\phi = 0.902/0.948 = 0.951$. Similarly, the values of $\phi$ at other time points can be calculated. Once $\phi$ is obtained, the value of $\eta$ can be calculated according to formula (7.4.3).

In the next step, we need to calculate $\theta$, which needs specification of hazard rates within each interval. First, we know before $t = 0.1$, all patients in control group staying active in treatment $(A_E)$ and all patients in the experimental group staying active in control $(A_C)$. According to our assumption, the hazard rates for the two groups are given by 1 and 0.5, respectively. Hence, $\theta = 2$. When $t = 0.2$, we know in the control group the proportion of patients experienced events is $0.181 - 0.095 = 0.086$. Hence the hazard rate can be obtained by $\log(1-0.086)/0.1$. Similarly, the hazard rate in the experimental groups is given by $\log(1 - (0.095 - 0.049))/0.1 = \log(1 - 0.046)/0.1$. Hence, the value of $\theta$ is given by $\log(1 - 0.086)/log(1 - 0.046) = 1.986$. The value of $\theta$ at other time points can be obtained similarly.

Finally, we need to calculate $\rho_i$. First, we can notice that the total events for the control and experimental groups are given by 0.837 and 0.627, respectively. The events experienced in the first interval ($t_i = 0.1$) for the two groups are given by 0.095 and 0.049, respectively. Hence, the value of $\rho$ when $t_i = 0.1$ is given by $(0.095+0.049)/(0.837+0.627) = 0.098$. When $t_i = 0.2$, the event experienced in control is given by $0.181 - 0.095 = 0.096$. The event experienced in experimental groups is given by $0.095 - 0.049 = 0.046$. Hence, the value of $\rho$ can be obtained by $(0.086 + 0.046)/(0.837 + 0.627) = 0.090$. The value of $\rho$ at other time points can be obtained similarly.

Due to rounding error, the readers may not be able to reproduce exactly the same number of the derived parameters ($\gamma$, $\eta$, $\rho$, $\theta$, $\phi$) as us by performing appropriate operation on the first eight columns in Table 7.4.1. However, by keeping enough decimal digits and following our instructions given above, one should be able to reproduce exactly the same number as us.

Once all the derived parameters are specified, we can caculate the desired number of events according to (7.4.4), which gives $d = 101.684 = 102$. On the other hand, we can notice that the overall event rate for control group is $P_C = 0.837$ and for experimental groups is $P_E = 0.627$. Hence, the total sample size needed is given by

$$n = \frac{2d}{P_E + P_C} = \frac{2 \times 102}{0.837 + 0.627} = 138.947 \approx 139.$$

## 7.5 Practical Issues

### 7.5.1 Binomial Versus Time-to-Event

In clinical trials, it is not common to define the so-called responder based on the study endpoints. For example, in cancer trials, we may define a subject as a responder based on his/her time to disease progression. We can then perform an analysis based on the response rate to evaluate the treatment effect. This analysis reduces to a two-sample problem for comparing proportions as described in the previous chapters. However, it should be noted that the analysis using the response rate, which is defined based on the time-to-event data, is not as efficient as the analysis using the time-to-event data, expecially when the underlying distribution for the time-to-event satisfies the exponential model or Cox's proportional hazards model.

### 7.5.2 Local Alternative Versus Fixed Alternative

The sample size calculation formulas for both Cox's proportional hazards model or exponential model are all based on the so-called local alternatives (see, Fleming and Harrington, 1991), which implies that the difference between treatment groups in terms of the parameters of interest (e.g., hazard function or survival function) decrease to 0 at the rate of $1/\sqrt{n}$, where $n$ is the total sample size. In practice, this is a dilemma because the alternative hypothesis is always fixed, which does not change as the sample size changes. However, the sample size estimation for Cox's proportional hazard model and the weighted log-rank test are derived based on local alternatives. As a result, further research in sample size estimation based on a fixed alternative is an interesting but challenging topic for statisticians in the pharmaceutical industry.

### 7.5.3 One-Sample Versus Historical Control

Historical control is often considered in survival analysis when the clinical trial involves only the test treatment. In practice, two approaches are commonly employed. First, it is to treat the parameters estimated from historical control (e.g., hazard rate, survival function, median survival time, etc.) as fixed reference (true) values. Then, the objective of the study is to compare the corresponding parameters of the test treatment with the reference values. This is analogous to the one-sample problem discussed in the previous chapters. Under the assumption that the time-to-event is exponentially distributed, formulas can be similarly derived. Another approach is to utilize the whole sample from the historical study. Then, the standard testing procedure (e.g., log-rank test) will be used to assess the treatment effects. Some discussion on sample size determination for this approach can be found in Emrich (1989) and Dixon and Simon (1988).

# Chapter 8

# Group Sequential Methods

Most clinical trials are longitudinal in nature. In practice, it is almost impossible to enroll and randomize all required subjects at the same time. Clinical data are accumulated sequentially over time. As a result, it is of interest to monitor the information for management of the study. In addition, it is of particular interest to obtain early evidence regarding efficacy, safety, and benefit/risk of the test drug under investigation for a possible early termination. Thus, it is not uncommon to employ a group sequential design with a number of planned interim analyses in a clinical trial. The rationale for interim analyses of accumulating data in clinical trials with group sequential designs have been well documented in the Greenberg Report (Heart Special Project Committee, 1988) more than three decades ago. Since then, the development of statistical methodology and decision processes for implementation of data monitoring and interim analyses for early termination has attracted a lot of attention from academia, the pharmaceutical industry, and health authorities (see, e.g., Jennison and Turnbull, 2000).

Sections 8.1-8.4 introduce Pocock's test, O'Brien and Fleming's test, Wang and Tsiatis' test, and the inner wedge test for clinical trials with group sequential designs, respectively. Also included in these sections are the corresponding procedures for sample size calculation. The application of these tests to discrete study endpoints such as binary responses and time-to-event data are discussed in Sections 8.5 and 8.6, respectively. In Section 8.7, the concept of alpha spending function in group sequential methods is outlined. Procedures for sample size re-estimation at a given interim analysis without unblinding are examined in Section 8.8. In Section

8.9, conditional powers at interim analyses are derived for the cases when comparing means and proportions. Some practical issues are discussed in the last section.

## 8.1 Pocock's Test

In clinical trials, a commonly employed statistical test for a group sequential design with a number of interim analyses is to analyze accumulating data at each interim analysis. This kind of test is referred to as a repeated significance test (Jennison and Turnbull, 2000). In this section, we introduce Pocock's test and the corresponding sample size calculation formula.

### 8.1.1 The Procedure

Pocock (1977) suggested performing a test at a constant nominal level to analyze accumulating data at each interim analysis over the course of the intended clinical trial. Suppose that the investigator is interested in conducting a clinical trial for comparing two treatment groups under a group sequential design with $K$ planned interim analyses. Let $x_{ij}$ be the observation from the $j$th subject in the $i$th treatment group, $i = 1, 2; j = 1, ..., n$. For a fixed $i$, it is assumed that $x_{ij}$'s are independent and identically distributed normal random variables with mean $\mu_i$ and variance $\sigma_i^2$. Denote by $n_k$ the information (or the number of subjects) accumulated at the $k$th ($k = 1, ..., K$) interim analysis. For simplicity, we further assume that at each interim analysis, the numbers of subjects accumulated in each treatment group are the same. Note that in practice, this assumption may not hold. How to deal with unequal numbers of subjects accumulated in each treatment group is challenging to clinical scientists. One solution to this problem is using Lan and DeMets' alpha spending function, which is discussed in Section 8.7.1. At each interim analysis, the following test statistic is usually calculated

$$Z_k = \frac{1}{\sqrt{n_k(\sigma_1^2 + \sigma_2^2)}} \left( \sum_{j=1}^{n_k} x_{1j} - \sum_{j=1}^{n_k} x_{2j} \right), \quad k = 1, ..., K.$$

Note that $\sigma_i^2$ is usually unknown and it is usually estimated by the data available up to the point of the interim analysis. At each interim analysis, $\sigma_i^2$ is usually replaced with its estimates. Denote by $C_P(K, \alpha)$ the critical value for having an overall type I error rate of $\alpha$. Pocock's test can be summarized as follows (see also Jennison and Turnbull, 2000):

## 8.1. Pocock's Test

(1) After group $k = 1, ..., K-1$,
   - if $|Z_k| > C_P(K, \alpha)$ then stop, reject $H_0$;
   - otherwise continue to group $k+1$.

(2) After group $K$,
   - if $|Z_K| > C_P(K, \alpha)$ then stop, rejct $H_0$;
   - otherwise stop, accept $H_0$.

As an example, one Pocock type boundary for the standardized test statistic is plotted in Figure 8.1.1.

As it can be seen that the critical value $C_P(K, \alpha)$ only depends upon the type I error $(\alpha)$ and the total number of planned interim analysis $(K)$, which is independent of the visit number $(k)$. In other words, for each planned interim analysis, the same critical value is used for comparing treatment difference using the standard test statistic $Z_k$. The value of $C_P(K, \alpha)$ is choosing in such a way that the above test procedure has an overall type I error rate of $\alpha$ under the null hypothesis that $\mu_1 - \mu_2 = 0$. Since there exists no explicit formula for calculation of $C_P(K, \alpha)$, a selection of various values of $C_P(K, \alpha)$ under different choices of parameters ($K$ and $\alpha$) is given in Table 8.1.1.

Table 8.1.1: $C_P(K, \alpha)$ for Two-Sided Tests with $K$ Interim Analyses

| $K$ | $\alpha = 0.01$ | $\alpha = 0.05$ | $\alpha = 0.10$ |
|---|---|---|---|
| 1  | 2.576 | 1.960 | 1.645 |
| 2  | 2.772 | 2.178 | 1.875 |
| 3  | 2.873 | 2.289 | 1.992 |
| 4  | 2.939 | 2.361 | 2.067 |
| 5  | 2.986 | 2.413 | 2.122 |
| 6  | 3.023 | 2.453 | 2.164 |
| 7  | 3.053 | 2.485 | 2.197 |
| 8  | 3.078 | 2.512 | 2.225 |
| 9  | 3.099 | 2.535 | 2.249 |
| 10 | 3.117 | 2.555 | 2.270 |
| 11 | 3.133 | 2.572 | 2.288 |
| 12 | 3.147 | 2.588 | 2.304 |
| 15 | 3.182 | 2.626 | 2.344 |
| 20 | 3.225 | 2.672 | 2.392 |

Figure 8.1.1: Pocock Type Stopping Rule

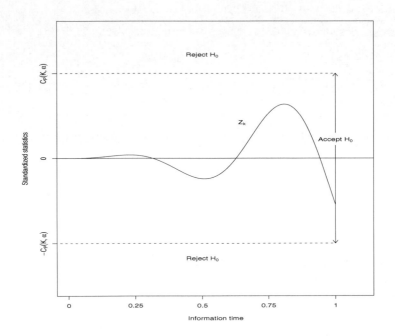

On the other hand, under the alternative hypothesis (i.e., $\theta \neq 0$), the power of the above test procedure can be determined by the total number of planned interim analysis ($K$), type I error rate ($\alpha$), and type II error rate ($\beta$), and the proportion between $\sigma^2$ and $\delta^2$ (i.e., $\sigma^2/\delta^2$), where $\delta = |\mu_1 - \mu_2|$. As discussed in the previous chapters, if there are no interim analyses planned (i.e., $K = 1$), then the sample size is proportional to $\sigma^2/\delta^2$. As a result, it is sufficient to specify the ratio $R_P(K, \alpha, \beta)$ of the maximum sample size of the group sequential test to the fixed sample size. The values of $R_P(K, \alpha, \beta)$ are given in Table 8.1.2. The maximum sample size needed for a group sequential trial with $K$ interim analyses can be obtained by first calculating the fixed sample size without interim analyses, and then multiplying it by $R_P(K, \alpha, \beta)$.

## 8.1.2 An Example

Suppose that an investigator is interested in conducting a clinical trial with 5 interim analyses for comparing a test drug (T) with a placebo (P). Based on information obtained from a pilot study, data from the test drug and

## 8.2. O'Brien and Fleming's Test

Table 8.1.2: $R_P(K,\alpha,\beta)$ for Two-Sided Tests with $K$ Interim Analyses

|   | $1-\beta=0.8$ | | | $1-\beta=0.9$ | | |
|---|---|---|---|---|---|---|
| $K$ | $\alpha=0.01$ | $\alpha=0.05$ | $\alpha=0.10$ | $\alpha=0.01$ | $\alpha=0.05$ | $\alpha=0.10$ |
| 1 | 1.000 | 1.000 | 1.000 | 1.000 | 1.000 | 1.000 |
| 2 | 1.092 | 1.110 | 1.121 | 1.084 | 1.100 | 1.110 |
| 3 | 1.137 | 1.166 | 1.184 | 1.125 | 1.151 | 1.166 |
| 4 | 1.166 | 1.202 | 1.224 | 1.152 | 1.183 | 1.202 |
| 5 | 1.187 | 1.229 | 1.254 | 1.170 | 1.207 | 1.228 |
| 6 | 1.203 | 1.249 | 1.277 | 1.185 | 1.225 | 1.249 |
| 7 | 1.216 | 1.265 | 1.296 | 1.197 | 1.239 | 1.266 |
| 8 | 1.226 | 1.279 | 1.311 | 1.206 | 1.252 | 1.280 |
| 9 | 1.236 | 1.291 | 1.325 | 1.215 | 1.262 | 1.292 |
| 10 | 1.243 | 1.301 | 1.337 | 1.222 | 1.271 | 1.302 |
| 11 | 1.250 | 1.310 | 1.348 | 1.228 | 1.279 | 1.312 |
| 12 | 1.257 | 1.318 | 1.357 | 1.234 | 1.287 | 1.320 |
| 15 | 1.272 | 1.338 | 1.381 | 1.248 | 1.305 | 1.341 |
| 20 | 1.291 | 1.363 | 1.411 | 1.264 | 1.327 | 1.367 |

the placebo seem to have a common variance, i.e., $\sigma^2 = \sigma_1^2 = \sigma_2^2 = 4$ with $\mu_T - \mu_P = 1$. Assuming these observed values are true, it is desirable to select a maximum sample size such that there is a 90% $(1-\beta=0.90)$ power for detecting such a difference between the test drug and the placebo at the 5% ($\alpha=0.05$) level of significance.

By the formula for sample size calculation given in Chapter 3, the required fixed sample size when there are no planned interim analyses is

$$n_{\text{fixed}} = \frac{(z_{\alpha/2}+z_\beta)^2(\sigma_1^2+\sigma_2^2)}{(\mu_1-\mu_2)^2} = \frac{(1.96+1.28)^2(4+4)}{1^2} \approx 84.$$

By Table 8.1.2, we have

$$R_P(5, 0.05, 0.1) = 1.207.$$

Hence, the maximum sample size needed for the group sequential trial is given by

$$n_{\max} = R_P(5, 0.05, 0.1)n_{\text{fixed}} = 1.207 \times 84 = 101.4.$$

Hence, it is necessary to have

$$n = n_{\max}/K = 101.4/5 = 20.3 \approx 21$$

subjects per group at each interim analysis.

## 8.2 O'Brien and Fleming's Test

Pocock's test is straightforward and simple. However, it is performed at a constant nominal level. As an alternative to Pocock's test, O'Brien and Fleming (1979) proposed a test, which is also based on the standardized statistics $Z_k$, by increasing the nominal significance level for rejecting $H_0$ at each analysis as the study progresses. As a result, it is difficult to reject the null hypothesis at early stages of the trial.

### 8.2.1 The Procedure

O'Brien and Fleming's test is carried out as follows (see, also Jennison and Turnbull, 2000):

(1) After group $k = 1, \cdots, K - 1$,
   - if $|Z_k| > C_B(K, \alpha)\sqrt{K/k}$ then stop, reject $H_0$;
   - otherwise continue to group $k + 1$.

(2) After group $K$,
   - if $|Z_K| > C_B(K, \alpha)$ then stop, reject $H_0$;
   - otherwise stop, accept $H_0$.

As an example, one O'Brien-Fleming type boundary is plotted in Figure 8.2.2. Note that the value of $C_B(K, \alpha)$ is chosen to ensure that the over type I error rate is $\alpha$. Like $C_P(K, \alpha)$, there exists no closed form for calculating $C_B(K, \alpha)$. For convenience, a selection of various values of $C_B(K, \alpha)$ under different choices of parameters are provided in Table 8.2.1.

Similar to the procedure for sample size calculation for Pocock's method, the maximum sample size needed in order to achieve a desired power at a given level of significance can be obtained by first calculating the sample size needed for a fixed sample size design, and then multiplying by a constant $R_B(K, \alpha, \beta)$. For various parameters, the values of $R_B(K, \alpha, \beta)$ are given in Table 8.2.2.

### 8.2.2 An Example

Consider the example described in Section 8.1.2. Suppose that the investigator wish to perform the same group sequential test using O'Brien and Fleming's test rather than Pocock's test. By Table 8.2.2,

$$R_B(5, 0.05, 0.1) = 1.026.$$

Figure 8.2.2: O'Brien-Fleming Type Stopping Rule

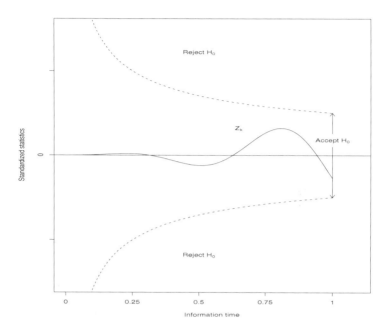

Since the required fixed sample size is given by $n_{\text{fixed}} = 84$, the maximum sample size needed for each treatment group is given by

$$n_{\max} = R_B(5, 0.05, 0.1) n_{\text{fixed}} = 1.026 \times 84 = 86.2 \approx 87.$$

Therefore, $n = n_{\max}/K = 87/5 = 17.4 \approx 18$ subjects per treatment group at each interim analysis is required for achieving a 90% power at the 5% level of significance.

## 8.3 Wang and Tsiatis' Test

In addition to Pocock's test and O'Brien and Fleming's test, Wang and Tsiatis (1987) proposed a family of two-sided tests indiced by the parameter of $\Delta$, which is also based on the standardized test statistic $Z_k$. Wang and Tsiatis' test include Pocock's and O'Brien-Fleming's boundaries as special cases.

Table 8.2.1: $C_B(K, \alpha)$ for Two-Sided Tests with $K$ Interim Analyses

| $K$ | $\alpha = 0.01$ | $\alpha = 0.05$ | $\alpha = 0.10$ |
|---|---|---|---|
| 1 | 2.576 | 1.960 | 1.645 |
| 2 | 2.580 | 1.977 | 1.678 |
| 3 | 2.595 | 2.004 | 1.710 |
| 4 | 2.609 | 2.024 | 1.733 |
| 5 | 2.621 | 2.040 | 1.751 |
| 6 | 2.631 | 2.053 | 1.765 |
| 7 | 2.640 | 2.063 | 1.776 |
| 8 | 2.648 | 2.072 | 1.786 |
| 9 | 2.654 | 2.080 | 1.794 |
| 10 | 1.660 | 2.087 | 1.801 |
| 11 | 2.665 | 2.092 | 1.807 |
| 12 | 2.670 | 2.098 | 1.813 |
| 15 | 2.681 | 2.110 | 1.826 |
| 20 | 2.695 | 2.126 | 1.842 |

Table 8.2.2: $R_B(K, \alpha, \beta)$ for Two-Sided Tests with $K$ Interim Analyses

| | $1 - \beta = 0.8$ | | | $1 - \beta = 0.9$ | | |
|---|---|---|---|---|---|---|
| $K$ | $\alpha = 0.01$ | $\alpha = 0.05$ | $\alpha = 0.10$ | $\alpha = 0.01$ | $\alpha = 0.05$ | $\alpha = 0.10$ |
| 1 | 1.000 | 1.000 | 1.000 | 1.000 | 1.000 | 1.000 |
| 2 | 1.001 | 1.008 | 1.016 | 1.001 | 1.007 | 1.014 |
| 3 | 1.007 | 1.017 | 1.027 | 1.006 | 1.016 | 1.025 |
| 4 | 1.011 | 1.024 | 1.035 | 1.010 | 1.022 | 1.032 |
| 5 | 1.015 | 1.028 | 1.040 | 1.014 | 1.026 | 1.037 |
| 6 | 1.017 | 1.032 | 1.044 | 1.016 | 1.030 | 1.041 |
| 7 | 1.019 | 1.035 | 1.047 | 1.018 | 1.032 | 1.044 |
| 8 | 1.021 | 1.037 | 1.049 | 1.020 | 1.034 | 1.046 |
| 9 | 1.022 | 1.038 | 1.051 | 1.021 | 1.036 | 1.048 |
| 10 | 1.024 | 1.040 | 1.053 | 1.022 | 1.037 | 1.049 |
| 11 | 1.025 | 1.041 | 1.054 | 1.023 | 1.039 | 1.051 |
| 12 | 1.026 | 1.042 | 1.055 | 1.024 | 1.040 | 1.052 |
| 15 | 1.028 | 1.045 | 1.058 | 1.026 | 1.042 | 1.054 |
| 20 | 1.030 | 1.047 | 1.061 | 1.029 | 1.045 | 1.057 |

## 8.3.1 The Procedure

Wang and Tsiatis' test can be summarized as follows (see also Jennison and Turnbull, 2000):

(1) After group $k = 1, \cdots, K - 1$,
   - if $|Z_k| > C_{WT}(K, \alpha, \Delta)(k/K)^{\Delta - 1/2}$ then stop, reject $H_0$;
   - otherwise continue to group $k + 1$.

(2) After group $K$,
   - if $|Z_K| > C_{WT}(K, \alpha, \Delta)$ then stop, reject $H_0$;
   - otherwise stop, accept $H_0$.

As an example, the Wang-Tsiatis type boundary when $\Delta = 0.25$ is given in Figure 8.3.3. As it can be seen that Wang and Tsiatis' test reduces to Pocock's test when $\Delta = 0.5$. When $\Delta = 0$, Wang and Tsiatis' test is the same as O'Brien and Fleming's test. As a result, values of $C_{WT}(K, \alpha, \Delta)$ with $\Delta = 0$ and 0.5 can be obtained from Tables 8.1.1 and 8.2.1. Values of $C_{WT}(K, \alpha, \Delta)$ when $\Delta = 0.1, 0.25$, and 0.4 are given in Table 8.3.1.

Table 8.3.1: $C_{WT}(K, \alpha, \Delta)$ for Two-Sided Tests with $K$ Interim Analyses and $\alpha = 0.05$

| $K$ | $\Delta = 0.10$ | $\Delta = 0.25$ | $\Delta = 0.40$ |
|---|---|---|---|
| 1 | 1.960 | 1.960 | 1.960 |
| 2 | 1.994 | 2.038 | 2.111 |
| 3 | 2.026 | 2.083 | 2.186 |
| 4 | 2.050 | 2.113 | 2.233 |
| 5 | 2.068 | 2.136 | 2.267 |
| 6 | 2.083 | 2.154 | 2.292 |
| 7 | 2.094 | 2.168 | 2.313 |
| 8 | 2.104 | 2.180 | 2.329 |
| 9 | 2.113 | 2.190 | 2.343 |
| 10 | 2.120 | 2.199 | 2.355 |
| 11 | 2.126 | 2.206 | 2.366 |
| 12 | 2.132 | 2.213 | 2.375 |
| 15 | 2.146 | 2.229 | 2.397 |
| 20 | 2.162 | 2.248 | 2.423 |

Figure 8.3.3: Wang-Tsiatis Type Stopping Rule with $\Delta = 0.25$

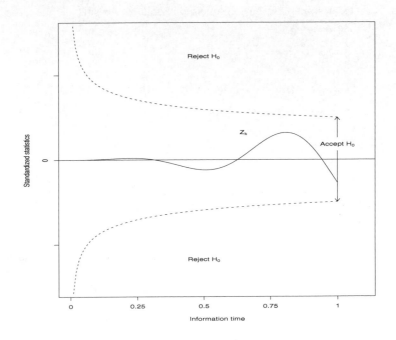

Sample size calculation for Wang and Tsiatis' test can be performed in a similar manner as those for Pocock's test and O'Brien and Fleming's test. First, we need to calculate the sample size for a fixed sample size design with given significance level and power. Then, we multiply this sample size by the constant of $R_{WT}(K, \alpha, \beta, \Delta)$ whose values are given in Table 8.3.2.

### 8.3.2 An Example

For illustration, consider the same example given in Section 8.1.2. Suppose that the investigator wishes to perform the same group sequential test using Wang and Tsiatis' test with $\Delta = 0.25$. By Table 8.3.2,

$$R_{WT}(5, 0.05, 0.1, 0.25) = 1.066.$$

Since the fixed sample size is given by $n_{\text{fixed}} = 84$, the maximum sample size needed for each treatment group is given by

$$n_{\max} = R_B(5, 0.05, 0.1)n_{\text{fixed}} = 1.066 \times 84 = 89.5 \approx 90.$$

## 8.4. Inner Wedge Test

Table 8.3.2: $R_{WT}(K, \alpha, \beta, \Delta)$ for Two-Sided Tests with $K$ Interim Analyses and $\alpha = 0.05$

| | $1 - \beta = 0.8$ | | | $1 - \beta = 0.9$ | | |
|---|---|---|---|---|---|---|
| $K$ | $\Delta = 0.01$ | $\Delta = 0.05$ | $\Delta = 0.10$ | $\Delta = 0.01$ | $\Delta = 0.05$ | $\Delta = 0.10$ |
| 1 | 1.000 | 1.000 | 1.000 | 1.000 | 1.000 | 1.000 |
| 2 | 1.016 | 1.038 | 1.075 | 1.014 | 1.034 | 1.068 |
| 3 | 1.027 | 1.054 | 1.108 | 1.025 | 1.050 | 1.099 |
| 4 | 1.035 | 1.065 | 1.128 | 1.032 | 1.059 | 1.117 |
| 5 | 1.040 | 1.072 | 1.142 | 1.037 | 1.066 | 1.129 |
| 6 | 1.044 | 1.077 | 1.152 | 1.041 | 1.071 | 1.138 |
| 7 | 1.047 | 1.081 | 1.159 | 1.044 | 1.075 | 1.145 |
| 8 | 1.050 | 1.084 | 1.165 | 1.046 | 1.078 | 1.151 |
| 9 | 1.052 | 1.087 | 1.170 | 1.048 | 1.081 | 1.155 |
| 10 | 1.054 | 1.089 | 1.175 | 1.050 | 1.083 | 1.159 |
| 11 | 1.055 | 1.091 | 1.178 | 1.051 | 1.085 | 1.163 |
| 12 | 1.056 | 1.093 | 1.181 | 1.053 | 1.086 | 1.166 |
| 15 | 1.059 | 1.097 | 1.189 | 1.055 | 1.090 | 1.172 |
| 20 | 1.062 | 1.101 | 1.197 | 1.058 | 1.094 | 1.180 |

Thus, at each interim analysis, sample size per treatment group required for achieving a 90% power at the 5% level of significance is given by

$$n = n_{\max}/K = 90/5 = 18.$$

## 8.4 Inner Wedge Test

As described above, the three commonly used group sequential methods allow early stop under the alternative hypothesis. In other words, the trial is terminated if there is substantial evidence of efficacy. In practice, however, if the trial demonstrates strong evidence that the test drug has no treatment effect, it is also of interest to stop the trial prematurely. For good medical practice, it may not be ethical to expose patients to a treatment with little or no efficacy but potential serious adverse effects. In addition, the investigator may want to put the resources on other promising drugs. To allow an early stop with either substantial evidence of efficacy or no efficacy, the most commonly used group sequential method is the so-called two-sided inner wedge test, which is also based on the standardized test statistics $Z_k$.

### 8.4.1 The Procedure

The inner wedge test can be carried out as follows (see also Jennison and Turnbull, 2000):

(1) After group $k = 1, ..., K - 1$,

- if $|Z_k| \geq b_k$ then stop and reject $H_0$;
- if $|Z_k| < a_k$ then stop and accept $H_0$;
- otherwise continue to group $k + 1$.

(2) After group $K$,

- if $|Z_k| \geq b_K$ then stop and reject $H_0$;
- if $|Z_k| < a_K$ then stop and accept $H_0$.

Figure 8.4.4: Inner Wedge Type Stopping Rule with $\Delta = 0.25$

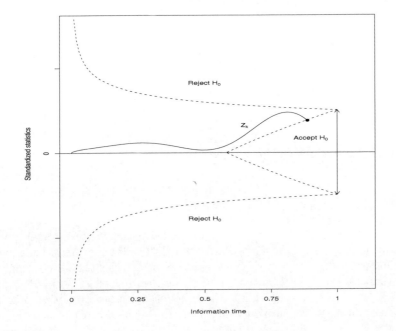

## 8.4. Inner Wedge Test

Table 8.4.1: Constants $C_{W1}(K, \alpha, \beta, \Delta)$, $C_{W2}(K, \alpha, \beta, \Delta)$, and $R_W(K, \alpha, \beta, \Delta)$ with $\alpha = 0.05$ and $1 - \beta = 0.8$

| $\Delta$ | $K$ | $C_{W1}$ | $C_{W2}$ | $R_W$ | $\Delta$ | $K$ | $C_{W1}$ | $C_{W2}$ | $R_W$ |
|---|---|---|---|---|---|---|---|---|---|
| $-0.50$ | 1 | 1.960 | 0.842 | 1.000 | $-0.25$ | 1 | 1.960 | 0.842 | 1.000 |
|  | 2 | 1.949 | 0.867 | 1.010 |  | 2 | 1.936 | 0.902 | 1.026 |
|  | 3 | 1.933 | 0.901 | 1.023 |  | 3 | 1.932 | 0.925 | 1.040 |
|  | 4 | 1.929 | 0.919 | 1.033 |  | 4 | 1.930 | 0.953 | 1.059 |
|  | 5 | 1.927 | 0.932 | 1.041 |  | 5 | 1.934 | 0.958 | 1.066 |
|  | 10 | 1.928 | 0.964 | 1.066 |  | 10 | 1.942 | 0.999 | 1.102 |
|  | 15 | 1.931 | 0.979 | 1.078 |  | 15 | 1.948 | 1.017 | 1.120 |
|  | 20 | 1.932 | 0.988 | 1.087 |  | 20 | 1.952 | 1.027 | 1.131 |
| 0.00 | 1 | 1.960 | 0.842 | 1.000 | 0.25 | 1 | 1.960 | 0.842 | 1.000 |
|  | 2 | 1.935 | 0.948 | 1.058 |  | 2 | 1.982 | 1.000 | 1.133 |
|  | 3 | 1.950 | 0.955 | 1.075 |  | 3 | 2.009 | 1.059 | 1.199 |
|  | 4 | 1.953 | 0.995 | 1.107 |  | 4 | 2.034 | 1.059 | 1.219 |
|  | 5 | 1.958 | 1.017 | 1.128 |  | 5 | 2.048 | 1.088 | 1.252 |
|  | 10 | 1.980 | 1.057 | 1.175 |  | 10 | 2.088 | 1.156 | 1.341 |
|  | 15 | 1.991 | 1.075 | 1.198 |  | 15 | 2.109 | 1.180 | 1.379 |
|  | 20 | 1.998 | 1.087 | 1.212 |  | 20 | 2.122 | 1.195 | 1.40 |

The constants $a_k$ and $b_k$ are given by

$$a_k = [C_{W1}(K, \alpha, \beta, \Delta) + C_{W2}(K, \alpha, \beta, \Delta)] * \sqrt{k/K}$$
$$\quad - C_{W2}(K, \alpha, \beta, \Delta)(k/K)^{\Delta - 1/2},$$
$$b_k = C_{W1}(K, \alpha, \beta, \Delta)(k/K)^{\Delta - 1/2}.$$

As an example, one inner wedge type boundary is given in Figure 8.4.4. For a given desired power $(1 - \beta)$, the sample size can be similarly determined. First, we calculate the sample size required for a fixed sample size design, denoted by $n_{\text{fixed}}$. Then, $n_{\text{fixed}}$ is multiplied by $R_W(K, \alpha, \beta, \Delta)$. Values of $C_{W1}(K, \alpha, \beta, \Delta)$, $C_{W2}(K, \alpha, \beta, \Delta)$, and $R_W(K, \alpha, \beta, \Delta)$ are given in Tables 8.4.1 and 8.4.2.

### 8.4.2 An Example

To illustrate sample size calculation based on the inner wedge test, consider the following example. A group sequential trial with 5 ($K = 5$) interim analyses is planned. The objective is to compare a test drug with a standard

Table 8.4.2: Constants $C_{W1}(K,\alpha,\beta,\Delta)$, $C_{W2}(K,\alpha,\beta,\Delta)$, and $R_W(K,\alpha,\beta,\Delta)$ with $\alpha = 0.05$ and $1-\beta = 0.9$

| $\Delta$ | $K$ | $C_{W1}$ | $C_{W2}$ | $R_W$ | $\Delta$ | $K$ | $C_{W1}$ | $C_{W2}$ | $R_W$ |
|---|---|---|---|---|---|---|---|---|---|
| −0.50 | 1 | 1.960 | 1.282 | 1.000 | −0.25 | 1 | 1.960 | 1.282 | 1.000 |
| | 2 | 1.960 | 1.282 | 1.000 | | 2 | 1.957 | 1.294 | 1.006 |
| | 3 | 1.952 | 1.305 | 1.010 | | 3 | 1.954 | 1.325 | 1.023 |
| | 4 | 1.952 | 1.316 | 1.016 | | 4 | 1.958 | 1.337 | 1.033 |
| | 5 | 1.952 | 1.326 | 1.023 | | 5 | 1.960 | 1.351 | 1.043 |
| | 10 | 1.958 | 1.351 | 1.042 | | 10 | 1.975 | 1.379 | 1.071 |
| | 15 | 1.963 | 1.363 | 1.053 | | 15 | 1.982 | 1.394 | 1.085 |
| | 20 | 1.967 | 1.370 | 1.060 | | 20 | 1.988 | 1.403 | 1.094 |
| 0.00 | 1 | 1.960 | 1.282 | 1.000 | 0.25 | 1 | 1.960 | 1.282 | 1.000 |
| | 2 | 1.958 | 1.336 | 1.032 | | 2 | 2.003 | 1.398 | 1.100 |
| | 3 | 1.971 | 1.353 | 1.051 | | 3 | 2.037 | 1.422 | 1.139 |
| | 4 | 1.979 | 1.381 | 1.075 | | 4 | 2.058 | 1.443 | 1.167 |
| | 5 | 1.990 | 1.385 | 1.084 | | 5 | 2.073 | 1.477 | 1.199 |
| | 10 | 2.013 | 1.428 | 1.127 | | 10 | 2.119 | 1.521 | 1.261 |
| | 15 | 2.026 | 1.447 | 1.148 | | 15 | 2.140 | 1.551 | 1.297 |
| | 20 | 2.034 | 1.458 | 1.160 | | 20 | 2.154 | 1.565 | 1.316 |

therapy through a parallel trial. A inner wedge test with $\Delta = 0.25$ is utilized. Based on a pilot study, the mean difference between the two treatments is 20% ($\mu_1 - \mu_2 = 0.2$) and the standard deviation is 1.00 for both treatments ($\sigma_1 = \sigma_2 = 1$). It is desirable to select a sample size to achieve an 80% ($1-\beta = 0.80$) power for detecting such a difference at the 5% ($\alpha = 0.05$) level of significance. The sample size needed for a fixed sample size design can be obtained as

$$n_{\text{fixed}} = \frac{(z_{0.975} + z_{0.80})^2(\sigma_1^2 + \sigma_2^2)}{(\mu_1 - \mu_2)^2} = \frac{(1.96 + 0.84)^2(1+1)}{0.2^2} = 392.$$

By Table 8.4.2,

$$n_{\max} = n_{\text{fixed}} R_W(5, 0.05, 0.2, 0.25) = 392 \times 1.199 = 470.$$

Hence, at each interim analysis, the sample size necessary per treatment group is given by

$$n = \frac{n_{\max}}{K} = \frac{470}{5} = 94.$$

## 8.5 Binary Variables

In this section we consider binary response variables.

### 8.5.1 The Procedure

Let $x_{ij}$ be the binary response from the $j$th subject in the $i$th treatment group. Within each treatment group (i.e., for a fixed $i$), $x_{ij}$'s are assumed to be independent and identically distributed with mean $p_i$. Suppose that there are $K$ planned interim analyses. Suppose also that at each interim analysis, equal number of subjects is accumulated in each treatment group. At each interim analysis, the following test statistic is usually considered:

$$Z_k = \frac{\sqrt{n_k}(\hat{p}_{1,k} - \hat{p}_{2,k})}{\sqrt{\hat{p}_{1,k}(1-\hat{p}_{1,k}) + \hat{p}_{2,k}(1-\hat{p}_{2,k})}},$$

where

$$\hat{p}_{i,k} = \frac{1}{n_{i,k}} \sum_{j=1}^{n_{i,k}} x_{ij}$$

and $n_k$ is the number of subjects accumulated by the time of the $k$th interim analysis. Since $Z_k$, $k = 1, ..., K$, are asymptotically normally distributed with the same distribution as that of $Z_k$'s for the continuous response, the repeated significance test procedures (e.g., Pocock, O'Brien-Fleming, and Wang-Tsiatis) can also be applied for binary responses. The resulting test procedure has an asymptotically type I error rate of $\alpha$.

### 8.5.2 An Example

Suppose that an investigator is interested in conducting a group sequential trial comparing a test drug with a placebo. The primary efficacy study endpoint is a binary response. Based on information obtained in a pilot study, the response rates for the test drug and the placebo are given by 60% ($p_1 = 0.60$) and 50% ($p_2 = 0.50$), respectively. Suppose that a total of 5 ($K = 5$) interim analyses are planned. It is desirable to select a maximum sample size in order to have an 80% ($1 - \beta = 0.80$) power at the 5% ($\alpha = 0.05$) level of significance. The sample size needed for a fixed sample size design is

$$\begin{aligned} n_{\text{fixed}} &= \frac{(z_{\alpha/2} + z_\beta)^2 (p_1(1-p_1) + p_2(1-p_2))}{(p_1 - p_2)^2} \\ &= \frac{(1.96 + 0.84)^2 (0.6(1-0.6) + 0.5(1-0.5))}{(0.6 - 0.5)^2} \\ &\approx 385. \end{aligned}$$

If Pocock's test is used, then by Table 8.1.2, we have

$$n_{\max} = n_{\text{fixed}} R_P(5, 0.05, 0.20) = 385 \times 1.229 \approx 474.$$

Hence, at each interim analysis, the sample size per treatment group is $474/5 = 94.8 \approx 95$.

On the other hand, if O'Brien and Fleming's method is employed, Table 8.2.2 gives

$$n_{\max} = n_{\text{fixed}} R_B(5, 0.05, 0.20) = 385 \times 1.028 \approx 396.$$

Thus, at each interim analysis, the sample size per treatment group is $396/5 = 79.2 \approx 80$.

Alternatively, if Wang and Tsitis' test with $\Delta = 0.25$ is considered, Table 8.3.2 leads to

$$n_{\max} = n_{\text{fixed}} R_{WT}(5, 0.05, 0.20, 0.25) = 385 \times 1.072 \approx 413.$$

As a result, at each interim analysis, the sample size per treatment group is given by $413/5 = 82.6 \approx 83$.

## 8.6 Time-to-Event Data

To apply the repeated significance test procedures to time-to-event data, for simplicity, we only consider Cox's proportional hazard model.

### 8.6.1 The Procedure

As indicated in Chapter 7, under the assumption of proportional hazards, the log-rank test is usually used to compare the two treatment groups. More specifically, let $h(t)$ be the hazard function of treatment group A and $e^\theta h(t)$ be the hazard function of treatment group B. Let $d_k$ denote the total number of uncensored failures observed when the $k$th interim analysis is conducted, $k = 1, ..., K$. For illustration purposes and without loss of generality, we assume that there are no ties. Let $\tau_{i,k}$ be the survival times of these subjects, $i = 1, ..., d_k$. Let $r_{iA,k}$ and $r_{iB,k}$ be the numbers of subjects who are still at risk at the $k$th interim analysis at time $\tau_{i,k}$ for treatment A and B, respectively. The log-rank test statistic at the $k$th interim analysis is then given by

$$S_k = \sum_{i=1}^{d_k} \left( \delta_{iB,k} - \frac{r_{iB,k}}{r_{iA,k} + r_{iB,k}} \right),$$

## 8.7. Alpha Spending Function

where $\delta_{iB,k} = 1$ if the failure at time $\tau_{i,k}$ is on treatment $B$ and 0 otherwise. Jennison and Turnbull (2000) proposed to use $N(\theta I_k, I_k)$ to approximate the distribution of $S_k$, where $I_k$ is the so-called observed information and is defined as

$$I_k = \sum_{i=1}^{d_k} \frac{r_{iA,k} r_{iB,k}}{(r_{iA,k} + r_{iB,k})^2}.$$

Then, the standardized test statistic can be calculated as

$$Z_k = \frac{S_k}{\sqrt{I_k}}.$$

As a result, $Z_k$ can be used to compare with the commonly used group sequential boundaries (e.g., Pocock, O'Brien-Fleming, and Wang-Tsiatis). Under the alternative hypothesis, the sample size can be determined by first finding the information needed for a fixed sample size design with the same significance level and power. Then, calculate the maximum information needed for a group sequential trial by multiplying appropriate constants from Tables 8.1.2, 8.2.2, and 8.3.2.

### 8.6.2 An Example

Suppose that an investigator is interested in conducting a survival trial with 5 ($K = 5$) planned interim analyses at the 5% level of significance ($\alpha = 0.05$) with an 80% ($1 - \beta = 0.80$) power. Assume that $\theta = 0.405$. As indicated by Jennison and Turnbull (2000), the information needed for a fixed sample size design is given by

$$I_{\text{fixed}} = \frac{(z_{\alpha/2} + z_\beta)^2}{\theta^2} = \frac{(1.96 + 0.84)^2}{0.405^2} = 47.8.$$

If O'Brien and Fleming boundaries are utilized as a stopping rule, then the maximum information needed in order to achieve the desired power can be calculated as

$$I_{\max} = I_{\text{fixed}} \times R_B(K, \alpha, \beta) = 47.8 \times 1.028 = 49.1,$$

where the value 1.028 of $R_B(5, 0.05, 0.2)$ is taken from Table 8.2.2. If $\theta$ is close to 0, which is true under the local alternative, it is expected that $r_{iA,k} \approx r_{iB,k}$ for each $i$. Hence, $I_k$ can be approximated by $0.25 d_k$. It follows that the number of events needed is given by

$$n_d = \frac{I_{\max}}{0.25} = 196.4 \approx 197.$$

Hence, a total number of 197 events are needed in order to achieve an 80% power for detecting a difference of $\theta = 0.405$ at the 5% level of significance. The corresponding sample size can be derived based on $n_d$ by adjusting for some other factors, such as competing risk, censoring, and dropouts.

## 8.7 Alpha Spending Function

One of the major disadvantages of the group sequential methods discussed in the previous sections is that they are designed for a fixed number of interim analyses with equally spaced information time. In practice, however, it is not uncommon that the interim analysis is actually planned based on calendar time. As a result, the information accumulated at each time point may not be equally spaced. The consequence is that the overall type I error may be far away from the target value.

As an alternative, Lan and DeMets (1983) proposed to distribute (or spend) the total probability of false positive risk as a continuous function of the information time in group sequential procedures for interim analyses. If the total information scheduled to accumulate over the maximum duration $T$ is known, the boundaries can be computed as a continuous function of the information time. This continuous function of the information time is referred to as the alpha spending function, denoted by $\alpha(s)$. The alpha spending function is an increasing function of information time. It is 0 when information time is 0; and is equal to the overall significance level when information time is 1. In other words, $\alpha(0) = 0$ and $\alpha(1) = \alpha$. Let $s_1$ and $s_2$ be two information times, $0 < s_1 < s_2 \leq 1$. Also, denote $\alpha(s_1)$ and $\alpha(s_2)$ as their corresponding value of alpha spending function at $s_1$ and $s_2$. Then, $0 < \alpha(s_1) < \alpha(s_2) \leq \alpha$. $\alpha(s_1)$ is the probability of type I error one wishes to spend at information time $s_1$. For a given alpha spending function $(\alpha(s))$ and a series of standardized test statistic $Z_k, k = 1, ..., K$. The corresponding boundaries $c_k, k = 1, ..., K$ are chosen such that under the null hypothesis

$$P(|Z_1| < c_1, ..., |Z_{k-1}| < c_{k-1}, |Z_k| \geq c_k) = \alpha\left(\frac{k}{K}\right) - \alpha\left(\frac{k-1}{K}\right).$$

Some commonly used alpha-spending functions are summarized in Table 8.7.1 and Figure 8.7.5 is used to illustrate a true alpha spending function.

Table 8.7.1: Various Alpha Spending Functions

| | |
|---|---|
| $\alpha_1(s) = 2\{1 - \Phi(z_{\alpha/2}/\sqrt{2})$ | O'Brien-Fleming |
| $\alpha_2(s) = \alpha \log[1 + (e-1)s]$ | Pocock |
| $\alpha_3(s) = \alpha s^\rho, \rho > 0$ | Lan-DeMets-Kim |
| $\alpha_4(s) = \alpha[(1 - e^{\zeta s})/(1 - e^{-\zeta})], \zeta \neq 0$ | Hwang-Shih |

## 8.7. Alpha Spending Function

Figure 8.7.5: The Alpha Spending Function $\alpha(s)$

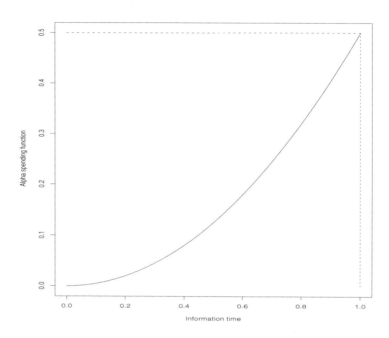

We now introduce the procedure for sample size calculation based on Lan-DeMets' alpha spending function, i.e.,

$$\alpha(s) = \alpha s^\rho, \rho > 0.$$

Although alpha spending function does not require a fixed maximum number and equal spaced interim analyses, it is necessary to make those assumptions in order to calculate the sample size under the alternative hypothesis. The sample size calculation can be performed in a similar manner. For a given significance level $\alpha$ and power $1 - \beta$, we can first calculate the sample size needed for a fixed sample size design and then multiply it by a constant $R_{LD}(K, \alpha, \beta, \rho)$. The values of $R_{LD}(K, \alpha, \beta, \rho)$ are tabulated in Table 8.7.2.

Consider the same example as discussed in Section 8.1. In order to achieve a 90% power at the 5% level of significance, it is necessary to have $n_{\text{fixed}} = 84$ subjects per treatment group. Then, the maximum sample size needed for achieving the desired power with 5 interim analyses using the Lan-DeMets type alpha spending function with $\rho = 2$ can be calculated as

$$n_{\max} = n_{\text{fixed}} \times R_{LD}(5, 0.05, 0.9, 2) = 84 \times 1.075 \approx 92.$$

Table 8.7.2: $R_{LD}(K, \alpha, \beta, \rho)$ for Two-Sided Tests with $K$ Interim Analyses and $\alpha = 0.05$

| | $1 - \beta = 0.8$ | | | $1 - \beta = 0.9$ | | |
|---|---|---|---|---|---|---|
| $K$ | $\rho = 0.01$ | $\rho = 0.05$ | $\rho = 0.10$ | $\rho = 0.01$ | $\rho = 0.05$ | $\rho = 0.10$ |
| 1 | 1.000 | 1.000 | 1.000 | 1.000 | 1.000 | 1.000 |
| 2 | 1.082 | 1.028 | 1.010 | 1.075 | 1.025 | 1.009 |
| 3 | 1.117 | 1.045 | 1.020 | 1.107 | 1.041 | 1.018 |
| 4 | 1.137 | 1.056 | 1.027 | 1.124 | 1.051 | 1.025 |
| 5 | 1.150 | 1.063 | 1.032 | 1.136 | 1.058 | 1.030 |
| 6 | 1.159 | 1.069 | 1.036 | 1.144 | 1.063 | 1.033 |
| 7 | 1.165 | 1.073 | 1.039 | 1.150 | 1.067 | 1.036 |
| 8 | 1.170 | 1.076 | 1.041 | 1.155 | 1.070 | 1.039 |
| 9 | 1.174 | 1.079 | 1.043 | 1.159 | 1.073 | 1.040 |
| 10 | 1.178 | 1.081 | 1.045 | 1.162 | 1.075 | 1.042 |
| 11 | 1.180 | 1.083 | 1.046 | 1.164 | 1.077 | 1.043 |
| 12 | 1.183 | 1.085 | 1.048 | 1.166 | 1.078 | 1.044 |
| 15 | 1.188 | 1.088 | 1.050 | 1.171 | 1.082 | 1.047 |
| 20 | 1.193 | 1.092 | 1.054 | 1.176 | 1.085 | 1.050 |

Thus, a total of 92 subjects per treatment group is needed in order to have a 90% power at the 5% level of significance.

## 8.8 Sample Size Re-Estimation

In clinical trials with planned interim analyses, it is desirable to perform sample size re-estimation at interim analyses. The objective is to determine whether the selected sample size is justifiable based on clinical data accumulated up to the time point of interim analysis. In practice, however, unblinding the treatment codes for sample size re-estimation may introduce bias to remaining clinical trials. Shih (1993) and Shih and Zhao (1997) proposed some procedures without unblinding for sample size re-estimation with interim data for double-blind clinical trials with binary outcomes.

### 8.8.1 The Procedure

Suppose that $y_i, i = 1, ..., n$ (treatment) and $y_j, j = n + 1, ..., N$ (control) are observations from a randomized, double-blind clinical trial. It is as-

## 8.8. Sample Size Re-Estimation

sumed that $y_i$ and $y_j$ are distributed as $B(1, p_1)$ and $B(1, p_2)$, respectively. Suppose that the hypotheses of interest are

$$H_0 : p_1 = p_2 \quad \text{versus} \quad H_a : p_1 \neq p_2.$$

Further, suppose that $N = 2n$ and a clinically meaningful difference is $\Delta = |p_1 - p_2|$. Then, as discussed in Chapter 4, the sample size required for achieving a desired power of $(1 - \beta)$ at $\alpha$ level of significance by an unconditional method is given by

$$n = \frac{(z_{\alpha/2} + z_\beta)^2 [p_1(1 - p_1) + p_2(1 - p_2)]}{\Delta^2}.$$

As discussed in Chapter 4, there are two methods available for comparing two proportions. They are, namely, conditional and unconditional methods. For illustration purposes, we only adopt the formula of unconditional method. However, the procedure introduced below can easily be generalized to the conditional method. The estimated sample size can be obtained by simply replacing $p_1$ and $p_2$ with their estimates. As a result, sample size re-estimation at an interim analysis without unblinding is to obtain estimates of $p_1$ and $p_2$ without revealing the treatment codes. For multi-center trials, Shih (1993) and Shih and Zhao (1997) suggested the following procedure for sample size re-estimation without unblinding when 50% of the subjects as originally planned in the study protocol complete the trial.

First, within each center, each subject is randomly assigned to a dummy stratum, i.e., either stratum A or stratum B. Note that this stratification is not based on any of the subjects' baseline characteristics. The use of dummy stratification is for sample size re-estimation at the interim stage and statistical inference should not be affected at the end of the trial. Now, subjects in stratum A are randomly allocated to the treatment group with probability $\pi$ and to the control group with probability $1 - \pi$, where $\pi \in (0, 0.5)$. Similarly, subjects in stratum B are randomly allocated to the treatment group with probability $1 - \pi$ and to the control group with probability $\pi$, where $\pi \in (0, 0.5)$. Based on the pooled events rates observed from each stratum, we then estimate $p_1$ and $p_2$ without unblinding the treatment codes as follows. We use the results from stratum A to estimate

$$\theta_1 = P(y_j = 1 | \text{subject } j \in \text{stratum } A) = \pi p_1 + (1 - \pi) p_2$$

and that of stratum B to estimate

$$\theta_2 = P(y_j = 1 | \text{subject } j \in \text{stratum } B) = (1 - \pi) p_1 + \pi p_2.$$

Based on the observed events rate $\theta_1$ from stratum A and the observed event rate $\theta_2$ from stratum B, $p_1$ and $p_2$ can be estimated by solving the following equations simultaneously:

$$\pi p_1 + (1-\pi)p_2 = \theta_1$$
$$(1-\pi)p_1 + \pi p_2 = \theta_2.$$

Thus, the estimates of $p_1$ and $p_2$ are given by

$$\hat{p}_1 = \frac{\pi\hat{\theta}_1 - (1-\pi)\hat{\theta}_2}{2\pi - 1}$$

and

$$\hat{p}_2 = \frac{\pi\hat{\theta}_2 - (1-\pi)\hat{\theta}_1}{2\pi - 1}.$$

Estimates $\hat{p}_1$ and $\hat{p}_2$ can then be used to update the sample size based on the formula for sample size calculation given above. Note that if the resultant sample size $n^*$ is greater than the originally planned sample size $n$ (i.e., $n^* > n$), it is suggested that an increase in sample size is necessary in order to achieve the desired power at the end of the trial. On the other hand, if $n^* < m$, a sample size reduction is justifiable. More details regarding sample size re-estimation without unblinding the treatment codes can be found in Shih and Zhao (1997).

## 8.8.2 An Example

Consider a cancer trial comparing the response rates (i.e., complete response plus partial response) of patients between two treatments (i.e., test and control). The trial was conducted in two centers (A and B) with 18 patients each. At center A, each patient is assigned to the test treatment group with a probability of 0.6 and the control group with a probability of 0.4. At center B, each patient is assigned to the test treatment group with a probability of 0.4 and the control group with a probability of 0.6. It follows that $\pi = 0.4$. One interim analysis was planned when half of patients (i.e., 9 patients per center) completed the trial. At the time of interim analysis, it is noted that the observed response rates for center A and B are given by 0.6 ($\theta_1 = 0.6$) and 0.5 ($\theta_2 = 0.5$), respectively. It follows that

$$0.4p_1 + 0.6p_2 = 0.6$$
$$0.6p_1 + 0.4p_2 = 0.5.$$

This gives $p_1 = 0.3$ and $p_2 = 0.8$. Hence, the sample size needed in order to achieve a 90% ($\beta = 0.10$) at the 5% ($\alpha = 0.05$) level of significance is given by

$$n = \frac{(z_{\alpha/2} + z_\beta)^2(p_1(1-p_1) + p_2(1-p_2))}{(p_1 - p_2)^2}$$

$$= \frac{(1.96 + 1.64)^2(0.3(1-0.3) + 0.8(1-0.8))}{(0.3 - 0.8)^2}$$

$$\approx 20.$$

Hence, a total of 40 patients are needed in order to achieve the desired power. This sample size re-estimation suggests that in addition to the planned 36 patients, four more patients are necessarily enrolled.

## 8.9 Conditional Power

Conditional power at a given interim analysis in group sequential trials is defined as the power of rejecting the null hypothesis at the end of the trial conditional on the observed data accumulated up to the time point of the planned interim analysis. For many repeated significance tests such as Pocock's test, O'Brien and Fleming's test, and Wang and Tsiatis' test, the trial can be terminated only under the alternative hypothesis. In practice, this is usually true if the test treatment demonstrates substantial evidence of efficacy. However, it should be noted that if the trial indicates a strong evidence of futility (lack of efficacy) during the interim analysis, it is unethical to continue the trial. Hence, the trial may also be terminated under the null hypothesis. However, except for the inner wedge test, most repeated significance tests are designed for early stop under the alternative hypothesis. In such a situation, the analysis of conditional power (or equivalently, futility analysis) can be used as a quantitative method for determining whether the trial should be terminated prematurely.

### 8.9.1 Comparing Means

Let $x_{ij}$ be the observation from the $j$th subject ($j = 1, ..., n_i$) in the $i$th treatment group ($i = 1, 2$). $x_{ij}, j = 1, ..., n_i$, are assumed to be independent and identically distributed normal random variables with mean $\mu_i$ and variance $\sigma_i^2$. At the time of interim analysis, it is assumed that the first $m_i$ of $n_i$ subjects in the $i$th treatment group have already been observed. The investigator may want to evaluate the power for rejection of the null hypothesis based on the observed data and appropriate assumption under the alternative hypothesis. More specifically, define

$$\bar{x}_{a,i} = \frac{1}{m_i}\sum_{j=1}^{m_i} x_{ij} \quad \text{and} \quad \bar{x}_{b,i} = \frac{1}{n_i - m_i}\sum_{j=m_i+1}^{n_i} x_{ij}.$$

At the end of the trial, the following $Z$ test statistic is calculated:

$$Z = \frac{\bar{x}_1 - \bar{x}_2}{\sqrt{s_1^2/n_1 + s_2^2/n_2}}$$

$$\approx \frac{\bar{x}_1 - \bar{x}_2}{\sqrt{\sigma_1^2/n_1 + \sigma_2^2/n_2}}$$

$$= \frac{(m_1\bar{x}_{a,1} + (n_1-m_1)\bar{x}_{b,1})/n_1 - (m_2\bar{x}_{a,2} + (n_2-m_2)\bar{x}_{b,2})/n_2}{\sqrt{\sigma_1^2/n_1 + \sigma_2^2/n_2}}.$$

Under the alternative hypothesis, we assume $\mu_1 > \mu_2$. Hence, the power for rejecting the null hypothesis can be approximated by

$$1 - \beta = P(Z > z_{\alpha/2})$$

$$= P\left(\frac{\frac{(n_1-m_1)(\bar{x}_{b,1}-\mu_1)}{n_1} - \frac{(n_2-m_2)(\bar{x}_{b,2}-\mu_2)}{n_2}}{\sqrt{\frac{(n_1-m_1)\sigma_1^2}{n_1^2} + \frac{(n_2-m_2)\sigma_2^2}{n_2^2}}} > \tau\right)$$

$$= 1 - \Phi(\tau),$$

where

$$\tau = \left[z_{\alpha/2}\sqrt{\sigma_1^2/n_1 + \sigma_2^2/n_2} - (\mu_1 - \mu_2)\right.$$

$$\left. - \left(\frac{m_1}{n_1}(\bar{x}_{a,1} - \mu_1) - \frac{m_2}{n_2}(\bar{x}_{a,2} - \mu_2)\right)\right]$$

$$\left[\frac{(n_1-m_1)\sigma_1^2}{n_1^2} + \frac{(n_2-m_2)\sigma_2^2}{n_2^2}\right]^{-1/2}.$$

As it can be seen from the above, the conditional power depends not only upon the assumed alternative hypothesis $(\mu_1, \mu_2)$ but also upon the observed values $(\bar{x}_{a,1}, \bar{x}_{a,2})$ and the amount of information that has been accumulated $(m_i/n_i)$ at the time of interim analysis.

### 8.9.2 Comparing Proportions

When the responses are binary, similar formulas can also be obtained. Let $x_{ij}$ be the binary response observed from the $j$th subject $(j = 1, ..., n_i)$ in the $i$th treatment group $(i = 1, 2)$. Again, $x_{ij}, j = 1, ..., n_i$, are assumed to be independent and identically distributed binary variables with mean $p_i$. At the time of interim analysis, it is also assumed that the first $m_i$ of $n_i$ subjects in the $i$th treatment group have been observed. Define

$$\bar{x}_{a,i} = \frac{1}{m_i}\sum_{j=1}^{m_i} x_{ij} \quad \text{and} \quad \bar{x}_{b,i} = \frac{1}{n_i - m_i}\sum_{j=m_i+1}^{n_i} x_{ij}.$$

At the end of the trial, the following $Z$ test statistic is calculated:

$$Z = \frac{\bar{x}_1 - \bar{x}_2}{\sqrt{\bar{x}_1(1-\bar{x}_1)/n_1 + \bar{x}_2(1-\bar{x}_2)/n_2}}$$

$$\approx \frac{\bar{x}_1 - \bar{x}_2}{\sqrt{p_1(1-p_1)/n_1 + p_2(1-p_2)/n_2}}$$

$$= \frac{(m_1\bar{x}_{a,1} + (n_1 - m_1)\bar{x}_{b,1})/n_1 - (m_2\bar{x}_{a,2} + (n_2 - m_2)\bar{x}_{b,2})/n_2}{\sqrt{p_1(1-p_1)/n_1 + p_2(1-p_2)/n_2}}.$$

Under the alternative hypothesis, we assume $p_1 > p_2$. Hence, the power for rejecting the null hypothesis can be approximated by

$$1 - \beta = P(Z > z_{\alpha/2})$$

$$= P\left( \frac{\frac{(n_1-m_1)(\bar{x}_{b,1}-\mu_1)}{n_1} - \frac{(n_2-m_2)(\bar{x}_{b,2}-\mu_2)}{n_2}}{\sqrt{\frac{(n_1-m_1)p_1(1-p_1)}{n_1^2} + \frac{(n_2-m_2)p_2(1-p_2)}{n_2^2}}} > \tau \right)$$

$$= 1 - \Phi(\tau),$$

where

$$\tau = \left[ z_{\alpha/2}\sqrt{p_1(1-p_1)/n_1 + p_2(1-p_2)/n_2} - (\mu_1 - \mu_2) \right.$$
$$\left. - \left( \frac{m_1}{n_1}(\bar{x}_{a,1} - \mu_1) - \frac{m_2}{n_2}(\bar{x}_{a,2} - \mu_2) \right) \right]$$
$$\left[ \frac{(n_1 - m_1)p_1(1-p_1)}{n_1^2} + \frac{(n_2 - m_2)p_2(1-p_2)}{n_2^2} \right]^{-1/2}.$$

Similarly, the conditional power depends not only upon the assumed alternative hypothesis $(p_1, p_2)$ but also upon the observed values $(\bar{x}_{a,1}, \bar{x}_{a,2})$ and the amount of information that has been accumulated $(m_i/n_i)$ at the time of interim analysis.

## 8.10 Practical Issues

The group sequential procedures for interim analyses are basically in the context of hypothesis testing which is aimed at pragmatic study objectives, i.e., which treatment is better. However, most new treatments such as cancer drugs are very expensive or very toxic or both. As a result, if the degree of the benefit provided by the new treatment exceeds some minimum clinically significant requirement, only then will it be considered for the treatment of the intended medical conditions. Therefore, an adequate well-controlled trial should be able to provide not only the qualitative evidence, whether the experimental treatment is effective, but also the quantitative evidence from the unbiased estimation of the size of the effectiveness or safety over placebo given by the experimental therapy. For a fixed sample design without interim analyses for early termination, it is possible to achieve both qualitative and quantitative goals with respect to the treatment effect. However, with group sequential procedure the size of benefit of the experimental treatment by the maximum likelihood method is usually overestimated because of the choice of stopping rule. Jennison and Turnbull (1990) pointed out that the sample mean might not even be contained in the final confidence interval. As a result, estimation of the size of treatment effect has received a lot of attention. Various estimation procedures have been proposed such as modified maximum likelihood estimator (MLE), median unbiased estimator (MUE) and the midpoint of the equal-tailed 90% confidence interval. For more details, see Cox (1952), Tsiatis et al., (1984), Kim and DeMets (1987), Kim (1989), Chang and O'Brien (1986), Chang et al. (1989), Chang (1989), Hughes and Pocock (1988), and Pocock and Hughes (1989).

The estimation procedures proposed in the above literature require extensive computation. On the other hand, simulation results (Kim, 1989; Hughes and Pocock, 1988) showed that the alpha spending function corresponding to the O'Brien-Fleming group sequential procedure is very concave and allocates only a very small amount of total nominal significance level to early stages of interim analyses, and hence, the bias, variance, and mean square error of the point estimator following O'Brien-Fleming procedure are also the smallest. Current research focuses mainly upon the estimation of the size of the treatment effect for the primary clinical endpoints on which the group sequential procedure is based. However, there are many other secondary efficacy and safety endpoints to be evaluated in the same trial. The impact of early termination of the trial based on the results from primary clinical endpoints on the statistical inference for these secondary clinical endpoints are unclear. In addition, group sequential methods and their followed estimation procedures so far are concentrated only on the population average. On the other hand, inference of variability is sometimes also of vital importance for certain classes of drug products and diseases. Research on estimation of variability following early termination is still lacking. Other areas of interest for interim analyses include clinical trials with more than 2 treatments and bioequivalence assessment. For group sequential procedures for the trials with multiple treatments, see Hughes (1993) and Proschan et al. (1994). For group sequential bioequivalence testing procedure, see Gould (1995).

In practice, one of the most commonly used methods for sample size estimation in group sequential trials is to consider the most conservative scenario. In other words, we assume that the trial will not be stopped

## 8.9. Conditional Power

prematurely. Let $C_K$ be the critical value for final analysis. Then, we reject the null hypothesis at the $\alpha$ level of significance if and only if $|Z_K| > C_K$. Under the null hypothesis, however, the type I error rate is no longer $\alpha$. Instead it becomes

$$\alpha^* = P(|Z_K| > C_K).$$

Hence, the sample size for achieving a desired power can be estimated by adjusting $\alpha$ to $\alpha^*$. This method has the merit of simplicity. Besides, it works well if $C_K \approx Z_{\alpha/2}$. However, if $C_K >> Z_{\alpha/2}$, the resulting sample size could be very conservative.

# Chapter 9

# Comparing Variabilities

In most clinical trials comparing a test drug and a control (e.g., a placebo control or an active control), treatment effect is usually established by comparing mean response change from the baseline of some primary study endpoints, assuming that their corresponding variabilities are comparable. In practice, however, variabilities associated with the test drug and the control could be very different. When the variability of the test drug is much larger than that of the reference drug, safety of the test drug could be a concern. Thus, in addition to comparing mean responses between treatments, it is also of interest to compare the variabilities associated with the responses between treatments.

In practice, the variabilities are usually classified into two categories, namely, the intra-subject (or within subject) variability and the inter-subject (or between subject) variability. Intra-subject variability refers to the variability observed from repeated measurements from the same subject under the same experimental conditions. On the other hand, inter-subject variability is the variability due to the heterogeneity among subjects. The total variability is simply the sum of the intra- and inter-subject variabilities. In practice, it is of interest to test for equality, non-inferiority/superiority, and similarity between treatments in terms of the intra-subject, inter-subject, and/or total variabilities. The problem of comparing intra-subject variabilities is well studied by Chinchilli and Esinhart (1996) through an F statistic under a replicated crossover model. A similar idea can also be applied to comparing total variabilities under a parallel design without replicates. However, how to compare inter-subject and total variabilities under a crossover design is still challenging to biostatisticians in clinical research.

The remainder of this chapter is organized as follows. In the next two sections, formulas for sample size calculation for comparing intra-subject variabilities and intra-subject CVs are derived, respectively, under both replicated crossover designs and parallel designs with replicates. Sections 9.3 and 9.4 provide formulas for sample size calculation for comparing inter-subject variabilities and total variabilities, respectively, under both crossover designs and parallel designs. Some practical issues are discussed in the last section.

## 9.1 Comparing Intra-Subject Variabilities

To assess intra-subject variability, replicates from the same subject are necessarily obtained. For this purpose, replicated crossover designs or parallel group designs with replicates are commonly employed. In what follows, statistical tests for comparing intra-subject variabilities under a parallel design with replicates and a replicated crossover design (e.g., a 2 × 4 replicated crossover design) are studied.

### 9.1.1 Parallel Design with Replicates

Let $x_{ijk}$ be the observation of the $k$th replicate ($k = 1, ..., m$) of the $j$th subject ($j = 1, ..., n_i$) from the $i$th treatment ($i =$ T, R). It is assumed that

$$x_{ijk} = \mu_i + S_{ij} + e_{ijk}, \qquad (9.1.1)$$

where $\mu_i$ is the treatment effect, $S_{ij}$ is the random effect due to the $j$th subject in the $i$th treatment group, and $e_{ijk}$ is the intra-subject variability under the $i$th treatment. It is assumed that for a fixed $i$, $S_{ij}$ are independent and identically distributed as normal random variables with mean 0 and variance $\sigma_{Bi}^2$, and $e_{ijk}, k = 1, ..., m$, are independent and identically distributed as a normal random variable with mean 0 and variance $\sigma_{Wi}^2$. Under this model, an unbiased estimator for $\sigma_{Wi}^2$ is given by

$$\hat{\sigma}_{Wi}^2 = \frac{1}{n_i(m-1)} \sum_{j=1}^{n_i} \sum_{k=1}^{m} (x_{ijk} - \bar{x}_{ij\cdot})^2, \qquad (9.1.2)$$

where

$$\bar{x}_{ij\cdot} = \frac{1}{m} \sum_{k=1}^{m} x_{ijk}. \qquad (9.1.3)$$

It can be seen that $n_i(m-1)\hat{\sigma}_{Wi}^2/\sigma_{Wi}^2$ is distributed as a $\chi^2_{n_i(m-1)}$ random variable.

## 9.1. Comparing Intra-Subject Variabilities

**Test for Equality**

In practice, it is often of interest to test whether two drug products have the same intra-subject variability. The following hypotheses are then of interest:
$$H_0: \sigma_{WT}^2 = \sigma_{WR}^2 \quad \text{versus} \quad H_a: \sigma_{WT}^2 \neq \sigma_{WR}^2.$$
A commonly used test statistic for testing the above hypotheses is given by
$$T = \frac{\hat{\sigma}_{WT}^2}{\hat{\sigma}_{WR}^2}.$$
Under the null hypothesis, $T$ is distributed as an $F$ random variable with $n_T(m-1)$ and $n_R(m-1)$ degrees of freedom. Hence, we reject the null hypothesis at the $\alpha$ level of significance if
$$T > F_{\alpha/2, n_T(m-1), n_R(m-1)}$$
or
$$T < F_{1-\alpha/2, n_T(m-1), n_R(m-1)},$$
where $F_{\alpha/2, n_T(m-1), n_R(m-1)}$ is the upper $(\alpha/2)$th quantile of an F distribution with $n_T(m-1)$ and $n_R(m-1)$ degrees of freedom. Under the alternative hypothesis, without loss of generality, we assume that $\sigma_{WT}^2 < \sigma_{WR}^2$. The power of the above test is

$$\begin{aligned}
\text{Power} &= P(T < F_{1-\alpha/2, n_T(m-1), n_R(m-1)}) \\
&= P(1/T > F_{\alpha/2, n_R(m-1), n_T(m-1)}) \\
&= P\left(\frac{\hat{\sigma}_{WR}^2/\sigma_{WR}^2}{\hat{\sigma}_{WT}^2/\sigma_{WT}^2} > \frac{\sigma_{WT}^2}{\sigma_{WR}^2} F_{\alpha/2, n_R(m-1), n_T(m-1)}\right) \\
&= P\left(F_{n_R(m-1), n_T(m-1)} > \frac{\sigma_{WT}^2}{\sigma_{WR}^2} F_{\alpha/2, n_R(m-1), n_T(m-1)}\right),
\end{aligned}$$

where $F_{a,b}$ denotes an F random variable with $a$ and $b$ degrees of freedom. Under the assumption that $n = n_R = n_T$ and with a fixed $\sigma_{WT}^2$ and $\sigma_{WR}^2$, the sample size needed in order to achieve a desired power of $1 - \beta$ can be obtained by solving the following equation for $n$:
$$\frac{\sigma_{WT}^2}{\sigma_{WR}^2} = \frac{F_{1-\beta, n(m-1), n(m-1)}}{F_{\alpha/2, n(m-1), n(m-1)}}.$$

**Test for Non-Inferiority/Superiority**

The problem of testing non-inferiority and superiority can be unified by the following hypotheses:
$$H_0: \frac{\sigma_{WT}}{\sigma_{WR}} \geq \delta \quad \text{versus} \quad H_a: \frac{\sigma_{WT}}{\sigma_{WR}} < \delta.$$

When $\delta < 1$, the rejection of the null hypothesis indicates the superiority of the test product over the reference in terms of the intra-subject variability. When $\delta > 1$, the rejection of the null hypothesis indicates the non-inferiority of the test product over the reference. The test statistic is given by

$$T = \frac{\hat{\sigma}_{WT}^2}{\delta^2 \hat{\sigma}_{WR}^2}.$$

Under the null hypothesis, $T$ is distributed as an F random variable with $n_T(m-1)$ and $n_R(m-1)$ degrees of freedom. Hence, we reject the null hypothesis at the $\alpha$ level of significance if

$$T < F_{1-\alpha, n_T(m-1), n_R(m-1)}.$$

Under the alternative hypothesis that $\sigma_{WT}^2/\sigma_{WR}^2 < \delta$, the power of the above test is

$$\begin{aligned}
\text{Power} &= P(T < F_{1-\alpha, n_T(m-1), n_R(m-1)}) \\
&= P(1/T > F_{\alpha, n_R(m-1), n_T(m-1)}) \\
&= P\left(\frac{\hat{\sigma}_{WR}^2/\sigma_{WR}^2}{\hat{\sigma}_{WT}^2/\sigma_{WT}^2} > \frac{\sigma_{WT}^2}{\delta \sigma_{WR}^2} F_{\alpha, n_R(m-1), n_T(m-1)}\right) \\
&= P\left(F_{n_R(m-1), n_T(m-1)} > \frac{\sigma_{WT}^2}{\delta^2 \sigma_{WR}^2} F_{\alpha, n_R(m-1), n_T(m-1)}\right).
\end{aligned}$$

Under the assumption that $n = n_T = n_R$, the sample size needed in order to achieve a desired power of $1 - \beta$ at the $\alpha$ level of significance can be obtained by solving the following equation for $n$:

$$\frac{\sigma_{WT}^2}{\delta^2 \sigma_{WR}^2} = \frac{F_{1-\beta, n(m-1), n(m-1)}}{F_{\alpha, n(m-1), n(m-1)}}.$$

**Test for Similarity**

For testing similarity, the following hypotheses are usually considered:

$$H_0 : \frac{\sigma_{WT}^2}{\sigma_{WR}^2} \geq \delta \text{ or } \frac{\sigma_{WT}^2}{\sigma_{WR}^2} \leq 1/\delta \quad \text{versus} \quad H_a : \frac{1}{\delta} < \frac{\sigma_{WT}^2}{\sigma_{WR}^2} < \delta,$$

where $\delta > 1$ is the similarity limit. The above hypotheses can be decomposed into the following two one-sided hypotheses:

$$H_{01} : \frac{\sigma_{WT}}{\sigma_{WR}} \geq \delta \quad \text{versus} \quad H_{a1} : \frac{\sigma_{WT}}{\sigma_{WR}} < \delta,$$

and

$$H_{02} : \frac{\sigma_{WT}}{\sigma_{WR}} \leq \frac{1}{\delta} \quad \text{versus} \quad H_{a2} : \frac{\sigma_{WT}}{\sigma_{WR}} > \frac{1}{\delta}.$$

## 9.1. Comparing Intra-Subject Variabilities

These two one-sided hypotheses can be tested by the following two test statistics:
$$T_1 = \frac{\hat{\sigma}_{WT}}{\delta \hat{\sigma}_{WR}} \quad \text{and} \quad T_2 = \frac{\delta \hat{\sigma}_{WT}}{\hat{\sigma}_{WR}}.$$

We then reject the null hypothesis and conclude similarity at the $\alpha$ level of significance if
$$T_1 < F_{1-\alpha, n_T(m-1), n_R(m-1)} \quad \text{and} \quad T_2 > F_{\alpha, n_T(m-1), n_R(m-1)}.$$

Assuming that $n = n_T = n_R$ and $\sigma^2_{WT} \leq \sigma^2_{WR}$, the power of the above test is

$$\begin{aligned}
\text{Power} &= P\left(\frac{F_{\alpha, n(m-1), n(m-1)}}{\delta^2} < \frac{\hat{\sigma}^2_{WT}}{\hat{\sigma}^2_{WR}} < \delta^2 F_{1-\alpha, n(m-1), n(m-1)}\right) \\
&= P\left(\frac{1}{F_{1-\alpha, n(m-1), n(m-1)} \delta^2} < \frac{\hat{\sigma}^2_{WT}}{\hat{\sigma}^2_{WR}} < \delta^2 F_{1-\alpha, n(m-1), n(m-1)}\right) \\
&\geq 1 - 2P\left(\frac{\hat{\sigma}^2_{WR}}{\hat{\sigma}^2_{WT}} > \delta^2 F_{1-\alpha, n(m-1), n(m-1)}\right) \\
&= 1 - 2P\left(F_{n(m-1), n(m-1)} > \frac{\delta^2 \sigma^2_{WT}}{\sigma^2_{WR}} F_{1-\alpha, n(m-1), n(m-1)}\right).
\end{aligned}$$

Thus, a conservative estimate for the sample size required for achieving a desired power of $1 - \beta$ can be obtained by solving the following equation for $n$:
$$\frac{\delta^2 \sigma^2_{WT}}{\sigma^2_{WR}} = \frac{F_{\beta/2, n(m-1), n(m-1)}}{F_{1-\alpha, n(m-1), n(m-1)}}.$$

**An Example**

Suppose that an investigator is interested in conducting a two-arm parallel trial with 3 ($m = 3$) replicates per subject to compare the variability of an inhaled formulation of a drug product (treatment) with a subcutaneous (SC) injected formulation (control) in terms of AUC. In practice, it is expected that the inhaled formulation has smaller intra-subject variability as compared to that of SC formulation. Based on PK data obtained from pilot studies, it is assumed the true standard deviation of treatment and control are given by 30% ($\sigma_{WT} = 0.30$) and 45% ($\sigma_{WR} = 0.45$), respectively. It is also believed that 10% ($\delta = 1.1$) of $\sigma_{WR}$ is of no clinical importance. Hence, for testing non-inferiority, the sample size per treatment needed in order to achieve an 80% power at the 5% level of significance can be obtained by solving the following equation:
$$\frac{0.30^2}{1.1^2 \times 0.45^2} = \frac{F_{0.80, 2n, 2n}}{F_{0.05, 2n, 2n}}.$$

The solution can be obtained by a standard numerical iteration technique, such as the simple grid search, which gives $n = 13$.

## 9.1.2 Replicated Crossover Design

Compared with the parallel design with replicates, the merit of a crossover design is the ability to make comparisons within subjects. In this section, without loss of generality, consider a $2 \times 2m$ replicated crossover design comparing two treatments. For convenience, we refer to the two treatments as a test formulation and a reference formulation. Under a $2 \times 2m$ replicated crossover design, in each sequence, each subject receives the test formulation $m$ times and the reference formulation $m$ times at different dosing periods. When $m = 1$, the $2 \times 2m$ replicated crossover design reduces to the standard two-sequence, two-period ($2 \times 2$) crossover design. When $m = 2$, the $2 \times 2m$ replicated crossover design becomes the $2 \times 4$ crossover design recommended by the FDA for assessment of population/individual bioequivalence (FDA, 2001).

Suppose that $n_1$ subjects are assigned to the first sequence and $n_2$ subjects are assigned to the second sequence. Let $x_{ijkl}$ be the observation from the $j$th subject ($j = 1, ..., n_i$) in the $i$th sequence ($i = 1, 2$) under the $l$th replicate ($l = 1, ..., m$) of the $k$th treatment ($k = T, R$). As indicated in Chinchilli and Esinhart (1996), the following mixed effects model can best describe data observed from the $2 \times 2m$ replicated crossover design:

$$x_{ijkl} = \mu_k + \gamma_{ikl} + S_{ijk} + \epsilon_{ijkl}, \qquad (9.1.4)$$

where $\mu_k$ is the treatment effect for formulation $k$, $\gamma_{ikl}$ is the fixed effect of the $l$th replicate on treatment $k$ in the $i$th sequence with constraint

$$\sum_{i=1}^{2} \sum_{l=1}^{m} \gamma_{ikl} = 0,$$

$S_{ijT}$ and $S_{ijR}$ are the random effects of the $j$th subject in the $i$th sequence, $(S_{ijT}, S_{ijR})'$'s are independent and identically distributed bivariate normal random vectors with mean $(0,0)'$ and covariance matrix

$$\Sigma_B = \begin{pmatrix} \sigma_{BT}^2 & \rho \sigma_{BT} \sigma_{BR} \\ \rho \sigma_{BT} \sigma_{BR} & \sigma_{BR}^2 \end{pmatrix},$$

$\epsilon_{ijkl}$'s are independent random variables from the normal distribution with mean 0 and variance $\sigma_{WT}^2$ or $\sigma_{WR}^2$, and the $(S_{ijT}, S_{ijR})'$ and $\epsilon_{ijkl}$ are independent. Note that $\sigma_{BT}^2$ and $\sigma_{BR}^2$ are the inter-subject variances and $\sigma_{WT}^2$ and $\sigma_{WR}^2$ are intra-subject variances.

## 9.1. Comparing Intra-Subject Variabilities

To obtain estimators of intra-subject variances, it is a common practice to use an orthogonal transformation, which is considered by Chinchilli and Esinhart (1996). A new random variable $z_{ijkl}$ can be obtained by using the orthogonal transformation

$$\mathbf{z}_{ijk} = \mathbf{P}'\mathbf{x}_{ijk} \qquad (9.1.5)$$

where

$$\mathbf{x}'_{ijk} = (x_{ijk1}, x_{ijk2}, \ldots, x_{ijkm}), \quad \mathbf{z}'_{ijk} = (z_{ijk1}, z_{ijk2}, \ldots, z_{ijkm})$$

and $\mathbf{P}$ is an $m \times m$ orthogonal matrix, i.e., $\mathbf{P}'\mathbf{P}$ is a $m \times m$ diagonal matrix. The first column of $\mathbf{P}$ is usually defined by the vector $(1, 1, \ldots, 1)'/\sqrt{m}$ to obtain $z_{ijk1} = \bar{x}_{ijk.}$. The other columns can be defined to satisfy the orthogonality of $\mathbf{P}$ and $\text{var}(z_{ijkl}) = \sigma_{Wk}^2$ for $l = 2, \ldots, m$. For example, in the $2 \times 4$ crossover design, the new random variable $z_{ijkl}$ can be defined as

$$z_{ijk1} = \frac{x_{ijk1} + x_{ijk2}}{2} = \bar{x}_{ijk.} \quad \text{and} \quad z_{ijk2} = \frac{x_{ijk1} - x_{ijk2}}{\sqrt{2}}.$$

Now, the estimator of intra-subject variance can be defined as

$$\hat{\sigma}_{WT}^2 = \frac{1}{(n_1 + n_2 - 2)(m-1)} \sum_{i=1}^{2} \sum_{j=1}^{n_i} \sum_{l=2}^{m} (z_{ijTl} - \bar{z}_{i.Tl})^2,$$

$$\hat{\sigma}_{WR}^2 = \frac{1}{(n_1 + n_2 - 2)(m-1)} \sum_{i=1}^{2} \sum_{j=1}^{n_i} \sum_{l=2}^{m} (z_{ijRl} - \bar{z}_{i.Rl})^2,$$

where

$$\bar{z}_{i.kl} = \frac{1}{n_i} \sum_{j=1}^{n_i} \bar{z}_{ijkl}.$$

It should be noted that $\hat{\sigma}_{WT}^2$ and $\hat{\sigma}_{WR}^2$ are independent.

**Test for Equality**

The following hypotheses are usually considered for testing equality in intra-subject variability:

$$H_0 : \sigma_{WT}^2 = \sigma_{WR}^2 \quad \text{versus} \quad H_a : \sigma_{WT}^2 \neq \sigma_{WR}^2.$$

Under the null hypothesis, the test statistic

$$T = \frac{\hat{\sigma}_{WT}^2}{\hat{\sigma}_{WR}^2}$$

is distributed as an $F$ random variable with $d$ and $d$ degrees of freedom, where $d = (n_1 + n_2 - 2)(m - 1)$. Hence, we reject the null hypothesis at the $\alpha$ level of significance if

$$T > F_{\alpha/2, d, d}$$

or

$$T < F_{1-\alpha/2}, d, d.$$

Under the alternative hypothesis, without loss of generality, we assume that $\sigma^2_{WT} < \sigma^2_{WR}$. The power of the above test is

$$\begin{aligned}
\text{power} &= P(T < F_{1-\alpha/2, d, d}) \\
&= P(1/T > F_{\alpha/2, d, d}) \\
&= P\left(\frac{\hat{\sigma}^2_{WR}/\sigma^2_{WR}}{\hat{\sigma}^2_{WT}/\sigma^2_{WT}} > \frac{\sigma^2_{WT}}{\sigma^2_{WR}} F_{\alpha/2, d, d}\right) \\
&= P\left(F_{(d,d)} > \frac{\sigma^2_{WT}}{\sigma^2_{WR}} F_{\alpha/2, d, d}\right).
\end{aligned}$$

Under the assumption that $n = n_1 = n_2$ and with fixed $\sigma^2_{WT}$ and $\sigma^2_{WR}$, the sample size needed in order to achieve a desired power of $1 - \beta$ can be obtained by solving the following equation for $n$:

$$\frac{\sigma^2_{WT}}{\sigma^2_{WR}} = \frac{F_{1-\beta, (2n-2)(m-1), (2n-2)(m-1)}}{F_{\alpha/2, (2n-2)(m-1), (2n-2)(m-1)}}.$$

### Test for Non-Inferiority/Superiority

The problem of testing non-inferiority and superiority can be unified by the following hypotheses:

$$H_0: \frac{\sigma_{WT}}{\sigma_{WR}} \geq \delta \quad \text{versus} \quad H_a: \frac{\sigma_{WT}}{\sigma_{WR}} < \delta.$$

When $\delta < 1$, the rejection of the null hypothesis indicates the superiority of test product over the reference in terms of the intra-subject variability. When $\delta > 1$, the rejection of the null hypothesis indicates the non-inferiority of the test product over the reference. Consider the following test statistic:

$$T = \frac{\hat{\sigma}^2_{WT}}{\delta^2 \hat{\sigma}^2_{WR}}.$$

Under the null hypothesis, $T$ is distributed as an F random variable with $d$ and $d$ degrees of freedom. Hence, we reject the null hypothesis at the $\alpha$ level of significance if

$$T < F_{1-\alpha, d, d}.$$

## 9.1. Comparing Intra-Subject Variabilities

Under the alternative hypothesis that $\sigma^2_{WT}/\sigma^2_{WR} < \delta$, the power of the above test is

$$\begin{aligned}
\text{Power} &= P(T < F_{1-\alpha,d,d}) \\
&= P(1/T > F_{\alpha,d,d}) \\
&= P\left(\frac{\hat{\sigma}^2_{WR}/\sigma^2_{WR}}{\hat{\sigma}^2_{WT}/\sigma^2_{WT}} > \frac{\sigma^2_{WT}}{\delta\sigma^2_{WR}}F_{\alpha,d,d}\right) \\
&= P\left(F_{(d,d)} > \frac{\sigma^2_{WT}}{\delta^2\sigma^2_{WR}}F_{\alpha,d,d}\right).
\end{aligned}$$

Thus, under the assumption that $n = n_1 = n_2$, the sample size needed in order to achieve a desired power of $1 - \beta$ at the $\alpha$ level of significance can be obtained by solving the following equation for $n$:

$$\frac{\sigma^2_{WT}}{\delta^2\sigma^2_{WR}} = \frac{F_{1-\beta,(2n-2)(m-1),(2n-2)(m-1)}}{F_{\alpha,(2n-2)(m-1),(2n-2)(m-1)}}.$$

**Test for Similarity**

For testing similarity, the hypotheses of interest are given by

$$H_0: \frac{\sigma_{WT}}{\sigma_{WR}} \geq \delta \text{ or } \frac{\sigma_{WT}}{\sigma_{WR}} \leq 1/\delta \quad \text{versus} \quad H_a: \frac{1}{\delta} < \frac{\sigma_{WT}}{\sigma_{WR}} < \delta,$$

where $\delta > 1$ is the equivalence limit. The above hypotheses can be decomposed into the following two one-sided hypotheses:

$$H_{01}: \frac{\sigma_{WT}}{\sigma_{WR}} \geq \delta \quad \text{versus} \quad H_{a1}: \frac{\sigma_{WT}}{\sigma_{WR}} < \delta,$$

and

$$H_{02}: \frac{\sigma_{WT}}{\sigma_{WR}} \leq \frac{1}{\delta} \quad \text{versus} \quad H_{a2}: \frac{\sigma_{WT}}{\sigma_{WR}} > \frac{1}{\delta}.$$

These two hypotheses can be tested by the following two test statistics:

$$T_1 = \frac{\hat{\sigma}^2_{WT}}{\delta^2\hat{\sigma}^2_{WR}} \quad \text{and} \quad T_2 = \frac{\delta^2\hat{\sigma}^2_{WT}}{\hat{\sigma}^2_{WR}}.$$

We then reject the null hypothesis and conclude similarity at the $\alpha$ level of significance if

$$T_1 < F_{1-\alpha,d,d} \quad \text{and} \quad T_2 > F_{\alpha,d,d}.$$

Assuming that $n = n_1 = n_2$, under the alternative hypothesis that $\sigma^2_{WT} \leq$

$\sigma_{WR}^2$, the power of the above test is

$$\text{Power} = P\left(\frac{F_{\alpha,d,d}}{\delta} < \frac{\hat{\sigma}_{WT}^2}{\hat{\sigma}_{WR}^2} < \delta F_{1-\alpha,d,d}\right)$$

$$= P\left(\frac{1}{F_{1-\alpha,d,d}\delta} < \frac{\hat{\sigma}_{WT}^2}{\hat{\sigma}_{WR}^2} < \delta F_{1-\alpha,d,d}\right)$$

$$\geq 1 - 2P\left(\frac{\hat{\sigma}_{WR}^2}{\hat{\sigma}_{WT}^2} > \delta^2 F_{1-\alpha,d,d}\right)$$

$$= 1 - 2P\left(F_{(d,d)} > \frac{\delta^2 \sigma_{WT}^2}{\sigma_{WR}^2}F_{1-\alpha,d,d}\right),$$

Hence, a conservative estimate for the sample size needed in order to achieve the power of $1 - \beta$ can be obtained by solving the following equation:

$$\frac{\delta^2 \sigma_{WT}^2}{\sigma_{WR}^2} = \frac{F_{\beta/2,(2n-2)(m-1),(2n-2)(m-1)}}{F_{1-\alpha,(2n-2)(m-1),(2n-2)(m-1)}}.$$

### An Example

Consider the same example regarding comparison of intra-subject variabilities between two formulations (i.e., inhaled and SC) of a drug product as described in the previous subsection. Suppose the intended study will be conducted under a 2 × 4 replicated crossover ($m = 2$) design rather than a parallel design with 3 replicates.

It is assumed that the true standard deviation of inhaled formulation and SC formulation are given by 30% ($\sigma_{WT} = 0.30$) and 45% ($\sigma_{WR} = 0.45$), respectively. It is also believed that 10% ($\delta = 1.10$) of $\sigma_{WR}$ is of no clinical importance. Hence, the sample size needed per sequence in order to achieve an 80% power in establishing non-inferiority at the 5% level of significance can be obtained by solving the following equation:

$$\frac{0.30^2}{1.1^2 \times 0.45^2} = \frac{F_{0.80,2n-2,2n-2}}{F_{0.05,2n-2,2n-2}}.$$

This gives $n = 14$.

## 9.2 Comparing Intra-Subject CVs

In addition to comparing intra-subject variances, it is often of interest to study the intra-subject CV, which is a relative standard deviation adjusted for mean. In recent years, the use of intra-subject CV has become increasingly popular. For example, the FDA defines highly variable drug products

## 9.2. Comparing Intra-Subject CVs

based on their intra-subject CVs. A drug product is said to be a highly variable drug if its intra-subject CV is greater than 30%. The intra-subject CV is also used as a measure for reproducibility of blood levels (or blood concentration-time curves) of a given formulation when the formulation is repeatedly adminstered at different dosing periods. In addition, the information regarding the intra-subject CV of a reference product is usually used for performing power analysis for sample size calculation in bioavailability and bioequivalence studies. In practice, two methods are commonly used for comparing intra-subject CVs. One is proposed by Chow and Tse (1990), which is referred to as conditional random effects model. The other one is suggested by Quan and Shih (1996), which is a simple one-way random effects model. In this section, these two models are introduced and the corresponding formulas for sample size calculation are derived.

### 9.2.1 Simple Random Effects Model

Quan and Shih (1996) developed a method to estimate the intra-subject CV based on a simple one-way random mixed effects model. Comparing this model with model (9.2.1), it can be noted that the mixed effects model assumes that the intra-subject variability is a constant. An intuitive unbiased estimator for $\mu_i$ is given by

$$\hat{\mu}_i = \frac{1}{n_i m} \sum_{j=1}^{n_i} \sum_{k=1}^{m} x_{ijk}.$$

Hence, an estimator of the intra-subject CV can be obtained as

$$\widehat{CV}_i = \frac{\hat{\sigma}_{Wi}}{\hat{\mu}_i}.$$

By Taylor's expansion, it follows that

$$\widehat{CV}_i - CV_i = \frac{\hat{\sigma}_{Wi}}{\hat{\mu}_i} - \frac{\sigma_{Wi}}{\mu_i}$$
$$\approx \frac{1}{2\mu_i \sigma_{Wi}}(\hat{\sigma}_{Wi}^2 - \sigma_{Wi}^2) - \frac{\sigma_{Wi}}{\mu_i^2}(\hat{\mu}_i - \mu_i).$$

Hence, by the Central Limit Theorem, $CV_i$ is asymptotically distributed as a normal random variable with mean $CV_i$ and variance $\sigma_i^{*2}/n_i$, where

$$\sigma_i^{*2} = \frac{\sigma_{Wi}^2}{2m\mu_i^2} + \frac{\sigma_{Wi}^4}{\mu_i^4} = \frac{1}{2m}CV_i^2 + CV_i^4.$$

An intuitive estimator of $\sigma_i^{*2}$ is given by

$$\hat{\sigma}_i^{*2} = \frac{1}{2m}\widehat{CV}_i^2 + \widehat{CV}_i^4.$$

## Test for Equality

The following hypotheses are usually considered for testing equality in intra-subject CVs:

$$H_0 : CV_T = CV_R \quad \text{versus} \quad H_a : CV_T \neq CV_R.$$

Under the null hypothesis, the test statistic

$$T = \frac{\widehat{CV_T} - \widehat{CV_R}}{\sqrt{\hat{\sigma}_T^{*2}/n_T + \hat{\sigma}_R^{*2}/n_R}}$$

is asymptotically distributed as a standard normal random variable. Hence, we reject the null hypothesis at the $\alpha$ level of significance if $|T| > z_{\alpha/2}$. Under the alternative hypothesis, without loss of generality, it is assumed that $CV_T > CV_R$. The distribution of $T$ can be approximated by a normal distribution with unit variance and mean

$$\frac{CV_T - CV_R}{\sqrt{\sigma_T^{*2}/n_T + \sigma_R^{*2}/n_R}}.$$

Thus, the power is approximately

$$P(|T| > z_{\alpha/2}) \approx P(T > z_{\alpha/2})$$

$$= 1 - \Phi\left(z_{\alpha/2} - \frac{CV_T - CV_R}{\sqrt{\sigma_T^{*2}/n_T + \sigma_R^{*2}/n_R}}\right).$$

Under the assumption that $n = n_1 = n_2$, the sample size needed in order to have a power of $1 - \beta$ can be obtained by solving the following equation:

$$z_{\alpha/2} - \frac{CV_T - CV_R}{\sqrt{\sigma_T^{*2}/n + \sigma_R^{*2}/n}} = -z_\beta.$$

This leads to

$$n = \frac{(\sigma_T^{*2} + \sigma_R^{*2})(z_{\alpha/2} + z_\beta)^2}{(CV_T - CV_R)^2}.$$

## Test for Non-Inferiority/Superiority

Similarly, the problem of testing non-inferiority and superiority can be unified by the following hypotheses:

$$H_0 : CV_R - CV_T < \delta \quad \text{versus} \quad H_a : CV_R - CV_T \geq \delta,$$

where $\delta$ is the non-inferiority/superiority margin. When $\delta > 0$, the rejection of the null hypothesis indicates the superiority of the test drug over the reference drug. When $\delta < 0$, the rejection of the null hypothesis indicates that non-inferiority of the test drug over the reference drug.

Under the null hypothesis, the test statistic

$$T = \frac{\widehat{CV}_T - \widehat{CV}_R - \delta}{\sqrt{\hat{\sigma}_T^{*2}/n_T + \hat{\sigma}_R^{*2}/n_R}}$$

is asymptotically distributed as a standard normal random variable. Hence, we reject the null hypothesis at the $\alpha$ level of significance if $T > z_\alpha$. Under the alternative hypothesis, the distribution of $T$ can be approximated by a normal distribution with unit variance and mean

$$\frac{CV_T - CV_R - \delta}{\sqrt{\sigma_T^{*2}/n_T + \sigma_R^{*2}/n_R}}.$$

Hence, the power is approximately

$$P(T > z_{\alpha/2}) = 1 - \Phi\left(z_{\alpha/2} - \frac{CV_T - CV_R - \delta}{\sqrt{\sigma_T^{*2}/n_T + \sigma_R^{*2}/n_R}}\right).$$

Under the assumption that $n = n_1 = n_2$, the sample size needed in order to have a power of $1 - \beta$ can be obtained by solving

$$z_{\alpha/2} - \frac{CV_T - CV_R - \delta}{\sqrt{\sigma_T^{*2}/n + \sigma_R^{*2}/n}} = -z_\beta.$$

This leads to

$$n = \frac{(\sigma_T^{*2} + \sigma_R^{*2})(z_{\alpha/2} + z_\beta)^2}{(CV_T - CV_R - \delta)^2}.$$

**Test for Similarity**

For testing similarity, the following hypotheses are usually considered:

$$H_0: |CV_T - CV_R| \geq \delta \quad \text{versus} \quad H_a: |CV_T - CV_R| < \delta.$$

The two drug products are concluded to be similar to each other if the null hypothesis is rejected at a given significance level. The null hypothesis is rejected at the $\alpha$ level of significance if

$$\frac{\widehat{CV}_T - \widehat{CV}_R + \delta}{\sqrt{\hat{\sigma}_T^{*2}/n_T + \hat{\sigma}_R^{*2}/n_R}} > z_\alpha \quad \text{and} \quad \frac{\widehat{CV}_T - \widehat{CV}_R - \delta}{\sqrt{\hat{\sigma}_T^{*2}/n_T + \hat{\sigma}_R^{*2}/n_R}} < -z_\alpha.$$

Under the alternative hypothesis that $|CV_T - CV_R| < \delta$, the power of the above test procedure is approximately

$$2\Phi\left(\frac{\delta - |CV_T - CV_R|}{\sqrt{\sigma_T^{*2}/n_T + \sigma_R^{*2}/n_R}} - z_\alpha\right) - 1.$$

Hence, under the assumption that $n = n_1 = n_2$, the sample size needed in order to achieve $1 - \beta$ power at the $\alpha$ level of significance can be obtained by solving

$$\frac{\delta - |CV_T - CV_R|}{\sqrt{\sigma_T^{*2}/n_T + \sigma_R^{*2}/n_R}} - z_\alpha = z_{\beta/2}.$$

This gives

$$n = \frac{(z_\alpha + z_{\beta/2})^2(\sigma_T^{*2} + \sigma_R^{*2})}{(\delta - |CV_T - CV_R|)^2}.$$

**An Example**

Consider the same example as described in the previous subsection. Suppose the investigator is interested in conducting a parallel trial to compare intra-subject CVs between the inhaled formulation and SC formulation of the drug product under investigation rather than comparing intra-subject variabilties. Based on information obtained form a pilot study, it is assumed that the true CV of the treatment and control are given by 50% and 70%, respectively. Assume that 10% difference in CV is of no clinical importance. The sample size needed per treatment group in order to establish non-inferiority can be obtained as follows:

$$\sigma_1^2 = 0.25 \times 0.50^2 + 0.50^4 = 0.125$$
$$\sigma_2^2 = 0.25 \times 0.70^2 + 0.70^4 = 0.363.$$

Hence, the sample size needed in order to achieve an 80% power for establishement of non-inferiority at the 5% level of significance is given by

$$n = \frac{(1.64 + 0.84)^2(0.125 + 0.363)}{(0.10 + 0.70 - 0.50)^2} \approx 34.$$

## 9.2.2 Conditional Random Effects Model

In practice, the variability of the observed response often increases as the mean increases. In many cases, the standard deviaiton of the intra-subject variability is approximately proportional to the mean value. To best describe this type of data, Chow and Tse (1990) proposed the following conditional random effects model:

$$x_{ijk} = A_{ij} + A_{ij}e_{ijk}, \qquad (9.2.1)$$

where $x_{ijk}$ is the observation from the $k$th replicate ($k = 1, ..., m$) of the $j$th subject ($j = 1, ..., n_i$) from the $i$th treatment ($i =$ T, R), and $A_{ij}$ is the random effect due to the $j$th subject in the $i$th treatment. It is assumed that $A_{ij}$ is normally distributed as a normal random variable with mean

## 9.2. Comparing Intra-Subject CVs

$\mu_i$ and variance $\sigma_{Bi}^2$ and $e_{ijk}$ is normally distributed as a normal random variable with mean 0 and variance $\sigma_{Wi}^2$. For a given subject with a fixed $A_{ij}$, $x_{ijk}$ is normally distributed as a normal random variable with mean $A_{ij}$ and variance $A_{ij}^2 \sigma_{Wi}^2$. Hence, the CV for this subject is given by

$$CV_i = \frac{|A_{ij}\sigma_{Wi}|}{|A_{ij}|} = \sigma_{Wi}.$$

As it can be seen, the conditional random effects model assumes the CV is constant across subjects.

Define

$$\bar{x}_{i..} = \frac{1}{nm}\sum_{j=1}^{n_i}\sum_{k=1}^{m} x_{ijk}$$

$$M_{i1} = \frac{m}{n_i - 1}\sum_{j=1}^{n_i}(\bar{x}_{ij.} - \bar{x}_{i..})^2$$

$$M_{i2} = \frac{1}{n_i(m_i - 1)}\sum_{j=1}^{n_i}\sum_{k=1}^{m}(x_{ijk} - \bar{x}_{ij.})^2.$$

It can be verified that

$$E(\bar{x}_{i..}) = \mu_i$$
$$E(M_{i1}) = (\mu_i^2 + \sigma_{BT}^2)\sigma_{Wi}^2 + m\sigma_{Bi}^2 = \tau_{i1}^2$$
$$E(M_{i2}) = (\mu_i^2 + \sigma_{BT}^2)\sigma_{Wi}^2 = \tau_{i2}^2.$$

It follows that

$$CV_i = \sigma_{Wi} = \sqrt{\frac{E(M_{i2})}{E^2(\bar{x}_{i..}) + (M_{i1} - M_{i2})}}.$$

Hence, an estimator of $CV_i$ is given by

$$\widehat{CV}_i = \sqrt{\frac{M_{i2}}{\bar{x}_{i..}^2 + (M_{i1} - M_{i2})/m}}.$$

By Taylor's expansion,

$$\widehat{CV}_i - CV_i \approx \frac{1}{\tau_{i1}\tau_{i2}}(M_{i2} - \tau_{i2}^2) - \frac{\mu_i \tau_{i2}}{\tau_{i1}^3}(\bar{x}_{i..} - \mu_i)$$
$$- \frac{\tau_{i2}}{2m\tau_{i1}^3}(M_{i1} - M_{i2} - (\tau_{i1}^2 - \tau_{i2}^2))$$
$$= k_0(\bar{x}_{i..} - \mu_i) + k_1(M_{i1} - \tau_{i1}^2) + k_2(M_{i2} - \tau_{i2}^2),$$

where

$$k_0 = -\frac{\mu_i \tau_{i2}}{\tau_{i1}^3}$$

$$k_1 = -\frac{\tau_{i2}}{2m\tau_{i1}^3}$$

$$k_2 = \left(\frac{1}{\tau_{i1}\tau_{i2}} + \frac{\tau_{i2}}{2m\tau_{i1}^3}\right).$$

As a result, the distribution of $\widehat{CV}_i$ can be approximated by a normal random variable with mean $CV_i$ and variance $\sigma_i^{*2}/n_i$, where

$$\sigma_i^{*2} = \text{var}\left[k_0 \bar{x}_{ij\cdot} + mk_1(\bar{x}_{ij\cdot} - \bar{x}_{i\cdot\cdot})^2 + \frac{k_2}{m-1}\sum_{k=1}^{m}(x_{ijk} - \bar{x}_{ij\cdot})^2\right].$$

An intuitive estimator for $\sigma_i^{*2}$ is the sample variance, denoted by $\hat{\sigma}_i^{*2}$, of

$$k_0 \bar{x}_{ij\cdot} + mk_1(\bar{x}_{ij\cdot} - \bar{x}_{i\cdot\cdot})^2 + \frac{k_2}{m-1}\sum_{k=1}^{m}(x_{ijk} - \bar{x}_{ij\cdot})^2, \quad j = 1, ..., n_i.$$

**Test for Equality**

For testing equality, the following hypotheses are of interest:

$$H_0 : CV_T = CV_R \quad \text{versus} \quad H_a : CV_T \neq CV_R.$$

Under the null hypothesis, test statistic

$$T = \frac{\widehat{CV}_T - \widehat{CV}_R}{\sqrt{\hat{\sigma}_T^{*2}/n_T + \hat{\sigma}_R^{*2}/n_R}}$$

is asymptotically distributed as a standard normal random variable. Hence, we reject the null hypothesis at the $\alpha$ level of significance if $|T| > z_{\alpha/2}$. Under the alternative hypothesis, without loss of generality, we assume that $CV_T > CV_R$. The distribution of $T$ can be approximated by a normal distribution with unit variance and mean

$$\frac{CV_T - CV_R}{\sqrt{\sigma_T^{*2}/n_T + \sigma_R^{*2}/n_R}}.$$

Hence, the power is approximately

$$P(|T| > z_{\alpha/2}) \approx P(T > z_{\alpha/2})$$

$$= 1 - \Phi\left(z_{\alpha/2} - \frac{CV_T - CV_R}{\sqrt{\sigma_T^{*2}/n_T + \sigma_R^{*2}/n_R}}\right).$$

## 9.2. Comparing Intra-Subject CVs

Under the assumption that $n = n_1 = n_2$, the sample size required for having a desired power of $1 - \beta$ can be obtained by solving

$$z_{\alpha/2} - \frac{CV_T - CV_R}{\sqrt{\sigma_T^{*2}/n + \sigma_R^{*2}/n}} = -z_\beta.$$

This leads to

$$n = \frac{(z_{\alpha/2} + z_\beta)^2(\sigma_T^{*2} + \sigma_R^{*2})}{(CV_T - CV_R)^2}.$$

### Test for Non-Inferiority/Superiority

The problem of testing non-inferiority and superiority can be unified by the following hypotheses:

$$H_0: CV_R - CV_T < \delta \quad \text{versus} \quad H_a: CV_R - CV_T \geq \delta,$$

where $\delta$ is the non-inferiority/superiority margin. When $\delta > 0$, the rejection of the null hypothesis indicates the superiority of the test drug over the reference drug. When $\delta < 0$, the rejection of the null hypothesis indicates non-inferiority of the test drug over the reference drug. Under the null hypothesis, test statistic

$$T = \frac{\widehat{CV}_T - \widehat{CV}_R - \delta}{\sqrt{\hat{\sigma}_T^{*2}/n_T + \hat{\sigma}_R^{*2}/n_R}}$$

is asymptotically distributed as a standard normal random variable. Hence, we reject the null hypothesis at the $\alpha$ level of significance if $T > z_\alpha$. Under the alternative hypothesis, the distribution of $T$ can be approximated by a normal distribution with unit variance and mean

$$\frac{CV_T - CV_R - \delta}{\sqrt{\sigma_T^{*2}/n_T + \sigma_R^{*2}/n_R}}.$$

Hence, the power is approximately

$$P(T > z_{\alpha/2}) = 1 - \Phi\left(z_{\alpha/2} - \frac{CV_T - CV_R - \delta}{\sqrt{\sigma_T^{*2}/n_T + \sigma_R^{*2}/n_R}}\right).$$

Under the assumption $n = n_1 = n_2$, the sample size needed in order to have the desired power $1 - \beta$ can be obtained by solving

$$z_{\alpha/2} - \frac{CV_T - CV_R - \delta}{\sqrt{\sigma_T^{*2}/n + \sigma_R^{*2}/n}} = -z_\beta.$$

This gives

$$n = \frac{(\sigma_T^{*2} + \sigma_R^{*2})(z_{\alpha/2} + z_\beta)^2}{(CV_T - CV_R - \delta)^2}.$$

**Test for Similarity**

For testing similarity, consider the following hypotheses:

$$H_0 : |CV_T - CV_R| \geq \delta \quad \text{versus} \quad H_a : |CV_T - CV_R| < \delta.$$

The two drug products are concluded to be similar to each other if the null hypothesis is rejected at a given significance level. The null hypothesis is rejected at $\alpha$ level of significance if

$$\frac{\widehat{CV}_T - \widehat{CV}_R + \delta}{\sqrt{\hat{\sigma}_T^{*2}/n_T + \hat{\sigma}_R^{*2}/n_R}} > z_\alpha \quad \text{versus} \quad \frac{\widehat{CV}_T - \widehat{CV}_R - \delta}{\sqrt{\hat{\sigma}_T^{*2}/n_T + \hat{\sigma}_R^{*2}/n_R}} < -z_\alpha.$$

Under the alternative hypothesis that $|CV_T - CV_R| < \delta$, the power of the above test procedure is approximately

$$2\Phi\left(\frac{\delta - |CV_T - CV_R|}{\sqrt{\sigma_T^{*2}/n_T + \sigma_R^{*2}/n_R}} - z_\alpha\right) - 1.$$

Hence, under the assumption that $n = n_1 = n_2$, the sample size needed in order to achieve $1 - \beta$ power at the $\alpha$ level of significance can be obtained by solving

$$\frac{\delta - |CV_T - CV_R|}{\sqrt{\sigma_T^{*2}/n_T + \sigma_R^{*2}/n_R}} - z_\alpha = z_{\beta/2}.$$

This gives

$$n = \frac{(z_\alpha + z_{\beta/2})^2(\sigma_T^{*2} + \sigma_R^{*2})}{(\delta - |CV_T - CV_R|)^2}.$$

**An Example**

Consider the same example as described in the previous subsection. Suppose it is found that the variability of the CV increases as the mean increases. In this case, the conditional random effects model is useful for comparing the two treatments. Again, we assume that CV of the test drug and the reference drug are given by 50% and 70%, respectively. Suppose it is also estimated from other studies that $\sigma_T^* = 0.30$ and $\sigma_R^* = 0.35$. Assume that 10% difference in CV is of no clinical importance. The sample size needed per treatment group in order to establish non-inferiority can be obtained as follows:

$$n = \frac{(1.64 + 0.84)^2(0.30^2 + 0.35^2)}{(0.10 + 0.70 - 0.50)^2} \approx 15.$$

As a result, 15 subjects per treatment group are needed in order to have an 80% power at the 5% level of significance.

**Remarks**

For comparing intra-subject variabilities and/or intra-subject CVs between treatment groups, replicates from the same subject are essential regardless of whether the study design is a parallel group design or a crossover design. In clinical research, data are often log-transformed before the analysis. It should be noted that the intra-subject standard deviation of log-transformed data is approximately equal to the intra-subject CV of the untransformed (raw) data. As a result, it is suggested that intra-subject variability be used when analyzing log-transformed data, while the intra-subject CV be considered when analyzing untransformed data.

## 9.3 Comparing Inter-Subject Variabilities

In addition to comparing intra-subject variabilities or intra-subject CVs, it is also of interest to compare inter-subject variabilities. In practice, it is not uncommon that clinical results may not be reproducible from subject to subject within the target population or from subjects within the target population to subjects within a similar but slightly different population due to the inter-subject variability. How to test a difference in inter-subject and total variability between two treatments is a challenging problem to clinical scientists, especially biostatisticians, due to the following factors. First, unbiased estimators of the inter-subject and total variabilities are usually not chi-square distributed under both parallel and crossover design with replicates. Second, the estimators for the inter-subject and total variabilities under different treatments are usually not independent under a crossover design. As a result, unlike tests for comparing intra-subject variabilities, the standard F test is not applicable. Tests for comparing inter-subject variabilities under a parallel design can be performed by using the method of a modified large sample (MLS) method. See Howe (1974); Graybill and Wang (1980); Ting et al. (1990); Hyslop et al. (2000). As indicated earlier, the MLS method is superior to many other approximation methods. Under crossover designs, however, the MLS method cannot be directly applied since estimators of variance components are not independent. Lee et al. (2002a) proposed an extension of the MLS method when estimators of variance components are not independent. In addition, tests for comparing inter-subject and total variabilities under crossover designs are studied by Lee et al. (2002b). Note that the MLS method by Hyslop et al. (2000) is recommended by the FDA (2001) as a statistical test for individual bioequivalence.

## 9.3.1 Parallel Design with Replicates

Under model (9.1.1), define

$$s_{Bi}^2 = \frac{1}{n_i - 1} \sum_{j=1}^{n_i} (\bar{x}_{ij\cdot} - \bar{x}_{i\cdot\cdot})^2, \qquad (9.3.1)$$

where

$$\bar{x}_{i\cdot\cdot} = \frac{1}{n_i} \sum_{j=1}^{n_i} \bar{x}_{ij\cdot}.$$

and $\bar{x}_{ij\cdot}$ is given in (9.1.3). Note that $E(s_{Bi}^2) = \sigma_{Bi}^2 + \sigma_{Wi}^2/m$. Therefore,

$$\hat{\sigma}_{Bi}^2 = s_{Bi}^2 - \frac{1}{m}\hat{\sigma}_{Wi}^2$$

are unbiased estimators for the inter-subject variances, where $\hat{\sigma}_{Wi}^2$ is defined in (9.1.2).

**Test for Equality**

For testing equality in inter-subject variability, the following hypotheses are usually considered:

$$H_0 : \frac{\sigma_{BT}}{\sigma_{BR}} = 1 \quad \text{versus} \quad H_a : \frac{\sigma_{BT}}{\sigma_{BR}} \neq 1.$$

Testing the above hypotheses is equivalent to testing the following hypotheses:

$$H_0 : \sigma_{BT}^2 - \sigma_{BR}^2 = 0 \quad \text{versus} \quad H_a : \sigma_{BT}^2 - \sigma_{BR}^2 \neq 0.$$

Let $\eta = \sigma_{BT}^2 - \sigma_{BR}^2$. An intuitive estimator of $\eta$ is given by

$$\hat{\eta} = \hat{\sigma}_{BR}^2 - \hat{\sigma}_{BT}^2$$
$$= s_{BT}^2 - s_{BR}^2 - \hat{\sigma}_{WT}^2/m + \hat{\sigma}_{WR}^2/m.$$

A $(1-\alpha)\times 100\%$ confidence interval for $\eta$ is given by $(\hat{\eta}_L, \hat{\eta}_U)$, where

$$\hat{\eta}_L = \hat{\eta} - \sqrt{\Delta_L}, \quad \hat{\eta}_U = \hat{\eta} + \sqrt{\Delta_U}$$

## 9.3. Comparing Inter-Subject Variabilities

and

$$\Delta_L = s_{BT}^4 \left(1 - \frac{n_T - 1}{\chi_{\alpha/2, n_T - 1}^2}\right)^2 + s_{BR}^4 \left(1 - \frac{n_R - 1}{\chi_{1-\alpha/2, n_R - 1}^2}\right)^2$$
$$+ \frac{\hat{\sigma}_{WT}^4}{m^2}\left(1 - \frac{n_T(m-1)}{\chi_{1-\alpha/2, n_T(m-1)}^2}\right)^2 + \frac{\hat{\sigma}_{WR}^4}{m^2}\left(1 - \frac{n_R(m-1)}{\chi_{\alpha/2, n_R(m-1)}^2}\right)^2$$

$$\Delta_U = s_{BT}^4 \left(1 - \frac{n_T - 1}{\chi_{1-\alpha/2, n_T - 1}^2}\right)^2 + s_{BR}^4 \left(1 - \frac{n_R - 1}{\chi_{\alpha/2, n_R - 1}^2}\right)^2$$
$$+ \frac{\hat{\sigma}_{WT}^4}{m^2}\left(1 - \frac{n_T(m-1)}{\chi_{\alpha/2, n_T(m-1)}^2}\right)^2 + \frac{\hat{\sigma}_{WR}^4}{m^2}\left(1 - \frac{n_R(m-1)}{\chi_{1-\alpha/2, n_R(m-1)}^2}\right)^2.$$

We reject the null hypothesis at the $\alpha$ level of significance if $0 \notin (\hat{\eta}_L, \hat{\eta}_U)$. Under the alternative hypothesis, without loss of generality, we assume that $\sigma_{BR}^2 > \sigma_{BT}^2$ and $n = n_T = n_R$. Thus, the power of the above test procedure can be approximated by

$$1 - \Phi\left(z_{\alpha/2} - \frac{\sqrt{n}(\sigma_{BT}^2 - \sigma_{BR}^2)}{\sigma^*}\right),$$

where

$$\sigma^{*2} = 2\left[\left(\sigma_{BT}^2 + \frac{\sigma_{WT}^2}{m}\right)^2 + \left(\sigma_{BR}^2 + \frac{\sigma_{WR}^2}{m}\right)^2 + \frac{\sigma_{WT}^4}{m^2(m-1)} + \frac{\sigma_{WR}^4}{m^2(m-1)}\right].$$

As a result, the sample size needed in order to achieve the desired power of $1 - \beta$ at the $\alpha$ level of significance can be obtained by solving

$$z_{\alpha/2} - \frac{\sqrt{n}(\sigma_{BT}^2 - \sigma_{BR}^2)}{\sigma^*} = -z_\beta.$$

This leads to

$$n = \frac{\sigma^{*2}(z_{\alpha/2} + z_\beta)^2}{(\sigma_{BT}^2 - \sigma_{BR}^2)^2}.$$

**Test for Non-Inferiority/Superiority**

Similar to testing intra-subject variabilities, the problem of testing non-inferiority/superiority can be unified by the following hypotheses:

$$H_0: \frac{\sigma_{BT}}{\sigma_{BR}} \geq \delta \quad \text{versus} \quad H_a: \frac{\sigma_{BT}}{\sigma_{BR}} < \delta.$$

Testing the above hypotheses is equivalent to testing the following hypotheses:
$$H_0: \sigma_{BT}^2 - \delta^2\sigma_{BR}^2 \geq 0 \quad \text{versus} \quad H_a: \sigma_{BT}^2 - \delta^2\sigma_{BT}^2 < 0.$$

Define
$$\eta = \sigma_{BT}^2 - \delta^2\sigma_{BR}^2.$$

For a given significance level $\alpha$, similarly, the $(1-\alpha) \times 100\%$th MLS upper confidence bound of $\eta$ can be constructed as
$$\hat{\eta}_U = \hat{\eta} + \sqrt{\Delta_U}$$

where $\Delta_U$ is given by
$$\Delta_U = s_{BT}^4 \left(1 - \frac{n_T - 1}{\chi_{1-\alpha,n_T-1}^2}\right)^2 + \delta^4 s_{BR}^4 \left(1 - \frac{n_R - 1}{\chi_{\alpha,n_R-1}^2}\right)^2$$
$$+ \frac{\hat{\sigma}_{WT}^4}{m^2}\left(1 - \frac{n_T(m-1)}{\chi_{\alpha,n_T(m-1)}^2}\right)^2 + \frac{\delta^4\hat{\sigma}_{WR}^4}{m^2}\left(1 - \frac{n_R(m-1)}{\chi_{1-\alpha,n_R(m-1)}^2}\right)^2.$$

We then reject the null hypothesis at the $\alpha$ level of significance if $\hat{\eta}_U < 0$. Under the assumption that $n = n_T = n_R$, using a similar argument to those in the previous section, the power of the above testing procedure can be approximated by
$$1 - \Phi\left(z_\alpha - \frac{\sqrt{n}(\sigma_{BT}^2 - \delta^2\sigma_{BR}^2)}{\sigma^*}\right),$$

where
$$\sigma^{*2} = 2\left[\left(\sigma_{BT}^2 + \frac{\sigma_{WT}^2}{m}\right)^2 + \delta^4\left(\sigma_{BR}^2 + \frac{\sigma_{WR}^2}{m}\right)^2 \right.$$
$$\left. + \frac{\sigma_{WT}^4}{m^2(m-1)} + \frac{\delta^4\sigma_{WR}^4}{m^2(m-1)}\right].$$

As a result, the sample size needed in order to achieve the power of $1-\beta$ at the $\alpha$ level of significance can be obtained by solving
$$z_\alpha - \frac{\sqrt{n}(\sigma_{BT}^2 - \delta^2\sigma_{BR}^2)^2}{\sigma^*} = -z_\beta.$$

This gives
$$n = \frac{\sigma^{*2}(z_\alpha + z_\beta)^2}{(\sigma_{BT}^2 - \delta^2\sigma_{BR}^2)^2}.$$

## 9.3. Comparing Inter-Subject Variabilities

### An Example

For illustration purposes, consider the same example as described in the previous subsection (i.e., a parallel design with 3 replicates). Suppose we are interested in testing difference in inter-subject variabilities. In this case, we assume

$$\sigma_{BT} = 0.30 \qquad \sigma_{BR} = 0.40$$
$$\sigma_{WT} = 0.20 \qquad \sigma_{WR} = 0.30.$$

Hence, the sample size needed in order to achieve an 80% power $(1 - \beta = 0.80)$ in establishing non-inferiority with a non-inferiority margin 0.10 ($\delta = 1.10$) at the 5% level of significance ($\alpha = 0.05$) can be obtained as

$$\sigma^{*2} = 2\left[\left(0.30^2 + \frac{0.20^2}{3}\right)^2 + 1.1^4 \times \left(0.40^2 + \frac{0.30^2}{3}\right)^2 \right.$$
$$\left. + \frac{0.20^4}{3^2(3-1)} + \frac{1.1^4 0.30^4}{3^2(3-1)}\right]$$
$$= 0.129.$$

Hence,

$$n = \frac{0.129(1.64 + 0.84)^2}{(0.30^2 - 1.1^2 \times 0.40^2)^2} \approx 74.$$

### 9.3.2 Replicated Crossover Design

Under model (9.1.4), estimators of inter-subject variances can be defined by

$$s_{BT}^2 = \frac{1}{n_1 + n_2 - 2} \sum_{i=1}^{2} \sum_{j=1}^{n_i} (\bar{x}_{ijT.} - \bar{x}_{i.T.})^2,$$

$$s_{BR}^2 = \frac{1}{n_1 + n_2 - 2} \sum_{i=1}^{2} \sum_{j=1}^{n_i} (\bar{x}_{ijR.} - \bar{x}_{i.R.})^2,$$

where

$$\bar{x}_{i.k.} = \frac{1}{n_i} \sum_{j=1}^{n_i} \bar{x}_{ijk.}.$$

Note that $E(s_{Bk}^2) = \sigma_{Bk}^2 + \sigma_{Wk}^2/m$ for $k = T, R$. Therefore, unbiased estimators for the inter-subject variance are given by

$$\hat{\sigma}_{BT}^2 = s_{BT}^2 - \frac{1}{m}\hat{\sigma}_{WT}^2 \qquad (9.3.2)$$

$$\hat{\sigma}_{BR}^2 = s_{BR}^2 - \frac{1}{m}\hat{\sigma}_{WR}^2. \qquad (9.3.3)$$

### Test for Equality

For testing the equality in inter-subject variability, the following hypotheses are considered:

$$H_0: \frac{\sigma_{BT}}{\sigma_{BR}} = 1 \quad \text{versus} \quad H_a: \frac{\sigma_{BT}}{\sigma_{BR}} \neq 1.$$

Testing the above hypotheses is equivalent to test the following hypotheses:

$$H_0: \sigma_{BT}^2 - \sigma_{BR}^2 = 0 \quad \text{versus} \quad H_a: \sigma_{BT}^2 - \sigma_{BR}^2 \neq 0.$$

Let $\eta = \sigma_{BT}^2 - \sigma_{BR}^2$. An intuitive estimator of $\eta$ is given by

$$\hat{\eta} = \hat{\sigma}_{BT}^2 - \hat{\sigma}_{BR}^2$$
$$= s_{BT}^2 - s_{BR}^2 - \hat{\sigma}_{WT}^2/m + \hat{\sigma}_{WR}^2/m,$$

where $\hat{\sigma}_{BT}^2$ and $\hat{\sigma}_{BR}^2$ are given in (9.3.2) and (9.3.3), respectively. Random vector $(\bar{x}_{ijT.}, \bar{x}_{ijR.})'$ for the $j$th subject in $i$th sequence has a bivariate normal distribution with covariance matrix given by

$$\Omega_B = \begin{pmatrix} \sigma_{BT}^2 + \sigma_{WT}^2/m & \rho\sigma_{BT}\sigma_{BR} \\ \rho\sigma_{BT}\sigma_{BR} & \sigma_{BR}^2 + \sigma_{WR}^2/m \end{pmatrix}. \quad (9.3.4)$$

An unbiased estimator of the covariance matrix $\Omega_B$ is

$$\hat{\Omega}_B = \begin{pmatrix} s_{BT}^2 & s_{BTR}^2 \\ s_{BTR}^2 & s_{BR}^2 \end{pmatrix}, \quad (9.3.5)$$

where

$$s_{BTR}^2 = \frac{1}{n_1 + n_2 - 2} \sum_{i=1}^{2} \sum_{j=1}^{n_i} (\bar{x}_{ijT.} - \bar{x}_{i.T.})(\bar{x}_{ijR.} - \bar{x}_{i.R.})$$

is the sample covariance between $\bar{x}_{ijT.}$ and $\bar{x}_{ijR.}$. Let $\lambda_i, i = 1, 2$, be the two eigenvalues of the matrix $\Theta\Omega_B$, where

$$\Theta = \begin{pmatrix} 1 & 0 \\ 0 & -1 \end{pmatrix}. \quad (9.3.6)$$

Hence, $\lambda_i$ can be estimated by

$$\hat{\lambda}_i = \frac{s_{BT}^2 - s_{BR}^2 \pm \sqrt{(s_{BT}^2 + s_{BR}^2)^2 - 4s_{BTR}^4}}{2} \quad \text{for } i = 1, 2.$$

Without loss of generality, it can be assumed that $\hat{\lambda}_1 < 0 < \hat{\lambda}_2$. In Lee et al. (2002b), a $(1 - \alpha) \times 100\%$ confidence interval of $\eta$ is given by $(\hat{\eta}_L, \hat{\eta}_U)$, where

$$\hat{\eta}_L = \hat{\eta} - \sqrt{\Delta_L}, \quad \hat{\eta}_U = \hat{\eta} + \sqrt{\Delta_U},$$

## 9.3. Comparing Inter-Subject Variabilities

$$\Delta_L = \hat{\lambda}_1^2 \left(1 - \frac{n_s - 1}{\chi^2_{\alpha/2, n_s - 1}}\right)^2 + \hat{\lambda}_2^2 \left(1 - \frac{n_s - 1}{\chi^2_{1-\alpha/2, n_s - 1}}\right)^2$$

$$+ \frac{\hat{\sigma}^4_{WT}}{m^2}\left(1 - \frac{n_s(m-1)}{\chi^2_{\alpha/2, n_s(m-1)}}\right)^2 + \frac{\hat{\sigma}^4_{WR}}{m^2}\left(1 - \frac{n_s(m-1)}{\chi^2_{1-\alpha/2, n_s(m-1)}}\right)^2$$

$$\Delta_U = \hat{\lambda}_1^2 \left(1 - \frac{n_s - 1}{\chi^2_{1-\alpha/2, n_s - 1}}\right)^2 + \hat{\lambda}_2^2 \left(1 - \frac{n_s - 1}{\chi^2_{\alpha/2, n_s - 1}}\right)^2$$

$$+ \frac{\hat{\sigma}^4_{WT}}{m^2}\left(1 - \frac{n_s(m-1)}{\chi^2_{1-\alpha/2, n_s(m-1)}}\right)^2 + \frac{\hat{\sigma}^4_{WR}}{m^2}\left(1 - \frac{n_s(m-1)}{\chi^2_{\alpha/2, n_s(m-1)}}\right)^2,$$

and $n_s = n_1 + n_2 - 2$. Then, we reject the null hypothesis at the $\alpha$ level of significance if $0 \notin (\hat{\eta}_L, \hat{\eta}_U)$.

Under the alternative hypothesis, the power of the above test can be approximated by

$$1 - \Phi\left(z_{\alpha/2} - \frac{\sqrt{n_s}(\sigma^2_{BT} - \sigma^2_{BR})}{\sigma^*}\right),$$

where

$$\sigma^{*2} = 2\left[\left(\sigma^2_{BT} + \frac{\sigma^2_{WT}}{m}\right)^2 + \left(\sigma^2_{BR} + \frac{\sigma^2_{WR}}{m}\right)^2 - 2\rho^2 \sigma^2_{BT} \sigma^2_{BR}\right.$$

$$\left. + \frac{\sigma^4_{WT}}{m^2(m-1)} + \frac{\sigma^4_{WR}}{m^2(m-1)}\right].$$

Thus, the sample size needed in order to achieve the power of $1 - \beta$ at the $\alpha$ level of significance can be obtained by solving

$$z_\alpha - \frac{\sqrt{n_s}(\sigma^2_{BT} - \sigma^2_{BR})}{\sigma^*} = -z_\beta.$$

This leads to

$$n_s = \frac{\sigma^{*2}(z_{\alpha/2} + z_\beta)^2}{(\sigma^2_{BT} - \sigma^2_{BR})^2}.$$

### Test for Non-Inferiority/Superiority

Similar to testing intra-subject variabilities, the problem of testing non-inferiority/superiority can be unified by the following hypotheses:

$$H_0: \frac{\sigma_{BT}}{\sigma_{BR}} \geq \delta \quad \text{versus} \quad H_a: \frac{\sigma_{BT}}{\sigma_{BR}} < \delta.$$

Testing the above hypotheses is equivalent to testing the following hypotheses:
$$H_0: \sigma_{BT}^2 - \delta^2\sigma_{BR}^2 \geq 0 \quad \text{versus} \quad H_a: \sigma_{BT}^2 - \delta^2\sigma_{BR}^2 < 0.$$

When $\delta < 1$, the rejection of the null hypothesis indicates the superiority of the test drug versus the reference drug. When $\delta > 1$, a rejection of the null hypothesis indicates the non-inferiority of the test drug versus the reference drug. Let $\eta = \sigma_{BT}^2 - \delta^2\sigma_{BR}^2$. For a given significance level of $\alpha$, similarly, the $(1-\alpha)$th upper confidence bound of $\eta$ can be constructed as

$$\hat{\eta}_U = \hat{\eta} + \sqrt{\Delta_U},$$

where $\Delta_U$ is given by

$$\Delta_U = \hat{\lambda}_1^2\left(1 - \frac{n_s - 1}{\chi_{1-\alpha/2, n_s - 1}^2}\right)^2 + \hat{\lambda}_2^2\left(1 - \frac{n_s - 1}{\chi_{\alpha/2, n_s - 1}^2}\right)^2$$
$$+ \frac{\hat{\sigma}_{WT}^4}{m^2}\left(1 - \frac{n_s(m-1)}{\chi_{1-\alpha/2, n_s(m-1)}^2}\right)^2 + \frac{\delta^4\hat{\sigma}_{WR}^4}{m^2}\left(1 - \frac{n_s(m-1)}{\chi_{\alpha/2, n_s(m-1)}^2}\right)^2,$$

$n_s = n_1 + n_2 - 2$, and

$$\hat{\lambda}_i = \frac{s_{BT}^2 - \delta^2 s_{BR}^2 \pm \sqrt{(s_{BT}^2 + \delta^2 s_{BR}^2)^2 - 4\delta^2 s_{BTR}^4}}{2}.$$

We then reject the null hypothesis at the $\alpha$ level of significance if $\hat{\eta}_U < 0$.

Using a similar argument to the previous section, the power of the above test procedure can be approximated by

$$1 - \Phi\left(z_\alpha - \frac{\sqrt{n_s}(\sigma_{BT}^2 - \delta^2\sigma_{BR}^2)}{\sigma^*}\right),$$

where

$$\sigma^{*2} = 2\left[\left(\sigma_{BT}^2 + \frac{\sigma_{WT}^2}{m}\right)^2 + \delta^4\left(\sigma_{BR}^2 + \frac{\sigma_{WR}^2}{m}\right)^2 - 2\delta^2\rho^2\sigma_{BT}^2\sigma_{BR}^2\right.$$
$$\left. + \frac{\sigma_{WT}^4}{m^2(m-1)} + \frac{\delta^4\sigma_{WR}^4}{m^2(m-1)}\right].$$

As a result, the sample size needed in order to achieve a power of $1-\beta$ at the $\alpha$ level of significance can be obtained by solving

$$z_\alpha - \frac{\sqrt{n_s}(\sigma_{BT}^2 - \delta^2\sigma_{BR}^2)}{\sigma^*} = -z_\beta.$$

This leads to

$$n_s = \frac{\sigma^{*2}(z_{\alpha/2} + z_\beta)^2}{(\sigma_{BT}^2 - \delta^2\sigma_{BR}^2)^2}.$$

## An Example

Suppose a $2 \times 4$ crossover design (ABAB,BABA) is used to compare two treatments (A and B) in terms of their inter-subject variabilities. Information from pilot studies indicates that $\rho = 0.75$, $\sigma_{BT} = 0.3$, $\sigma_{BR} = 0.4$, $\sigma_{WT} = 0.2$, and $\sigma_{WR} = 0.3$. The objective is to establish non-inferiority with a margin of 10% ($\delta = 1.10$). It follows that

$$\sigma^{*2} = 2\left[\left(0.30^2 + \frac{0.20^2}{2}\right)^2 + 1.1^4 \times \left(0.40^2 + \frac{0.30^2}{2}\right)^2 \right.$$
$$\left. -2 \times 1.1^2(0.75 \times 0.3 \times 0.4)^2 + \frac{0.20^4}{2^2} + \frac{1.1^4 \times 0.30^4}{2^2}\right]$$
$$= 0.115.$$

Hence, the sample size needed in order to achieve an 80% power ($1 - \beta = 0.80$) for establishment of non-inferiority at the 5% level of significance ($\alpha = 0.05$) is given by

$$n_s = \frac{0.115(1.64 + 0.84)^2}{(0.30^2 - 1.1^2 \times 0.40^2)^2} \approx 66.$$

Since $n_s = n_1 + n_2 - 2$, approximately 29 subjects per sequence are required for achieving an 80% power at the 5% level of significance.

## 9.4 Comparing Total Variabilities

In practice, it may also be of interest to compare total variabilities between drug products. For example, comparing total variability is required in assessing drug prescribability (FDA, 2001). Total variability can be estimated under a parallel-group design with and without replicates and under various crossover designs (e.g., a $2 \times 2$ standard crossover design or a $2 \times 2m$ replicated crossover design). In this section, we focus on sample size calculation under a parallel-group design with and without replicates, the standard $2 \times 2$ crossover design, and the $2 \times 2m$ replicated crossover design.

### 9.4.1 Parallel Designs Without Replicates

For parallel design without replicates, the model in (9.1.1) is reduced to

$$x_{ij} = \mu_i + \epsilon_{ij},$$

where $x_{ij}$ is the observation from the $j$th subject in the $i$th treatment group. Also, we assume that the random variable $\epsilon_{ij}$ has normal distribution with mean 0 and variance $\sigma_{Ti}^2$ for $i = T, R$. Hence, the total variability can be estimated by

$$\hat{\sigma}_{Ti}^2 = \frac{1}{n_i - 1} \sum_{j=1}^{n_i} (x_{ij} - \bar{x}_{i\cdot})^2,$$

where

$$\bar{x}_{i\cdot} = \frac{1}{n_i} \sum_{j=1}^{n_i} x_{ij}.$$

**Test for Equality**

For testing equality in total variability, the following hypotheses are considered:

$$H_0 : \sigma_{TT}^2 = \sigma_{TR}^2 \quad \text{versus} \quad H_a : \sigma_{TT}^2 \neq \sigma_{TR}^2.$$

Under the null hypothesis, the test statistic

$$T = \frac{\hat{\sigma}_{TT}^2}{\hat{\sigma}_{TR}^2}.$$

is distributed as an F random variable with $n_T - 1$ and $n_R - 1$ degrees of freedom. Hence, we reject the null hypothesis at the $\alpha$ level of significance if

$$T > F_{\alpha/2, n_T - 1, n_R - 1}$$

or

$$T < F_{1 - \alpha/2, n_T - 1, n_R - 1}.$$

Under the alternative hypothesis (without loss of generality, we assume that $\sigma_{TT}^2 < \sigma_{TR}^2$), the power of the above test procedure is

$$\begin{aligned}
\text{Power} &= P(T < F_{1-\alpha/2, n_T-1, n_R-1}) \\
&= P(1/T > F_{\alpha/2, n_R-1, n_T-1}) \\
&= P\left( \frac{\hat{\sigma}_{TR}^2/\sigma_{TR}^2}{\hat{\sigma}_{TT}^2/\sigma_{TT}^2} > \frac{\sigma_{TT}^2}{\sigma_{TR}^2} F_{\alpha/2, n_R-1, n_T-1} \right) \\
&= P\left( F_{n_R, n_T} > \frac{\sigma_{TT}^2}{\sigma_{TR}^2} F_{\alpha/2, n_R-1, n_T-1} \right).
\end{aligned}$$

Under the assumption that $n = n_R = n_T$ and with a fixed $\sigma_{TT}^2$ and $\sigma_{TR}^2$, the sample size needed in order to achieve a desired power of $1 - \beta$ can be obtained by solving the following equation for $n$:

$$\frac{\sigma_{TT}^2}{\sigma_{TR}^2} = \frac{F_{1-\beta, n-1, n-1}}{F_{\alpha/2, n-1, n-1}}.$$

## 9.4. Comparing Total Variabilities

### Test for Non-Inferiority/Superiority

The problem of testing non-inferiority and superiority can be unified by the following hypotheses:

$$H_0 : \frac{\sigma_{TT}}{\sigma_{TR}} \geq \delta \quad \text{versus} \quad \frac{\sigma_{TT}}{\sigma_{TR}} < \delta.$$

When $\delta < 1$, the rejection of the null hypothesis indicates the superiority of test product over the reference in terms of the total variability. When $\delta > 1$, the rejection of the null hypothesis indicates the non-inferiority of the test product over the reference. The test statistic is given by

$$T = \frac{\hat{\sigma}_{TT}^2}{\delta^2 \hat{\sigma}_{TR}^2}.$$

Under the null hypothesis, $T$ is distributed as an F random variable with $n_T$ and $n_R$ degrees of freedom. Hence, we reject the null hypothesis at the $\alpha$ level of significance if

$$T < F_{1-\alpha, n_T, n_R}.$$

Under the alternative hypothesis that $\sigma_{TT}^2 / \sigma_{TR}^2 < \delta^2$, the power of the above test procedure is

$$\begin{aligned}
\text{Power} &= P(T < F_{1-\alpha, n_R-1, n_T-1}) \\
&= P(1/T > F_{\alpha, n_R-1, n_T-1}) \\
&= P\left( \frac{\hat{\sigma}_{TR}^2 / \sigma_{TR}^2}{\hat{\sigma}_{TT}^2 / \sigma_{TT}^2} > \frac{\sigma_{TT}^2}{\delta^2 \sigma_{TR}^2} F_{\alpha, n_R-1, n_T-1} \right) \\
&= P\left( F_{n_R, n_T} > \frac{\sigma_{TT}^2}{\delta^2 \sigma_{TR}^2} F_{\alpha, n_R-1, n_T-1} \right).
\end{aligned}$$

Under the assumption that $n = n_T = n_R$, the sample size needed in order to achieve a desired power of $1 - \beta$ at the $\alpha$ level of significance can be obtained by solving

$$\frac{\sigma_{TT}^2}{\delta^2 \sigma_{TR}^2} = \frac{F_{1-\beta, n-1, n-1}}{F_{\alpha, n-1, n-1}}.$$

### Test for Similarity

For testing similarity, the hypotheses of interest are given by

$$H_0 : \frac{\sigma_{TT}}{\sigma_{TR}} \geq \delta \text{ or } \frac{\sigma_{TT}}{\sigma_{TR}} \leq 1/\delta \quad \text{versus} \quad H_a : \frac{1}{\delta} < \frac{\sigma_{TT}}{\sigma_{TR}} < \delta,$$

where $\delta > 1$ is the similarity limit. The above hypotheses can be decomposed into the following two one-sided hypotheses

$$H_{01}: \frac{\sigma_{TT}}{\sigma_{TR}} \geq \delta \quad \text{versus} \quad H_{a1}: \frac{\sigma_{TT}}{\sigma_{TR}} < \delta,$$

and

$$H_{02}: \frac{\sigma_{TT}}{\sigma_{TR}} \leq \frac{1}{\delta} \quad \text{versus} \quad H_{a2}: \frac{\sigma_{TT}}{\sigma_{TR}} > \frac{1}{\delta}.$$

These two hypotheses can be tested by the following two test statistics:

$$T_1 = \frac{\hat{\sigma}_{TT}^2}{\delta^2 \hat{\sigma}_{TR}^2} \quad \text{and} \quad T_2 = \frac{\delta^2 \hat{\sigma}_{TT}^2}{\hat{\sigma}_{TR}^2}.$$

We reject the null hypothesis and conclude similarity at the $\alpha$ level of significance if

$$T_1 < F_{1-\alpha, n_T, n_R} \quad \text{and} \quad T_2 > F_{\alpha, n_T, n_R}.$$

Assuming that $n = n_T = n_R$, under the alternative hypothesis that $\sigma_{TT}^2 \leq \sigma_{TR}^2$, the power of the above test is

$$\text{Power} = P\left(\frac{F_{\alpha, n-1, n-1}}{\delta^2} < \frac{\hat{\sigma}_{TT}^2}{\hat{\sigma}_{TR}^2} < \delta^2 F_{1-\alpha, n-1, n-1}\right)$$

$$= P\left(\frac{1}{F_{\alpha, n-1, n-1} \delta^2} < \frac{\hat{\sigma}_{TT}^2}{\hat{\sigma}_{TR}^2} < \delta^2 F_{1-\alpha, n-1, n-1}\right)$$

$$\geq 1 - 2P\left(\frac{\hat{\sigma}_{TT}^2}{\hat{\sigma}_{TR}^2} > \frac{\delta^2 \sigma_{TT}^2}{\sigma_{TR}^2} F_{1-\alpha, n-1, n-1}\right)$$

$$= 1 - 2P\left(F_{n-1, n-1} > \frac{\delta^2 \sigma_{TT}^2}{\sigma_{TR}^2} F_{1-\alpha, n-1, n-1}\right).$$

Hence, a conservative estimate for the sample size needed in order to achieve the desired power of $1-\beta$ can be obtained by solving the following equation for $n$:

$$\frac{\delta^2 \sigma_{TT}^2}{\sigma_{TR}^2} = \frac{F_{\beta/2, n-1, n-1}}{F_{1-\alpha, n-1, n-1}}.$$

**An Example**

Consider the example discussed in the previous subsections. Suppose a parallel-group design without replicates is to be conducted for comparing total variabilities between a test drug and a reference drug. It is assumed that $\sigma_{TT} = 0.55$ and $\sigma_{TR} = 0.75$. The sample size needed in order to achieve an 80% power $(1-\beta = 0.80)$ at the 5% level of significance ($\alpha =$

## 9.4. Comparing Total Variabilities

0.05) in establishing non-inferiority with the non-inferiority margin $\delta = 1.1$ can be obtained by solving

$$\frac{0.55^2}{1.10^2 \times 0.75^2} = \frac{F_{0.20, n-1, n-1}}{F_{0.05, n-1, n-1}}.$$

This gives $n = 40$.

### 9.4.2 Parallel Design with Replicates

In practice, parallel design with replicates can also be used to assess total variability. The merit of the parallel design with replicates is that it can serve more than just one purpose. For example, it can not only assess total variabilities, but also inter-subject and intra-subject variablities. Model (9.1.1) can be used to represent data here. Unbiased estimators for total variabilities are given by

$$\hat{\sigma}_{Ti}^2 = s_{Bi}^2 + \frac{m-1}{m}\hat{\sigma}_{Wi}^2,$$

where $s_{Bi}^2$ is defined in 9.3.1.

**Test for Equality**

Let $\eta = \sigma_{TT}^2 - \sigma_{TR}^2$; hence, a natural estimator for $\eta$ is given by

$$\hat{\eta} = \hat{\sigma}_{TT}^2 - \hat{\sigma}_{TR}^2.$$

For testing equality in total variability, the following hypotheses are considered:

$$H_0 : \sigma_{TT}^2 = \sigma_{TR}^2 \quad \text{versus} \quad H_a : \sigma_{TT}^2 \neq \sigma_{TR}^2.$$

A $(1-\alpha) \times 100\%$ confidence interval of $\eta$ is given by $(\hat{\eta}_L, \hat{\eta}_U)$, where

$$\hat{\eta}_L = \hat{\eta} - \sqrt{\Delta_L}, \quad \hat{\eta}_U = \hat{\eta} + \sqrt{\Delta_U},$$

$$\Delta_L = s_{BT}^4 \left(1 - \frac{n_T - 1}{\chi^2_{\alpha/2, n_T - 1}}\right)^2 + s_{BR}^4 \left(1 - \frac{n_R - 1}{\chi^2_{1-\alpha/2, n_R - 1}}\right)^2$$

$$+ \frac{(m-1)^2 \hat{\sigma}_{WT}^4}{m^2} \left(1 - \frac{n_T(m-1)}{\chi^2_{1-\alpha/2, n_T(m-1)}}\right)^2$$

$$+ \frac{(m-1)^2 \hat{\sigma}_{WR}^4}{m^2} \left(1 - \frac{n_R(m-1)}{\chi^2_{\alpha/2, n_R(m-1)}}\right)^2,$$

and

$$\Delta_U = s_{BT}^4 \left(1 - \frac{n_T - 1}{\chi^2_{1-\alpha/2, n_T-1}}\right)^2 + s_{BR}^4 \left(1 - \frac{n_R - 1}{\chi^2_{\alpha/2, n_R-1}}\right)^2$$
$$+ \frac{(m-1)^2 \hat{\sigma}_{WT}^4}{m^2}\left(1 - \frac{n_T(m-1)}{\chi^2_{\alpha/2, n_T(m-1)}}\right)^2$$
$$+ \frac{(m-1)^2 \hat{\sigma}_{WR}^4}{m^2}\left(1 - \frac{n_R(m-1)}{\chi^2_{1-\alpha/2, n_R(m-1)}}\right)^2.$$

We reject the null hypothesis at the $\alpha$ level of significance if $0 \notin (\hat{\eta}_L, \hat{\eta}_U)$. Under the alternative hypothesis and assume that $n = n_T = n_R$, the power of the above test procedure can be approximated by

$$\Phi\left(z_{\alpha/2} - \frac{\sqrt{n}(\sigma_{TT}^2 - \sigma_{TR}^2)}{\sigma^*}\right),$$

where

$$\sigma^{*2} = 2\left[\left(\sigma_{BT}^2 + \frac{\sigma_{WT}^2}{m}\right)^2 + \left(\sigma_{BR}^2 + \frac{\sigma_{WR}^2}{m}\right)^2\right.$$
$$\left. + \frac{(m-1)\sigma_{WT}^4}{m^2} + \frac{(m-1)\sigma_{WR}^4}{m^2}\right].$$

As a result, the sample size needed in order to achieve $1 - \beta$ power at the $\alpha$ level of significance can be obtained by solving

$$z_{\alpha/2} - \frac{\sqrt{n}(\sigma_{TT}^2 - \sigma_{TR}^2)}{\sigma^*} = -z_\beta.$$

This gives

$$n = \frac{\sigma^{*2}(z_{\alpha/2} + z_\beta)^2}{(\sigma_{TT}^2 - \sigma_{TR}^2)^2}.$$

### Test for Non-Inferiority/Superiority

The problem of testing non-inferiority/superiority can be unified by the following hypotheses:

$$H_0: \frac{\sigma_{TT}}{\sigma_{TR}} \geq \delta \quad \text{versus} \quad H_a: \frac{\sigma_{TT}}{\sigma_{TR}} < \delta.$$

Testing the above hypotheses is equivalent to testing the following hypotheses:

$$H_0: \sigma_{TT}^2 - \delta^2 \sigma_{TR}^2 \geq 0 \quad \text{versus} \quad H_a: \sigma_{TT}^2 - \delta^2 \sigma_{TR}^2 < 0.$$

## 9.4. Comparing Total Variabilities

When $\delta < 1$, the rejection of the null hypothesis indicates the superiority of the test drug versus the reference drug. When $\delta > 1$, the rejection of the null hypothesis indicates the non-inferiority of the test drug versus the reference drug. Let $\eta = \sigma_{TT}^2 - \delta^2 \sigma_{TR}^2$. For a given significance level of $\alpha$, the $(1-\alpha)$th upper confidence bound of $\eta$ can be constructed as

$$\hat{\eta}_U = \hat{\eta} + \sqrt{\Delta_U}$$

where $\hat{\eta} = \hat{\sigma}_{TT}^2 - \delta^2 \hat{\sigma}_{TR}^2$ and $\Delta_U$ is given by

$$\Delta_U = s_{BT}^4 \left(1 - \frac{n_T - 1}{\chi_{1-\alpha, n_T-1}^2}\right)^2 + \delta^4 s_{BR}^4 \left(1 - \frac{n_R - 1}{\chi_{\alpha, n_R-1}^2}\right)^2$$
$$+ \frac{(m-1)^2 \hat{\sigma}_{WT}^4}{m^2} \left(1 - \frac{n_T(m-1)}{\chi_{\alpha, n_T(m-1)}^2}\right)^2$$
$$+ \frac{\delta^4 (m-1)^2 \hat{\sigma}_{WR}^4}{m^2} \left(1 - \frac{n_R(m-1)}{\chi_{1-\alpha, n_R(m-1)}^2}\right)^2.$$

We then reject the null hypothesis at the $\alpha$ level of significance if $\hat{\eta}_U < 0$. Using a similar argument to the previous section, the power of the above testing procedure can be approximated by

$$1 - \Phi\left(z_\alpha - \frac{\sqrt{n}(\sigma_{TT}^2 - \delta^2 \sigma_{TR}^2)}{\sigma^*}\right),$$

where

$$\sigma^{*2} = 2\left[\left(\sigma_{BT}^2 + \frac{\sigma_{WT}^2}{m}\right)^2 + \delta^4 \left(\sigma_{BR}^2 + \delta^4 \frac{\sigma_{WR}^2}{m}\right)^2 \right.$$
$$\left. + \frac{(m-1)\sigma_{WT}^4}{m^2} + \delta^4 \frac{(m-1)\sigma_{WR}^4}{m^2}\right].$$

As a result, the sample size needed in order to achieve the desired power of $1 - \beta$ at the $\alpha$ level of significance can be obtained by solving

$$z_\alpha - \frac{\sqrt{n}(\sigma_{TT}^2 - \delta^2 \sigma_{TR}^2)}{\sigma^{*2}} = -z_\beta.$$

This gives

$$n = \frac{\sigma^{*2}(z_\alpha + z_\beta)^2}{(\sigma_{TT}^2 - \delta^2 \sigma_{TR}^2)^2}.$$

## An Example

Consider the same example discussed in the previous subsection. Suppose a trial with a parallel design with 3 replicates ($m = 3$) is conducted to compare total variabilities between treatment groups. It is assumed that $\sigma_{BT} = 0.30$, $\sigma_{BR} = 0.40$, $\sigma_{WT} = 0.20$, and $\sigma_{WR} = 0.30$. The objective is to establish the non-inferiority with $\delta = 1.1$. It follows that

$$\sigma^{*2} = 2\left[\left(0.30^2 + \frac{0.20^2}{3}\right)^2 + 1.1^4\left(0.4^2 + \frac{0.3^2}{3}\right)^2 \right.$$
$$\left. + \frac{(3-1)0.20^4}{3^2} + 1.1^4\frac{(3-1)0.3^4}{3^2}\right]$$
$$= 0.133.$$

As a result, the sample size needed per treatment group in order to achieve an 80% ($1 - \beta = 0.80$) power at the 5% ($\alpha = 0.05$) level of significance is given by

$$n = \frac{0.133(1.64 + 0.84)^2}{(0.30^2 + 0.20^2 - 1.1^2(0.4^2 + 0.3^2))^2} \approx 28.$$

### 9.4.3 The Standard $2 \times 2$ Crossover Design

Under the standard $2 \times 2$ crossover design, model (9.1.4) is still useful. We omitted the subscript $l$ since there are no replicates.

Intuitive estimators for the total variabilities are given by

$$\hat{\sigma}_{TT}^2 = \frac{1}{n_1 + n_2 - 2}\sum_{i=1}^{2}\sum_{j=1}^{n_i}(x_{ijT} - \bar{x}_{i\cdot T})^2$$

and

$$\hat{\sigma}_{TR}^2 = \frac{1}{n_1 + n_2 - 2}\sum_{i=1}^{2}\sum_{j=1}^{n_i}(x_{ijR} - \bar{x}_{i\cdot R})^2,$$

where

$$\bar{x}_{i\cdot T} = \frac{1}{n_i}\sum_{j=1}^{n_i}x_{ijT}, \quad \text{and} \quad \bar{x}_{i\cdot R} = \frac{1}{n_i}\sum_{j=1}^{n_i}x_{ijR}.$$

**Test for Equality**

For testing the equality in total variability, again consider the following hypotheses:

$$H_0: \frac{\sigma_{TT}^2}{\sigma_{TR}^2} = 1 \quad \text{versus} \quad H_a: \frac{\sigma_{TT}^2}{\sigma_{TR}^2} \neq 1.$$

## 9.4. Comparing Total Variabilities

Testing the above hypotheses is equivalent to testing the following hypotheses:
$$H_0 : \sigma_{TT}^2 - \sigma_{TR}^2 = 0 \quad \text{versus} \quad H_a : \sigma_{TT}^2 - \sigma_{TR}^2 \neq 0.$$
Let $\eta = \sigma_{TT}^2 - \sigma_{TR}^2$. An intuitive estimator of $\eta$ is given by
$$\hat{\eta} = \hat{\sigma}_{TT}^2 - \hat{\sigma}_{TR}^2.$$
Let
$$\sigma_{BTR}^2 = \frac{1}{n_1 + n_2 - 2} \sum_{i=1}^{2} \sum_{j=1}^{n_i} (x_{ijT} - \bar{x}_{i.T})(x_{ijR} - \bar{x}_{i.R}).$$
Define $\hat{\lambda}_i, i = 1, 2$, by
$$\hat{\lambda}_i = \frac{\hat{\sigma}_{TT}^2 - \hat{\sigma}_{TR}^2 \pm \sqrt{(\hat{\sigma}_{TT}^2 + \hat{\sigma}_{TR}^2)^2 - 4\hat{\sigma}_{BTR}^4}}{2}.$$
Assume that $\hat{\lambda}_1 < 0 < \hat{\lambda}_2$. In Lee et al. (2002b), a $(1-\alpha) \times 100\%$ confidence interval of $\eta$ is given by $(\hat{\eta}_L, \hat{\eta}_U)$, where
$$\hat{\eta}_L = \hat{\eta} - \sqrt{\Delta_L}, \quad \hat{\eta}_U = \hat{\eta} + \sqrt{\Delta_U},$$
$$\Delta_L = \hat{\lambda}_1^2 \left(1 - \frac{n_1 + n_2 - 2}{\chi_{1-\alpha/2, n_1+n_2-2}^2}\right)^2 + \hat{\lambda}_2^2 \left(1 - \frac{n_1 + n_2 - 2}{\chi_{\alpha/2, n_1+n_2-2}^2}\right)^2$$
$$\Delta_U = \hat{\lambda}_1^2 \left(1 - \frac{n_1 + n_2 - 2}{\chi_{\alpha/2, n_1+n_2-2}^2}\right)^2 + \hat{\lambda}_2^2 \left(1 - \frac{n_1 + n_2 - 2}{\chi_{1-\alpha/2, n_1+n_2-2}^2}\right)^2.$$
We reject the null hypothesis at the $\alpha$ level of significance if $0 \notin (\hat{\eta}_L, \hat{\eta}_U)$.

Under the alternative hypothesis, without loss of generality, we assume $\sigma_{TR}^2 > \sigma_{TT}^2$. Let $n_s = n_1 + n_2 - 2$. The power of the above test can be approximated by
$$1 - \Phi\left(z_{\alpha/2} - \frac{\sqrt{n_s}(\sigma_{TT}^2 - \sigma_{TR}^2)}{\sigma^*}\right),$$
where
$$\sigma^{*2} = 2(\sigma_{TT}^4 + \sigma_{TR}^4 - 2\rho^2 \sigma_{BT}^2 \sigma_{BR}^2).$$
Hence, the sample size needed in order to achieve the power of $1-\beta$ power at the $\alpha$ level of significance can be obtained by solving the following equation:
$$z_{\alpha/2} - \frac{\sqrt{n_s}(\sigma_{TT}^2 - \sigma_{TR}^2)}{\sigma^*} = -z_\beta,$$
which implies that
$$n_s = \frac{\sigma^{*2}(z_{\alpha/2} + z_\beta)^2}{(\sigma_{TT}^2 - \sigma_{TR}^2)^2}.$$

## Test for Non-Inferiority/Superiority

The problem of testing non-inferiority/superiority can be unified by the following hypotheses:

$$H_0 : \frac{\sigma_{TT}}{\sigma_{TR}} \geq \delta \quad \text{versus} \quad H_a : \frac{\sigma_{TT}}{\sigma_{TR}} < \delta.$$

Testing the above hypotheses is equivalent to testing the following hypotheses:

$$H_0 : \sigma_{TT}^2 - \delta^2 \sigma_{TR}^2 \geq 0 \quad \text{versus} \quad H_a : \sigma_{TT}^2 - \delta^2 \sigma_{TR}^2 < 0.$$

When $\delta < 1$, the rejection of the null hypothesis indicates the superiority of the test drug versus the reference drug. When $\delta > 1$, the rejection of the null hypothesis indicates the non-inferiority of the test drug versus the reference drug. Let $\eta = \sigma_{TT}^2 - \delta^2 \sigma_{TR}^2$. For a given significance level of $\alpha$, similarly, the $(1-\alpha)$th upper confidence bound of $\eta$ can be constructed as

$$\hat{\eta}_U = \hat{\eta} + \sqrt{\Delta_U}$$

where $\Delta_U$ is given by

$$\Delta_U = \hat{\lambda}_1^2 \left( \frac{n_1 + n_2 - 2}{\chi^2_{\alpha, n_1+n_2-2}} - 1 \right)^2 + \hat{\lambda}_2^2 \left( \frac{n_1 + n_2 - 2}{\chi^2_{1-\alpha, n_1+n_2-2}} - 1 \right)^2,$$

and $\hat{\lambda}_i, i = 1, 2$, are given by

$$\hat{\lambda}_i = \frac{\hat{\sigma}_{TT}^2 - \delta^4 \hat{\sigma}_{TR}^2 \pm \sqrt{(\hat{\sigma}_{TT}^2 + \delta^4 \hat{\sigma}_{TR}^2)^2 - 4\delta^2 \hat{\sigma}_{BTR}^4}}{2}.$$

We reject the null hypothesis at the $\alpha$ level of significance if $\hat{\eta}_U < 0$. Under the alternative hypothesis, the power of the above test procedure can be approximated by

$$\Phi \left( z_\alpha - \frac{\sqrt{n}(\sigma_{TT}^2 - \delta^2 \sigma_{TR}^2)}{\sigma^*} \right),$$

where

$$\sigma^{*2} = 2(\sigma_{TT}^4 + \delta^4 \sigma_{TR}^4 - 2\delta^2 \rho^2 \sigma_{BT}^2 \sigma_{BR}^2).$$

Hence, the sample size needed in order to achieve $1 - \beta$ power at $\alpha$ level of significance can be obtained by solving

$$z_\alpha - \frac{\sqrt{n_s}(\sigma_{TT}^2 - \delta^2 \sigma_{TR}^2)}{\sigma^*} = -z_\beta.$$

This gives

$$n_s = \frac{\sigma^{*2}(z_\alpha + z_\beta)^2}{(\sigma_{TT}^2 - \delta^2 \sigma_{TR}^2)^2}.$$

## 9.4. Comparing Total Variabilities

**An Example**

Consider the same example discussed in the previous subsection. Under the standard $2 \times 2$ crossover design, it is assumed that $\rho = 1$, $\sigma_{BT} = 0.30$, $\sigma_{BR} = 0.40$, $\sigma_{WT} = 0.20$, and $\sigma_{WR} = 0.30$. The objective is to establish non-inferiority with a margin $\delta = 1.1$. It follows that

$$\begin{aligned}\sigma^{*2} &= 2[(0.30^2 + 0.20^2)^2 + 1.1^4(0.4^2 + 0.3^2)^2 \\ &\quad -2 \times 1.1^2 \times 0.30^2 \times 0.4^2] = 0.147.\end{aligned}$$

As a result, the sample size needed in order to achieve an 80% $(1 - \beta = 0.80)$ power at the 5% $(\alpha = 0.05)$ level of significance is given by

$$n_s = \frac{(0.153)(1.64 + 0.84)^2}{(0.30^2 + 0.20^2 - 1.1^2 \times (0.4^2 + 0.3^2))^2} \approx 31.$$

Since $n_s = n_1 + n_2 - 2$, approximately 17 subjects should be assigned to each sequence to achieve an 80% $(1 - \beta = 0.80)$ power.

### 9.4.4 Replicated $2 \times 2m$ Crossover Design

We can use a similar argument for test of inter-subject variabilities under model (9.1.4) with the estimators

$$\hat{\sigma}_{Tk}^2 = s_{Bk}^2 + \frac{m-1}{m}\hat{\sigma}_{Wk}^2, \quad k = T, R.$$

**Test for Equality**

For testing the equality in total variability, consider the following hypotheses:

$$H_0 : \frac{\sigma_{TT}^2}{\sigma_{TR}^2} = 1 \quad \text{versus} \quad H_a : \frac{\sigma_{TT}^2}{\sigma_{TR}^2} \neq 1.$$

Testing the above hypotheses is equivalent to testing the following hypotheses:

$$H_0 : \sigma_{TT}^2 - \sigma_{TR}^2 = 0 \quad \text{versus} \quad H_a : \sigma_{TT}^2 - \sigma_{TR}^2 \neq 0.$$

Let $\hat{\eta} = \hat{\sigma}_{TT}^2 - \hat{\sigma}_{TR}^2$. In Lee et al. (2002b), a $(1 - \alpha) \times 100\%$ confidence interval of $\eta$ is given by $(\hat{\eta}_L, \hat{\eta}_U)$, where

$$\hat{\eta}_L = \hat{\eta} - \sqrt{\Delta_L}, \quad \hat{\eta}_U = \hat{\eta} + \sqrt{\Delta_U},$$

$$\Delta_L = \hat{\lambda}_1^2\left(1 - \frac{n_s-1}{\chi^2_{1-\alpha/2,n_s-1}}\right)^2 + \hat{\lambda}_2^2\left(1 - \frac{n_s-1}{\chi^2_{\alpha/2,n_s-1}}\right)^2$$

$$+ \frac{(m-1)^2\hat{\sigma}^4_{WT}}{m^2}\left(1 - \frac{n_s(m-1)}{\chi^2_{\alpha/2,n_s(m-1)}}\right)^2$$

$$+ \frac{(m-1)^2\hat{\sigma}^4_{WR}}{m^2}\left(1 - \frac{n_s(m-1)}{\chi^2_{1-\alpha/2,n_s(m-1)}}\right)^2$$

$$\Delta_U = \hat{\lambda}_1^2\left(1 - \frac{n_s-1}{\chi^2_{\alpha/2,n_s-1}}\right)^2 + \hat{\lambda}_2^2\left(1 - \frac{n_s-1}{\chi^2_{1-\alpha/2,n_s-1}}\right)^2$$

$$+ \frac{(m-1)^2\hat{\sigma}^4_{WT}}{m^2}\left(1 - \frac{n_s(m-1)}{\chi^2_{1-\alpha/2,n_s(m-1)}}\right)^2$$

$$+ \frac{(m-1)^2\hat{\sigma}^4_{WR}}{m^2}\left(1 - \frac{n_s(m-1)}{\chi^2_{\alpha/2,n_s(m-1)}}\right)^2,$$

and $\hat{\lambda}_i$'s are the same as those used for the test of equality for inter-subject variabilities. We reject the null hypothesis at the $\alpha$ level of significance if $0 \notin (\hat{\eta}_L, \hat{\eta}_U)$.

Under the alternative hypothesis, without loss of generality, we assume $\sigma^2_{TR} > \sigma^2_{TT}$ and $n = n_T = n_R$. The power of the above test can be approximated by

$$1 - \Phi\left(z_{\alpha/2} - \frac{\sqrt{n}(\sigma^2_{TT} - \sigma^2_{TR})}{\sigma^*}\right),$$

where

$$\sigma^{*2} = 2\left[\left(\sigma^2_{BT} + \frac{\sigma^2_{WT}}{m}\right)^2 + \left(\sigma^2_{BR} + \frac{\sigma^2_{WR}}{m}\right)^2 - 2\rho^2\sigma^2_{BT}\sigma^2_{BR}\right.$$

$$\left. + \frac{(m-1)\sigma^4_{WT}}{m^2} + \frac{(m-1)\sigma^4_{WR}}{m^2}\right].$$

Hence, the sample size needed in order to achieve the power of $1-\beta$ at the $\alpha$ level of significance can be obtained by solving the following equation:

$$z_{\alpha/2} - \frac{\sqrt{n}(\sigma^2_{TT} - \sigma^2_{TR})}{\sigma^*} = z_\beta.$$

This leads to

$$n = \frac{\sigma^{*2}(z_{\alpha/2} + z_\beta)^2}{(\sigma^2_{TT} - \sigma^2_{TR})^2}.$$

## Test for Non-Inferiority/Superiority

The problem of testing non-inferiority/superiority can be unified by the following hypotheses:

$$H_0 : \frac{\sigma_{TT}}{\sigma_{TR}} \geq \delta \quad \text{versus} \quad H_a : \frac{\sigma_{TT}}{\sigma_{TR}} < \delta,$$

which is equivalent to

$$H_0 : \sigma_{TT}^2 - \delta^2 \sigma_{TR}^2 \geq 0 \quad \text{versus} \quad H_a : \sigma_{TT}^2 - \delta^2 \sigma_{TR}^2 < 0.$$

When $\delta < 1$, the rejection of the null hypothesis indicates the superiority of the test drug versus the reference drug. When $\delta > 1$, the rejection of the null hypothesis indicates the non-inferiority of the test drug versus the reference drug. Let $\hat{\eta} = \hat{\sigma}_{TT}^2 - \delta^2 \hat{\sigma}_{TR}^2$. For a given significance level of $\alpha$, similarly, the $(1-\alpha)$th upper confidence bound of $\eta$ can be constructed as

$$\hat{\eta}_U = \hat{\eta} + \sqrt{\Delta_U}$$

where $\hat{\eta} = \hat{\sigma}_{TT}^2 - \delta^2 \hat{\sigma}_{TR}^2$,

$$\Delta_U = \hat{\lambda}_1^2 \left(1 - \frac{n_s - 1}{\chi^2_{\alpha, n_s - 1}}\right)^2 + \hat{\lambda}_2^2 \left(1 - \frac{n_s - 1}{\chi^2_{1-\alpha, n_s - 1}}\right)^2$$
$$+ \frac{(m-1)^2 \hat{\sigma}_{WT}^4}{m^2} \left(1 - \frac{n_s(m-1)}{\chi^2_{1-\alpha, n_s(m-1)}}\right)^2$$
$$+ \frac{(m-1)^2 \hat{\sigma}_{WR}^4}{m^2} \left(1 - \frac{n_s(m-1)}{\chi^2_{\alpha, n_s(m-1)}}\right)^2,$$

and $\hat{\lambda}_i$'s are same as those used for the test of non-inferiority for inter-subject variabilities. We then reject the null hypothesis at the $\alpha$ level of significance if $\hat{\eta}_U < 0$. Using a similar argument to the previous section, the power of the above testing procedure can be approximated by

$$1 - \Phi\left(z_\alpha - \frac{\sqrt{n_s}(\sigma_{TT}^2 - \delta^2 \sigma_{TR}^2)}{\sigma^*}\right),$$

where

$$\sigma^{*2} = 2\left[\left(\sigma_{BT}^2 + \frac{\sigma_{WT}^2}{m}\right)^2 + \delta^4 \left(\sigma_{BR}^2 + \frac{\sigma_{WR}^2}{m}\right)^2 - 2\delta^2 \rho^2 \sigma_{BT}^2 \sigma_{BR}^2 \right.$$
$$\left. + \frac{(m-1)\sigma_{WT}^4}{m^2} + \frac{\delta^4(m-1)\sigma_{WR}^4}{m^2}\right].$$

Hence, the sample size needed in order to achieve the power of $1-\beta$ at the $\alpha$ level of significance can be obtained by solving the following equation:

$$z_{\alpha/2} - \frac{\sqrt{n_s}(\sigma_{TT}^2 - \delta^2\sigma_{TR}^2)}{\sigma^*} = z_\beta.$$

This leads to

$$n_s = \frac{\sigma^{*2}(z_{\alpha/2} + z_\beta)^2}{(\sigma_{TT}^2 - \delta^2\sigma_{TR}^2)^2}.$$

**An Example**

Suppose a $2 \times 4$ crossover design (ABAB,BABA) is used to compare two treatments (A and B) in terms of their total variabilities. Information from pilot studies indicates that $\rho = 0.75$, $\sigma_{BT}^2 = 0.3, \sigma_{BR}^2 = 0.4, \sigma_{WT}^2 = 0.2$, and $\sigma_{WR}^2 = 0.3$. The objective is to establish non-inferiority with a margin $\delta = 1.1$. It follows that

$$\sigma^{*2} = 2\left[\left(0.30^2 + \frac{0.20^2}{2}\right)^2 + 1.1^4\left(0.40^2 + \frac{0.30^2}{2}\right)^2\right.$$
$$-2 \times 1.1^2 \times (0.75 \times 0.3 \times 0.4)^2$$
$$\left. + \frac{0.20^4}{2^2} + \frac{1.1^4 \times 0.30^4}{2^2}\right]$$
$$= 0.106.$$

Hence, the sample size needed in order to achieve an 80% power $(1-\beta = 0.80)$ at the 5% level of significance $(\alpha = 0.05)$ is given by

$$n_s = \frac{(0.106)(1.64+0.84)^2}{(0.3^2 + 0.2^2 - 1.1^2 \times (0.4^2 + 0.3^2))^2} \approx 22.$$

Since $n_s = n_1 + n_2 - 2$, approximately 12 subjects per sequence are required for achieving an 80% power at the 5% level of significance.

## 9.5 Practical Issues

In recent years, the assessment of reproducibility in terms of intra-subject variability or intra-subject CV in clinical research has received much attention. Shao and Chow (2002) defined reproducibility of a study drug as a collective term that encompasses consistency, similarity, and stability (control) within the therapeutic index (or window) of a subject's clinical status (e.g., clinical response of some primary study endpoint, blood levels, or blood concentration-time curve) when the study drug is repeatedly

## 9.5. Practical Issues

administered at different dosing periods under the same experimental conditions. Reproducibility of clinical results observed from a clinical study can be quantitated through the evaluation of the so-called reproducibility probability, which will be briefly introduced in Chapter 12 (see also Shao and Chow, 2002).

For assessment of inter-subject variability and/or total variability, Chow and Tse (1991) indicated that the usual analysis of variance models could lead to negative estimates of the variance components, especially the inter-subject variance component. In addition, the sum of the best estimates of the intra-subject variance and the inter-subject variance may not lead to the best estimate for the total variance. Chow and Shao (1988) proposed an estimation procedure for variance components which will not only avoid negative estimates but also provide a better estimate as compare to the maximum likelihood estimates. For estimation of total variance, Chow and Tse (1991) proposed a method as an alternative to the sum of estimates of individual variance components. These ideas could be applied to provide a better estimate of sample sizes for studies comparing variabilities between treatment groups.

# Chapter 10
# Bioequivalence Testing

When a brand-name drug is going off-patent, generic drug companies may file abbreviated new drug applications for generic drug approval. An approved generic drug can be used as a substitute for the brand-name drug. In 1984, the FDA was authorized to approve generic drugs through *bioavailability* and *bioequivalence* studies under the Drug Price and Patent Term Restoration Act. Bioequivalence testing is usually considered as a surrogate for clinical evaluation of drug products based on the *Fundamental Bioequivalence Assumption* that when two formulations of the reference product (e.g., a brand-name drug) and and the test product (a generic copy) are equivalent in bioavailability, they will reach the same therapeutic effect. *In vivo* bioequivalence testing is commonly conducted with a crossover design on healthy volunteers to assess bioavailability through pharmacokinetic (PK) responses such as area under the blood or plasma concentration-time curve (AUC) and maximum concentration ($C_{\max}$). For some locally acting drug products such as nasal aerosols (e.g., metered-dose inhalers) and nasal sprays (e.g., metered-dose spray pumps) that are not intended to be absorbed into the bloodstream, bioavailability may be assessed by measurements intended to reflect the rate and extent to which the active ingredient or active moiety becomes available at the site of action. Bioequivalence related to these products is called *in vitro* bioequivalence and is usually studied under a parallel design. Statistical procedures for some types of bioequivalence studies are described in the FDA guidances (FDA, 2000, 2001). Chow and Shao (2002) provided a review of statistical procedures for bioequivalence studies that are not provided by the FDA.

In Section 10.1, we introduce various bioequivalence criteria. Section 10.2 introduces sample size calculation for the average bioequivalence. Sample size formulas for population bioequivalence and individual bioequivalence are provided in Sections 10.3 and 10.4, respectively. Section 10.5

focuses on sample size calculation for *in vitro* bioequivalence.

## 10.1 Bioequivalence Criteria

In 1992, the FDA published its first guidance on statistical procedures for *in vivo* bioequivalence studies (FDA, 1992). The 1992 FDA guidance requires that the evidence of bioequivalence in average bioavailability in PK responses between the two drug products be provided. Let $y_R$ and $y_T$ denote PK responses (or log-PK responses if appropriate) of the reference and test formulations, respectively, and let $\delta = E(y_T) - E(y_R)$. Under the 1992 FDA guidance, two formulations are said to be bioequivalent if $\delta$ falls in the interval $(\delta_L, \delta_U)$ with 95% assurance, where $\delta_L$ and $\delta_U$ are given limits specified in the FDA guidance. Since only the averages $E(y_T)$ and $E(y_R)$ are concerned in this method, this type of bioequivalence is usually referred to as *average bioequivalence* (ABE). In 2000, the FDA issued a guidance on general considerations of bioavailability and bioequivalence studies for orally administered drug products, which replaces the 1992 FDA guidance (FDA, 2000). Statistical design and analysis for assessment of ABE as described in the 2000 FDA guidance are the same as those given in the 1992 FDA guidance.

The ABE approach for bioequivalence, however, has limitations for addressing drug interchangeability, since it focuses only on the comparison of population averages between the test and reference formulations (Chen, 1997a). Drug interchangeability can be classified as either drug prescribability or drug switchability. Drug prescribability is referred to as the physician's choice for prescribing an appropriate drug for his/her new patients among the drug products available, while drug switchability is related to the switch from a drug product to an alternative drug product within the same patient whose concentration of the drug product has been titrated to a steady, efficacious, and safe level. To assess drug prescribability and switchability, *population bioequivalence* (PBE) and *individual bioequivalence* (IBE) are proposed, respectively (see Anderson and Hauck, 1990; Esinhart and Chinchilli, 1994; Sheiner, 1992; Schall and Luus, 1993; Chow and Liu, 1995; and Chen, 1997a). The concepts of PBE and IBE are described in the 1999 FDA draft guidance (FDA, 1999a) and the 2001 FDA guidance for industry (FDA, 2001). Let $y_T$ be the PK response from the test formulation, $y_R$ and $y'_R$ be two identically distributed PK responses from the reference formulation, and

$$\theta = \frac{E(y_R - y_T)^2 - E(y_R - y'_R)^2}{\max\{\sigma_0^2, E(y_R - y'_R)^2/2\}}, \qquad (10.1.1)$$

where $\sigma_0^2$ is a given constant specified in the 2001 FDA guidance. If $y_R$,

## 10.2. Average Bioequivalence

$y_R'$ and $y_T$ are independent observations from different subjects, then the two formulations are PBE when $\theta < \theta_{PBE}$, where $\theta_{PBE}$ is an equivalence limit for assessment of PBE as specified in the 2001 FDA guidance. If $y_R$, $y_R'$ and $y_T$ are from the same subject ($E(y_R - y_R')^2/2$ is then the within-subject variance), then the two formulations are IBE when $\theta < \theta_{IBE}$, where $\theta_{IBE}$ is an equivalence limit for IBE as specified in the 2001 FDA guidance. Note that $\theta$ in (10.1.1) is a measure of the relative difference between the mean squared errors of $y_R - y_T$ and $y_R - y_R'$. When $y_R$, $y_R'$ and $y_T$ are from the same individual, it measures the drug switchability within the same individual. On the other hand, it measures drug prescribability when $y_R$, $y_R'$, and $y_T$ are from different subjects. Thus, IBE addresses drug switchability, whereas PBE addresses drug prescribability. According to the 2001 FDA guidance, IBE or PBE can be claimed if a 95% upper confidence bound for $\theta$ is smaller than $\theta_{IBE}$ or $\theta_{PBE}$, provided that the observed ratio of geometric means is within the limits of 80% and 125%.

For locally acting drug products such as nasal aerosols (e.g., metered-dose inhalers) and nasal sprays (e.g., metered-dose spray pumps) that are not intended to be absorbed into the bloodstream, the FDA indicates that bioequivalence may be assessed, with suitable justification, by *in vitro* bioequivalence studies alone (21 CFR 320.24). In the 1999 FDA guidance, *in vitro* bioequivalence can be established through six *in vitro* bioequivalence tests, which are for dose or spray content uniformity through container life, droplet or particle size distribution, spray pattern, plume geometry, priming and repriming, and tail off distribution. The FDA classifies statistical methods for assessment of the six *in vitro* bioequivalence tests for nasal aerosols and sprays as either the nonprofile analysis or the profile analysis. For the nonprofile analysis, the FDA adopts the criterion and limit of the PBE. For the profile analysis, bioequivalence may be assessed by comparing the profile variation between test product and reference product bottles with the profile variation between reference product bottles.

## 10.2 Average Bioequivalence

It should be noted that testing ABE is a special case of testing equivalence. As a result, the formulas derived in Chapter 3 for testing equivalence under various designs are still valid for testing ABE. In practice, the most commonly used design for ABE is a standard two-sequence and two-period crossover design. Hence, for the sake of convenience, the sample size formula for ABE under such a design is presented here. Details regarding more general designs can be found in Chapter 3.

For the ABE, a standard two-sequence, two-period ($2 \times 2$) crossover design is recommended by the FDA guidances. In a standard $2 \times 2$ crossover design, subjects are randomly assigned to one of the two sequences of formulations. In the first sequence, $n_1$ subjects receive treatments in the order of TR (T = test formulation, R = reference formulation) at two different dosing periods, whereas in the second sequence, $n_2$ subjects receive treatments in the order of RT at two different dosing periods. A sufficient length of washout between dosing periods is usually applied to wear off the possible residual effect that may be carried over from one dosing period to the next dosing period. Let $y_{ijk}$ be the original or the log-transformation of the PK response of interest from the $i$th subject in the $k$th sequence at the $j$th dosing period. The following statistical model is considered:

$$y_{ijk} = \mu + F_l + P_j + Q_k + S_{ikl} + e_{ijk}, \qquad (10.2.1)$$

where $\mu$ is the overall mean; $P_j$ is the fixed effect of the $j$th period ($j = 1, 2$, and $P_1 + P_2 = 0$); $Q_k$ is the fixed effect of the $k$th sequence ($k = 1, 2$, and $Q_1 + Q_2 = 0$); $F_l$ is the fixed effect of the $l$th formulation (when $j = k$, $l = T$; when $j \neq k$, $l = R$; $F_T + F_R = 0$); $S_{ikl}$ is the random effect of the $i$th subject in the $k$th sequence under formulation $l$ and $(S_{ikT}, S_{ikR})$, $i = 1, ..., n_k$, $k = 1, 2$, are independent and identically distributed bivariate normal random vectors with mean 0 and an unknown covariance matrix

$$\begin{pmatrix} \sigma_{BT}^2 & \rho\sigma_{BT}\sigma_{BR} \\ \rho\sigma_{BT}\sigma_{BR} & \sigma_{BR}^2 \end{pmatrix};$$

$e_{ijk}$'s are independent random errors distributed as $N(0, \sigma_{Wl}^2)$; and $S_{ikl}$'s and $e_{ijk}$'s are mutually independent. Note that $\sigma_{BT}^2$ and $\sigma_{BR}^2$ are between-subject variances and $\sigma_{WT}^2$ and $\sigma_{WR}^2$ are within-subject variances, and that $\sigma_{TT}^2 = \sigma_{BT}^2 + \sigma_{WT}^2$ and $\sigma_{TR}^2 = \sigma_{BR}^2 + \sigma_{WR}^2$ are the total variances for the test and reference formulations, respectively. Under model (10.2.1), the ABE parameter $\delta$ defined in Section 10.1 is equal to $\delta = F_T - F_R$. According to the 2000 FDA guidance, ABE is claimed if the following null hypothesis $H_0$ is rejected at the 5% level of significance:

$$H_0 : \delta \leq \delta_L \text{ or } \delta \geq \delta_U \quad \text{versus} \quad H_1 : \delta_L < \delta < \delta_U, \qquad (10.2.2)$$

where $\delta_L$ and $\delta_U$ are given bioequivalence limits. Under model (10.2.1),

$$\hat{\delta} = \frac{\bar{y}_{11} - \bar{y}_{12} - \bar{y}_{21} + \bar{y}_{22}}{2} \sim N\left(\delta, \frac{\sigma_{1,1}^2}{4}\left(\frac{1}{n_1} + \frac{1}{n_2}\right)\right), \qquad (10.2.3)$$

where $\bar{y}_{jk}$ is the sample mean of the observations in the $k$th sequence at the $j$th period and $\sigma_{1,1}^2$ is

$$\sigma_{a,b}^2 = \sigma_D^2 + a\sigma_{WT}^2 + b\sigma_{WR}^2 \qquad (10.2.4)$$

## 10.2. Average Bioequivalence

with $a = 1$ and $b = 1$. Let

$$\hat{\sigma}_{1,1}^2 = \frac{1}{n_1 + n_2 - 2} \sum_{k=1}^{2} \sum_{i=1}^{n_k} (y_{i1k} - y_{i2k} - \bar{y}_{1k} + \bar{y}_{2k})^2. \qquad (10.2.5)$$

Then $\hat{\sigma}_{1,1}^2$ is independent of $\hat{\delta}$ and

$$(n_1 + n_2 - 2)\hat{\sigma}_{1,1}^2 \sim \sigma_{1,1}^2 \chi_{n_1+n_2-2}^2,$$

where $\chi_r^2$ is the chi-square distribution with $r$ degrees of freedom. Thus, the limits of a 90% confidence interval for $\delta$ are given by

$$\hat{\delta}_{\pm} = \hat{\delta} \pm t_{0.05, n_1+n_2-2} \frac{\hat{\sigma}_{1,1}}{2} \sqrt{\frac{1}{n_1} + \frac{1}{n_2}},$$

where $t_{0.05,r}$ is the upper 5th quantile of the t-distribution with $r$ degrees of freedom. According to the 2000 FDA guidance, ABE can be claimed if and only if the 90% confidence interval falls within $(-\delta_L, \delta_U)$, i.e., $\delta_L < \hat{\delta}_- < \hat{\delta}_+ < \delta_U$. Note that this is based on the two one-sided tests procedure proposed by Schuirmann (1987). The idea of Schuirmann's two one-sided tests is to decompose $H_0$ in (10.2.2) into the following two one-sided hypotheses:

$$H_{01} : \delta \leq \delta_L \quad \text{and} \quad H_{02} : \delta \geq \delta_U.$$

Apparently, both $H_{01}$ and $H_{02}$ are rejected at the 5% significance level if and only if $\delta_L < \hat{\delta}_- < \hat{\delta}_+ < \delta_U$. Schuirmann's two one-sided tests procedure is a test of size 5% (Berger and Hsu, 1996, Theorem 2).

Assume without loss of generality that $n_1 = n_2 = n$. Under the alternative hypothesis that $|\epsilon| < \delta$, the power of the above test is approximately

$$2\Phi\left(\frac{\sqrt{2n}(\delta - |\epsilon|)}{\sigma_{1,1}} - t_{\alpha, 2n-2}\right) - 1.$$

As a result, the sample size needed for achieving a power of $1 - \beta$ can be obtained by solving

$$\frac{\sqrt{2n}(\delta - |\epsilon|)}{\sigma_{1,1}} - t_{\alpha, 2n-2} = t_{\beta/2, 2n-2}.$$

This leads to

$$n \geq \frac{(t_{\alpha, 2n-2} + t_{\beta/2, 2n-2})^2 \sigma_{1,1}^2}{2(\delta - |\epsilon|)^2}. \qquad (10.2.6)$$

Since the above equations do not have an explicit solution, for convenience, for $2 \times 2$ crossover design, the total sample size needed to achieve a power

Table 10.2.1: Sample Size for Assessment of Equivalence
Under a $2 \times 2$ Crossover Design ($m = 1$)

|  | Power = 80% | | | | Power=90 | | | |
| --- | --- | --- | --- | --- | --- | --- | --- | --- |
| $\epsilon =$ | 0% | 5% | 10% | 15% | 0% | 5% | 10% | 15% |
| $\sigma_{1,1} = 0.10$ | 3 | 3 | 4 | 9 | 3 | 4 | 5 | 12 |
| 0.12 | 3 | 4 | 6 | 13 | 3 | 4 | 7 | 16 |
| 0.14 | 3 | 4 | 7 | 17 | 4 | 5 | 9 | 21 |
| 0.16 | 4 | 5 | 9 | 22 | 4 | 6 | 11 | 27 |
| 0.18 | 4 | 6 | 11 | 27 | 5 | 7 | 13 | 34 |
| 0.20 | 5 | 7 | 13 | 33 | 6 | 9 | 16 | 42 |
| 0.22 | 6 | 8 | 15 | 40 | 7 | 10 | 19 | 51 |
| 0.24 | 6 | 10 | 18 | 48 | 8 | 12 | 22 | 60 |
| 0.26 | 7 | 11 | 20 | 56 | 9 | 14 | 26 | 70 |
| 0.28 | 8 | 13 | 24 | 64 | 10 | 16 | 29 | 81 |
| 0.30 | 9 | 14 | 27 | 74 | 11 | 18 | 34 | 93 |
| 0.32 | 10 | 16 | 30 | 84 | 13 | 20 | 38 | 105 |
| 0.34 | 11 | 18 | 34 | 94 | 14 | 22 | 43 | 119 |
| 0.36 | 13 | 20 | 38 | 105 | 16 | 25 | 48 | 133 |
| 0.38 | 14 | 22 | 42 | 117 | 17 | 28 | 53 | 148 |
| 0.40 | 15 | 24 | 47 | 130 | 19 | 30 | 59 | 164 |

Note: (1) the bioequivalence limit $\delta$ is 22.3%; (2) sample size calculation was performed based on log-transformed data.

of 80% or 90% at 5% level of significance with various combinations of $\epsilon$ and $\delta$ is given in Table 10.2.1.

When sample size is sufficiently large, equation (10.2.6) can be further simplified into

$$n = \frac{(z_\alpha + z_{\beta/2})^2 \sigma_{1,1}^2}{2(\delta - |\epsilon|)^2}.$$

**An Example**

Suppose an investigator is interested in conducting a clinical trial with $2 \times 2$ crossover design to establish ABE between an inhaled formulation of a drug product (test) and a subcutaneous (SC) injected formulation (reference) in terms of log-transformed AUC. Based on PK data obtained from pilot studies, the mean difference of AUC can be assumed to be 5% ($\delta = 0.05$). Also it is assumed the standard deviation for intra-subject comparison is 0.40. By referring to Table 10.2.1, a total of 24 subjects per sequence is needed in order to achieve an 80% power at the 5% level of significance. On the other side, if we use normal approximation, the sample size needed can be obtained as

$$n = \frac{(z_{0.05} + z_{0.10})^2 \sigma_{1,1}^2}{2(\delta - |\epsilon|)^2} = \frac{(1.96 + 0.84)^2 \times 0.40^2}{2(0.223 - 0.05)^2} \approx 21.$$

## 10.3 Population Bioequivalence

PBE can be assessed under the $2 \times 2$ crossover design described in Section 10.2. Under model (10.2.1), the parameter $\theta$ in (10.1.1) for PBE is equal to

$$\theta = \frac{\delta^2 + \sigma_{TT}^2 - \sigma_{TR}^2}{\max\{\sigma_0^2, \sigma_{TR}^2\}}. \tag{10.3.1}$$

In view of (10.3.1), PBE can be claimed if the null hypothesis in

$$H_0 : \lambda \geq 0 \quad \text{versus} \quad H_1 : \lambda < 0$$

is rejected at the 5% significance level provided that the observed ratio of geometric means is within the limits of 80% and 125%, where

$$\lambda = \delta^2 + \sigma_{TT}^2 - \sigma_{TR}^2 - \theta_{PBE} \max\{\sigma_0^2, \sigma_{TR}^2\}$$

and $\theta_{PBE}$ is a constant specified in FDA (2001).

Under model (10.2.1), an unbiased estimator of $\delta$ is $\hat{\delta}$ given in (10.2.3). Commonly used unbiased estimators of $\sigma_{TT}^2$ and $\sigma_{TR}^2$ are respectively

$$\hat{\sigma}_{TT}^2 = \frac{1}{n_1 + n_2 - 2} \left[ \sum_{i=1}^{n_1} (y_{i11} - \bar{y}_{11})^2 + \sum_{i=1}^{n_2} (y_{i22} - \bar{y}_{22})^2 \right]$$

$$\sim \frac{\sigma_{TT}^2 \chi_{n_1+n_2-2}^2}{n_1 + n_2 - 2}$$

and

$$\hat{\sigma}_{TR}^2 = \frac{1}{n_1 + n_2 - 2} \left[ \sum_{i=1}^{n_1} (y_{i21} - \bar{y}_{21})^2 + \sum_{i=1}^{n_2} (y_{i12} - \bar{y}_{12})^2 \right]$$

$$\sim \frac{\sigma_{TR}^2 \chi_{n_1+n_2-2}^2}{n_1 + n_2 - 2}.$$

Applying linearization to the moment estimator

$$\hat{\lambda} = \hat{\delta}^2 + \hat{\sigma}_{TT}^2 - \hat{\sigma}_{TR}^2 - \theta_{PBE} \max\{\sigma_0^2, \hat{\sigma}_{TR}^2\},$$

Chow, Shao, and Wang (2003a) obtained the following approximate 95% upper confidence bound for $\lambda$. When $\sigma_{TR}^2 \geq \sigma_0^2$,

$$\hat{\lambda}_U = \hat{\delta}^2 + \hat{\sigma}_{TT}^2 - (1 + \theta_{PBE})\hat{\sigma}_{TR}^2 + t_{0.05, n_1+n_2-2}\sqrt{V}, \qquad (10.3.2)$$

where $V$ is an estimated variance of $\hat{\delta}^2 + \hat{\sigma}_{TT}^2 - (1 + \theta_{PBE})\hat{\sigma}_{TR}^2$ of the form

$$V = \left(2\hat{\delta}, 1, -(1+\theta_{PBE})\right) C \left(2\hat{\delta}, 1, -(1+\theta_{PBE})\right)',$$

and $C$ is an estimated variance-covariance matrix of $(\hat{\delta}, \hat{\sigma}_{TT}^2, \hat{\sigma}_{TR}^2)$. Since $\hat{\delta}$ and $(\hat{\sigma}_{TT}^2, \hat{\sigma}_{TR}^2)$ are independent,

$$C = \begin{pmatrix} \frac{\hat{\sigma}_{1,1}^2}{4}\left(\frac{1}{n_1} + \frac{1}{n_2}\right) & (0,0) \\ (0,0)' & \frac{(n_1-1)C_1}{(n_1+n_2-2)^2} + \frac{(n_2-1)C_2}{(n_1+n_2-2)^2} \end{pmatrix},$$

where $\hat{\sigma}_{1,1}^2$ is defined by (10.2.5), $C_1$ is the sample covariance matrix of $((y_{i11} - \bar{y}_{11})^2, (y_{i21} - \bar{y}_{21})^2)$, $i = 1, ..., n_1$, and $C_2$ is the sample covariance matrix of $((y_{i22} - \bar{y}_{22})^2, (y_{i12} - \bar{y}_{12})^2)$, $i = 1, ..., n_2$.

When $\sigma_{TR}^2 < \sigma_0^2$, the upper confidence bound for $\lambda$ should be modified to

$$\hat{\lambda}_U = \hat{\delta}^2 + \hat{\sigma}_{TT}^2 - \hat{\sigma}_{TR}^2 - \theta_{PBE}\sigma_0^2 + t_{0.05, n_1+n_2-2}\sqrt{V_0}, \qquad (10.3.3)$$

where

$$V_0 = \left(2\hat{\delta}, 1, -1\right) C \left(2\hat{\delta}, 1, -1\right)'.$$

The confidence bound $\hat{\lambda}_U$ in (10.3.2) is referred to as the confidence bound under the reference-scaled criterion, whereas $\hat{\lambda}_U$ in (10.3.3) is referred to as the confidence bound under the constant-scaled criterion. In practice, whether $\sigma_{TR}^2 \geq \sigma_0^2$ is usually unknown. Hyslop, Hsuan, and Holder (2000) recommend using the reference-scaled criterion or the constant-scaled criterion according to $\hat{\sigma}_{TR}^2 \geq \sigma_0^2$ or $\hat{\sigma}_{TR}^2 < \sigma_0^2$, which is referred to as the estimation method. Alternatively, we may test the hypothesis of $\sigma_{TR}^2 \geq \sigma_0^2$ versus $\sigma_{TR}^2 < \sigma_0^2$ to decide which confidence bound should be used; i.e., if $\hat{\sigma}_{TR}^2(n_1+n_2-2) \geq \sigma_0^2 \chi_{0.95, n_1+n_2-2}^2$, then $\hat{\lambda}_U$ in (10.3.2) should be used; otherwise $\hat{\lambda}_U$ in (10.3.3) should be used, where $\chi_{\alpha, r}^2$ denotes the $\alpha$th upper quantile of the chi-square distribution with $r$ degrees of freedom. This is referred to as the test method and is more conservative than the estimation method.

Based on an asymptotic analysis, Chow, Shao, and Wang (2003a) derived the following formula for sample size determination assuming that $n_1 = n_2 = n$:

$$n \geq \frac{\zeta(z_{0.05} + z_\beta)^2}{\lambda^2}, \qquad (10.3.4)$$

where
$$\zeta = 2\delta^2\sigma_{1,1}^2 + \sigma_{TT}^4 + (1+a)^2\sigma_{TR}^4 - 2(1+a)\rho^2\sigma_{BT}^2\sigma_{BR}^2,$$

$\delta$, $\sigma_{1,1}^2$, $\sigma_{TT}^2$, $\sigma_{TR}^2$, $\sigma_{BT}^2$, $\sigma_{BR}^2$ and $\rho$ are given initial values, $z_t$ is the upper $t$th quantile of the standard normal distribution, $1 - \beta$ is the desired power, $a = \theta_{PBE}$ if $\sigma_{TR} \geq \sigma_0$ and $a = 0$ if $\sigma_{TR} < \sigma_0$.

Sample sizes $n$ selected using (10.3.4) with $1 - \beta = 80\%$ and the power $P_n$ of the PBE test based on 10,000 simulations (assuming that the initial parameter values are the true parameter values) are listed in Table 10.3.1. It can be seen from Table 10.3.1 that the actual power $P_n$ corresponding to each selected $n$ is larger than the target value of 80%, although the sample size obtained by formula (10.3.4) is conservative since $P_n$ is much larger than 80% in some cases.

**An Example**

Suppose an investigator is interested in conducting a clinical trial with $2 \times 2$ crossover design to establish PBE between an inhaled formulation of a drug product (test) and a subcutaneous (SC) injected formulation (reference) in terms of log-transformed AUC. Based on PK data obtained from pilot studies, the mean difference of AUC can be assumed to be 5% ($\delta = 0.00$). Also it is assumed that the inter-subject variability under the test and the reference are given by 0.40 and 0.40, respectively. The inter-subject correlation coefficient ($\rho$) is assumed to be 0.75. It is further assumed that the intra-subject variability under the test and the reference are given by 0.10 and 0.10, respectively. The sample size needed in order to achieve an 80% power at the 5% level of significance is given by 12 subjects per sequence according to Table 10.3.1.

## 10.4 Individual Bioequivalence

For the IBE, the standard $2 \times 2$ crossover design is not useful because each subject receives each formulation only once and, hence, it is not possible to obtain unbiased estimators of within-subject variances. To obtain unbiased estimators of the within-subject variances, FDA (2001) suggested that the following $2 \times 4$ crossover design be used. In the first sequence, $n_1$ subjects receive treatments at four periods in the order of TRTR (or TRRT), while in the second sequence, $n_2$ subjects receive treatments at four periods in the order of RTRT (or RTTR). Let $y_{ijk}$ be the observed response (or log-response) of the $i$th subject in the $k$th sequence at $j$th period, where $i = 1, ..., n_k$, $j = 1, ..., 4$, $k = 1, 2$. The following statistical model is assumed:

$$y_{ijk} = \mu + F_l + W_{ljk} + S_{ikl} + e_{ijk}, \quad (10.4.1)$$

Table 10.3.1: Sample Size $n$ Selected Using (10.3.4) with $1 - \beta = 80\%$ and the Power $P_n$ of the PBE Test Based on 10,000 Simulations

| | | Parameter | | | | $\rho = .75$ | | $\rho = 1$ | |
|---|---|---|---|---|---|---|---|---|---|
| $\sigma_{BT}$ | $\sigma_{BR}$ | $\sigma_{WT}$ | $\sigma_{WR}$ | $\delta$ | $\lambda$ | $n$ | $P_n$ | $n$ | $P_n$ |
| .1 | .1 | .1 | .4 | .4726 | $-.2233$ | 37 | .8447 | 36 | .8337 |
| | | | | .4227 | $-.2679$ | 24 | .8448 | 24 | .8567 |
| | | | | .2989 | $-.3573$ | 12 | .8959 | 12 | .9035 |
| | | | | .0000 | $-.4466$ | 7 | .9863 | 7 | .9868 |
| .1 | .4 | .1 | .1 | .4726 | $-.2233$ | 34 | .8492 | 32 | .8560 |
| | | | | .3660 | $-.3127$ | 16 | .8985 | 15 | .8970 |
| | | | | .2113 | $-.4020$ | 9 | .9560 | 8 | .9494 |
| .1 | .1 | .4 | .4 | .2983 | $-.2076$ | 44 | .8123 | 43 | .8069 |
| | | | | .1722 | $-.2670$ | 23 | .8381 | 23 | .8337 |
| | | | | .0000 | $-.2966$ | 17 | .8502 | 17 | .8531 |
| .1 | .4 | .4 | .4 | .5323 | $-.4250$ | 36 | .8305 | 35 | .8290 |
| | | | | .4610 | $-.4958$ | 25 | .8462 | 24 | .8418 |
| | | | | .2661 | $-.6375$ | 13 | .8826 | 13 | .8872 |
| | | | | .0000 | $-.7083$ | 10 | .9318 | 10 | .9413 |
| .1 | .4 | .6 | .4 | .3189 | $-.4066$ | 39 | .8253 | 38 | .8131 |
| | | | | .2255 | $-.4575$ | 29 | .8358 | 28 | .8273 |
| | | | | .0000 | $-.5083$ | 22 | .8484 | 22 | .8562 |
| .1 | .4 | .6 | .6 | .6503 | $-.6344$ | 44 | .8186 | 44 | .8212 |
| | | | | .4598 | $-.8459$ | 22 | .8424 | 22 | .8500 |
| | | | | .3252 | $-.9515$ | 16 | .8615 | 16 | .8689 |
| | | | | .0000 | $-1.057$ | 12 | .8965 | 12 | .9000 |
| .4 | .4 | .1 | .1 | .3445 | $-.1779$ | 37 | .8447 | 22 | .8983 |
| | | | | .2436 | $-.2373$ | 20 | .8801 | 12 | .9461 |
| | | | | .1722 | $-.2670$ | 15 | .8951 | 9 | .9609 |
| | | | | .0000 | $-.2966$ | 12 | .9252 | 7 | .9853 |
| .4 | .4 | .1 | .4 | .5915 | $-.3542$ | 44 | .8354 | 38 | .8481 |
| | | | | .4610 | $-.4958$ | 21 | .8740 | 18 | .8851 |
| | | | | .2661 | $-.6375$ | 12 | .9329 | 11 | .9306 |
| | | | | .0000 | $-.7083$ | 9 | .9622 | 9 | .9698 |
| .4 | .4 | .6 | .4 | .0000 | $-.3583$ | 46 | .8171 | 43 | .8213 |
| .4 | .4 | .6 | .6 | .5217 | $-.6351$ | 41 | .8246 | 39 | .8252 |
| | | | | .3012 | $-.8166$ | 22 | .8437 | 21 | .8509 |
| | | | | .0000 | $-.9073$ | 17 | .8711 | 16 | .8755 |
| .4 | .6 | .4 | .4 | .6655 | $-.6644$ | 33 | .8374 | 30 | .8570 |
| | | | | .5764 | $-.7751$ | 23 | .8499 | 21 | .8709 |
| | | | | .3328 | $-.9965$ | 13 | .9062 | 12 | .9258 |
| | | | | .0000 | $-1.107$ | 10 | .9393 | 9 | .9488 |
| .4 | .6 | .4 | .6 | .9100 | $-.8282$ | 45 | .8403 | 42 | .8447 |
| | | | | .7049 | $-1.159$ | 21 | .8684 | 20 | .8874 |
| | | | | .4070 | $-1.491$ | 11 | .9081 | 11 | .9295 |
| | | | | .0000 | $-1.656$ | 9 | .9608 | 8 | .9577 |
| .6 | .4 | .1 | .4 | .3905 | $-.3558$ | 41 | .8334 | 32 | .8494 |
| | | | | .3189 | $-.4066$ | 30 | .8413 | 24 | .8649 |
| | | | | .2255 | $-.4575$ | 23 | .8584 | 18 | .8822 |
| | | | | .0000 | $-.3583$ | 17 | .8661 | 14 | .9009 |
| .6 | .4 | .4 | .4 | .0000 | $-.3583$ | 42 | .8297 | 35 | .8403 |
| .6 | .6 | .1 | .4 | .7271 | $-.5286$ | 47 | .8335 | 36 | .8584 |
| | | | | .5632 | $-.7401$ | 23 | .8785 | 18 | .9046 |
| | | | | .3252 | $-.9515$ | 13 | .9221 | 10 | .9474 |
| | | | | .0000 | $-1.057$ | 10 | .9476 | 8 | .9780 |
| .6 | .6 | .4 | .4 | .6024 | $-.5444$ | 47 | .8246 | 38 | .8455 |
| | | | | .3012 | $-.8166$ | 19 | .8804 | 15 | .8879 |
| | | | | .0000 | $-.9073$ | 14 | .8903 | 12 | .9147 |

## 10.4. Individual Bioequivalence

where $\mu$ is the overall mean; $F_l$ is the fixed effect of the $l$th formulation ($l = T, R$ and $F_T + F_R = 0$); $W_{ljk}$'s are fixed period, sequence, and interaction effects ($\sum_k \bar{W}_{lk} = 0$, where $\bar{W}_{lk}$ is the average of $W_{ljk}$'s with fixed $(l,k)$, $l = T, R$); and $S_{ikl}$'s and $e_{ijk}$'s are similarly defined as those in (10.2.1). Under model (10.4.1), $\theta$ in (10.1.1) for IBE is equal to

$$\theta = \frac{\delta^2 + \sigma_D^2 + \sigma_{WT}^2 - \sigma_{WR}^2}{\max\{\sigma_0^2, \sigma_{WR}^2\}}, \quad (10.4.2)$$

where $\sigma_D^2 = \sigma_{BT}^2 + \sigma_{BR}^2 - 2\rho\sigma_{BT}\sigma_{BR}$ is the variance of $S_{ikT} - S_{ikR}$, which is referred to as the variance due to the subject-by-formulation interaction. Then, IBE is claimed if the null hypothesis $H_0 : \theta \geq \theta_{IBE}$ is rejected at the 5% level of significance provided that the observed ratio of geometric means is within the limits of 80% and 125%, where $\theta_{IBE}$ is the IBE limit specified in the 2001 FDA guidance. From (10.4.2), we need a 5% level test for

$$H_0 : \gamma \geq 0 \quad \text{versus} \quad H_1 : \gamma < 0,$$

where

$$\gamma = \delta^2 + \sigma_D^2 + \sigma_{WT}^2 - \sigma_{WR}^2 - \theta_{IBE}\max\{\sigma_0^2, \sigma_{WR}^2\}.$$

Therefore, it suffices to find a 95% upper confidence bound $\hat{\gamma}_U$ for $\gamma$. IBE is concluded if $\hat{\gamma}_U < 0$.

The confidence bound $\hat{\gamma}_U$ recommended in FDA (2001) is proposed by Hyslop, Hsuan, and Holder (2000), which can be described as follows. For subject $i$ in sequence $k$, let $x_{ilk}$ and $z_{ilk}$ be the average and the difference, respectively, of two observations from formulation $l$, and let $\bar{x}_{lk}$ and $\bar{z}_{lk}$ be respectively the sample mean based on $x_{ilk}$'s and $z_{ilk}$'s. Under model (10.4.1), an unbiased estimator of $\delta$ is

$$\hat{\delta} = \frac{\bar{x}_{T1} - \bar{x}_{R1} + \bar{x}_{T2} - \bar{x}_{R2}}{2} \sim N\left(\delta, \frac{\sigma_{0.5,0.5}^2}{4}\left(\frac{1}{n_1} + \frac{1}{n_2}\right)\right);$$

an unbiased estimator of $\sigma_{0.5,0.5}^2$ is

$$\hat{\sigma}_{0.5,0.5}^2 = \frac{(n_1-1)s_{d1}^2 + (n_2-1)s_{d2}^2}{n_1+n_2-2} \sim \frac{\sigma_{0.5,0.5}^2 \chi_{n_1+n_2-2}^2}{n_1+n_2-2},$$

where $s_{dk}^2$ is the sample variance based on $x_{iTk} - x_{iRk}$, $i = 1,...,n_k$; an unbiased estimator of $\sigma_{WT}^2$ is

$$\hat{\sigma}_{WT}^2 = \frac{(n_1-1)s_{T1}^2 + (n_2-1)s_{T2}^2}{2(n_1+n_2-2)} \sim \frac{\sigma_{WT}^2 \chi_{n_1+n_2-2}^2}{n_1+n_2-2},$$

where $s_{Tk}^2$ is the sample variance based on $z_{iTk}$, $i = 1, ..., n_k$; and an unbiased estimator of $\sigma_{WR}^2$ is

$$\hat{\sigma}_{WR}^2 = \frac{(n_1 - 1)s_{R1}^2 + (n_2 - 1)s_{R2}^2}{2(n_1 + n_2 - 2)} \sim \frac{\sigma_{WR}^2 \chi_{n_1+n_2-2}^2}{n_1 + n_2 - 2},$$

where $s_{Rk}^2$ is the sample variance based on $z_{iRk}$, $i = 1, ..., n_k$. Furthermore, estimators $\hat{\delta}$, $\hat{\sigma}_{0.5,0.5}^2$, $\hat{\sigma}_{WT}^2$ and $\hat{\sigma}_{WR}^2$ are independent. When $\sigma_{WR}^2 \geq \sigma_0^2$, an approximate 95% upper confidence bound for $\gamma$ is

$$\hat{\gamma}_U = \hat{\delta}^2 + \hat{\sigma}_{0.5,0.5}^2 + 0.5\hat{\sigma}_{WT}^2 - (1.5 + \theta_{IBE})\hat{\sigma}_{WR}^2 + \sqrt{U}, \quad (10.4.3)$$

where $U$ is the sum of the following four quantities:

$$\left[\left(|\hat{\delta}| + t_{0.05,n_1+n_2-2}\frac{\hat{\sigma}_{0.5,0.5}}{2}\sqrt{\frac{1}{n_1} + \frac{1}{n_2}}\right)^2 - \hat{\delta}^2\right]^2,$$

$$\hat{\sigma}_{0.5,0.5}^4 \left(\frac{n_1 + n_2 - 2}{\chi_{0.95,n_1+n_2-2}^2} - 1\right)^2,$$

$$0.5^2 \hat{\sigma}_{WT}^4 \left(\frac{n_1 + n_2 - 2}{\chi_{0.95,n_1+n_2-2}^2} - 1\right)^2,$$

and

$$(1.5 + \theta_{IBE})^2 \hat{\sigma}_{WR}^4 \left(\frac{n_1 + n_2 - 2}{\chi_{0.05,n_1+n_2-2}^2} - 1\right)^2. \quad (10.4.4)$$

When $\sigma_0^2 > \sigma_{WR}^2$, an approximate 95% upper confidence bound for $\gamma$ is

$$\hat{\gamma}_U = \hat{\delta}^2 + \hat{\sigma}_{0.5,0.5}^2 + 0.5\hat{\sigma}_{WT}^2 - 1.5\hat{\sigma}_{WR}^2 - \theta_{IBE}\sigma_0^2 + \sqrt{U_0}, \quad (10.4.5)$$

where $U_0$ is the same as $U$ except that the quantity in (10.4.4) should be replaced by

$$1.5^2 \hat{\sigma}_{WR}^4 \left(\frac{n_1 + n_2 - 2}{\chi_{0.05,n_1+n_2-2}^2} - 1\right)^2.$$

The estimation or test method for PBE described in Section 10.3 can be applied to decide whether the reference-scaled bound $\hat{\gamma}_U$ in (10.4.3) or the constant-scaled bound $\hat{\gamma}_U$ in (10.4.5) should be used.

Although the 2 × 2 crossover design and the 2 × 4 crossover design have the same number of subjects, the 2 × 4 crossover design yields four observations, instead of two, from each subject. This may increase the overall cost substantially. As an alternative to the 2 × 4 crossover design, Chow, Shao, and Wang (2002) recommended a 2 × 3 extra-reference design,

## 10.4. Individual Bioequivalence

in which $n_1$ subjects in sequence 1 receive treatments at three periods in the order of TRR, while $n_2$ subjects in sequence 2 receive treatments at three periods in the order of RTR. The statistical model under this design is still given by (10.4.1). An unbiased estimator of $\delta$ is

$$\hat{\delta} = \frac{\bar{x}_{T1} - \bar{x}_{R1} + \bar{x}_{T2} - \bar{x}_{R2}}{2} \sim N\left(\delta, \frac{\sigma^2_{1,0.5}}{4}\left(\frac{1}{n_1} + \frac{1}{n_2}\right)\right),$$

where $\sigma^2_{a,b}$ is given by (10.2.4); an unbiased estimator of $\sigma^2_{1,0.5}$ is

$$\hat{\sigma}^2_{1,0.5} = \frac{(n_1-1)s^2_{d1} + (n_2-1)s^2_{d2}}{n_1 + n_2 - 2} \sim \frac{\sigma^2_{1,0.5}\chi^2_{n_1+n_2-2}}{n_1 + n_2 - 1};$$

an unbiased estimator of $\sigma^2_{WR}$ is

$$\hat{\sigma}^2_{WR} = \frac{(n_1-1)s^2_{R1} + (n_2-1)s^2_{R2}}{2(n_1 + n_2 - 2)} \sim \frac{\sigma^2_{WR}\chi^2_{n_1+n_2-2}}{n_1 + n_2 - 2};$$

and estimators $\hat{\delta}$, $\hat{\sigma}^2_{1,0.5}$, and $\hat{\sigma}^2_{WR}$ are independent, since $x_{iT1} - x_{iR1}$, $x_{iT2} - x_{iR2}$, $z_{iR1}$, and $z_{iR2}$ are independent. Chow, Shao, and Wang (2002) obtained the following approximate 95% upper confidence bound for $\gamma$. When $\sigma^2_{WR} \geq \sigma^2_0$,

$$\hat{\gamma}_U = \hat{\delta}^2 + \hat{\sigma}^2_{1,0.5} - (1.5 + \theta_{IBE})\hat{\sigma}^2_{WR} + \sqrt{U},$$

where $U$ is the sum of the following three quantities:

$$\left[\left(|\hat{\delta}| + t_{0.05,n_1+n_2-2}\frac{\hat{\sigma}_{1,0.5}}{2}\sqrt{\frac{1}{n_1} + \frac{1}{n_2}}\right)^2 - \hat{\delta}^2\right]^2,$$

$$\hat{\sigma}^4_{1,0.5}\left(\frac{n_1 + n_2 - 2}{\chi^2_{0.95,n_1+n_2-2}} - 1\right)^2,$$

and

$$(1.5 + \theta_{IBE})^2 \hat{\sigma}^4_{WR}\left(\frac{n_1 + n_2 - 2}{\chi^2_{0.05,n_1+n_2-2}} - 1\right)^2. \quad (10.4.6)$$

When $\sigma^2_{WR} < \sigma^2_0$,

$$\hat{\gamma}_U = \hat{\delta}^2 + \hat{\sigma}^2_{1,0.5} - 1.5\hat{\sigma}^2_{WR} - \theta_{IBE}\sigma^2_0 + \sqrt{U_0},$$

where $U_0$ is the same as $U$ except that the quantity in (10.4.6) should be replaced by

$$1.5^2 \hat{\sigma}^4_{WR}\left(\frac{n_1 + n_2 - 2}{\chi^2_{0.05,n_1+n_2-2}} - 1\right)^2.$$

Again, the estimation or test method for PBE described in Section 10.3 can be applied to decide which bound should be used.

To determine sample sizes $n_1$ and $n_2$, we would choose $n_1 = n_2 = n$ so that the power of the IBE test reaches a given level $1-\beta$ when the unknown parameters are set at some initial guessing values $\delta$, $\sigma_D^2$, $\sigma_{WT}^2$, and $\sigma_{WR}^2$. For the IBE test based on the confidence bound $\hat{\gamma}_U$, its power is given by

$$P_n = P(\hat{\gamma}_U < 0)$$

when $\gamma < 0$. Consider first the case where $\sigma_{WR}^2 > \sigma_0^2$. Let $U$ be given in the definition of the reference-scaled bound $\hat{\gamma}_U$ and $U_\beta$ be the same as $U$ but with 5% and 95% replaced by $\beta$ and $1-\beta$, respectively. Since

$$P(\hat{\gamma}_U < \gamma + \sqrt{U} + \sqrt{U_{1-\beta}}) \approx 1-\beta,$$

the power $P_n$ is approximately larger than $\beta$ if

$$\gamma + \sqrt{U} + \sqrt{U_{1-\beta}} \leq 0.$$

Let $\tilde{\gamma}$, $\tilde{U}$ and $\tilde{U}_{1-\beta}$ be $\gamma$, $U$ and $U_{1-\beta}$, respectively, with parameter values and their estimators replaced by the initial values $\delta$, $\sigma_D^2$, $\sigma_{WT}^2$, and $\sigma_{WR}^2$. Then, the required sample size $n$ to have approximately power $1-\beta$ is the smallest integer satisfying

$$\tilde{\gamma} + \sqrt{\tilde{U}} + \sqrt{\tilde{U}_{1-\beta}} \leq 0, \tag{10.4.7}$$

assuming that $n_1 = n_2 = n$ and the initial values are the true parameter values. When $\sigma_{WR}^2 < \sigma_0^2$, the previous procedure can be modified by replacing $U$ by $U_0$ in the definition of constant-scaled bound $\hat{\gamma}_U$. If $\tilde{\sigma}_{WR}^2$ is equal or close to $\sigma_0^2$, then we recommend the use of $U$ instead of $U_0$ to produce a more conservative sample size and the use of the test approach in the IBE test.

This procedure can be applied to either the $2 \times 3$ design or the $2 \times 4$ design.

Since the IBE tests are based on the asymptotic theory, $n$ should be reasonably large to ensure the asymptotic convergence. Hence, we suggest that the solution greater than 10 from (10.4.7) be used. In other words, a sample size of more than $n=10$ per sequence that satisfies (10.4.7) is recommended.

Sample sizes $n_1 = n_2 = n$ selected using (10.4.7) with $1-\beta = 80\%$ and the power $P_n$ of the IBE test based on 10,000 simulations are listed in Table 10.4.1 for both the $2 \times 3$ extra-reference design and $2 \times 4$ crossover design. For each selected $n$ that is smaller than 10, the power of the IBE test using $n^* = \max(n, 10)$ as the sample size, which is denoted by $P_{n^*}$, is also included. It can be seen from Table 10.4.1 that the actual power $P_n$ is larger than the target value of 80% in most cases and only in a few cases where $n$ determined from (10.4.7) is very small, the power $P_n$ is lower than 75%. Using $n^* = \max(n, 10)$ as the sample size produces better results when selected by (10.4.7) is very small, but in most cases it results in a power much larger than 80%.

**An Example**

Suppose an investigator is interested in conducting a clinical trial with $2 \times 4$ crossover design to establish IBE between an inhaled formulation of a drug product (test) and a subcutaneous (SC) injected formulation (reference) in terms of log-transformed AUC. Based on PK data obtained from pilot studies, the mean difference of AUC can be assumed to be 0%. Also it is assumed the intra-subject standard deviation of test and reference are given by 60% and 40%, respectively. It is further assumed that the inter-subject standard deviation of test and reference are given by 10% and 40%, respectively. The inter-subject correlation coefficient ($\rho$) is assumed to be 0.75. According to Table 10.4.1, a total of 22 subjects per sequence is needed in order to achieve an 80% power at the 5% level of significance.

## 10.5 In Vitro Bioequivalence

Statistical methods for assessment of *in vitro* bioequivalence testing for nasal aerosols and sprays can be classified as the nonprofile analysis and the profile analysis. In this section, we consider sample size calculation for nonprofile analysis.

The nonprofile analysis applies to tests for dose or spray content uniformity through container life, droplet size distribution, spray pattern, and priming and repriming. The FDA adopts the criterion and limit of the PBE for assessment of *in vitro* bioequivalence in the nonprofile analysis. Let $\theta$ be defined in (10.1.1) with independent *in vitro* bioavailabilities $y_T$, $y_R$, and $y'_R$, and let $\theta_{BE}$ be the bioequivalence limit. Then, the two formulations are *in vitro* bioequivalent if $\theta < \theta_{BE}$. Similar to the PBE, *in vitro* bioequivalence can be claimed if the hypothesis that $\theta \geq \theta_{BE}$ is rejected at the 5% level of significance provided that the observed ratio of geometric means is within the limits of 90% and 110%.

Suppose that $m_T$ and $m_R$ canisters (or bottles) from respectively the test and the reference products are randomly selected and one observation from each canister is obtained. The data can be described by the following model:

$$y_{jk} = \mu_k + \varepsilon_{jk}, \quad j = 1, ..., m_k, \qquad (10.5.1)$$

Table 10.4.1: Sample Size $n$ Selected Using (10.4.7) with $1-\beta = 80\%$ and the Power $P_n$ of the IBE Test Based on 10,000 Simulations

| Parameter | | | | $2 \times 3 extra-reference$ | | | | $2 \times 4 crossover$ | | | |
|---|---|---|---|---|---|---|---|---|---|---|---|
| $\sigma_D$ | $\sigma_{WT}$ | $\sigma_{WR}$ | $\delta$ | $n$ | $P_n$ | $n^*$ | $P_{n*}$ | $n$ | $P_n$ | $n^*$ | $P_{n*}$ |
| 0 | .15 | .15 | 0 | 5 | .7226 | 10 | .9898 | 4 | .7007 | 10 | .9998 |
| | | | .1 | 6 | .7365 | 10 | .9572 | 5 | .7837 | 10 | .9948 |
| | | | .2 | 13 | .7718 | 13 | | 9 | .7607 | 10 | .8104 |
| 0 | .2 | .15 | 0 | 9 | .7480 | 10 | .8085 | 7 | .7995 | 10 | .9570 |
| | | | .1 | 12 | .7697 | 12 | | 8 | .7468 | 10 | .8677 |
| | | | .2 | 35 | .7750 | 35 | | 23 | .7835 | 23 | |
| 0 | .15 | .2 | 0 | 9 | .8225 | 10 | .8723 | 8 | .8446 | 10 | .9314 |
| | | | .1 | 12 | .8523 | 12 | | 10 | .8424 | 10 | |
| | | | .2 | 26 | .8389 | 26 | | 23 | .8506 | 23 | |
| 0 | .2 | .2 | 0 | 15 | .8206 | 15 | | 13 | .8591 | 13 | |
| | | | .1 | 20 | .8373 | 20 | | 17 | .8532 | 17 | |
| | | | .2 | 52 | .8366 | 52 | | 44 | .8458 | 44 | |
| 0 | .3 | .2 | 0 | 91 | .8232 | 91 | | 71 | .8454 | 71 | |
| .2 | .15 | .15 | 0 | 20 | .7469 | 20 | | 17 | .7683 | 17 | |
| | | | .1 | 31 | .7577 | 31 | | 25 | .7609 | 25 | |
| .2 | .15 | .2 | 0 | 31 | .8238 | 31 | | 28 | .8358 | 28 | |
| | | | .1 | 43 | .8246 | 43 | | 39 | .8296 | 39 | |
| .2 | .2 | .2 | 0 | 59 | .8225 | 59 | | 51 | .8322 | 51 | |
| | | | .2 | 91 | .8253 | 91 | | 79 | .8322 | 79 | |
| 0 | .15 | .3 | 0 | 7 | .8546 | 10 | .9607 | 6 | .8288 | 10 | .9781 |
| | | | .1 | 7 | .8155 | 10 | .9401 | 7 | .8596 | 10 | .9566 |
| | | | .2 | 10 | .8397 | 10 | | 9 | .8352 | 10 | .8697 |
| | | | .3 | 16 | .7973 | 16 | | 15 | .8076 | 15 | |
| | | | .4 | 45 | .8043 | 45 | | 43 | .8076 | 43 | |
| 0 | .3 | .3 | 0 | 15 | .7931 | 15 | | 13 | .8162 | 13 | |
| | | | .1 | 17 | .7942 | 17 | | 14 | .8057 | 14 | |
| | | | .2 | 25 | .8016 | 25 | | 21 | .8079 | 21 | |
| | | | .3 | 52 | .7992 | 52 | | 44 | .8009 | 44 | |
| 0 | .2 | .5 | 0 | 6 | .8285 | 10 | .9744 | 6 | .8497 | 10 | .9810 |
| | | | .1 | 6 | .8128 | 10 | .9708 | 6 | .8413 | 10 | .9759 |
| | | | .2 | 7 | .8410 | 10 | .9505 | 7 | .8600 | 10 | .9628 |
| | | | .3 | 8 | .8282 | 10 | .9017 | 8 | .8548 | 10 | .9239 |
| | | | .4 | 10 | .8147 | 10 | | 10 | .8338 | 10 | |
| | | | .5 | 14 | .8095 | 14 | | 14 | .8248 | 14 | |
| | | | .6 | 24 | .8162 | 24 | | 23 | .8149 | 23 | |
| | | | .7 | 51 | .8171 | 51 | | 49 | .8170 | 49 | |
| 0 | .5 | .5 | 0 | 15 | .7890 | 15 | | 13 | .8132 | 13 | |
| | | | .1 | 16 | .8000 | 16 | | 13 | .7956 | 13 | |
| | | | .2 | 18 | .7980 | 18 | | 15 | .8033 | 15 | |
| | | | .3 | 23 | .8002 | 23 | | 19 | .8063 | 19 | |
| | | | .5 | 52 | .7944 | 52 | | 44 | .8045 | 44 | |
| .2 | .2 | .3 | 0 | 13 | .7870 | 13 | | 12 | .7970 | 12 | |
| | | | .1 | 15 | .8007 | 15 | | 14 | .8144 | 14 | |
| | | | .2 | 21 | .7862 | 21 | | 20 | .8115 | 20 | |
| | | | .3 | 43 | .8037 | 43 | | 40 | .8034 | 40 | |
| .2 | .3 | .3 | 0 | 26 | .7806 | 26 | | 22 | .7877 | 22 | |
| | | | .1 | 30 | .7895 | 30 | | 26 | .8039 | 26 | |
| .2 | .3 | .5 | 0 | 9 | .8038 | 10 | .8502 | 8 | .8050 | 10 | .8947 |
| | | | .1 | 9 | .7958 | 10 | .8392 | 9 | .8460 | 10 | .8799 |
| | | | .2 | 10 | .7966 | 10 | | 9 | .7954 | 10 | .8393 |
| | | | .3 | 12 | .7929 | 12 | | 11 | .8045 | 11 | |
| | | | .4 | 16 | .7987 | 16 | | 15 | .8094 | 15 | |

$n^* = \max(n, 10)$

## 10.5. In Vitro Bioequivalence

where $k = T$ for the test product, $k = R$ for the reference product, $\mu_T$ and $\mu_R$ are fixed product effects, and $\varepsilon_{jk}$'s are independent random measurement errors distributed as $N(0, \sigma_k^2)$, $k = T, R$. Under model (10.5.1), the parameter $\theta$ in (10.1.1) is equal to

$$\theta = \frac{(\mu_T - \mu_R)^2 + \sigma_T^2 - \sigma_R^2}{\max\{\sigma_0^2, \sigma_R^2\}} \qquad (10.5.2)$$

and $\theta < \theta_{BE}$ if and only if $\zeta < 0$, where

$$\zeta = (\mu_T - \mu_R)^2 + \sigma_T^2 - \sigma_R^2 - \theta_{BE} \max\{\sigma_0^2, \sigma_R^2\}. \qquad (10.5.3)$$

Under model (10.5.1), the best unbiased estimator of $\delta = \mu_T - \mu_R$ is

$$\hat{\delta} = \bar{y}_T - \bar{y}_R \sim N\left(\delta, \frac{\sigma_T^2}{m_T} + \frac{\sigma_R^2}{m_R}\right),$$

where $\bar{y}_k$ is the average of $y_{jk}$ over $j$ for a fixed $k$. The best unbiased estimator of $\sigma_k^2$ is

$$s_k^2 = \frac{1}{m_k - 1} \sum_{j=1}^{m_k} (y_{jk} - \bar{y}_k)^2 \sim \frac{\sigma_k^2 \chi_{m_k-1}^2}{m_k - 1}, \qquad k = T, R.$$

Using the method for IBE testing (Section 10.4), an approximate 95% upper confidence bound for $\zeta$ in (10.5.3) is

$$\tilde{\zeta}_U = \hat{\delta}^2 + s_T^2 - s_R^2 - \theta_{BE} \max\{\sigma_0^2, s_R^2\} + \sqrt{U_0},$$

where $U_0$ is the sum of the following three quantities:

$$\left[\left(|\hat{\delta}| + z_{0.05}\sqrt{\frac{s_T^2}{m_T} + \frac{s_R^2}{m_R}}\right)^2 - \hat{\delta}^2\right]^2,$$

$$s_T^4 \left(\frac{m_T - 1}{\chi_{0.95, m_T-1}^2} - 1\right)^2,$$

and

$$(1 + c\theta_{BE})^2 s_R^4 \left(\frac{m_R - 1}{\chi_{0.05, m_R-1}^2} - 1\right)^2,$$

and $c = 1$ if $s_R^2 \geq \sigma_0^2$ and $c = 0$ if $s_R^2 < \sigma_0^2$. Note that the estimation method for determining the use of the reference-scaled criterion or the constant-scaled criterion is applied here. *In vitro* bioequivalence can be claimed if $\tilde{\zeta}_U < 0$. This procedure is recommended by the FDA guidance.

To ensure that the previously described test has a significant level close to the nominal level 5% with a desired power, the FDA requires that at least 30 canisters of each of the test and reference products be tested. However, $m_k = 30$ may not be enough to achieve a desired power of the bioequivalence test in some situations (see Chow, Shao, and Wang, 2003b). Increasing $m_k$ can certainly increase the power, but in some situations, obtaining replicates from each canister may be more practical, and/or cost-effective. With replicates from each canister, however, the previously described test procedure is necessarily modified in order to address the between- and within-canister variabilities.

Suppose that there are $n_k$ replicates from each canister for product $k$. Let $y_{ijk}$ be the $i$th replicate in the $j$th canister under product $k$, $b_{jk}$ be the between-canister variation, and $e_{ijk}$ be the within-canister measurement error. Then

$$y_{ijk} = \mu_k + b_{jk} + e_{ijk}, \quad i = 1, ..., n_k, \ j = 1, ..., m_k, \quad (10.5.4)$$

where $b_{jk} \sim N(0, \sigma_{Bk}^2)$, $e_{ijk} \sim N(0, \sigma_{Wk}^2)$, and $b_{jk}$'s and $e_{ijk}$'s are independent. Under model (10.5.4), the total variances $\sigma_T^2$ and $\sigma_R^2$ in (10.5.2) and (10.5.3) are equal to $\sigma_{BT}^2 + \sigma_{WT}^2$ and $\sigma_{BR}^2 + \sigma_{WR}^2$, respectively, i.e., the sums of between-canister and within-canister variances. The parameter $\theta$ in (10.1.1) is still given by (10.5.2) and $\theta < \theta_{BE}$ if and only if $\zeta < 0$, where $\zeta$ is given in (10.5.3).

Under model (10.5.4), the best unbiased estimator of $\delta = \mu_T - \mu_R$ is

$$\hat{\delta} = \bar{y}_T - \bar{y}_R \sim N\left(\delta, \ \frac{\sigma_{BT}^2}{m_T} + \frac{\sigma_{BR}^2}{m_R} + \frac{\sigma_{WT}^2}{m_T n_T} + \frac{\sigma_{WR}^2}{m_R n_R}\right),$$

where $\bar{y}_k$ is the average of $y_{ijk}$ over $i$ and $j$ for a fixed $k$.

To construct a confidence bound for $\zeta$ in (10.5.3) using the approach in IBE testing, we need to find independent, unbiased, and chi-square distributed estimators of $\sigma_T^2$ and $\sigma_R^2$. These estimators, however, are not available when $n_k > 1$. Note that

$$\sigma_k^2 = \sigma_{Bk}^2 + n_k^{-1}\sigma_{Wk}^2 + (1 - n_k^{-1})\sigma_{Wk}^2, \quad k = T, R;$$

$\sigma_{Bk}^2 + n_k^{-1}\sigma_{Wk}^2$ can be estimated by

$$s_{Bk}^2 = \frac{1}{m_k - 1}\sum_{j=1}^{m_k}(\bar{y}_{jk} - \bar{y}_k)^2 \sim \frac{(\sigma_{Bk}^2 + n_k^{-1}\sigma_{Wk}^2)\chi_{m_k-1}^2}{m_k - 1},$$

where $\bar{y}_{jk}$ is the average of $y_{ijk}$ over $i$; $\sigma_{Wk}^2$ can be estimated by

$$s_{Wk}^2 = \frac{1}{m_k(n_k - 1)}\sum_{j=1}^{m_k}\sum_{i=1}^{n_k}(y_{ijk} - \bar{y}_{jk})^2 \sim \frac{\sigma_{Wk}^2\chi_{m_k(n_k-1)}^2}{m_k(n_k - 1)};$$

## 10.5. In Vitro Bioequivalence

and $\hat{\delta}$, $s^2_{Bk}$, $s^2_{Wk}$, $k = T, R$, are independent. Thus, an approximate 95% upper confidence bound for $\zeta$ in (10.5.3) is

$$\hat{\zeta}_U = \hat{\delta}^2 + s^2_{BT} + (1 - n_T^{-1})s^2_{WT} - s^2_{BR} - (1 - n_R^{-1})s^2_{WR}$$
$$- \theta_{BE} \max\{\sigma_0^2, s^2_{BR} + (1 - n_R^{-1})s^2_{WR}\} + \sqrt{U},$$

where $U$ is the sum of the following five quantities,

$$\left[\left(|\hat{\delta}| + z_{0.05}\sqrt{\frac{s^2_{BT}}{m_T} + \frac{s^2_{BR}}{m_R}}\right)^2 - \hat{\delta}^2\right]^2,$$

$$s^4_{BT}\left(\frac{m_T - 1}{\chi^2_{0.95, m_T - 1}} - 1\right)^2,$$

$$(1 - n_T^{-1})^2 s^4_{WT}\left(\frac{m_T(n_T - 1)}{\chi^2_{0.95, m_T(n_T - 1)}} - 1\right)^2,$$

$$(1 + \theta_{BE})^2 s^4_{BR}\left(\frac{m_R - 1}{\chi^2_{0.05, m_R - 1}} - 1\right)^2,$$

and

$$(1 + c\theta_{BE})^2 (1 - n_R^{-1})^2 s^4_{WR}\left(\frac{m_R(n_R - 1)}{\chi^2_{0.05, m_R(n_R - 1)}} - 1\right)^2,$$

and $c = 1$ if $s^2_{BR} + (1 - n_R^{-1})s^2_{WR} \geq \sigma_0^2$ and $c = 0$ if $s^2_{BR} + (1 - n_R^{-1})s^2_{WR} < \sigma_0^2$. In vitro bioequivalence can be claimed if $\hat{\zeta}_U < 0$ provided that the observed ratio of geometric means is within the limits of 90% and 110%.

Note that the minimum sample sizes required by the FDA are $m_k = 30$ canisters and $n_k = 1$ observation from each canister. To achieve a desired power, Chow, Shao, and Wang (2003b) proposed the following procedure of sample size calculation. Assume that $m = m_T = m_R$ and $n = n_T = n_R$. Let $\psi = (\delta, \sigma^2_{BT}, \sigma^2_{BR}, \sigma^2_{WT}, \sigma^2_{WR})$ be the vector of unknown parameters under model (10.5.4). Let $U$ be given in the definition of $\hat{\zeta}_U$ and $U_{1-\beta}$ be the same as $U$ but with 5% and 95% replaced by $\beta$ and $1 - \beta$, respectively, where $1 - \beta$ is a given power. Let $\tilde{U}$ and $\tilde{U}_{1-\beta}$ be $U$ and $U_{1-\beta}$, respectively, with $(\hat{\delta}, s^2_{BT}, s^2_{BR}, s^2_{WT}, s^2_{WR})$ replaced by $\tilde{\psi}$, an initial guessing value for which the value of $\zeta$ (denoted by $\tilde{\zeta}$) is negative. From the results in Chow, Shao, and Wang (2003b), it is advantageous to have a large $m$ and a small $n$ when $mn$, the total number of observations for one treatment, is fixed. Thus, the sample sizes $m$ and $n$ can be determined as follows.

Table 10.5.1: Selected Sample Sizes $m_*$ and $n_*$
and the Actual Power $p$ (10,000 Simulations)

| $\sigma_{BT}$ | $\sigma_{BR}$ | $\sigma_{WT}$ | $\sigma_{WR}$ | $\delta$ | Step 1 $p$ | Step 2 $m_*, n_*$ | Step 2 $p$ | Step 2' $m_*, n_*$ | Step 2' $p$ |
|---|---|---|---|---|---|---|---|---|---|
| 0 | 0 | .25 | .25 | .0530 | .4893 | 55, 1 | .7658 | 30, 2 | .7886 |
|   |   |   |   | 0     | .5389 | 47, 1 | .7546 | 30, 2 | .8358 |
|   |   | .25 | .50 | .4108 | .6391 | 45, 1 | .7973 | 30, 2 | .8872 |
|   |   |   |   | .2739 | .9138 | -- | -- | -- | -- |
|   |   | .50 | .50 | .1061 | .4957 | 55, 1 | .7643 | 30, 2 | .7875 |
|   |   |   |   | 0     | .5362 | 47, 1 | .7526 | 30, 2 | .8312 |
| .25 | .25 | .25 | .25 | .0750 | .4909 | 55, 1 | .7774 | 30, 3 | .7657 |
|   |   |   |   | 0     | .5348 | 47, 1 | .7533 | 30, 2 | .7323 |
|   |   | .25 | .50 | .4405 | .5434 | 57, 1 | .7895 | 30, 3 | .8489 |
|   |   |   |   | .2937 | .8370 | -- | -- | -- | -- |
|   |   | .50 | .50 | .1186 | .4893 | 55, 1 | .7683 | 30, 2 | .7515 |
|   |   |   |   | 0     | .5332 | 47, 1 | .7535 | 30, 2 | .8091 |
| .50 | .25 | .25 | .50 | .1186 | .4903 | 55, 1 | .7660 | 30, 4 | .7586 |
|   |   |   |   | 0     | .5337 | 47, 1 | .7482 | 30, 3 | .7778 |
| .25 | .50 | .25 | .25 | .2937 | .8357 | -- | -- | -- | -- |
|   |   | .50 | .25 | .1186 | .5016 | 55, 1 | .7717 | 30, 4 | .7764 |
|   |   |   |   | 0     | .5334 | 47, 1 | .7484 | 30, 3 | .7942 |
|   |   | .25 | .50 | .5809 | .6416 | 45, 1 | .7882 | 30, 2 | .7884 |
|   |   |   |   | .3873 | .9184 | -- | -- | -- | -- |
|   |   | .50 | .50 | .3464 | .6766 | 38, 1 | .7741 | 30, 2 | .8661 |
|   |   |   |   | .1732 | .8470 | -- | -- | -- | -- |
| .50 | .50 | .25 | .50 | .3464 | .6829 | 38, 1 | .7842 | 30, 2 | .8045 |
|   |   |   |   | .1732 | .8450 | -- | -- | -- | -- |
|   |   | .50 | .50 | .1500 | .4969 | 55, 1 | .7612 | 30, 3 | .7629 |
|   |   |   |   | 0     | .5406 | 47, 1 | .7534 | 30, 2 | .7270 |

In step 1, $m_* = 30$, $n_* = 1$

Step 1. Set $m = 30$ and $n = 1$. If

$$\tilde{\zeta} + \sqrt{\tilde{U}} + \sqrt{\tilde{U}_{1-\beta}} \leq 0 \qquad (10.5.5)$$

holds, stop and the required sample sizes are $m = 30$ and $n = 1$; otherwise, go to step 2.

Step 2. Let $n = 1$ and find a smallest integer $m_*$ such that (10.5.5) holds. If $m_* \leq m_+$ (the largest possible number of canisters in a given problem), stop and the required sample sizes are $m = m_*$ and $n = 1$; otherwise, go to step 3.

Step 3. Let $m = m_+$ and find a smallest integer $n_*$ such that (10.5.5) holds. The required sample sizes are $m = m_+$ and $n = n_*$.

If in practice it is much easier and inexpensive to obtain more replicates than to sample more canisters, then Steps 2-3 in the previous procedure can be replaced by

## 10.5. In Vitro Bioequivalence

**Step 2′.** Let $m = 30$ and find a smallest integer $n_*$ such that (10.5.5) holds. The required sample sizes are $m = 30$ and $n = n_*$.

Table 10.5.1 contains selected $m_*$ and $n_*$ according to Steps 1-3 or Steps 1 and 2′ with $1 - \beta = 80\%$ and the simulated power $p$ of the *in vitro* bioequivalence test using these sample sizes.

### An Example

Suppose an investigator is interested in conducting a clinical trial with a parallel design with no replicates to establish *in vitro* bioequivalence between a generic drug product (test) and a brand name drug product (reference) in terms of *in vitro* bioavailability. Based on data obtained from pilot studies, the mean difference can be assumed to be 0% ($\delta = 0.00$). Also, it is assumed the intra-subject standard deviation of test and reference are given by 50% and 50%, respectively. It is further assumed that the inter-subject standard deviation of the test and the reference are given by 50% and 50%, respectively. According to Table 10.5.1, 47 subjects per treatment group are needed in order to yield an 80% power at the 5% level of significance.

# Chapter 11

# Dose Response Studies

As indicated in 21 CFR 312.21, the primary objectives of phase I clinical investigation are to (i) determine the metabolism and pharmacological activities of the drug, the side effects associated with increasing dose and early evidence in effectiveness and (ii) obtain sufficient information regarding the drug's pharmacokinetics and pharmacological effects to permit the design of well controlled and scientifically valid phase II clinical studies. Thus, phase I clinical investigation includes studies of drug metabolism, bioavailibility, dose ranging and multiple dose. The primary objectives of phase II studies are not only to initially evaluate the effectiveness of a drug based on clinical endpoints for a particular indication or indications in patients with disease or condition under study but also to determine the dosing ranges and doses for phase III studies and common short-term side effects and risks associated with the drug. In practice, the focus of phase I dose response studies is safety, while phase II dose response studies emphasize the efficacy.

When studying the dose response relationship of an investigational drug, a randomized, parallel-group trial involving a number of dose levels of the investigational drug and a control is usually conducted. Ruberg (1995a, 1995b) indicated that some questions dictating design and analysis are necessarily addressed. These questions include (i) Is there any evidence of the drug effect? (ii) What does exhibit a response different from the control response? (iii) What is the nature of the dose-response? (iv) What is the optimal dose? The first question is usually addressed by the analysis of variance. The second question can be addressed by the Williams' test for minimum effective dose (MED). The third question can be addressed by model-based approaches, either frequentist or Bayesian. The last question is a multiple dimensional issue involving efficacy as well as tolerability and safety such as the determination of maximum tolerable dose (MTD). In this chapter, we will limit our discussion to the sample size calculations for addressing the above questions.

In the next three sections, formulas for sample size calculation for continuous, binary response, and time-to-event study endpoints under a multiple-arm dose response trial are derived, respectively. Section 11.4 provides sample size formula for determination of minimum effective dose (MED) based on Williams' test. A sample size formula based on Cocharan-Armitage's trend test for binary response is given in Section 11.5. In Section 11.6, sample size estimation and related operating characteristics of phase I dose escalation trials are discussed. A brief concluding remark is given in the last section.

## 11.1 Continuous Response

To characterize the response curve, a multi-arm design including a control group and $K$ active dose groups is usually considered. This multi-arm trial is informative for the drug candidates with a wide therapeutic window. The null hypothesis of interest is then given by

$$H_0 : \mu_0 = \mu_1 = ... = \mu_K, \qquad (11.1.1)$$

where $\mu_0$ is mean response for the control group and $\mu_i$ is mean response for the $i$th dose group. The rejection of hypothesis (11.1.1) indicated that there is a treatment effect. The dose response relationship can then be examined under appropriate alternative hypothesis. Under a specific alternative hypothesis, the required sample size per dose group can then be obtained. Spriet and Dupin-Spriet (1992) identified the following eight alternative hypotheses ($H_a$) for dose responses:

(1) $\mu_0 < \mu_1 < ... < \mu_{K-1} < \mu_K$;

(2) $\mu_0 < ... < \mu_i = ... = \mu_j > ... > \mu_K$;

(3) $\mu_0 < ... < \mu_i = ... = \mu_K$;

(4) $\mu_0 = ... = \mu_i < ... < \mu_K$;

(5) $\mu_0 < \mu_1 < ... = \mu_i = ... = \mu_K$;

(6) $\mu_0 = \mu_1 = ... = \mu_i < ... < \mu_{K-1} < \mu_K$;

(7) $\mu_0 = \mu_1 < ... < \mu_i = ... = \mu_K$;

(8) $\mu_0 = ... = \mu_i < ... < \mu_{K-1} = \mu_K$.

## 11.1. Continuous Response

In the subsequent sections, we will derive sample size formulas for various study endpoints such as continuous response, binary response, and time-to-event data under a multi-arm dose response design, respectively.

### 11.1.1 Linear Contrast Test

Under a multi-arm dose response design, a linear contrast test is commonly employed. Consider the following one-sided hypotheses:

$$H_o : L(\mu) = \sum_{i=0}^{K} c_i \mu_i \leq 0 \text{ vs. } H_a : L(\mu) = \sum_{i=0}^{K} c_i \mu_i = \varepsilon > 0,$$

where $\mu_i$ could be mean, proportion, or ranking score in the ith arm, $c_i$ are the contrast coefficients satisfying $\sum_{i=0}^{K} c_i = 0$, and $\varepsilon$ is a constant. The test statistics under the null hypothesis and the alternative hypothesis can be expressed as

$$T(H) = \frac{L(\widehat{\boldsymbol{\mu}})}{\sqrt{var(L(\widehat{\boldsymbol{\mu}})|H_o)}}; \ H \in H_o \cup H_a.$$

Under the alternative hypothesis, we have $\varepsilon = E(L(\widehat{\boldsymbol{\mu}})|H_a)$. Denote $v_o^2 = var(L(\widehat{\boldsymbol{\mu}})|H_o)$ and $v_a^2 = var(L(\widehat{\boldsymbol{\mu}})|H_a)$. Then, under the null hypothesis, for large sample, we have

$$T(H_o) = \frac{L(\widehat{\boldsymbol{\mu}}; \delta)|H_o}{v_o} \sim N(0, 1).$$

Similarly, under the alternative hypothesis, it can be verified that

$$T(H_a) = \frac{L(\widehat{\boldsymbol{\mu}}; \delta)}{v_o} \sim N(\frac{\varepsilon}{v_o}, \frac{v_a^2}{v_o^2})$$

for large sample, where

$$v_o^2 = var(L(\widehat{\boldsymbol{\mu}}; \delta)|H_o) = \sum_{i=0}^{k} c_i^2 var(\widehat{\mu}_i|H_o) = \sigma_o^2 \sum_{i=0}^{K} \frac{c_i^2}{n_i}$$

$$v_a^2 = var(L(\widehat{\boldsymbol{\mu}}; \delta)|H_a) = \sum_{i=0}^{k} c_i^2 var(\widehat{\mu}_i|H_o) = \sum_{i=0}^{K} \frac{c_i^2 \sigma_i^2}{n_i}$$

That is,

$$\begin{cases} v_o^2 = \frac{\sigma_o^2}{n} \sum_{i=0}^{K} \frac{c_i^2}{f_i} \\ v_a^2 = \frac{1}{n} \sum_{i=0}^{K} \frac{c_i^2 \sigma_i^2}{f_i} \end{cases}, \quad (11.1.2)$$

where the size fraction $f_i = \frac{n_i}{n}$ with $N = \sum_{i=0}^{K} n_i$. Note that $\sigma_o$ and $\sigma_a$ are the standard deviation of the response under $H_0$ and $H_a$, respectively. Let $\mu_i$ be the population mean for group i. The null hypothesis of no treatment effects can be written as follows

$$H_o : L(\mu) = \sum_{i=0}^{K} c_i \mu_i = 0, \qquad (11.1.3)$$

where $\sum_{i=0}^{K} c_i = 0$. Under the following alternative hypothesis

$$H_a : L(\mu) = \sum_{i=0}^{K} c_i \mu_i = \varepsilon, \qquad (11.1.4)$$

and the assumption of homogeneous variances, the sample size can be obtained as

$$N = \left[ \frac{(z_{1-\alpha} + z_{1-\beta})\sigma}{\varepsilon} \right]^2 \sum_{i=0}^{k} \frac{c_i^2}{f_i},$$

where $f_i$ is the sample size fraction for the $i$th group and the population parameter $\sigma$. Note that, in practice, for the purpose of sample size calculation, one may use the pooled standard deviation if prior data are available.

**An Example**

Suppose that a pharmaceutical company is interested in conducting a dose response study for a test drug developed for treating patients with asthma. A 4-arm design consisting of a placebo control and three active dose levels (0, 20mg, 40mg, and 60mg) of the test drug is proposed. The primary efficacy endpoint is percent change from baseline in FEV1. Based on data collected from pilot studies, it is expected that there are 5% improvement for the control group, 12%, 14%, and 16% improvement over baseline in the 20mg, 40mg, and 60mg dose groups, respectively. Based on the data from the pilot studies, the homogeneous standard deviation for the FEV1 change from baseline is assumed to be $\sigma = 22\%$. Thus, we may consider the following contrasts for sample size calculation:

$$c_0 = -6, \ c_1 = 1, \ c_2 = 2, \ c_3 = 3.$$

Note that $\sum c_i = 0$. Moreover, we have $\varepsilon = \sum_{i=0}^{3} c_i \mu_i = 58\%$. For simplicity, consider the balanced case (i.e., $f_i = 1/4$ for $i = 0, 1, ..., 3$) with one-sided at $\alpha = 0.05$, the sample size required for detecting the difference of $\varepsilon = 0.58$ with an 80% power is then given by

## 11.2. Binary Response

$$\begin{aligned}
N &= \left[\frac{(z_{1-\alpha} + z_{1-\beta})\sigma}{\varepsilon}\right]^2 \sum_{i=0}^{K} \frac{c_i^2}{f_i} \\
&= \left[\frac{(1.645 + 0.842)0.22}{0.58}\right]^2 4((-6)^2 + 1^2 + 2^2 + 3^2) \\
&= 178.
\end{aligned}$$

In other words, approximately 45 subjects per dose group is required for achieving an 80% power for detecting the specified clinical difference at the 5% level of significance.

### Remark

Table 11.1.1 provide five different dose response curves and the corresponding contrasts.

Sample sizes required for different dose response curves and contrasts are given in Table 11.1.2. It can be seen from Table 11.1.2 that when the dose response curve and the contrasts have the same shape, a minimum sample size is required. If an inappropriate set of contrasts is used, the sample size could be 30 times larger than the optimal design.

Table 11.1.1: Response and Contrast Shapes

| Shape | $\mu_0$ | $\mu_1$ | $\mu_2$ | $\mu_3$ | $c_0$ | $c_1$ | $c_2$ | $c_3$ |
|---|---|---|---|---|---|---|---|---|
| Linear | 0.1 | 0.3 | 0.5 | 0.7 | -3.00 | -1.00 | 1.00 | 3.00 |
| Step | 0.1 | 0.4 | 0.4 | 0.7 | -3.00 | 0.00 | 0.00 | 3.00 |
| Umbrella | 0.1 | 0.4 | 0.7 | 0.5 | -3.25 | -0.25 | 2.75 | 0.75 |
| Convex | 0.1 | 0.1 | 0.1 | 0.6 | -1.25 | -1.25 | -1.25 | 3.75 |
| Concave | 0.1 | 0.6 | 0.6 | 0.6 | -3.75 | 1.25 | 1.25 | 1.25 |

Table 11.1.2: Sample Size Per Group for Various Contrasts

| Response | Contrast | | | | |
|---|---|---|---|---|---|
|  | Linear | Step | Umbrella | Convex | Concave |
| Linear | 31 | 35 | 52 | 52 | 52 |
| Step | 39 | 35 | 81 | 52 | 52 |
| Umbrella | 55 | 74 | 33 | 825 | 44 |
| Convex | 55 | 50 | 825 | 33 | 297 |
| Concave | 55 | 50 | 44 | 297 | 33 |

Note: $\sigma = 1$, one-sided $\alpha = 0.05$.

## 11.2 Binary Response

Denote $p_i$ the proportion of response in the $i$th group. Consider testing the following null hypothesis

$$H_o : p_0 = p_1 = ... = p_k \quad (11.2.5)$$

against the alternative hypothesis of

$$H_a : L(\mathbf{p}) = \sum_{i=0}^{k} c_i p_i = \varepsilon, \quad (11.2.6)$$

where $c_i$ are the contrasts satisfying $\sum_{i=1}^{k} c_i = 0$.

Similarly, by applying the linear contrast approach described above, the sample size required for achieving an 80% power for detecting a clinically significant difference of $\varepsilon$ at the 5% level of significance can be obtained as

$$N \geq \left[ \frac{z_{1-\alpha}\sqrt{\sum_{i=0}^{k} \frac{c_i^2}{f_i} \bar{p}(1-\bar{p})} + z_{1-\beta}\sqrt{\sum_{i=0}^{k} \frac{c_i^2}{f_i} p_i(1-p_i)}}{\varepsilon} \right]^2, \quad (11.2.7)$$

where $\bar{p}$ is the average of $p_i$.

**Remark**

Table 11.2.1 provides sample sizes required for different dose response curves and contrasts. As it can be seen from Table 11.2.1, an appropriate selection of contrasts (i.e., it can reflect the dose response curve) yields a minimum sample size required for achieving the desired power.

Table 11.2.1: Total Sample Size Comparisons for Binary Data

| Response | Contrast | | | | |
|---|---|---|---|---|---|
| | Linear | Step | Umbrella | Convex | Concave |
| Linear | 26 | 28 | 44 | 48 | 44 |
| Step | 28 | 28 | 68 | 48 | 40 |
| Umbrella | 48 | 68 | 28 | 792 | 36 |
| Convex | 28 | 36 | 476 | 24 | 176 |
| Concave | 36 | 44 | 38 | 288 | 28 |

Note: One-sided $\alpha = 0.05$, $\sigma_o^2 = \bar{p}(1-\bar{p})$, $\bar{p} = \sum_{i=0}^{k} f_i \hat{p}_i$

## 11.3 Time-to-Event Endpoint

Under an exponential survival model, the relationship between hazard ($\lambda$), median ($T_{median}$) and mean ($T_{mean}$) survival time can be described as follows

$$T_{Median} = \frac{\ln 2}{\lambda} = (\ln 2) T_{mean}. \qquad (11.3.8)$$

Let $\lambda_i$ be the population hazard rate for group $i$. The contrast test for multiple survival curves can be written as

$$H_o : L(\mu) = \sum_{i=0}^{k} c_i \lambda_i = 0 \text{ vs. } L(\mu) = \sum_{i=0}^{k} c_i \lambda_i = \varepsilon > 0,$$

where contrasts satisfy the condition that $\sum_{i=0}^{k} c_i = 0$.

Similar to the continuous and binary endpoints, the sample size required for achieving the desired power of $1 - \beta$ is given by

$$N \geq \left[ \frac{z_{1-\alpha} \sigma_o \sqrt{\sum_{i=0}^{k} \frac{c_i^2}{f_i}} + z_{1-\beta} \sqrt{\sum_{i=0}^{k} \frac{c_i^2}{f_i} \sigma_i}}{\varepsilon} \right]^2. \qquad (11.3.9)$$

where the variance $\sigma_i^2$ can be derived in several different ways. For simplicity, we may consider Lachin and Foulkes's maximum likelihood approach (Lachin and Foulkes, 1986).

Suppose we design a clinical trial with k groups. Let $T_0$ and T be the accrual time period and the total trial duration, respectively. We can then prove that the variance for uniform patient entry is given by

$$\sigma^2(\lambda_i) = \lambda_i^2 \left[ 1 + \frac{e^{-\lambda_i T}(1 - e^{\lambda_i T_0})}{T_0 \lambda_i} \right]^{-1}. \qquad (11.3.10)$$

### An Example

In a four arm (the active control, lower dose of test drug, higher dose of test drug and combined therapy) phase II oncology trial, the objective is to determine if there is treatment effect with time-to-progression as the primary endpoint. Patient enrollment duration is estimated to be $T_0 = 9$ months and the total trial duration $T = 16$ months. The estimated median time for the four groups are 14, 20, 22, and 24 months (corresponding hazard rates of 0.0495, 0.0347, 0.0315, and 0.0289/month, respectively). For this phase II design, we use one-sided $\alpha = 0.05$ and power = 80%. In order to achieve the most efficient design (i.e., minimum sample size), sample sizes from different contrasts and various designs (balanced or unbalanced) are compared. Table 11.3.1 are the sample sizes for the balanced design. Table 11.3.2 provides sample sizes for unbalanced design with specific sample size ratios, i.e., (Control : control, lower dose: Control, higher dose : control, and Combined : control) =(1, 2, 2, 2). This type of design is often seen in clinical trials where patients are assigned to the test group more than the control group due to the fact that the investigators are usually more interested in the response in the test groups. However, this unbalanced design is usually not an efficient design. An optimal design, i.e., minimum variance design, where the number of patients assigned to each group is proportional to the variance of the group, is studied (Table 11.3.3). It can be seen from Table 11.3.2 that the optimal designs with sample size ratios (1, 0.711, 0.634, 0.574) are generally most powerful and requires fewer patients regardless the shape of the contrasts. In all cases, the contrasts with a trend in median time or the hazard rate works well. The contrasts with linear trend also works well in most cases under assumption of this particular trend of response (hazard rate). Therefore, the minimum variance design seems attractive with total sample sizes 525 subjects, i.e., 180, 128, 114, 103 for the active control, lower dose, higher dose, and combined therapy groups, respectively. In practice, if more patients assigned to the control group is a concern and it is desirable to obtain more information on the test groups, a balanced design should be chosen with a total sample size 588 subjects or 147 subjects per group.

Table 11.3.1: Sample Sizes for Different Contrasts (Balanced Design)

| Scenario | Contrast | | | | Total n |
|---|---|---|---|---|---|
| Average dose effect | -3 | 1 | 1 | 1 | 666 |
| Linear response trend | -6 | 1 | 2 | 3 | 603 |
| Median time trend | -6 | 0 | 2 | 4 | 588 |
| Hazard rate trend | 10.65 | -0.55 | -3.75 | -6.35 | 589 |

Note: sample size ratios to the control group: 1, 1, 1, 1.

Table 11.3.2: Sample Sizes for Different Contrasts (Unbalanced Design)

| Scenario | Contrast | | | | Total n |
|---|---|---|---|---|---|
| Average dose effect | -3 | 1 | 1 | 1 | 1036 |
| Linear dose response | -6 | 1 | 2 | 3 | 924 |
| Median time shape | -6 | 0 | 2 | 4 | 865 |
| Hazard rate shape | 10.65 | -0.55 | -3.75 | -6.35 | 882 |

Note: sample size ratios to the control group: 1, 2 ,2, 2.

Table 11.3.3: Sample Sizes for Different Contrasts
(Minimum Variance Design)

| Scenario | Contrast | | | | Total n |
|---|---|---|---|---|---|
| Average dose effect | -3 | 1 | 1 | 1 | 548 |
| Linear dose response | -6 | 1 | 2 | 3 | 513 |
| Median time shape | -6 | 0 | 2 | 4 | 525 |
| Hazard rate shape | 10.65 | -0.55 | -3.75 | -6.35 | 516 |

Note: sample size ratios (proportional to the variances): 1, 0.711, 0.634, 0.574.

## 11.4 Williams' Test for Minimum Effective Dose (MED)

Under the assumption of monotonicity in dose response, Williams (1971, 1972) proposed a test to determine the lowest dose level at which there is evidence for a difference from control. Williams considered the following alternative hypothesis:

$$H_a : \mu_0 = \mu_1 = ... = \mu_{i-1} < \mu_i \leq \mu_{i+1} \leq ... \leq \mu_K$$

and proposed the following test statistic:

$$T_i = \frac{\hat{\mu}_i - \hat{Y}_0}{\hat{\sigma}\sqrt{\frac{1}{n_i} + \frac{1}{n_0}}},$$

where $\hat{\sigma}^2$ is an unbiased estimate of $\sigma^2$, which is independent of $\hat{Y}_i$ and is distributed as $\sigma^2 \chi_v^2 / v$ and $\hat{\mu}_i$ is the maximum likelihood estimate of $\mu_i$ which is given by

$$\hat{\mu}_i = \max_{1 \leq u \leq i} \min_{i \leq v \leq K} \left\{ \frac{\sum_{j=u}^{v} n_j \hat{Y}_j}{\sum_{j=1}^{v} n_j} \right\}.$$

When $n_i = n$ for $i = 0, 1, ..., K$, this test statistic can be simplified as

$$T_i = \frac{\hat{\mu}_i - \bar{Y}_0}{s\sqrt{2/n}},$$

which can be approximated by $(X_i - Z_0)/s$, where $s^2$ is an unbiased estimate of $\sigma^2$,

$$X_i = \max_{1 \leq u \leq i} \sum_{j=u}^{i} \frac{Z_j}{i - u + 1}.$$

and $Z_j$ follows a standard normal distribution. We then reject the null hypothesis of no treatment difference and conclude that the $i$th dose level is the minimum effective dose if

$$T_j > t_j(\alpha) \text{ for all } j \geq i,$$

where $t_j(\alpha)$ is the upper $\alpha th$ percentile of the distribution of $T_j$. The critical values of $t_j(\alpha)$ are given in the Tables 11.4.1-11.4.4.

Since the power function of the above test is rather complicated, as an alternative, consider the following approximation to obtain the required sample size per dose group:

$$\begin{aligned} power &= \Pr\{reject\} H_o | \mu_i \geq \mu_0 + \Delta \text{ for some i}\} \\ &> \{\Pr\{reject\} H_o | \mu_0 = \mu_1 = ... = \mu_K = \mu_0 + \Delta\} \\ &\geq \Pr\left\{\frac{\hat{Y}_K - \hat{Y}_0}{\sigma\sqrt{2/n}} > t_K(\alpha) | \mu_K = \mu_0 + \Delta\right\} \\ &= 1 - \Phi\left(t_K(\alpha) - \frac{\Delta}{\sigma\sqrt{2/n}}\right), \end{aligned}$$

where $\Delta$ is the clinically meaningful minimal difference. To have a power of $1 - \beta$, required sample size per group can be obtained by solving

$$\beta = \Phi\left(t_K(\alpha) + \frac{\Delta}{\sigma\sqrt{2/n}} z_\beta\right).$$

Thus, we have

$$n = \frac{2\sigma^2 [t_k(\alpha) + z_\beta]^2}{\Delta^2}, \tag{11.4.11}$$

where values of $t_K(\alpha)$ can be obtained from Tables 11.4.1-11.4.4. It should be noted that this approach is conservative.

### An Example

We consider the previous example of an asthma trial with $power = 80\%$, $\sigma = 0.22$, one-sided $\alpha = 0.05$. (Note that there is no two-sided William's test.) Since the critical value $t_k(\alpha)$ is dependent on the degree of freedom $\nu$ that is related to the sample size $n$, iterations are usually needed. However, for the current case we know that $\nu > 120$ or $\infty$, which leads to $t_3(0.05) = 1.75$. Thus the sample size for 11% (16%-9%) treatment improvement over placebo in FEV1 is given by

$$n = \frac{2(0.22)^2(1.75 + 0.8415)}{0.11^2} = 53 \text{ per group}.$$

## 11.4. Williams' Test for Minimum Effective Dose (MED)

Table 11.4.1: Upper 5 Percentile $t_k(\alpha)$ for $T_k$

| | \multicolumn{9}{c}{$k$ = Number of Dose Levels} |
|---|---|---|---|---|---|---|---|---|---|
| $df/v$ | 2 | 3 | 4 | 5 | 6 | 7 | 8 | 9 | 10 |
| 5 | 2.14 | 2.19 | 2.21 | 2.22 | 2.23 | 2.24 | 2.24 | 2.25 | 2.25 |
| 6 | 2.06 | 2.10 | 2.12 | 2.13 | 2.14 | 2.14 | 2.15 | 2.15 | 2.15 |
| 7 | 2.00 | 2.04 | 2.06 | 2.07 | 2.08 | 2.09 | 2.09 | 2.09 | 2.09 |
| 8 | 1.96 | 2.00 | 2.01 | 2.02 | 2.03 | 2.04 | 2.04 | 2.04 | 2.04 |
| 9 | 1.93 | 1.96 | 1.98 | 1.99 | 2.00 | 2.00 | 2.01 | 2.01 | 2.01 |
| 10 | 1.91 | 1.94 | 1.96 | 1.97 | 1.97 | 1.98 | 1.98 | 1.98 | 1.98 |
| 11 | 1.89 | 1.92 | 1.94 | 1.94 | 1.95 | 1.95 | 1.96 | 1.96 | 1.96 |
| 12 | 1.87 | 1.90 | 1.92 | 1.93 | 1.93 | 1.94 | 1.94 | 1.94 | 1.94 |
| 13 | 1.86 | 1.89 | 1.90 | 1.91 | 1.92 | 1.92 | 1.93 | 1.93 | 1.93 |
| 14 | 1.85 | 1.88 | 1.89 | 1.90 | 1.91 | 1.91 | 1.91 | 1.92 | 1.92 |
| 15 | 1.84 | 1.87 | 1.88 | 1.89 | 1.90 | 1.90 | 1.90 | 1.90 | 1.91 |
| 16 | 1.83 | 1.86 | 1.87 | 1.88 | 1.89 | 1.89 | 1.89 | 1.90 | 1.90 |
| 17 | 1.82 | 1.85 | 1.87 | 1.87 | 1.88 | 1.88 | 1.89 | 1.89 | 1.89 |
| 18 | 1.82 | 1.85 | 1.86 | 1.87 | 1.87 | 1.88 | 1.88 | 1.88 | 1.88 |
| 19 | 1.81 | 1.84 | 1.85 | 1.86 | 1.87 | 1.87 | 1.87 | 1.87 | 1.88 |
| 20 | 1.81 | 1.83 | 1.85 | 1.86 | 1.86 | 1.86 | 1.87 | 1.87 | 1.87 |
| 22 | 1.80 | 1.83 | 1.84 | 1.85 | 1.85 | 1.85 | 1.86 | 1.86 | 1.86 |
| 24 | 1.79 | 1.81 | 1.82 | 1.83 | 1.84 | 1.84 | 1.84 | 1.84 | 1.85 |
| 26 | 1.79 | 1.81 | 1.82 | 1.83 | 1.84 | 1.84 | 1.84 | 1.84 | 1.85 |
| 28 | 1.78 | 1.81 | 1.82 | 1.83 | 1.83 | 1.83 | 1.84 | 1.84 | 1.84 |
| 30 | 1.78 | 1.80 | 1.81 | 1.82 | 1.83 | 1.83 | 1.83 | 1.83 | 1.83 |
| 35 | 1.77 | 1.79 | 1.80 | 1.81 | 1.82 | 1.82 | 1.82 | 1.82 | 1.83 |
| 40 | 1.76 | 1.79 | 1.80 | 1.80 | 1.81 | 1.81 | 1.81 | 1.82 | 1.82 |
| 60 | 1.75 | 1.77 | 1.78 | 1.79 | 1.79 | 1.80 | 1.80 | 1.80 | 1.80 |
| 120 | 1.73 | 1.75 | 1.77 | 1.77 | 1.78 | 1.78 | 1.78 | 1.78 | 1.78 |
| $\infty$ | 1.739 | 1.750 | 1.756 | 1.760 | 1.763 | 1.765 | 1.767 | 1.768 | 1.768 |

Table 11.4.2: Upper 2.5 Percentile $t_k(\alpha)$ for $T_k$

| $df/v$ | \multicolumn{7}{c}{$k$ = Number of Dose Levels} | | | | | | |
|---|---|---|---|---|---|---|---|
| | 2 | 3 | 4 | 5 | 6 | 8 | 10 |
| 5 | 2.699 | 2.743 | 2.766 | 2.779 | 2.788 | 2.799 | 2.806 |
| 6 | 2.559 | 2.597 | 2.617 | 2.628 | 2.635 | 2.645 | 2.650 |
| 7 | 2.466 | 2.501 | 2.518 | 2.528 | 2.535 | 2.543 | 2.548 |
| 8 | 2.400 | 2.432 | 2.448 | 2.457 | 2.463 | 2.470 | 2.475 |
| 9 | 2.351 | 2.381 | 2.395 | 2.404 | 2.410 | 2.416 | 2.421 |
| 10 | 2.313 | 2.341 | 2.355 | 2.363 | 2.368 | 2.375 | 2.379 |
| 11 | 2.283 | 2.310 | 2.323 | 2.330 | 2.335 | 2.342 | 2.345 |
| 12 | 2.258 | 2.284 | 2.297 | 2.304 | 2.309 | 2.315 | 2.318 |
| 13 | 2.238 | 2.263 | 2.275 | 2.282 | 2.285 | 2.292 | 2.295 |
| 14 | 2.220 | 2.245 | 2.256 | 2.263 | 2.268 | 2.273 | 2.276 |
| 15 | 2.205 | 2.229 | 2.241 | 2.247 | 2.252 | 2.257 | 2.260 |
| 16 | 2.193 | 2.216 | 2.227 | 2.234 | 2.238 | 2.243 | 2.246 |
| 17 | 2.181 | 2.204 | 2.215 | 2.222 | 2.226 | 2.231 | 2.234 |
| 18 | 2.171 | 2.194 | 2.205 | 2.211 | 2.215 | 2.220 | 2.223 |
| 19 | 2.163 | 2.185 | 2.195 | 2.202 | 2.205 | 2.210 | 2.213 |
| 20 | 2.155 | 2.177 | 2.187 | 2.193 | 2.197 | 2.202 | 2.205 |
| 22 | 2.141 | 2.163 | 2.173 | 2.179 | 2.183 | 2.187 | 2.190 |
| 24 | 2.130 | 2.151 | 2.161 | 2.167 | 2.171 | 2.175 | 2.178 |
| 26 | 2.121 | 2.142 | 2.151 | 2.157 | 2.161 | 2.165 | 2.168 |
| 28 | 2.113 | 2.133 | 2.143 | 2.149 | 2.152 | 2.156 | 2.159 |
| 30 | 2.106 | 2.126 | 2.136 | 2.141 | 2.145 | 2.149 | 2.151 |
| 35 | 2.093 | 2.112 | 2.122 | 2.127 | 2.130 | 2.134 | 2.137 |
| 40 | 2.083 | 2.102 | 2.111 | 2.116 | 2.119 | 2.123 | 2.126 |
| 60 | 2.060 | 2.078 | 2.087 | 2.092 | 2.095 | 2.099 | 2.101 |
| 120 | 2.037 | 2.055 | 2.063 | 2.068 | 2.071 | 2.074 | 2.076 |
| $\infty$ | 2.015 | 2.032 | 2.040 | 2.044 | 2.047 | 2.050 | 2.052 |

## 11.4. Williams' Test for Minimum Effective Dose (MED)

Table 11.4.3: Upper 1 Percentile $t_k(\alpha)$ for $T_k$

| | \multicolumn{9}{c}{$k =$ Number of Dose Levels} |
|---|---|---|---|---|---|---|---|---|---|
| $df/v$ | 2 | 3 | 4 | 5 | 6 | 7 | 8 | 9 | 10 |
| 5 | 3.50 | 3.55 | 3.57 | 3.59 | 3.60 | 3.60 | 3.61 | 3.61 | 3.61 |
| 6 | 3.26 | 3.29 | 3.31 | 3.32 | 3.33 | 3.34 | 3.34 | 3.34 | 3.35 |
| 7 | 3.10 | 3.13 | 3.15 | 3.16 | 3.16 | 3.17 | 3.17 | 3.17 | 3.17 |
| 8 | 2.99 | 3.01 | 3.03 | 3.04 | 3.04 | 3.05 | 3.05 | 3.05 | 3.05 |
| 9 | 2.90 | 2.93 | 2.94 | 2.95 | 2.95 | 2.96 | 2.96 | 2.96 | 2.96 |
| 10 | 2.84 | 2.86 | 2.88 | 2.88 | 2.89 | 2.89 | 2.89 | 2.90 | 2.90 |
| 11 | 2.79 | 2.81 | 2.82 | 2.83 | 2.83 | 2.84 | 2.84 | 2.84 | 2.84 |
| 12 | 2.75 | 2.77 | 2.78 | 2.79 | 2.79 | 2.79 | 2.80 | 2.80 | 2.80 |
| 13 | 2.72 | 2.74 | 2.75 | 2.75 | 2.76 | 2.76 | 2.76 | 2.76 | 2.76 |
| 14 | 2.69 | 2.71 | 2.72 | 2.72 | 2.72 | 2.73 | 2.73 | 2.73 | 2.73 |
| 15 | 2.66 | 2.68 | 2.69 | 2.70 | 2.70 | 2.70 | 2.71 | 2.71 | 2.71 |
| 16 | 2.64 | 2.66 | 2.67 | 2.68 | 2.68 | 2.68 | 2.68 | 2.68 | 2.69 |
| 17 | 2.63 | 2.64 | 2.65 | 2.66 | 2.66 | 2.66 | 2.66 | 2.67 | 2.67 |
| 18 | 2.61 | 2.63 | 2.64 | 2.64 | 2.64 | 2.65 | 2.65 | 2.65 | 2.65 |
| 19 | 2.60 | 2.61 | 2.62 | 2.63 | 2.63 | 2.63 | 2.63 | 2.63 | 2.63 |
| 20 | 2.58 | 2.60 | 2.61 | 2.61 | 2.62 | 2.62 | 2.62 | 2.62 | 2.62 |
| 22 | 2.56 | 2.58 | 2.59 | 2.59 | 2.59 | 2.60 | 2.60 | 2.60 | 2.60 |
| 24 | 2.55 | 2.56 | 2.57 | 2.57 | 2.57 | 2.58 | 2.58 | 2.58 | 2.58 |
| 26 | 2.53 | 2.55 | 2.55 | 2.56 | 2.56 | 2.56 | 2.56 | 2.56 | 2.56 |
| 28 | 2.52 | 2.53 | 2.54 | 2.54 | 2.55 | 2.55 | 2.55 | 2.55 | 2.55 |
| 30 | 2.51 | 2.52 | 2.53 | 2.53 | 2.54 | 2.54 | 2.54 | 2.54 | 2.54 |
| 35 | 2.49 | 2.50 | 2.51 | 2.51 | 2.51 | 2.51 | 2.52 | 2.52 | 2.52 |
| 40 | 2.47 | 2.48 | 2.49 | 2.49 | 2.50 | 2.50 | 2.50 | 2.50 | 2.50 |
| 60 | 2.43 | 2.45 | 2.45 | 2.46 | 2.46 | 2.46 | 2.46 | 2.46 | 2.46 |
| 120 | 2.40 | 2.41 | 2.42 | 2.42 | 2.42 | 2.42 | 2.42 | 2.42 | 2.43 |
| $\infty$ | 2.366 | 2.377 | 2.382 | 2.385 | 2.386 | 2.387 | 2.388 | 2.389 | 2.389 |

Table 11.4.4: Upper 0.5 Percentile $t_k(\alpha)$ for $T_k$

| $df/v$ | \multicolumn{7}{c}{$k$ = Number of Dose Levels} |
|---|---|---|---|---|---|---|---|
| | 2 | 3 | 4 | 5 | 6 | 8 | 10 |
| 5 | 4.179 | 4.229 | 4.255 | 4.270 | 4.279 | 4.292 | 4.299 |
| 6 | 3.825 | 3.864 | 3.883 | 3.895 | 3.902 | 3.912 | 3.197 |
| 7 | 3.599 | 3.631 | 3.647 | 3.657 | 3.663 | 3.670 | 3.674 |
| 8 | 3.443 | 3.471 | 3.484 | 3.492 | 3.497 | 3.504 | 3.507 |
| 9 | 3.329 | 3.354 | 3.366 | 3.373 | 3.377 | 3.383 | 3.886 |
| 10 | 3.242 | 3.265 | 3.275 | 3.281 | 3.286 | 3.290 | 3.293 |
| 11 | 3.173 | 3.194 | 3.204 | 3.210 | 3.214 | 3.218 | 3.221 |
| 12 | 3.118 | 3.138 | 3.147 | 3.152 | 3.156 | 3.160 | 3.162 |
| 13 | 3.073 | 3.091 | 3.100 | 3.105 | 3.108 | 3.112 | 3.114 |
| 14 | 3.035 | 3.052 | 3.060 | 3.065 | 3.068 | 3.072 | 3.074 |
| 15 | 3.003 | 3.019 | 3.027 | 3.031 | 3.034 | 3.037 | 3.039 |
| 16 | 2.957 | 2.991 | 2.998 | 3.002 | 3.005 | 3.008 | 3.010 |
| 17 | 2.951 | 2.955 | 2.973 | 2.977 | 2.980 | 2.938 | 2.984 |
| 18 | 2.929 | 2.944 | 2.951 | 2.955 | 2.958 | 2.960 | 2.962 |
| 19 | 2.911 | 2.925 | 2.932 | 2.936 | 2.938 | 2.941 | 2.942 |
| 20 | 2.894 | 2.903 | 2.915 | 2.918 | 2.920 | 2.923 | 2.925 |
| 22 | 2.866 | 2.879 | 2.855 | 2.889 | 2.891 | 2.893 | 2.895 |
| 24 | 2.842 | 2.855 | 2.861 | 2.864 | 2.866 | 2.869 | 2.870 |
| 26 | 2.823 | 2.835 | 2.841 | 2.844 | 2.846 | 2.848 | 2.850 |
| 28 | 2.806 | 2.819 | 2.824 | 2.827 | 2.829 | 2.831 | 2.832 |
| 30 | 2.792 | 2.804 | 2.809 | 2.812 | 2.814 | 2.816 | 2.817 |
| 35 | 2.764 | 2.775 | 2.781 | 2.783 | 2.785 | 2.787 | 2.788 |
| 40 | 2.744 | 2.755 | 2.759 | 2.762 | 2.764 | 2.765 | 2.766 |
| 60 | 2.697 | 2.707 | 2.711 | 2.713 | 2.715 | 2.716 | 2.717 |
| 120 | 2.651 | 2.660 | 2.664 | 2.666 | 2.667 | 2.669 | 2.669 |
| $\infty$ | 2.607 | 2.615 | 2.618 | 2.620 | 2.621 | 2.623 | 2.623 |

Note that this sample size formulation has a minimum difference from that based on the two sample t-test with the maximum treatment difference as the treatment difference. For the current example, $n = 54$ from the two sample t-test.

## 11.5 Cochran-Armitage's Test for Trend

Cochran-Armitage test (Cochran 1954, and Amitage 1955) is a widely used test for monotonic trend with binary response since it is more powerful than the chi-square homogeneity test in identifying a monotonic trend (Nam 1987). This test requires preassigned fixed dose scores. Equally spaced scores are most powerful for linear response. When the true dose-response relationship is not linear, equally-spaced scores may not be the best choice. Generally, single contrast-based test attains its greatest power when the dose-coefficient relationship has the same shape as the true dose-response relationship. Otherwise, it loses its power. Due to limited information at the design stage of a dose-response trial, it is risky to use single contrast test. Note that the rejection of the null hypothesis does not mean the dose-response is linear or monotonic. It means that based on the data it is unlikely the dose-response is flat or all doses have the same response.

The test for monotonic trend with binary response, we consider the following hypotheses:

$$H_o : p_0 = p_1 = ... = p_k \qquad (11.5.12)$$
$$\text{vs.} \quad H_a : p_0 \leq p_1 \leq ... \leq p_k \text{ with } p_0 < p_k.$$

Cochran (1954) and Amitage (1955) proposed the following test statistic

$$T_{CA} = \sqrt{\frac{N}{(N-X)X}} \frac{\sum_{i=1}^{k}(x_i - \frac{n_i X}{N})c_i}{\sqrt{\sum_{i=0}^{k}\frac{n_i c_i^2}{N} - \left(\sum_{i=0}^{k}\frac{n_i c_i}{N}\right)^2}}, \qquad (11.5.13)$$

where $c_i$ is the predetermined scores ($c_0 < c_1 < ... < c_k$). $x_i$ is the number of responses in group $i$ ($i = 0$ for the control group), and $p_i$ is the response rate in group $i$. $n_i$ is the sample size for group $i$, where $X = \sum_{i=0}^{k} x_i$ and $N = \sum_{i=0}^{k} n_i$.

Note that the test (one-sided test) by Portier and Hoel (1984) was the modification (Neuhauser and Hothorn, 1999) from Armitages' (1955) original two-sided test, which is asymptotically distributed as a standard normal variable under the null hypothesis.

Asymptotic power of test for linear trend and sample size calculation can be found in Nam (1998), which are briefly outlined below:

Let $x_i$ be the $k+1$ mutually independent binomial variates representing the number of responses among $n_i$ subjects at dose level $d_i$ for $i = 0, 1, ..., k$. Define average response rate $p_i = \frac{1}{N}\sum_i x_i$, $\bar{q} = 1 - \bar{p}$, and $\bar{d} = \frac{1}{N}\sum n_i d_i$. $U = \sum_i x_i(d_i - \bar{d})$.

Assume that the probability of response follows a linear trend in logistic scale

$$p_i = \frac{e^{\gamma + \lambda d_i}}{1 + e^{\gamma + \lambda d_i}}$$

An approximate test with continuity correction based on the asymptotically normal deviate is given by

$$z = \frac{(U - \frac{\Delta}{2})}{\sqrt{var(U|H_0 : \lambda = 0)}} = \frac{(U - \frac{\Delta}{2})}{\sqrt{\bar{p}\bar{q}}\sum_i \left[\sum_i n_i(d_i - \bar{d})^2\right]},$$

where $\Delta/2 = (d_i - d_{i-1})/2$ is the continuity correction for equally spaced doses. However, there is no constant $\Delta$ for unequally spaced doses.

The unconditional power is given by

$$\Pr(z \geq z_{1-\alpha}|H_a) = 1 - \Phi(u),$$

where

$$u = E(U - \frac{\Delta}{2}) + z_{1-\alpha}\frac{\sqrt{var(U|H_o)}}{\sqrt{var(U|H_a)}}.$$

Thus, we have

$$E(U) - \frac{\Delta}{2} + z_{1-\alpha}\sqrt{var(U|H_o)} + z_{1-\beta}\sqrt{var(U|H_a)}.$$

For $\Delta = 0$, i.e., without continuity correction, the sample size is given by

$$n_0^* = \frac{1}{A^2}\left\{z_{1-\alpha}\sqrt{pq\left[\sum r_i(d_i - \bar{d})^2\right]} + z_{1-\beta}\sqrt{\left[\sum p_i q_i r_i(d_i - \bar{d})^2\right]}\right\}^2, \quad (11.5.14)$$

where $A = \sum r_i p_i(d_i - \bar{d})$, $p = \frac{1}{N}\sum n_i p_i$, $q = 1 - p$, and $r_i = n_i/n_0$ is the sample size ratio between the ith group and the control.

On the other hand, sample size with continuity correction is given by

$$n_0 = \frac{n_0^*}{4}\left[1 + \sqrt{1 + 2\frac{\Delta}{An_0^*}}\right]^2. \quad (11.5.15)$$

Note that the actual power of the test depends on the specified alternative. Thus, the sample size formula holds for any monotonic increasing alternative, i.e., $p_{i-1} < p_i$, $i = 1, ..., k$.

## 11.5. Cochran-Armitage's Test for Trend

For balance design with equal size in each group, the formula for sample size per group is reduced to

$$n = \frac{n^*}{4}\left[1 + \sqrt{1 + \frac{2}{Dn^*}}\right]^2, \qquad (11.5.16)$$

where

$$n^* = \left\{z_{1-\alpha}\sqrt{k(k^2-1)pq} + z_{1-\beta}\sqrt{\sum b_i^2 p_i q_i}\right\}^2 \qquad (11.5.17)$$

and $b_i = i - 0.5k$, and $D = \sum b_i p_i$.

Note that the above formula is based on one-sided test at the $\alpha$ level. For two-sided test, the Type I error rate is controlled at the $2\alpha$ level. For equally spaced doses: 1, 2, 3, and 4, the sample sizes required for the five different sets of contracts are given in Table 11.5.1.

Table 11.5.1: Sample size from Nam Formula

| Dose | 1 | 2 | 3 | 4 | Total $n$ |
|---|---|---|---|---|---|
| | 0.1 | 0.3 | 0.5 | 0.7 | 26 |
| | 0.1 | 0.4 | 0.4 | 0.7 | 32 |
| Response | 0.1 | 0.4 | 0.7 | 0.5 | 48 |
| | 0.1 | 0.1 | 0.1 | 0.6 | 37 |
| | 0.1 | 0.6 | 0.6 | 0.6 | 49 |

Table 11.5.2: Power Comparisons with Cochran-Armitage Test

| Shape | Equal spaced scores | Convex scores | Concave scores | MERT |
|---|---|---|---|---|
| No diff | 0.03 | 0.03 | 0.03 | 0.03 |
| Linear | 0.91 | 0.82 | 0.89 | 0.92 |
| Step | 0.84 | 0.80 | 0.87 | 0.90 |
| Umbrella | 0.68 | 0.24 | 0.86 | 0.62 |
| Convex | 0.81 | 0.91 | 0.48 | 0.83 |
| Concave | 0.67 | 0.34 | 0.91 | 0.74 |

Source: Neuhauser and Hothorn (1999); $n_i = 10$, $\alpha = 0.05$.

Neuhauser and Hothorn (1999) studied the power of Cochran–Armitage test under different true response shape through simulations (Table 11.5.2). These simulation results confirm that the most powerful test is achieved when contrast shape is consistent with the response shape.

Gastwirth (1985) and Podgor, et al. (1996) proposed a single maximum efficiency robust test (MERT) statistic based on prior correlations between different contrasts, while Neuhauser and Hothorn (1999) proposed a maximum test among two or more contrasts and claim a gain in power.

## 11.6 Dose Escalation Trials

For non-life-threatening diseases, since the expected toxicity is mild and can be controlled without harm, phase I trials are usually conducted on healthy or normal volunteers. In life-threatening diseases such as cancer and AIDS, phase I studies are conducted with limited numbers of patients due to (i) the aggressiveness and possible harmfulness of treatments, (ii) possible systemic treatment effects, and (iii) the high interest in the new drug's efficacy in those patients directly.

Drug toxicity is considered as tolerable if the toxicity is manageable and reversible. The standardization of the level of drug toxicity is the Common Toxicity Criteria (CTC) of the United States National Cancer Institute (NCI). Any adverse event (AE) related to treatment from the CTC category of Grade 3 and higher is often considered a dose limiting toxicity (DLT). The maximum tolerable dose (MTD) is defined as the maximum dose level with toxicity rates occuring no more than a predetermined value.

There are usually 5 to 10 predetermined dose levels in a dose escalation study. A commonly used dose sequence is the so called modified Fibonacci sequence. Patients are treated with lowest dose first and then gradually escalated to higher doses if there is no major safety concern. The rules for dose escalation are predetermined. The commonly employed dose escalation rules are the traditional escalation rules (TER), also known as *the "3 + 3" rule*. The "3 + 3" rule is to enter three patients at a new dose level and enter another 3 patients when one toxicity is observed. The assessment of the six patients will be performed to determine whether the trial should be stopped at that level or to increase the dose. Basically, there are two types of the "3 + 3" rules, namely, TER and strict TER (or STER). TER does not allow dose de-escalation, but STER does when 2 of 3 patients have DLTs. The "3+3" STER can be generalized to the A+B TER and STER escalation rules. To introduce the traditional $A + B$ escalation rule, let $A, B, C, D,$ and E be integers. The notation $A/B$ indicates that there are $A$ toxicity incidences out of $B$ subjects and $> A/B$ means that there are more than A toxicity incidences out of $B$ subjects. We assume that there are n predefined doses with increasing levels and let $p_i$ be the probability of observing a DLT at dose level $i$ for $1 \leq i \leq n$. In what follows, general A+B designs without and with dose de-escalation will be described. The closed forms of sample size calculation by Lin and Shih (2001) are briefly reviewed.

## 11.6.1 The A + B Escalation Design without Dose De-escalation

The general A + B designs without dose de-escalation can be described as follows. Suppose that there are A patients at dose level $i$. If less than C/A patients have DLTs, then the dose is escalated to the next dose level $i + 1$. If more than D/A (where $D \geq C$) patients have DLTs, then the previous dose $i - 1$ will be considered the MTD. If no less than C/A but no more than D/A patients have DLTs, B more patients are treated at this dose level $i$. If no more than E (where $E \geq D$) of the total of A + B patients have DLTs, then the dose is escalated. If more than E of the total of A + B patients have DLT, then the previous dose $i - 1$ will be considered the MTD. It can be seen that the traditional "3 + 3" design without dose de-escalation is a special case of the general $A + B$ design with $A = B = 3$ and $C = D = E = 1$.

Under the general A+B design without dose-escalation, the probability of concluding that MTD has reached at dose $i$ is given by

$$P(MTD = \text{dose } i) = P\left(\begin{array}{c}\text{escalation at dose } \leq i \text{ and}\\ \text{stop escalation at dose } i+1\end{array}\right)$$

$$= (1 - P_0^{i+1} - Q_0^{i+1})\left(\prod_{j=1}^{i}(P_0^j + Q_0^j)\right), \quad 1 \leq i < n,$$

where

$$P_0^j = \sum_{k=0}^{C-1} \binom{A}{k} p_j^k (1 - p_j)^{A-k},$$

and

$$Q_0^j = \sum_{k=C}^{D} \sum_{m=0}^{E-k} \binom{A}{k} p_j^k (1 - p_j)^{A-k} \binom{B}{m} p_j^m (1 - p_j)^{B-m},$$

in which

$$N_{ji} = \begin{cases} \frac{AP_0^j + (A+B)Q_0^j}{P_0^j + Q_0^j} & \text{if } j < i+1 \\ \frac{A(1-P_0^j-P_1^j)+(A+B)(P_1^j-Q_0^j)}{1-P_0^j-Q_0^j} & \text{if } j = i+1 \\ 0 & \text{if } j > i+1 \end{cases}.$$

An overshoot is defined as an attempt to escalate to a dose level at the highest level planned, while a undershoot is referred to as an attempt to de-escalate to a dose level at a lower dose than the starting dose level. Thus, the probability of undershoot is given by

$$P_1^* = P(MTD < dose\ 1) = (1 - P_0^1 - Q_0^1), \qquad (11.6.18)$$

and probability of overshoot is given by

$$P_n^* = P(MTD \geq dose\ n) = \Pi_{j=1}^n (P_0^j + Q_0^j). \qquad (11.6.19)$$

The expected number of patients at dose level $j$ is given by

$$N_j = \sum_{i=0}^{n-1} N_{ji} P_i^*. \qquad (11.6.20)$$

Note that without consideration of undershoots and overshoots, the expected number of DLTs at dose $i$ can be obtained as $N_i p_i$. As a result, the total expected number DLTs for the trial is given by $\sum_{i=1}^n N_i p_i$.

We can use (11.6.20) to calculate the expected sample size at dose level for given toxicity rate at each dose level. We can also conduct a Monte Carlo study to simulate the trial and sample size required. Table 11.6.1 summarizes the simulation results. One can do two stage design and Bayesian adaptive and other advanced design with the software.

Table 11.6.1: Simulation results with 3+3 TER

| Dose level | 1 | 2 | 3 | 4 | 5 | 6 | 7 | Total |
|---|---|---|---|---|---|---|---|---|
| Dose | 10 | 15 | 23 | 34 | 51 | 76 | 114 | |
| DLT rate | 0.01 | 0.014 | 0.025 | 0.056 | 0.177 | 0.594 | 0.963 | |
| Expected $n$ | 3.1 | 3.2 | 3.2 | 3.4 | 3.9 | 2.8 | 0.2 | 19.7 |

Note: True MTD = 50, mean simulated MTD =70, mean number of DLTs =2.9

## 11.6.2 The A + B Escalation Design with Dose De-escalation

Basically, the general A + B design with dose de-escalation is similar to the design without dose de-escalation. However, it permits more patients to be treated at a lower dose (i.e. dose de-escalation) when excessive DLT incidences occur at the current dose level. The dose de-escalation occurs when more than $D/A$ (where $D \geq C$) or more than $E/(A+B)$ patients have DLTs at dose level $i$. In this case, $B$ more patients will be treated at dose level $i-1$ provided that only $A$ patients have been treated previously at this prior dose. If more than $A$ patients have already been treated previously, then dose $i-1$ is the MTD. The de-escalation may continue to the next dose level $i-2$ and so on if necessary. For this design, the MTD is the dose level at which no more than $E/(A+B)$ patients experience DLTs, and more than $D/A$ or (no less than $C/A$ and no more than $D/A$) if more than $E/(A+B)$ patients treated with the next higher dose have DLTs.

Similarly, under the general A+B design with dose de-escalation, the probability of concluding that MTD has been reached at dose $i$ is given by

$$P_i^* = P(MTD = dose\ i) = P\left( \begin{array}{c} \text{escalation at dose } \leq i \text{ and} \\ \text{stop escalation at dose } i+1 \end{array} \right)$$

$$= \sum_{k=i+1}^{n} p_{ik},$$

where

$$p_{ik} = (Q_0^i + Q_0^i)(1 - P_0^k - Q_0^k) \left( \prod_{j=1}^{i-1} (P_0^j + Q_0^j) \right) \prod_{j=i+1}^{k-1} Q_2^j,$$

and

$$P_1^j = \sum_{i=C}^{D} \binom{A}{k} p_j^k (1-p_j)^{A-k},$$

$$Q_1^j = \sum_{k=0}^{C-1} \sum_{m=0}^{E-k} \binom{A}{k} p_j^k (1-p_j)^{A-k} \binom{B}{m} p_j^m (1-p_j)^{B-m},$$

$$Q_2^j = \sum_{k=0}^{C-1} \sum_{m=E+1-k}^{E-k} \binom{A}{k} p_j^k (1-p_j)^{A-k} \binom{B}{m} p_j^m (1-p_j)^{B-m},$$

$$N_{jn} = \frac{AP_0^j + (A+B)Q_0^j}{P_0^j + Q_0^j},$$

Also, the probability of undershoot is given by

$$P_1^* = P(MTD < dose\ 1) = \sum_{k=1}^{n}\{\left(\Pi_{j=1}^{k-1}Q_2^j\right)(1 - P_0^k - Q_0^k)\},$$

and the probability of overshooting is

$$P_n^* = P(MTD \geq dose\ n) = \Pi_{j=1}^{n}(P_0^j + Q_0^j).$$

The expected number of patients at dose level $j$ is given by

$$N_j = N_{jn}P_n^* + \sum_{i=0}^{n-1}\sum_{k=i+1}^{n} N_{jik}p_{ik},$$

where

$$N_{jik} = \begin{cases} \frac{AP_0^j + (A+B)Q_0^j}{P_0^j + Q_0^j} & \text{if} \quad j < i \\ A + B & \text{if} \quad i \leq j < k \\ \frac{A(1-P_0^j-P_1^j)+(A+B)(P_1^j-Q_0^j)}{1-P_0^j-Q_0^j} & \text{if} \quad j = k \\ 0 & \text{if} \quad j > k \end{cases}.$$

Consequently, the total number of expected DLTs is given by $\sum_{i=1}^{n} N_i p_i$.

Table 11.6.2 is another example as in Table 11.6.1, but the simulation results are from STER rather than TER. In this example, we can see that the MTD is underestimated and the average sample size is 23 with STER, 3 patients more than that with TER. The excepted DLTs also increase with STER in this case. Note that the actual sample size varies from trial to trial. However, simulations will help in choosing the best escalation algorithm or optimal design based on the operating characteristics, such as accuracy and precision of the predicted MTD, expected DLTs and sample size, overshoots, undershoots, and the number of patients treated above MTD.

Table 11.6.2: Simulation results with 3+3 STER

| Dose level | 1 | 2 | 3 | 4 | 5 | 6 | 7 | Total |
|---|---|---|---|---|---|---|---|---|
| Dose | 10 | 15 | 23 | 34 | 51 | 76 | 114 | |
| DLT rate | 0.01 | 0.014 | 0.025 | 0.056 | 0.177 | 0.594 | 0.963 | |
| Expected $n$ | 3.1 | 3.2 | 3.5 | 4.6 | 5.5 | 3 | 0.2 | 23 |

Note: True MTD = 50, mean simulated MTD = 41. Mean number of DLTs = 3.3

## 11.7 Concluding Remarks

In general, linear contrast tests are useful in detecting specific shapes of the dose response curve. However, the selection of contrasts should be practically meaningful. It should be noted that the power of a linear contrast test is sensitive to the actual shape of the dose response curve Bretz and Hothorn, 2002). Alternatively, one may consider a slope approach to detect the shape of the dose response curve (Cheng, Chow, and Wang, 2006).

Williams' test is useful for identifying the minimum effective dose in the case of continuous response. Williams' test has a strong assumption of monotonic dose response. The test may not be statistically valid if the assumption is violated. It should be noted that Williams' test is not a test for monotonicity. The sample size formula given in (11.4.11) is rather conservative.

Nam's and Cochran-Armitage's methods are equivalent. Their methods are useful when the response is binary. Basically, both methods are regression-based methods for testing a monotonic trend. However, they are not rigorous tests for monotonicity. Testing to true monotonic response is practically difficult without extra assumptions (Chang and Chow, 2005).

The dose escalation trials are somewhat different because the sample size is not determined based on the error rates. Instead, it is determined by the escalation algorithm and dose response (toxicity) relationship and pre-determined dose levels. For the A+B escalation rules, the sample size has a closed form as given in Section 11.6. For other designs, sample size will have to be estimated through computer simulations. It should be noted that the escalation algorithm and dose intervals not only have an impact on the sample size, but also affect other important operating characteristics such as the accuracy and precision of the estimation of the MTD and the number of DLTs.

# Chapter 12

# Microarray Studies

One of the primary study objectives for microarray studies is to have a high probability of declaring genes to be differentially expressed if they are truly expressed, while keeping the probability of making false declarations of expression acceptably low (Lee and Whitmore, 2002). Traditional statistical testing approaches such as the two-sample t-test or Wilcoxon test, are often used for evaluating statistical significance of informative expressions but require adjustment for large-scale multiplicity. It is recognized that if a type I error rate of $\alpha$ is employed at each testing, then the probability to reject any hypothesis will exceed the overall $\alpha$ level. To overcome this problem, two approaches for controlling false discovery rate ($FDR$) and family-wise error rate ($FWER$) are commonly employed. In this chapter, formulas or procedures for sample size calculation for microarray studies derived under these two approaches are discussed.

In the next section, a brief literature review is given. Section 12.2 gives a brief definition of false discovery rate and introduces formulas and/or procedures for sample size calculation for the $FDR$ approach given in Jung (2005). Also included in this section are some examples with and without constant effect sizes based on two-sided tests. Section 12.3 reviews multiple testing procedures and gives procedures for sample size calculation for microarray studies for the $FWER$ approach (Jung, Bang, and Young, 2005). Also included in this section is an application to leukemia data given in Golub et al. (1999). A brief concluding remark is given in the last section of this chapter.

## 12.1 Literature Review

Microarray methods have been widely used for identifying differentially expressing genes in subjects with different types of disease. Sample size calculation plays an important role at the planning stage of a microarray study. Commonly considered standard microarray designs include a matched-pairs design, a completely randomized design, an isolated-effect design, and a replicated design. For a given microarray study, formulas and/or procedures for sample size calculation can be derived following the steps as described in previous chapters. Several procedures for sample size calculation have been proposed in the literature in the microarray context (see, e.g. Simon et al., 2002). Most of these procedures focused on exploratory and approximate relationships among statistical power, sample size (or the number of replicates), and effect size (often, in terms of fold-change), and used the most conservative Bonferroni adjustment for controlling family-wise error rate ($FWER$) without taking into consideration of the underlying correlation structure (see, e.g., Wolfinger et al., 2001; Black and Doerge, 2002; Pan et al., 2002; Cui and Churchill, 2003). Jung et al. (2005) incorporated the correlation structure to derive a sample size formula, which is able to control the $FWER$ efficiently.

As an alternative to the $FWER$ approach, many researchers have proposed the use of so-called false discovery rate ($FDR$) (see, e.g., Benjamini and Hochberg, 1995; Storey, 2002). It is believed that controlling $FDR$ would relax the multiple testing criteria compared to controlling the $FWER$. Consequently, controlling FDR would increase the number of declared significant genes. Some operating and numerical characteristics of $FDR$ are elucidated in recent publications (Genovese and Wasserman, 2002; Dudoit et al., 2003).

Lee and Whitmore (2002) considered multiple group cases, including the two-sample case, using ANOVA models and derived the relation between the effect sizes and the $FDR$ based on a Bayesian perspective. Their power analysis approach, however, does not consider the issue of multiplicity. Müller et al. (2004) chose a pair of testing errors, including $FDR$, and minimized one while controlling the other one at a specified level using a Bayesian decision rule. Müller et al. (2004) proposed using an algorithm to demonstrate the relationship between sample size and the chosen testing errors based on some asymptotic results for large samples. This approach, however, requires specification of complicated parametric models for prior and data distributions, and extensive computing for the Baysian simulations. Note that Lee and Whitmore (2002) and Gadbury et al. (2004) modelled a distribution of p-values from pilot studies to produce sample size estimates but did not provide an explicit sample size formula. Most of the existing methods for controlling $FDR$ in microarray studies fail to show

Table 12.2.1: Outcomes of $m$ multiple tests

| True hypothesis | Accepted hypothesis | | Total |
|---|---|---|---|
| | Null | Alternative | |
| Null | $A_0$ | $R_0$ | $m_0$ |
| Alternative | $A_1$ | $R_1$ | $m_1$ |
| Total | $A$ | $R$ | $m$ |

the explicit relationship between sample size and effect sizes because due to various reasons. To overcome this problem, Jung (2005) proposed a sample size estimation procedure for controlling $FDR$, which will be introduced in the following section.

In this chapter, our emphasis will be placed on formulas or procedures for sample size calculation derived based on two approaches for controlling false discovery rate ($FDR$) and family-wise error rate ($FWER$).

## 12.2 False Discovery Rate (FDR) Control

Benjamini and Hochberg (1995) define the $FDR$ as the expected value of the proportion of the non-prognostic genes among the discovered genes It is then suggested that sample size should be selected to control the $FDR$ at a prespecified level of significance.

### Model and Assumptions

Suppose that we conduct $m$ multiple tests, of which the null hypotheses are true for $m_0$ tests and the alternative hypotheses are true for $m_1 (= m - m_0)$ tests. The tests declare that, of the $m_0$ null hypotheses, $A_0$ hypotheses are null (true negative) and $R_0$ hypotheses are alternative (i.e., false rejection, false discovery or false positive). Among the $m_1$ alternative hypotheses, $A_1$ are declared null (i.e., false negative) and $R_0$ are declared alternative (i.e., true rejection, true discovery or true positive). Table 12.2.1 summarizes the outcome of $m$ hypothesis tests.

According to the definition by Benjamini and Hochberg (1995), the FDR is given by

$$FDR = E\left(\frac{R_0}{R}\right). \qquad (12.2.1)$$

Note that this expression is undefined if $\Pr(R = 0) > 0$. To avoid this issue,

Benjamini and Hochberg (1995) modified the definition of FDR as

$$FDR = \Pr(R > 0) E\left(\frac{R_0}{R} \Big| R > 0\right). \qquad (12.2.2)$$

These two definitions are identical if $\Pr(R = 0) = 0$, in which case we have $FDR = E(R_0/R|R > 0)$. Note that if $m = m_0$, then $FDR = 1$ for any critical value with $\Pr(R = 0) = 0$. As a result, Storey (2003) referred to the second term in the right hand side of (12.2.2) as $pFDR$, i.e.,

$$pFDR = E\left(\frac{R_0}{R} \Big| R > 0\right)$$

and proposed controlling this quantity instead of $FDR$. Storey (2002) indicated that $\Pr(R > 0) \approx 1$ with a large $m$. In this case, $pFDR$ is equivalent to $FDR$. Thus, throughout this chapter, we do not distinguish between $FDR$ and $pFDR$. Hence, definitions (12.2.1) and (12.2.2) are considered to be equivalent. Benjamini and Hochberg (1995) proposed a multi-step procedure to control the $FDR$ at a specified level. Their methods, however, are conservative and the conservativeness increases as $m_0$ increases (Storey et al., 2004).

Suppose that, in the $j$th testing, we reject the null hypothesis $H_j$ if the $p$-value $p_j$ is smaller than or equal to $\alpha \in (0, 1)$. Assuming independence of the $m$ $p$-values, we have

$$R_0 = \sum_{j=1}^{m} I(H_j \text{ true}, H_j \text{ rejected})$$

$$= \sum_{j=1}^{m} \Pr(H_j \text{ true}) \Pr(H_j \text{ rejected}|H_j) + o_p(m),$$

which equals $m_0 \alpha$, where $m^{-1} o_p(m) \to 0$ in probability as $m \to \infty$ (Storey, 2002). Ignoring the error term, we have

$$FDR(\alpha) = \frac{m_0 \alpha}{R(\alpha)}, \qquad (12.2.3)$$

where $R(\alpha) = \sum_{j=1}^{m} I(p_j \leq \alpha)$. Note that for a given $\alpha$, the estimation of $FDR$ by (12.2.3) requires the estimation of $m_0$.

For the estimation of $m_0$, Storey (2002) considered that the histogram of $m$ $p$-values is a mixture of (i) $m_0$ $p$-values that are corresponding to the true null hypotheses and following $U(0, 1)$ distribution, and (ii) $m_1$ $p$-values that are corresponding to the alternative hypotheses and expected to be close to 0. Consequently, for a chosen constant $\lambda$ away from 0, none

## 12.2. False Discovery Rate (FDR) Control

(or few, if any) of the $m_1$ p-values will fall above $\lambda$, so that the number of p-values above $\lambda$, $\sum_{j=1}^{m} I(p_j > \lambda)$, can be approximated by the expected frequency among the $m_0$ p-values above $\lambda$ from $U(0,1)$ distribution, i.e. $m_0/(1-\lambda)$. Hence, for a given $\lambda$, $m_0$ can be estimated by

$$\hat{m}_0(\lambda) = \frac{\sum_{j=1}^{m} I(p_j > \lambda)}{1 - \lambda}.$$

By combining this $m_0$ estimator with (12.2.3), Storey (2002) obtained the following estimator for $FDR(\alpha)$

$$\widehat{FDR}(\alpha) = \frac{\alpha \times \hat{m}_0(\lambda)}{R(\alpha)} = \frac{\alpha \sum_{j=1}^{m} I(p_j > \lambda)}{(1-\lambda) \sum_{j=1}^{m} I(p_j \leq \alpha)}.$$

For an observed p-value $p_j$, Storey (2002) defined the minimum FDR level at which we reject $H_j$ as q-value, which is given by

$$q_j = \inf_{\alpha \geq p_j} \widehat{FDR}(\alpha).$$

When $FDR(\alpha)$ is strictly increasing in $\alpha$, the above formula can be reduced to

$$q_j = \widehat{FDR}(p_j).$$

It can be verified that this assumption holds if the power function of the individual tests is concave in $\alpha$, which is the case when the test statistics follow a standard normal distribution under the null hypotheses. We would reject $H_j$ (or, equivalently, discovered gene $j$) if $q_j$ is smaller than or equal to the prespecified $FDR$ level.

Note that the primary assumption of independence among $m$ test statistics was relaxed to independence only among $m_0$ test statistics corresponding to the null hypotheses by Storey and Tibshirani (2001), and to weak independence among all $m$ test statistics by Storey (2003) and Story et al. (2004).

### 12.2.1 Sample Size Calculation

In this subsection, formulas and/or procedures for sample size calcuation based on the approach for controlling FDR proposed by Jung (2005) will be introduced. Let $\mathcal{M}_0$ and $\mathcal{M}_1$ denote the set of genes for which the null and alternative hypotheses are true, respectively. Note that the cardinalities of $\mathcal{M}_0$ and $\mathcal{M}_1$ are $m_0$ and $m_1$, respectively. Since the estimated FDR is invariant to the order of the genes, we may rearrange the genes and set $\mathcal{M}_1 = \{1, ..., m_1\}$ and $\mathcal{M}_0 = \{m_1 + 1, ..., m\}$.

By Storey (2002) and Storey and Tibshirani (2001), for large $m$ and under independence (or weak dependence) among the test statistics, we have

$$R(\alpha) = E(R_0(\alpha)) + E(R_1(\alpha)) + o_p(m)$$
$$= m_0\alpha + \sum_{j \in \mathcal{M}_1} \xi_j(\alpha) + o_p(m),$$

where $R_h(\alpha) = \sum_{j \in \mathcal{M}_h} I(p_j \leq \alpha)$ for $h = 0, 1$, $\xi_j(\alpha) = P(p_j \leq \alpha)$ is the marginal power of the single $\alpha$-test applied to gene $j \in \mathcal{M}_1$. From (12.2.3), we have

$$FDR(\alpha) = \frac{m_0\alpha}{m_0\alpha + \sum_{j \in \mathcal{M}_1} \xi_j(\alpha)} \qquad (12.2.4)$$

by omitting the error term.

Let $X_{ij}$ ($Y_{ij}$) denote the expression level of gene $j$ for subject $i$ in group 1 (and group 2, respectively) with common variance $\sigma_j^2$. For simplicity, we consider two-sample $t$-tests,

$$T_j = \frac{\bar{X}_j - \bar{Y}_j}{\hat{\sigma}_j \sqrt{n_1^{-1} + n_2^{-1}}},$$

for hypothesis $j$ ($= 1, ..., m$), where $n_k$ is the number of subjects in group $k$ ($= 1, 2$), $\bar{X}_j$ and $\bar{Y}_j$ are sample means of $\{X_{ij}, i = 1, ..., n_1\}$ and $\{Y_{ij}, i = 1, ..., n_2\}$, respectively, and $\hat{\sigma}_j^2$ is the pooled sample variance. We assume a large sample (i.e. $n_k \to \infty$), so that $T_j \sim N(0, 1)$ for $j \in \mathcal{M}_0$. Let $n = n_1 + n_2$ denote the total sample size, and $a_k = n_k/n$ the allocation proportion for group $k$.

Let $\delta_j$ denote the effect size for gene $j$ in the fraction of its standard error, i.e.

$$\delta_j = \frac{E(X_j) - E(Y_j)}{\sigma_j}.$$

At the moment, we consider one-sided tests, $H_j : \delta_j = 0$ against $\bar{H}_j : \delta_j > 0$, by assuming $\delta_j > 0$ for $j \in \mathcal{M}_1$ and $\delta_j = 0$ for $j \in \mathcal{M}_0$. Note that, for large $n$,

$$T_j \sim N(\delta_j \sqrt{na_1 a_2}, 1)$$

for $j \in \mathcal{M}_1$. Thus, we have

$$\xi_j(\alpha) = \bar{\Phi}(z_\alpha - \delta_j \sqrt{na_1 a_2}),$$

where $\bar{\Phi}(\cdot)$ denotes the survivor function and $z_\alpha = \bar{\Phi}^{-1}(\alpha)$ is the upper $100\alpha$-th percentile of $N(0, 1)$. Hence, (12.2.2) is expressed as

$$FDR(\alpha) = \frac{m_0 \alpha}{m_0 \alpha + \sum_{j \in \mathcal{M}_1} \bar{\Phi}(z_\alpha - \delta_j \sqrt{na_1 a_2})}. \qquad (12.2.5)$$

## 12.2. False Discovery Rate (FDR) Control

From (12.2.5), $FDR$ is decreasing in $\delta_j$, $n$ and $|a_1 - 1/2|$. Further, FDR is increasing in $\alpha$. To verify this, it suffices to show that, for $j \in \mathcal{M}_1$, $g(\alpha) = \xi_j(\alpha)/\alpha$ is decreasing in $\alpha$, or $g'(\alpha) = \alpha^{-1}\{\xi_j'(\alpha) - \alpha^{-1}\xi_j(\alpha)\}$ is negative for all $\alpha \in (0,1)$. Note that the latter condition holds if $\xi_j(\alpha)$ is concave in $\alpha$. For this purpose, we assume that the test statistics follow the standard normal distribution under the null hypotheses. Let $\phi(z) = 1/\sqrt{2\pi} \exp(-z^2/2)$ and $\bar{\Phi}(z) = \int_z^\infty \phi(t)dt$ denote the probability density function and the survivor function of the standard normal distribution, respectively. Noting that $\xi_j(\alpha) = \bar{\Phi}(z_\alpha - \delta_j\sqrt{na_1 a_2})$ and $z_\alpha = \bar{\Phi}^{-1}(\alpha)$, we have

$$g'(\alpha) = \frac{\alpha\phi(\bar{\Phi}^{-1}(\alpha) - \delta_j\sqrt{na_1 a_2})/\phi(\bar{\Phi}^{-1}(\alpha)) - \bar{\Phi}(\bar{\Phi}^{-1}(\alpha) - \delta_j\sqrt{na_1 a_2})}{\alpha^2}$$

$$= \frac{\bar{\Phi}(z_\alpha)\phi(z_\alpha - \delta_j\sqrt{na_1 a_2})/\phi(z_\alpha) - \bar{\Phi}(z_\alpha - \delta_j\sqrt{na_1 a_2})}{\alpha^2}.$$

Showing $g'(\alpha) < 0$ is equivalent to showing

$$\frac{\phi(z_\alpha - \delta_j\sqrt{na_1 a_2})}{\bar{\Phi}(z_\alpha - \delta_j\sqrt{na_1 a_2})} < \frac{\phi(z_\alpha)}{\bar{\Phi}(z_\alpha)},$$

which holds since $\delta_j > 0$ and $\phi(z)/\bar{\Phi}(z)$ is an increasing function by the following lemma.

**Lemma 12.2.1.** $\phi(z)/\bar{\Phi}(z)$ is an increasing function.
Proof: Let's show that

$$\ell(z) \equiv \log\{\phi(z)/\bar{\Phi}(z)\} = -\frac{z^2}{2} - \log\int_z^\infty \exp(-\frac{t^2}{2})dt$$

is an increasing function. Since

$$\ell'(z) = -z + \frac{\exp(-z^2/2)}{\int_z^\infty \exp(-t^2/2)dt},$$

$\ell'(z) > 0$ for $z \leq 0$. For $z > 0$, $\ell'(z) > 0$ if and only if

$$L(z) \equiv \frac{1}{z}\exp(-z^2/2) - \int_z^\infty \exp(-t^2/2)dt$$

is positive. We have

$$L'(z) = -\frac{1}{z^2}\exp(-z^2/2) - \exp(-z^2/2) + \exp(-z^2/2)$$

$$= -\frac{1}{z^2}\exp(-z^2/2) < 0.$$

Hence, for $z > 0$, $L$ is a decreasing function, and $\lim_{z \to 0} L(z) = \infty$ and $\lim_{z \to \infty} L(z) = 0$, so that $L(z)$ is positive. This completes the proof.

Note that if the effect sizes are equal among the prognostic genes, $FDR$ is increasing in $\pi_0 = m_0/m$. It can be verified that $FDR$ increases from 0 to $m_0/m$ as $\alpha$ increases from 0 to 1. At the design stage of a microarray study, $m$ is usually determined by the microarray chips chosen for experiment and $m_1$, $\{\delta_j, j \in \mathcal{M}_1\}$ and $a_1$ are projected based on past experience or data from pilot studies if any. The only variables undecided in (12.2.5) are $\alpha$ and $n$. With all other design parameters fixed, $FDR$ is controlled at a certain level by the chosen $\alpha$ level. Thus, Jung (2005) proposed choosing the sample size $n$ such that it will guarantee a certain number, say $r_1 (\leq m_1)$, of true rejections with $FDR$ controlled at a specified level $f$. Along this line, Jung (2005) derived a formula for sample size calculation as follows.

In (12.2.5), the expected number of true rejections is

$$E\{R_1(\alpha)\} = \sum_{j \in \mathcal{M}_1} \bar{\Phi}(z_\alpha - \delta_j \sqrt{n a_1 a_2}). \qquad (12.2.6)$$

In multiple testing controlling $FDR$, $E(R_1)/m_1$ plays the role of the power of a conventional testing, see Lee and Whitmore (2002) and van den Oord and Sullivan (2003). With $E(R_1)$ and the $FDR$ level set at $r_1$ and $f$, respectively, (12.2.5) is then expressed as

$$f = \frac{m_0 \alpha}{m_0 \alpha + r_1}.$$

By solving this equation with respect to $\alpha$, we obtain

$$\alpha^* = \frac{r_1 f}{m_0 (1 - f)}.$$

Given $m_0$, $\alpha^*$ is the marginal type I error level for $r_1$ true rejections with the $FDR$ controlled at $f$. With $\alpha$ and $E(R_1)$ replaced by $\alpha^*$ and $r_1$, respectively, (12.2.6) yields an equation $h(n) = 0$, where

$$h(n) = \sum_{j \in \mathcal{M}_1} \bar{\Phi}(z_{\alpha^*} - \delta_j \sqrt{n a_1 a_2}) - r_1. \qquad (12.2.7)$$

We can then obtain the sample size by solving this equation. Jung (2005) recommended solving the equation $h(n) = 0$ using the following bisection method:

(a) Choose $s_1$ and $s_2$ such that $0 < s_1 < s_2$ and $h_1 h_2 < 0$, where $h_k = h(s_k)$ for $k = 1, 2$. (If $h_1 h_2 > 0$ and $h_1 > 0$, then choose a smaller $s_1$; if $h_1 h_2 > 0$ and $h_2 < 0$, then choose a larger $s_2$.)

(b) For $s_3 = (s_1 + s_2)/2$, calculate $h_3 = h(s_3)$.

## 12.2. False Discovery Rate (FDR) Control

(c) If $h_1 h_3 < 0$, then replace $s_2$ and $h_2$ with $s_3$ and $h_3$, respectively. Else, replace $s_1$ and $h_1$ with $s_3$ and $h_3$, respectively. Go to (b).

(d) repeat (b) and (c) until $|s_1 - s_3| < 1$ and $|h_3| < 1$, and obtain the required sample size $n = [s_3] + 1$, where $[s]$ is the largest integer smaller than $s$.

If we do not have prior information on the effect sizes, we may want to assume equal effect sizes $\delta_j = \delta$ ($> 0$) for $j \in \mathcal{M}_1$. In this case, (12.2.7) is reduced to
$$h(n) = m_1 \bar{\Phi}(z_{\alpha^*} - \delta\sqrt{na_1 a_2}) - r_1$$
and, by solving $h(n) = 0$, we obtain the following formula:
$$n = \left[\frac{(z_{\alpha^*} + z_{\beta^*})^2}{a_1 a_2 \delta^2}\right] + 1, \qquad (12.2.8)$$
where $\alpha^* = r_1 f / \{m_0(1-f)\}$ and $\beta^* = 1 - r_1/m_1$. Note that formula (12.2.8) is equivalent to the conventional sample size formula for detecting an effect size of $\delta$ with a desired power of $1 - \beta^*$ while controlling the type I error level at $\alpha^*$.

As a result, the procedure for sample size calculation based on the approach of controlling FDR proposed by Jung (2005) can be summarized as follows.

- Step 1: Specify the input parameters:
  $f$ = FDR level
  $r_1$ = number of true rejections
  $a_k$ = allocation proportion for group $k (= 1, 2)$
  $m$ = total number of genes for testing
  $m_1$ = number of prognostic genes ($m_0 = m - m_1$)
  $\{\delta_j, j \in \mathcal{M}_1\}$ = effect sizes for prognostic genes

- Stpe 2: Obtain the required sample size:
  If the effect sizes are constant $\delta_j = \delta$ for $j \in \mathcal{M}_1$,
  $$n = \left[\frac{(z_{\alpha^*} + z_{\beta^*})^2}{a_1 a_2 \delta^2}\right] + 1,$$
  where $\alpha^* = r_1 f / \{m_0(1-f)\}$ and $\beta^* = 1 - r_1/m_1$.
  Otherwise, solve $h(n) = 0$ using the bisection method, where
  $$h(n) = \sum_{j \in \mathcal{M}_1} \bar{\Phi}(z_{\alpha^*} - \delta_j \sqrt{na_1 a_2}) - r_1$$
  and $\alpha^* = r_1 f / \{m_0(1-f)\}$.

## Remarks

Note that for given sample sizes $n_1$ and $n_2$, one may want to check how many true rejections are expected as if we want to check the power in a conventional testing. In this case, we may solve the equations for $r_1$. For example, when the effect sizes are constant, $\delta_j = \delta$ for $j \in \mathcal{M}_1$, we solve the equation

$$z_{\alpha^*(r_1)} + z_{\beta^*(r_1)} = \delta\sqrt{n_1^{-1} + n_2^{-1}}$$

with respect to $r_1$, where $\alpha^*(r_1) = r_1 f / \{m_0(1-f)\}$ and $\beta^*(r_1) = 1 - r_1/m_1$.

## Examples

To illustrate the procedure for sample size calculation under the approach for controlling $FDR$ proposed by Jung (2005), the examples based on one-sided tests with constant effect sizes and varied effect sizes described in Jung (2005) are used.

**Example 1: One-Sided Tests and Constant Effect Sizes.** Suppose that we want to design a microarray study on $m = 4000$ candidate genes, among which about $m_1 = 40$ genes are expected to be differentially expressing between two patient groups. Note that $m_0 = m - m_1 = 3960$. Constant effect sizes, $\delta_j = \delta = 1$, for the $m_1$ prognostic genes are projected. About equal number of patients are expected to enter the study from each group, i.e. $a_1 = a_2 = .5$. We want to discover $r_1 = 24$ prognostic genes by one-sided tests with the FDR controlled at $f = 1\%$ level. Then

$$\alpha^* = \frac{24 \times 0.01}{3960 \times (1 - 0.01)} = 0.612 \times 10^{-4}$$

and $\beta^* = 1 - 24/40 = 0.4$, so that $z_{\alpha^*} = 3.841$ and $z_{\beta^*} = 0.253$. Hence, from (12.2.8), the required sample size is given as

$$n = \left[\frac{(3.841 + 0.253)^2}{0.5 \times 0.5 \times 1^2}\right] + 1 = 68,$$

or $n_1 = n_2 = 34$.

**Example 2: One-Sided Tests and Varying Effect Sizes.** We assume $(m, m_1, a_1, r_1, f) = (4000, 40, 0.5, 24, 0.01)$, $\delta_j = 1$ for $1 \leq j \leq 20$ and $\delta_j = 1/2$ for $21 \leq j \leq 40$. Then

$$\alpha^* = \frac{24 \times 0.01}{3960 \times (1 - 0.01)} = 0.612 \times 10^{-4}$$

## 12.2. False Discovery Rate (FDR) Control

Table 12.2.2: The bisection procedure for Example 2.

| Step | $s_1$ | $s_2$ | $s_3$ | $h_1$ | $h_2$ | $h_3$ |
|---|---|---|---|---|---|---|
| 1 | 100.0 | 200.0 | 150.0 | −4.67 | 3.59 | 0.13 |
| 2 | 100.0 | 150.0 | 125.0 | −4.67 | 0.13 | −1.85 |
| 3 | 125.0 | 150.0 | 137.5 | −1.85 | 0.13 | −0.80 |
| 4 | 137.5 | 150.0 | 143.8 | −0.80 | 0.13 | −0.32 |
| 5 | 143.8 | 150.0 | 146.9 | −0.32 | 0.13 | −0.09 |
| 6 | 146.9 | 150.0 | 148.4 | −0.09 | 0.13 | 0.02 |
| 7 | 146.9 | 148.4 | 147.7 | −0.09 | 0.02 | −0.04 |

Source: Jung et al. (2005).

and $z_{\alpha^*} = 3.841$, so that we have

$$h(n) = 20\bar{\Phi}(3.841 - \sqrt{n/4}) + 20\bar{\Phi}(3.841 - .5\sqrt{n/4}) - 24$$

Table 12.2.2 displays the bisection procedure with starting values $s_1 = 100$ and $s_2 = 200$. The procedure stops after 7 iterations and gives $n = \lfloor 147.7 \rfloor + 1 = 148$.

### Two-Sided Tests

Suppose one wants to test $H_j : \delta_j = 0$ against $\bar{H}_j : \delta_j \neq 0$. We reject $H_j$ if $|T_j| > z_{\alpha/2}$ for a certain $\alpha$ level, and obtain the power function $\xi_j(\alpha) = \bar{\Phi}(z_{\alpha/2} - |\delta_j|\sqrt{na_1a_2})$. In this case, $\alpha^*$ is the same as that for one-sided test case, i.e.,

$$\alpha^* = \frac{r_1 f}{m_0(1-f)},$$

but (12.2.7) is changed to

$$h(n) = \sum_{j \in \mathcal{M}_1} \bar{\Phi}(z_{\alpha^*/2} - |\delta_j|\sqrt{na_1a_2}) - r_1. \quad (12.2.9)$$

If the effect sizes are constant, i.e. $\delta_j = \delta$ for $j \in \mathcal{M}_1$, then we have a closed form formula

$$n = \left\lceil \frac{(z_{\alpha^*/2} + z_{\beta^*})^2}{a_1 a_2 \delta^2} \right\rceil + 1, \quad (12.2.10)$$

where $\alpha^* = r_1 f / \{m_0(1-f)\}$ and $\beta^* = 1 - r_1/m_1$.

Now we derive the relationship between the sample size for one-sided test case and that for two-sided test case. Suppose that the input parameters $m$, $m_1$, $a_1$ and $\{\delta_j, j \in \mathcal{M}_1\}$ are fixed and we want $r_1$ true rejections in both cases. Without loss of generality, we assume that the effect sizes are nonnegative. The only difference between the two cases is the parts of $\alpha^*$ in (12.2.7) and $\alpha^*/2$ in (12.2.9). Let $f_1$ and $f_2$ denote the $FDR$ levels for one- and two-sided testing cases, respectively. Then, the two formulas will give exactly the same sample size as far as these two parts are identical, i.e.

$$\frac{r_1 f_1}{m_0(1-f_1)} = \frac{r_1 f_2}{2m_0(1-f_2)},$$

which yields $f_1 = f_2/(2-f_2)$. In other words, with all other parameters fixed, the sample size for two-sided tests to control the $FDR$ at $f$ can be obtained using the sample size formula for one-sided tests (12.2.7) by setting the target $FDR$ level at $f/(2-f)$. Note that this value is slightly larger than $f/2$. The same relationship holds when the effect sizes for prognostic genes are constant.

To illustrate the above procedure for sample size calculation under the approach for controlling $FDR$ proposed by Jung (2005), the following example based on two-sided tests with constant effect sizes described in Jung (2005) is considered.

**Example 3: Two-sided Tests and Constant Effect Sizes.** Jung (2005) considered $(m, m_1, \delta, a_1, r_1, f) = (4000, 40, 1, 0.5, 24, 0.01)$ as those given in Example 1, but use two-sided tests. Then

$$\alpha^* = \frac{24 \times 0.01}{3960 \times (1-0.01)} = 0.612 \times 10^{-4}$$

and $\beta^* = 1 - 24/40 = 0.4$, so that $z_{\alpha^*/2} = 4.008$ and $z_{\beta^*} = 0.253$. Hence, from (12.2.10), the required sample size is given as

$$n = \left[ \frac{(4.008 + 0.253)^2}{0.5 \times 0.5 \times 1^2} \right] + 1 = 73.$$

By the above argument, we obtain exactly the same sample size using formula (12.2.8) and $f = .01/(2 - .01) = 0.005025$. Note that this sample size is slightly larger than $n = 68$ which was obtained for one-sided tests in Example 1.

### Exact Formula Based on t-Distribution

Jung (2005) indicated that if the gene expression level, or its transformation, is a normal random variable and the available resources are so limited that only a small sample size can be considered, then one may want to use the exact formula based on $t$-distributions, rather than that based on normal approximation. In one-sided testing case, Jung (2005) suggested modifying (12.2.5) as follows

$$FDR(\alpha) = \frac{m_0 \alpha}{m_0 \alpha + \sum_{j \in \mathcal{M}_1} T_{n-2, \delta_j \sqrt{n a_1 a_2}}(t_{n-2,\alpha})},$$

where $T_{\nu,\eta}(t)$ is the survivor function for the non-central t-distribution with $\nu$ degrees of freedom and non-centrality parameter $\eta$, and $t_{\nu,\alpha} = T_{\nu,0}^{-1}(\alpha)$ is the upper $100\alpha$-th percentile of the central t-distribution with $\nu$ degrees of freedom. The required sample size $n$ for $r_1$ true rejections with the $FDR$ controlled at $f$ solves $h_T(n) = 0$, where

$$h_T(n) = \sum_{j \in \mathcal{M}_1} T_{n-2, \delta_j \sqrt{n a_1 a_2}}(t_{n-2,\alpha^*}) - r_1$$

and $\alpha^* = r_1 f / \{m_0(1 - f)\}$. If the effect sizes are constant among the prognostic genes, then the equation reduces to

$$T_{n-2, \delta \sqrt{n a_1 a_2}}(t_{n-2,\alpha^*}) = r_1/m_1,$$

but, contrary to the normal approximation case, we do not have a closed form sample size formula since $n$ is included in both the degrees of freedom and the non-centrality parameter of the $t$-distribution functions.

Similarly, the sample size for two-sided $t$-tests can be obtained by solving $h_T(n) = 0$, where

$$h_T(n) = \sum_{j \in \mathcal{M}_1} T_{n-2, |\delta_j| \sqrt{n a_1 a_2}}(t_{n-2,\alpha^*/2}) - r_1$$

and $\alpha^* = r_1 f / \{m_0(1 - f)\}$. Note that the sample size for $FDR = f$ with two-sided testings is the same as that for $FDR = f/(2 - f)$ with one-sided testings as in the testing based on normal approximation.

## 12.3 Family-wise Error Rate (FWER) Control

Microarray studies usually involve screening and monitoring of expression levels in cells for thousands of genes simultaneously for studying the association of the expression levels and an outcome or other risk factor of interest (Golub et al., 1999; Alizadeh and Staudt, 2000; Sander, 2000). A primary aim is often to reveal the association of the expression levels and an outcome or other risk factor of interest. Traditional statistical testing procedures, such as two-sample $t$-tests or Wilcoxon rank sum tests, are often used to determine statistical significance of the difference in gene expression patterns. These approaches, however, encounter a serious problem of multiplicity as a very large number—possibly 10,000 or more—of hypotheses are to be tested, while the number of studied experimental units is relatively small— tens to a few hundreds (West et al., 2001).

If we consider a per comparison type I error rate $\alpha$ in each test, the probability of rejecting any null hypothesis when all null hypotheses are true, which is called the family-wise error rate $(FWER)$, will be greatly inflated. So as to avoid this pitfall, the Bonferroni test is used most commonly in this field despite its well-known conservativeness. Although Holm (1979) and Hochberg (1988) improved upon such conservativeness by devising multi-step testing procedures, they did not exploit the dependency of the test statistics and consequently the resulting improvement is often minor. Westfall and Young (1989, 1993) proposed adjusting $p$-values in a state-of-the-art step-down manner using simulation or resampling method, by which dependency among test statistics is effectively incorporated. Westfall and Wolfinger (1997) derived exact adjusted p-values for a step-down method for discrete data. Recently, the Westfall and Young's permutation-based test was introduced to microarray data analyses and strongly advocated by Dudoit and her colleagues. Troendle, Korn, and McShane (2004) favor permutation test over bootstrap resampling due to slow convergence in high dimensional data. Various multiple testing procedures and error control methods applicable to microarray experiments are well documented in Dudoit et al. (2003). Which test to use among a bewildering variety of choices should be judged by relevance to research questions, validity (of underlying assumptions), type of control (strong or weak), and computability. Jung, Bang, and Young (2005) showed that the single-step test provides a simple and accurate method for sample size determination and that can also be used for multi-step tests.

### 12.3.1 Multiple Testing Procedures

In this subsection, commonly employed single-step and multi-step testing procedures are briefly described.

#### Single-Step vs. Multi-Step

Suppose that there are $n_1$ subjects in group 1 and $n_2$ subjects in group 2. Gene expression data for $m$ genes are measured from each subject. Furthermore, suppose that we would like to identify the informative genes, i.e., those that are differentially expressed between the two groups. Let $(X_{1i1}, ..., X_{1im})$ and $(X_{2i1}, ..., X_{2im})$ denote the gene expression levels obtained from subject $i$ ($= 1, ..., n_1$) in group 1 and subject $i$ ($= 1, ..., n_2$) in group 2, respectively. Let $\boldsymbol{\mu}_1 = (\mu_{11}, ..., \mu_{1m})$ and $\boldsymbol{\mu}_2 = (\mu_{21}, ..., \mu_{2m})$ represent the respective mean vectors. In order to test whether gene $j$ ($= 1, ..., m$) is not differentially expressed between the two conditions, i.e., $H_j : \mu_{1j} - \mu_{2j} = 0$, the following $t$-test statistic is commonly considered:

$$T_j = \frac{\bar{X}_{1j} - \bar{X}_{2j}}{S_j \sqrt{n_1^{-1} + n_2^{-1}}},$$

where $\bar{X}_{kj}$ is the sample mean in group $k$ ($= 1, 2$) and $S_j^2 = \{\sum_{i=1}^{n_1}(X_{1ij} - \bar{X}_{1j})^2 + \sum_{i=1}^{n_2}(X_{2ij} - \bar{X}_{2j})^2\}/(n_1 + n_2 - 2)$ is the pooled sample variance for the $j$-th gene.

Suppose that our interest is to identify any genes that are overexpressed in group 1. This can be formulated as multiple one-sided tests of $H_j$ vs. $\bar{H}_j : \mu_{1j} > \mu_{2j}$ for $j = 1, ..., m$. In this case, a single-step procedure, which adopts a common critical value $c$ to reject $H_j$ (in favor of $\bar{H}_j$, when $T_j > c$) is commonly employed. For this single-step procedure, the $FWER$ fixed at $\alpha$ is given by

$$\alpha = P(T_1 > c \text{ or } T_2 > c, ..., \text{ or } T_m > c | H_0) = P(\max_{j=1,...,m} T_j > c | H_0),$$
(12.3.11)

where $H_0 : \mu_{1j} = \mu_{2j}$ for all $j = 1, ..., m$, or equivalently $H_0 = \cap_{j=1}^{m} H_j$, is the complete null hypothesis and the relevant alternative hypothesis is $H_a = \cup_{j=1}^{m} \bar{H}_j$. In order to control $FWER$ at the nominal level $\alpha$, the method of Bonferroni uses $c = c_\alpha = t_{n_1+n_2-2, \alpha/m}$, the upper $\alpha$-quantile for the $t$-distribution with $n_1 + n_2 - 2$ degrees of freedom imposing normality for the expression data, or $c = z_{\alpha/m}$, the upper $\alpha$-quantile for the standard normal distribution based on asymptotic normality. If gene expression levels are not normally distributed, the assumption of $t$-distribution may be violated. Furthermore, $n_1$ and $n_2$ usually may not be large enough to warrant a normal approximation. Note that the Bonferroni procedure is conservative for correlated data even when the assumed conditions are met. In practice, microarray data are collected from the same individuals and experience co-regulation. Thus, they are expected to be correlated. To take into consideration the correlation structure under (12.3.11), Jung, Bang, and Young (2005) derived the distribution of $W = \max_{j=1,...,m} T_j$ under $H_0$ using the method permutation. Their method is briefly described below.

For a given total sample size $n$, there are $B = \binom{n}{n_1}$ different ways of partitioning the pooled sample of size $n = n_1 + n_2$ into two groups of sizes $n_1$ and $n_2$. The number of possible permutations $B$ can be very large even with a small sample size. For the observed test statistic $t_j$ of $T_j$ from the original data, the unadjusted (or raw) $p$-values can be approximated by

$$p_j \approx B^{-1} \sum_{b=1}^{B} I(t_j^{(b)} \geq t_j)$$

where $I(A)$ is an indicator function of event $A$. For gene-specific inference, Jung, Bang, and Young (2005) define an adjusted $p$-value for gene $j$ as the minimum $FWER$ for which $H_j$ will be rejected, i.e.,

$$\tilde{p}_j = P(\max_{j'=1,\ldots,m} T_{j'} \geq t_j | H_0).$$

This probability can be estimated by the following algorithms for permutation distribution:

## Algorithm 1 (Single-step procedure)

(A) Compute the test statistics $t_1, \ldots, t_m$ from the original data.

(B) For the $b$-th permutation of the original data $(b = 1, \ldots, B)$, compute the test statistics $t_1^{(b)}, \ldots, t_m^{(b)}$ and $w_b = \max_{j=1,\ldots,m} t_j^{(b)}$.

(C) Estimate the adjusted p-values by $\tilde{p}_j = \sum_{b=1}^{B} I(w_b \geq t_j)/B$ for $j = 1, \ldots, m$.

(D) Reject all hypotheses $H_j$ $(j = 1, \ldots, m)$ such that $\tilde{p}_j < \alpha$.

Alternatively, with steps (C) and (D) replaced, the cut-off value $c_\alpha$ can be determined:

## Algorithm 1'

(C') Sort $w_1, \ldots, w_B$ to obtain the order statistics $w_{(1)} \leq \cdots \leq w_{(B)}$ and compute the critical value $c_\alpha = w_{([B(1-\alpha)+1])}$, where $[a]$ is the largest integer no greater than $a$. If there exist ties, $c_\alpha = w_{(k)}$ where $k$ is the smallest integer such that $w_{(k)} \geq w_{([B(1-\alpha)+1])}$.

(D') Reject all hypotheses $H_j$ $(j = 1, \ldots, m)$ for which $t_j > c_\alpha$.

Below is a step-down analog suggested by Dudoit et al. (2002, 2003), originally proposed by Westfall and Young (1989, 1993):

## Algorithm 2 (Step-down procedure)

(A) Compute the test statistics $t_1, \ldots, t_m$ from the original data.

## 12.3. Family-wise Error Rate (FWER) Control

(A1) Sort $t_1, ..., t_m$ to obtain the ordered test statistics $t_{r_1} \geq \cdots \geq t_{r_m}$, where $H_{r_1}, ..., H_{r_m}$ are the corresponding hypotheses.

(B) For the $b$-th permutation of the original data ($b = 1, ..., B$), compute the test statistics $t_{r_1}^{(b)}, ..., t_{r_m}^{(b)}$ and $u_{b,j} = \max_{j'=j,...,m} t_{r_{j'}}^{(b)}$ for $j = 1, ..., m$.

(C) Estimate the adjusted p-values by $\tilde{p}_{r_j} = \sum_{b=1}^{B} I(u_{b,j} \geq t_{r_j})/B$ for $j = 1, ..., m$.

(C1) Enforce monotonicity by setting $\tilde{p}_{r_j} \leftarrow \max(\tilde{p}_{r_{j-1}}, \tilde{p}_{r_j})$ for $j = 2, ..., m$.

(D) Reject all hypotheses $H_{r_j}$ ($j = 1, ..., m$) for which $\tilde{p}_{r_j} < \alpha$.

**Remarks**

Note that as indicated by Westfall and Young (1993), two-sided tests can be fulfilled by replacing $t_j$ by $|t_j|$ in steps (B) and (C) in Algorithm 1. It can be shown that a single-step procedure, controlling the $FWER$ weakly as in (12.3.11), also controls the $FWER$ strongly under the condition of subset pivotality.

### 12.3.2 Sample Size Calculation

Jung, Bang, and Young (2005) derived a procedure for sample size calculation using the single-step procedure. As indicated by Jung, Bang, and Young (2005), the calculated sample size is also applied to the step-down procedure since the two procedures have the same global power. In what follows, the procedure proposed by Jung, Bang, and Young (2005) using the single-step procedure is briefly described.

**Algorithms for sample size calculation**

Suppose that one wishes to choose a sample size for achieving a desired global power of $1 - \beta$. Assuming that the gene expression data

$$\{(X_{ki1}, ..., X_{kim}), \text{ for } i = 1, .., n_k, k = 1, 2\}$$

are random samples from an unknown distribution with $E(X_{kij}) = \mu_{kj}$, $Var(X_{kij}) = \sigma_j^2$ and $Corr(X_{kij}, X_{kij'}) = \rho_{jj'}$. Let $\boldsymbol{R} = (\rho_{jj'})_{j,j'=1,...,m}$ be the $m \times m$ correlation matrix. Under $H_a$, the effect size is given by $\delta_j = (\mu_{1j} - \mu_{2j})/\sigma_j$. At the planning stage of a microarray study, we usually project the number of predictive genes $D$ and set an equal effect size among them, i.e.,

$$\begin{aligned} \delta_j &= \delta \text{ for } j = 1, ..., D \\ &= 0 \text{ for } j = D+1, ..., m. \end{aligned} \quad (12.3.12)$$

It can be verified that for large $n_1$ and $n_2$, $(T_1, ..., T_m)$ has approximately the same distribution as

$$(e_1, ..., e_m) \sim N(\mathbf{0}, \mathbf{R})$$

under $H_0$ and $(e_j + \delta_j \sqrt{npq}, j = 1, ..., m)$ under $H_a$, where $p = n_1/n$ and $q = 1 - p$. Hence, at FWER $= \alpha$, the common critical value $c_\alpha$ is given as the upper $\alpha$ quantile of $\max_{j=1,...,m} e_j$ from (12.3.11). Similarly, the global power as a function of $n$ is given by

$$h_a(n) = P\{\max_{j=1,...,m}(e_j + \delta_j\sqrt{npq}) > c_\alpha\}.$$

Thus, a given FWER $= \alpha$, the sample size $n$ required for detecting the specified effect sizes $(\delta_1, ..., \delta_m)$ with a global power $1 - \beta$ can be obtained as the solution to $h_a(n) = 1 - \beta$. Note that analytic calculation of $c_\alpha$ and $h_a(n)$ is feasible only when the distributions of $\max_j e_j$ and $\max_j(e_j + \delta_j\sqrt{npq})$ are available in simple forms. With a large $m$, however, it is almost impossible to derive the distributions. To avoid the difficulty, Jung, Bang, and Young suggested the following simulation be considered.

A simulation can be conducted to approximate $c_\alpha$ and $h_a(\cdot)$ by generating random vectors $(e_1, ..., e_m)$ from $N(\mathbf{0}, \mathbf{R})$. For simplicity, Jung, Bang, and Young (2005) suggested generating the random numbers assuming a simple, but realistic, correlation structure for the gene expression data such as block compound symmetry (BCS) or CS (i.e., with only 1 block). Suppose that $m$ genes are partitioned into $L$ blocks, and $\mathcal{B}_l$ denotes the set of genes belonging to block $l$ ($l = 1, ..., L$). We may assume that $\rho_{jj'} = \rho$ if $j, j' \in \mathcal{B}_l$ for some $l$, and $\rho_{jj'} = 0$ otherwise. Under the BCS structure, $(e_1, ..., e_m)$ can be generated as a function of i.i.d. standard normal random variates $u_1, ..., u_m, b_1, ..., b_L$:

$$e_j = u_j\sqrt{1-\rho} + b_l\sqrt{\rho} \text{ for } j \in \mathcal{B}_l. \quad (12.3.13)$$

As a result, the algorithm for sample size calculation can be summarized as follows:

(a) Specify FWER ($\alpha$), global power ($1 - \beta$), effect sizes ($\delta_1, ..., \delta_m$) and correlation structure ($\mathbf{R}$).

(b) Generate $K$ (say, $10,000$) i.i.d. random vectors $\{(e_1^{(k)}, ..., e_m^{(k)}), k = 1, ..., K\}$ from $N(\mathbf{0}, \mathbf{R})$. Let $\bar{e}_k = \max_{j=1,...,m} e_j^{(k)}$.

## 12.3. Family-wise Error Rate (FWER) Control

(c) Approximate $c_\alpha$ by $\bar{e}_{[(1-\alpha)K+1]}$, the $[(1-\alpha)K+1]$-th order statistic of $\bar{e}_1, ..., \bar{e}_K$.

(d) Calculate $n$ by solving $\hat{h}_a(n) = 1 - \beta$ by the bisection method (Press et al., 1996), where $\hat{h}_a(n) = K^{-1} \sum_{k=1}^{K} I\{\max_{j=1,...,m}(e_j^{(k)} + \delta_j \sqrt{npq}) > c_\alpha\}$.

Mathematically put, step (d) is equivalent to finding $n^* = \min\{n : \hat{h}_a(n) \geq 1 - \beta\}$.

Note that the permutation procedure may alter the correlation structure among the test statistics under $H_a$. Suppose that there are $m_1$ genes in block 1, among which the first $D$ are predictive. Then, under (12.3.13) and BCS, we have:

$$Corr(T_j, T_{j'}) \approx \begin{cases} (\rho + pq\delta^2)/(1 + pq\delta^2) \equiv \rho_1 & \text{if } 1 \leq j < j' \leq D \\ \rho/\sqrt{1 + pq\delta^2} \equiv \rho_2 & \text{if } 1 \leq j \leq D < j' \leq m_1 \\ \rho & \text{if } D < j < j' \leq m_1 \\ \rho & \text{or } j, j' \in \mathcal{B}_l, l \geq 2 \end{cases}$$
(12.3.14)

where the approximation is with respect to large $n$.

Let $\tilde{R}$ denote the correlation matrix with these correlation coefficients. Note that $\tilde{R} = R$ under $H_0 : \delta = 0$, so that calculation of $c_\alpha$ is the same as in the naive method. However, $h_a(n)$ should be modified to

$$\tilde{h}_a(n) = P\{\max_{j=1,...,m}(\tilde{e}_j + \delta_j\sqrt{npq}) > c_\alpha\}$$

where random samples of $(\tilde{e}_1, ..., \tilde{e}_m)$ can be generated using

$$\tilde{e}_j = \begin{cases} u_j\sqrt{1-\rho_1} + b_1\sqrt{\rho_2} + b_{-1}\sqrt{\rho_1 - \rho_2} & \text{if } 1 \leq j \leq D \\ u_j\sqrt{1-\rho} + b_1\sqrt{\rho_2} + b_0\sqrt{\rho - \rho_2} & \text{if } D < j \leq m_1 \\ u_j\sqrt{1-\rho} + b_l\sqrt{\rho} & \text{if } j \in \mathcal{B}_l \text{ for } l \geq 2 \end{cases}$$

with $u_1, ..., u_m, b_{-1}, b_0, b_1, ..., b_L$ independently from $N(0,1)$. Then, $\{(\tilde{e}_1^{(k)}, ..., \tilde{e}_m^{(k)}), k = 1, ..., K\}$ are i.i.d. random vectors from $N(\mathbf{0}, \tilde{R})$, and

$$\hat{\tilde{h}}_a(n) = K^{-1} \sum_{k=1}^{K} I\{\max_{j=1,...,m}(\tilde{e}_j^{(k)} + \delta_j\sqrt{npq}) > c_\alpha\}.$$

The sample size can be obtained by solving $\hat{\tilde{h}}_a(n) = 1 - \beta$.

**Remarks**

Note that the methods discussed above are different from a pure simulation method in the sense that it does not require generating the raw data and then calculating test statistics. Thus, the computing time is not of an order of $n \times m$, but of $m$. Furthermore, we can share the random numbers $u_1, ..., u_m, b_{-1}, b_0, b_1, ..., b_L$ in the calculation of $c_\alpha$ and $n$. We do not need to generate a new set of random numbers at each replication of the bisection procedures either. If the target $n$ is not large, the large sample approximation may not perform well. In our simulation study, we examine how large $n$ needs to be for an adequate approximation. If the target $n$ is so small that the approximation is questionable, then we have to use a pure simulation method by generating raw data.

### 12.3.3 Leukemia Example

To illustrate the use of the procedure described above, the leukemia data from Golub et al. (1999) are reanalyzed. There are $n_{all} = 27$ patients with acute lymphoblastic leukemia (ALL) and $n_{aml} = 11$ patients with acute myeloid leukemia (AML) in the training set, and expression patterns in $m = 6,810$ human genes are explored. Note that, in general, such expression measures are subject to preprocessing steps such as image analysis and normalization, and also to *a priori* quality control. Supplemental information and dataset can be found at the website http://www.genome.wi.mit.edu /MPR.

Gene-specific significance was ascertained for alternative hypotheses $\bar{H}_{1,j} : \mu_{ALL,j} \neq \mu_{AML,j}$, $\bar{H}_{2,j} : \mu_{ALL,j} < \mu_{AML,j}$, and $\bar{H}_{3,j} : \mu_{ALL,j} > \mu_{AML,j}$ by SDP and SSP. Jung, Bang, and Young (2005) implemented their algorithm as well as PROC MULTTEST in SAS with $B = 10,000$ permutations (Westfall, Zaykin and Young, 2001). Due to essentially identical results, we report the results from SAS. Table 12.3.1 lists 41 genes with two-sided adjusted p-values that are smaller than 0.05. Although adjusted p-values by SDP are slightly smaller than SSP, the results are extremely similar, confirming the findings from our simulation study. Note that Golub et al. (1999) and we identified 1,100 and 1,579 predictive genes without accounting for multiplicity, respectively. A Bonferroni adjustment declared 37 significant genes. This is not so surprising because relatively low correlations among genes were observed in this data. We do not show the results for $\bar{H}_{3,j}$; only four hypotheses are rejected. Note that the two-sided p-value is smaller than twice of the smaller one-sided p-value as theory predicts and that the difference is not often negligible (Shaffer, 2002).

In Table 12.3.1, adjusted p-values from 2-sided hypothesis less than .05 are listed in increasing order among total $m=6,810$ genes investigated. The

## 12.3. Family-wise Error Rate (FWER) Control

Table 12.3.3: Reanalysis of the leukemia data from Golub et al. (1999)

| Gene index (description) | Alternative hypothesis | | | |
|---|---|---|---|---|
| | $\mu_{all} \neq \mu_{aml}$ | | $\mu_{all} < \mu_{aml}$ | |
| | SDP | SSP | SDP | SSP |
| 1701 (FAH Fumarylacetoacetate) | .0003 | .0003 | .0004 | .0004 |
| 3001 (Leukotriene C4 synthase) | .0003 | .0003 | .0004 | .0004 |
| 4528 (Zyxin) | .0003 | .0003 | .0004 | .0004 |
| 1426 (LYN V-yes-1 Yamaguchi) | .0004 | .0004 | .0005 | .0005 |
| 4720 (LEPR Leptin receptor) | .0004 | .0004 | .0005 | .0005 |
| 1515 (CD33 CD33 antigen) | .0006 | .0006 | .0006 | .0006 |
| 402 (Liver mRNA for IGIF) | .0010 | .0010 | .0009 | .0009 |
| 3877 (PRG1 Proteoglycan 1) | .0012 | .0012 | .0010 | .0010 |
| 1969 (DF D component of complement) | .0013 | .0013 | .0011 | .0011 |
| 3528 (GB DEF) | .0013 | .0013 | .0010 | .0010 |
| 930 (Induced Myeloid Leukemia Cell) | .0016 | .0016 | .0013 | .0013 |
| 5882(IL8 Precursor) | .0016 | .0016 | .0013 | .0013 |
| 1923 (PEPTIDYL-PROLYL CIS-TRANS Isomerase) | .0017 | .0017 | .0014 | .0014 |
| 2939 (Phosphotyrosine independent ligand p62) | .0018 | .0018 | .0014 | .0014 |
| 1563 (CST3 Cystatin C) | .0026 | .0026 | .0021 | .0021 |
| 1792 (ATP6C Vacuolar H+ ATPase proton channel subunit) | .0027 | .0027 | .0023 | .0023 |
| 1802 (CTSD Cathepsin D) | .0038 | .0038 | .0032 | .0032 |
| 5881 (Interleukin 8) | .0041 | .0041 | .0036 | .0036 |
| 6054 (ITGAX Integrin) | .0056 | .0055 | .0042 | .0041 |
| 6220 (Epb72 gene exon 1) | .0075 | .0075 | .0062 | .0062 |
| 1724 (LGALS3 Lectin) | .0088 | .0088 | .0071 | .0071 |
| 2440 (Thrombospondin-p50) | .0091 | .0091 | .0073 | .0073 |
| 6484 (LYZ Lysozyme) | .0101 | .0100 | .0081 | .0080 |
| 1355 (FTL Ferritin) | .0107 | .0106 | .0086 | .0085 |
| 2083 (Azurocidin) | .0107 | .0106 | .0086 | .0085 |
| 1867 (Protein MAD3) | .0114 | .0113 | .0092 | .0091 |
| 6057 (PFC Properdin P factor) | .0143 | .0142 | .0108 | .0107 |
| 3286 (Lysophospholipase homolog) | .0168 | .0167 | .0126 | .0125 |
| 6487 (Lysozyme) | .0170 | .0169 | .0127 | .0126 |
| 1510 (PPGB Protective protein) | .0178 | .0177 | .0133 | .0132 |
| 6478 (LYZ Lysozyme) | .0193 | .0191 | .0144 | .0142 |
| 6358 (HOX 2.2) | .0210 | .0208 | .0160 | .0158 |
| 3733 (Catalase EC 1.11.1.6) | .0216 | .0214 | .0162 | .0160 |
| 1075 (FTH1 Ferritin heavy chain) | .0281 | .0279 | .0211 | .0209 |
| 6086 (CD36 CD36 antigen) | .0300 | .0298 | .0224 | .0222 |
| 189 (ADM) | .0350 | .0348 | .0260 | .0258 |
| 1948 (CDC25A Cell division cycle) | .0356 | .0354 | .0263 | .0261 |
| 5722 (APLP2 Amyloid beta precursor-like protein) | .0415 | .0413 | .0306 | .0304 |
| 5686 (TIMP2 Tissue inhibitor of metalloproteinase) | .0425 | .0423 | .0314 | .0312 |
| 5453 (C-myb) | .0461 | .0459 | 1.000 | 1.000 |
| 6059 (NF-IL6-beta protein mRNA) | .0482 | .0480 | .0350 | .0348 |

Source: Golub et al. (1999) and Jung et al. (2005).

total number of studied subjects $n$ was 38 ($n_{all} = 27$ and $n_{aml} = 11$). $B = 10,000$ times of permutation were used. Note that C-myb gene has p-value of 0.015 against the hypothesis $\mu_{all} > \mu_{aml}$. Although some gene descriptions are identical, gene accession numbers are different.

Suppose that we would like to design a prospective study to identify predictive genes overexpressing in AML based on observed parameter values. So we assume $m = 6,810$, $p = 0.3 (\approx 11/38)$, $D = 10$ or 100, $\delta = 0.5$ or 1, and BCS with block size 100 or CS with a common correlation coefficient of $\rho = 0.1$ or 0.4. We calculated the sample size using the modified formula under each parameter setting for FWER $\alpha = 0.05$ and a global power $1 - \beta = 0.8$ with $K = 5,000$ replications. For $D = 10$ and $\delta = 1$, the minimal sample size required for BCS/CS are 59/59 and 74/63 for $\rho = 0.1$ and 0.4, respectively. If a larger number of genes, say $D = 100$, are anticipated to overexpress in AML with the same effect size, the respective sample sizes reduce to 34/34 and 49/41 in order to maintain the same power. With $\delta = 0.5$, the required sample size becomes nearly 3.5 to 4 times that for $\delta = 1$. Note that, with the same $\rho$, BCS tends to require a larger sample size than CS.

An interesting question is raised regarding the accuracy of the sample size formula when the gene expression data have distributions other than the multivariate normal distributions. We considered the setting $\alpha = 0.05$, $1 - \beta = 0.8$, $\delta = 1$, $D = 100$, $\rho = 0.1$ with CS structure, which results in the smallest sample size, $n = 34$, in the above sample size calculation. Gene expression data were generated from a correlated asymmetric distribution:

$$X_{kj} = \mu_{kj} + (e_{kj} - 2)\sqrt{\rho/4} + (e_{k0} - 2)\sqrt{(1-\rho)/4}$$

for $1 \leq j \leq m$ and $k = 1, 2$. Here, $\mu_{1j} = \delta_j$ and $\mu_{2j} = 0$, and $e_{k0}, e_{k1}, ..., e_{km}$ are i.i.d. random variables from a $\chi^2$ distribution with 2 degrees of freedom. Note that $(X_{k1}, ..., X_{km})$ have means $(\mu_{k1}, ..., \mu_{km})$, marginal variances 1, and a compound symmetry correlation structure with $\rho = 0.1$. In this case, we obtained an empirical $FWER$ of 0.060 and an empirical global power of 0.832 which are close to the nominal $\alpha = 0.05$ and $1 - \beta = 0.8$, respectively, from a simulation with $B = N = 1,000$.

## 12.4 Concluding Remarks

Microarray has been a major high-throughput assay method to display DNA or RNA abundance for a large number of genes concurrently. Discovery of the prognostic genes should be made taking multiplicity into account, but also with enough statistical power to identify important genes successfully. Due to the costly nature of microarray experiments, however, often only a small sample size is available and the resulting data analysis does

## 12.4. Concluding Remarks

not give reliable answers to the investigators. If the findings from a small study look promising, a large scale study may be developed to confirm the findings using appropriate statistical tools. As a result, sample size calculation plays an important role in the design stage of such a confirmatory study. It can be used to check the statistical power, $r_1/m_1$, of a small scale pilot study as well.

In recent years, many researchers have proposed the new concepts for controlling errors such as $FDR$ and positive-$FDR$ (i.e., $pFDR$), which control the expected proportion of type I error among the rejected hypotheses (Benjamini and Hochberg, 1995; Storey, 2002). Controlling these quantities relaxes the multiple testing criteria compared to controlling $FWER$ in general and increase the number of declared significant genes. In particular, $pFDR$ is motivated by Bayesian perspective and inherits the idea of single-step in constructing $q$-values, which are the counterpart of the adjusted $p$-values in this case (Ge et al., 2003). In practice, it is of interest to compare sample sizes obtained using the methods for controlling $FDR$, $pFDR$ and $FWER$. $FWER$ is important as a benchmark because the re-examination of Golub et al.'s data reveals that classical FWER control (along with global power) may not necessarily be as exceedingly conservative as many researchers thought and carries clear conceptual and practical interpretations.

The formula and/or procedure for the $FDR$ approach described in this chapter is to calculate the sample size for a specified number of true rejections (or the expected number of true rejections given a sample size) while controlling the $FDR$ at a given level. The input variables to be pre-specified are total number of genes for testing $m$, projected number of prognostic genes $m_1$, allocation proportions $a_k$ between groups, and effect sizes for the prognostic genes. When the effect sizes among the prognostic genes are the same, a closed form formula for sample size calculation is available.

It should be noted that although there are many research publications on sample size estimation in the microarray context, none examined the accuracy of their estimates. Most of them focused on exploratory and approximate relationships among statistical power, sample size (or the number of replicates) and effect size (often, in terms of fold-change), and used the most conservative Bonferroni adjustment without any attempt to incorporate underlying correlation structure (Witte, Elston and Cardon, 2000; Wolfinger et al., 2001; Black and Doerge, 2002; Lee and Whitmore, 2002; Pan et al., 2002; Simon, Radmacher and Dobbin, 2002; Cui and Churchill, 2003). By comparing empirical power resulting from naive and modified methods, Jung, Bang, and Young (2005) showed that an ostensibly similar but incorrect choice of sample size ascertainment could cause considerable underestimation of required sample size. Thus. Jung, Bang, and Young recommended that the assessment of bias in empirical power (compared to nominal power) should be done as a conventional step in the research of sample size calculation.

# Chapter 13

# Bayesian Sample Size Calculation

During the past decade, the approach for sample size determination originating from Bayesian's point of view has received much attention from academia, industry, and government. Although there are still debates between frequentist and Bayesian, Berger, Boukai and Wang (1997, 1999) have successfully reconciled the merits from both frequentist and Bayesian approaches. However, no specific discussions regarding sample size determination for clinical trials at the planning stage are provided from Bayesian's point of view. Their work has stimulated research on sample size calculation using Bayesian's approach thereafter. The increasing popularity of sample size calculation using Bayesian's approach may be due to the following reason. The traditional sample size calculation based on the concept of frequencist assumes that the values of the true parameters under the alternative hypothesis are known. This is a strong assumption that can never be true in reality. In practice, these parameters are usually unknown and hence have to be estimated based on limited data from a pilot study. This raises an important question: how to control the uncertainty of the parameter from the pilot study (Wang, Chow, and Chen, 2005). Note that the relatively small pilot study may not be the only source of the parameter uncertainty. In some situations, the magnitude of the non-centrality parameter may be obtained simply from subjective clinical opinions (Spiegelhalter and Freedman, 1986). In such a situation, the true parameter specification uncertainty seems to be even severe. Some related works can be found in Joseph and Bélisle (1997), Joseph, Wolfson and du Berger (1995), Lindley (1997), and Pham-Gia (1997).

Many other researchers (e.g., Lee and Zelen, 2000) questioned the basic (frequentist) testing approach, which has been widely used in practice. More specifically, they argued that instead of using the frequentist type I and type II error rates for determining the needed sample size, it is more appropriate to use the posterior error rates from Bayesian's perspective. In other words, the Bayesian's approach concerns "If the trial is significant, what is the probability that the treatment is effective?" It has been argued that by ignoring these fundamental considerations, the frequentist's approach may result in positive harm due to inappropriate use of the error rates (Lee and Zelen, 2000). In this chapter, we summarize current Bayesian's sample size calculations into two categories. One category considers making use of Bayesian's framework to reflect investigator's belief regarding the uncertainty of the true parameters, while the traditional frequentist's testing procedure is still used for analyzing the data. The other category considers determining the required sample size when a Bayesian's testing procedure is used. We consider both categories important and useful methodologies for biopharmaceutical research and development. Hence, in this chapter, we will focus on research work done in these categories. On the other hand, we do believe the effort done thus far is far less than enough for providing a comprehensive overview of Bayesian's sample size calculations. Therefore, practice issues and possible future research topics will also be discussed whenever possible.

In the next section, we introduce the procedure proposed by Joseph and Bélisle (1997). In Section 13.2, the important work by Lee and Zelen (2000) is summarized. Lee and Zelen (2000) proposed a procedure for sample size calculation based on the concept for achieving a desired posterior error probability. The method is simple and yet very general. In Section 13.3, an alternative approach, which is referred to as the bootstrap-median approach, is proposed. This chapter is concluded with a brief discussion, where some practical issues and possible future research topics are briefly outlined.

## 13.1 Posterior Credible Interval Approach

In their early work, Joseph and Bélisle (1997) had studied the procedure for sample size calculation from Bayesian's point of view. As it can be seen from Chapter 3, for a one-sample two-sided hypotheses, the sample size needed to achieve the error rate of $(\alpha, \beta)$ is given by

$$n \geq \frac{4\sigma^2 z_{1-\alpha/2}}{l^2}. \tag{13.1.1}$$

Joseph and Bélisle (1997) indicated that such a commonly used (frequentist) formula may suffer the following drawbacks:

## 13.1. Posterior Credible Interval Approach

(1). The value of the standard deviation $\sigma$ is usually unknown and yet it plays a critical role in determination of the final sample size. Consequently, the resultant sample size estimate could be very sensitive to the choice of $\sigma$ value.

(2). In practice, statistical inference is made based on the observed data at the end of the study regardless of the unknown $\sigma$ value in 13.1.1. At the planning stage, the investigator will have to determine the sample size with many uncertainties such as the unknown $\sigma$ and the final observed data.

(3). In some situations, prior information regarding the mean difference $\epsilon$ may be available. Ignoring this important prior information may lead to an unnecessarily large sample size, which could be a huge waste of the limited resources.

In order to overcome the above-mentioned limitations, Joseph and Bélisle (1997) provided three elegant solutions from Bayesian's perspective. Specifically, three different criteria are proposed for sample size estimation. They are (i) the *average coverage criterion*, (ii) *average length criterion*, and (iii) *worst outcome criterion*, which will be discussed in details in the following sections.

### 13.1.1 Three Selection Criteria

Under the Bayesian framework, let $\theta \in \Theta$ denote a generic parameter and its associated parameter space. Then, prior information regarding the value of $\theta$ is described by a prior distribution $f(\theta)$. Consider $x = (x_1, \cdots, x_n)$ a generic data set with $n$ independent and identically distributed random observations. It is assumed that $x \in \mathcal{S}$, where $\mathcal{S}$ is the associated sample space. Then, the marginal distribution of $x$ is given by

$$f(x) = \int_{\Theta} f(x|\theta) f(\theta) d\theta,$$

where $f(x|\theta)$ denote the conditional distribution of $x$ given the parameter $\theta$. Then, the posterior distribution of $\theta$ given $x$ is given by

$$f(\theta|x) = \frac{f(x|\theta) f(\theta)}{f(x)}.$$

Based on the above Bayesian framework, the following three criteria can be used to select the optimal sample size.

## Average Coverage Criterion

Consider the situation where a fixed posterior interval length $l$ is pre-specified for an acceptable precision of an estimate. Thus, the concept of the *average coverage criterion* (ACC) is to select the minimum sample size $n$ such that the average coverage probability of such an interval is at least $(1 - \alpha)$, where $\alpha$ is a pre-specified level of significance. More specifically, ACC selects the minimum sample size by solving the following inequality

$$\int_{\mathcal{S}} \left\{ \int_{a}^{a+l} f(\theta|x,n)d\theta \right\} f(x)dx \geq 1 - \alpha,$$

where $a$ is some statistic to be determined by the data. Adcock (1988) first proposed to choose the interval $(a, a+l)$ so that it is symmetric about the mean. On the other hand, Joseph, et al. (1995) proposed to select $(a, a+l)$ to be a highest posterior density interval. Note that for a symmetric distribution like normal, both methods of Adcock (1988) and Joseph, et al. (1995) lead to the same solution. However, for a general asymmetric distribution, the two methods may lead to different results.

## Average Length Criterion

Note that the ACC criterion fixed the posterior credible interval length $l$ but optimize the sample size to achieve a desired coverage probability at the level of $(1 - \alpha)$. Following an idea similar to ACC, another possible solution is to fix the coverage probability of the posterior credible interval, then select the sample size so that the resulting posterior credible interval has a desired length $l$ on average. Such a sample size selection criterion is referred to as *average length criterion* (ALC). More specifically, ALC select the smallest sample size so that

$$\int_{\mathcal{S}} l'(x,n)f(x)dx \leq l,$$

where $l'(x,n)$ is the length of the $100(1-\alpha)\%$ posterior credible interval for data x, which determined by solving

$$\int_{a}^{a+l'(x,n)} f(\theta|x,n)d\theta = 1 - \alpha.$$

As before, different methods exist for the selection of $a$. For example, $a$ can be chosen to be the highest posterior density interval or some meaningful symmetric intervals.

## 13.1. Posterior Credible Interval Approach

**Worst Outcome Criterion**

In practice, the investigators may not be satisfied with the average based criterion due to its conservativeness. For example, the sample size selected by the ALC only ensures that the *average* of the posterior credible interval length will be no larger than $l$. On the other hand, one may wish to select a sample size such that the expected posterior credible interval length is as close to $l$ as possible. Thus, we may expect about a 50% chance that the resultant interval length is larger than $l$, which may not be desirable due to its conservativeness.

In this situation, the following *worst outcome criterion* (WOC) may be useful. More specifically, WOC selects the smallest sample size by solving the following inequality

$$\inf_{x \in \mathcal{S}_0} \left\{ \int_a^{a+l(x,n)} f(\theta|x,n) d\theta \right\} \geq 1 - \alpha,$$

where $\mathcal{S}_0$ is an appropriately selected subset of the original sample space $\mathcal{S}$. For example, we may consider $\mathcal{S}_0$ to be a region contains 95% of the sample $\mathcal{S}$. Then, WOC ensures that the length of the posterior credible length will be at most $l$ for any possible $x \in \mathcal{S}_0$.

### 13.1.2 One Sample

We first consider a one-sample problem. Let $x = (x_1, \ldots, x_n)$ be $n$ independent and identically distributed observations from $N(\mu, \sigma^2)$, where both $\mu$ and $\sigma^2 > 0$ are unknown parameters. Furthermore, we define precision $\lambda = \sigma^{-2}$, then we are able to utilize the following conjugate prior

$$\lambda \sim \Gamma(v, \beta)$$
$$\mu|\lambda \sim N(\mu_0, n_0 \lambda),$$

where $\mu_0$ and $n_0$ are hyperparameters. For a more detailed discussion for many standard Bayesian results used in this section, one may refer to Bernardo and Smith (1994).

**Known Precision**

When $\lambda$ is known, it can be shown that the posterior distribution of $\mu$ given $x$ is $N(\mu_n, \lambda_n)$, where

$$\lambda_n = (n + n_0)\lambda$$
$$\mu_n = \frac{n_0 \mu_0 + n\bar{x}}{n_0 + n},$$

where $\bar{x}$ is the usual sample mean. Note that the posterior precision depends only on the sample size $n$ and is independent of the value of the observed $x$. Consequently, all three criteria (ACC, ALC and WOC) lead to the same solution, which is also equivalent to that of Adcock (1988):

$$n \geq \frac{4z_{1-\alpha/2}^2}{\lambda l^2} - n_0. \qquad (13.1.2)$$

Note that if a non-informative prior with $n_0 = 0$ is used, then the above formula reduces to the usual formula for sample size calculation. Furthermore, by comparing (13.1.2) with (13.1.1), it can be seen that the sample size obtained from the Bayesian's approach is smaller than that of the traditional frequentist estimate by a number $n_0$. This simply reflects the effect of the usefulness of the prior information.

**Unknown Precision**

If the precision parameter $\lambda$ is unknown, then the posterior distribution of $\mu$ given the observed $x$ is given by

$$\mu|x \sim t_{2v+n}\sqrt{\frac{\beta_n}{(n+n_0)(v+n/s)}} + \mu_n,$$

where

$$\mu_n = \frac{n_0\mu_0 + n\bar{x}}{n + n_0},$$
$$\beta_n = \beta + \frac{1}{2}ns^2 + \frac{nn_0}{2(n+n_0)}(\bar{x} - \mu_0)^2,$$

where $s^2 = n^{-1}\sum(x_i - \bar{x})^2$ and $t_d$ represents a $t$-distribution with $d$ degrees of freedom. As it can be seen, for such a situation, the posterior precision varies with the value of $x$. Hence, different selection criteria will lead to different sample size estimations.

(1) *Average Coverage Criterion.* Adock (1988) showed that the ACC sample size can be obtained as follows

$$n = \frac{4\beta}{vl^2}t_{2v,1-\alpha/2}^2 - n_0.$$

Note that the above formula is very similar to (13.1.2) in the sense that (i) the precision $\lambda$ is replaced by the mean precision $v/\beta$ as specified in the prior, and (ii) the normal quantile is replaced by an appropriate $t$-quantile. However, it should be noted that the degrees of freedom used in the $t$-quantile does not increase as the sample size increases. Consequently, the resultant sample size could be very different from the frequentist estimator (13.1.1).

## 13.1. Posterior Credible Interval Approach

(2) *Average Length Criterion.* Consider the same Bayesian set up as for ACC. Then, the minimum sample size selected by ALC can be obtained by solving the following inequality

$$2t_{n+2v,1-\alpha/2}\sqrt{\frac{2\beta}{(n+2v)(n+n_0)}}\frac{\Gamma\left(\frac{n+2v}{2}\right)\Gamma\left(\frac{2v-1}{2}\right)}{\Gamma\left(\frac{n+2v-1}{2}\right)\Gamma(v)} \leq l. \quad (13.1.3)$$

Unfortunately, there exists no explicit solution for the above inequality. Since the left hand side can be calculated with a given sample size $n$, a bisectional searching algorithm could be useful in finding the optimal sample size. However, in the case where the sample size $n$ is large, the numerical evaluation of $\Gamma(0.5n+v)$ and $\Gamma(0.5n+v-0.5)$ could be very unstable. According to Graham *et. al.* (1994, Math-World), we have

$$\frac{\Gamma\left(\frac{n+2v}{2}\right)}{\Gamma\left(\frac{n+2v-1}{2}\right)} = \sqrt{0.5n}\{1+o(1)\}.$$

Then, the inequality (13.1.3) can be approximated by the following

$$\sqrt{2n}t_{n+2v,1-\alpha/2}\sqrt{\frac{2\beta}{(n+2v)(n+n_0)}}\frac{\Gamma\left(\frac{2v-1}{2}\right)}{\Gamma(v)} \leq l. \quad (13.1.4)$$

Note that the above formula (13.1.4) does provide an adequate approximation to (13.1.3).

(3) *Worst Outcome Criterion.* Let $\mathcal{S}_0 \subset \mathcal{S}$ be the subset of the sample space such that

$$\int_{\mathcal{S}_0} f(x)dx = 1 - w,$$

for some probability $w > 0$. Also, assume that $f(x) \geq f(y)$ for any $x \in \mathcal{S}$ and $y \notin \mathcal{S}$. Thus, the sample size needed can be approximated by

$$\frac{l^2(n+2v)(n+n_0)}{8\beta\{1+(n/2v)F_{n,2v,1-w}\}} \geq t^2_{n+2v,1-\alpha/2},$$

where $F_{d_1,d_2,1-\alpha}$ is the $(1-\alpha)$th quantile of the $F$-distribution with $(d_1, d_2)$ degrees of freedom. Note that the subsample space $\mathcal{S}_0$ cannot be exactly the same as $\mathcal{S}$. In this case, we have $w = 0$, hence $F_{n,2v,1-w} = \infty$. As a result, the sample size is not well defined.

Table 13.1.1: One-Sample Sample Sizes with Unknown Precision and $v = 2$

| $\beta$ | $n_0$ | $l$ | $\alpha$ | FREQ | ACC | ALC | WOC(90%) | WOC(95%) |
|---|---|---|---|---|---|---|---|---|
| 2 | 10 | 0.2 | 0.20 | 165 | 226 | 247 | 608 | 915 |
|   |    |     | 0.10 | 271 | 445 | 414 | 1008 | 1513 |
|   |    |     | 0.05 | 385 | 761 | 593 | 1436 | 2153 |
|   |    |     | 0.01 | 664 | 2110 | 1034 | 2488 | 3727 |
|   |    | 0.5 | 0.20 | 27 | 28 | 2 | 89 | 138 |
|   |    |     | 0.10 | 44 | 63 | 57 | 154 | 234 |
|   |    |     | 0.05 | 62 | 114 | 86 | 223 | 337 |
|   |    |     | 0.01 | 107 | 330 | 158 | 392 | 590 |
|   | 50 | 0.2 | 0.20 | 165 | 186 | 206 | 568 | 874 |
|   |    |     | 0.10 | 271 | 405 | 374 | 968 | 1473 |
|   |    |     | 0.05 | 385 | 721 | 553 | 1396 | 2113 |
|   |    |     | 0.01 | 664 | 2070 | 994 | 2448 | 3687 |
|   |    | 0.5 | 0.20 | 27 | 0 | 2 | 48 | 97 |
|   |    |     | 0.10 | 44 | 23 | 2 | 113 | 194 |
|   |    |     | 0.05 | 62 | 74 | 2 | 183 | 297 |
|   |    |     | 0.01 | 107 | 290 | 118 | 352 | 550 |
| 5 | 10 | 0.2 | 0.20 | 165 | 578 | 634 | 1534 | 2301 |
|   |    |     | 0.10 | 271 | 1127 | 1052 | 2535 | 3797 |
|   |    |     | 0.05 | 385 | 1918 | 1498 | 3603 | 5396 |
|   |    |     | 0.01 | 664 | 5290 | 2597 | 6231 | 9328 |
|   |    | 0.5 | 0.20 | 27 | 85 | 92 | 237 | 360 |
|   |    |     | 0.10 | 44 | 172 | 159 | 398 | 600 |
|   |    |     | 0.05 | 62 | 299 | 231 | 569 | 856 |
|   |    |     | 0.01 | 107 | 838 | 408 | 991 | 1486 |
|   | 50 | 0.2 | 0.20 | 165 | 538 | 594 | 1494 | 2261 |
|   |    |     | 0.10 | 271 | 1087 | 1012 | 2495 | 3757 |
|   |    |     | 0.05 | 385 | 1878 | 1458 | 3563 | 5356 |
|   |    |     | 0.01 | 664 | 5250 | 2557 | 6191 | 9288 |
|   |    | 0.5 | 0.20 | 27 | 45 | 2 | 197 | 320 |
|   |    |     | 0.10 | 44 | 132 | 118 | 358 | 560 |
|   |    |     | 0.05 | 62 | 259 | 191 | 529 | 816 |
|   |    |     | 0.01 | 107 | 798 | 368 | 951 | 1446 |

## 13.1. Posterior Credible Interval Approach

Table 13.1.2: One-Sample Sample Sizes with Unknown Precision and $v = 5$

| $\beta$ | $n_0$ | $l$ | $\alpha$ | FREQ | ACC | ALC | WOC(90%) | WOC(95%) |
|---|---|---|---|---|---|---|---|---|
| 2 | 10 | 0.2 | 0.20 | 165 | 66 | 2 | 124 | 155 |
|   |    |     | 0.10 | 271 | 122 | 110 | 212 | 264 |
|   |    |     | 0.05 | 385 | 189 | 164 | 306 | 380 |
|   |    |     | 0.01 | 664 | 392 | 297 | 537 | 665 |
|   |    | 0.5 | 0.20 | 27 | 3 | 2 | 10 | 15 |
|   |    |     | 0.10 | 44 | 12 | 2 | 25 | 33 |
|   |    |     | 0.05 | 62 | 22 | 2 | 41 | 52 |
|   |    |     | 0.01 | 107 | 55 | 2 | 79 | 99 |
|   | 50 | 0.2 | 0.20 | 165 | 26 | 2 | 83 | 114 |
|   |    |     | 0.10 | 271 | 82 | 2 | 172 | 224 |
|   |    |     | 0.05 | 385 | 149 | 2 | 266 | 340 |
|   |    |     | 0.01 | 664 | 352 | 2 | 497 | 625 |
|   |    | 0.5 | 0.20 | 27 | 0 | 2 | 2 | 2 |
|   |    |     | 0.10 | 44 | 0 | 2 | 2 | 2 |
|   |    |     | 0.05 | 62 | 0 | 2 | 2 | 2 |
|   |    |     | 0.01 | 107 | 15 | 2 | 39 | 59 |
| 5 | 10 | 0.2 | 0.20 | 165 | 179 | 175 | 327 | 406 |
|   |    |     | 0.10 | 271 | 319 | 301 | 546 | 676 |
|   |    |     | 0.05 | 385 | 487 | 435 | 780 | 965 |
|   |    |     | 0.01 | 664 | 995 | 764 | 1355 | 1675 |
|   |    | 0.5 | 0.20 | 27 | 21 | 2 | 43 | 55 |
|   |    |     | 0.10 | 44 | 43 | 2 | 79 | 99 |
|   |    |     | 0.05 | 62 | 70 | 2 | 117 | 146 |
|   |    |     | 0.01 | 107 | 151 | 109 | 210 | 261 |
|   | 50 | 0.2 | 0.20 | 165 | 139 | 2 | 286 | 365 |
|   |    |     | 0.10 | 271 | 279 | 2 | 506 | 636 |
|   |    |     | 0.05 | 385 | 447 | 394 | 740 | 925 |
|   |    |     | 0.01 | 664 | 955 | 724 | 1316 | 1635 |
|   |    | 0.5 | 0.20 | 27 | 0 | 2 | 2 | 2 |
|   |    |     | 0.10 | 44 | 3 | 2 | 37 | 57 |
|   |    |     | 0.05 | 62 | 30 | 2 | 76 | 105 |
|   |    |     | 0.01 | 107 | 111 | 2 | 170 | 221 |

## Mixed Bayesian Likelihood

In practice, although many investigators may acknowledge the usefulness and importance of the prior information, they will still make final inference based on the likelihood of the data. For example, the investigator may want to report the 95% confidence interval in the final analysis. In such a situation, the sample size needed by ACC can also be found based on the 95% confidence interval. Consider the case where the confidence interval is symmetric about $\bar{x}$. It follows that

$$(a, a+l) = (\bar{x} - l/2, \bar{x} + l/2)$$

$$\mu|x \sim \bar{x} + t_{n-1}\sqrt{\frac{ns^2}{n(n-1)}}$$

$$\int_{\bar{x}-l/2}^{\bar{x}+l/2} f(\mu|x)d\mu = 2p_t\left(\frac{l}{2}\sqrt{\frac{n(n-1)}{ns^2}}, n-1\right),$$

where $p_t(c, d)$ is the area between 0 and $c$ under a $t$-density with $d$ degrees of freedom. Note that the area only depends on the data via $ns^2$. Hence, the following algorithm can be used to obtain an approximate solution

(a) Select an initial estimate of the sample size $n$.

(b) Generate $m$ values of the random variables $ns^2$. Note that $ns^2|\lambda \sim \Gamma((n-1)/2, \lambda/2)$ and $\lambda$ from $\Gamma(v, \beta)$. Then, marginally $ns^2$ follows a gamma-gamma distribution with parameter $(v, 2\beta, (n-1)/2)$. Note that a random variable $x$ follows a gamma-gamma distribution if its density is given by

$$f(x|v, \beta, n) = \frac{\Gamma(v+n)\beta^v}{\Gamma(v)\Gamma(n)} \frac{x^{n-1}}{(\beta+x)^{v+n}}$$

for $x > 0$, $v > 0$, $\beta > 0$, and $n > 0$. For more details, one can refer to Bernardo and Smith (1994), p.p., 430.

(c) For each of the $m$ values of $ns_i^2$, $i = 1, 2, \cdots, m$ in step (b), calculate

$$\text{coverage}(ns_i^2) = 2p_i\left(\frac{l}{2}\sqrt{\frac{n(n-1)}{ns_i^2}}, n-1\right).$$

(d) Then, compute

$$\frac{1}{m}\sum_{i=1}^{m} \text{coverage}(ns_i^2)$$

as an approximate to the average coverage probability.

## 13.1. Posterior Credible Interval Approach

Repeating steps (b)-(d) for values of $n$ in conjunction with a bisectional search procedure will lead to an approximate sample size.

Similarly, the WOC sample size can be obtained by solving the following inequality

$$2p_t\left(\frac{l}{2}\sqrt{\frac{n(n-1)}{ns_i^2}}, n-1\right) \geq 1-\alpha$$

for about 95% or 99% (for example) of the $ns_i^2$ values with a fixed sample size $n$. On the other hand, the sample size needed by ALC is given by

$$2t_{n-1,1-\alpha/2}\sqrt{\frac{2\beta}{n(n-1)}}\frac{\Gamma(0.5n)}{\Gamma(0.5n-0.5)}\frac{\Gamma(v-0.5)}{\Gamma(v)} \leq l.$$

Therefore, finding the smallest sample size $n$ satisfying the above inequality provides an estimate for the sample size selected by ALC.

### 13.1.3 Two-Sample with Common Precision

Similarly, we can apply the idea of ACC, ALC, and WOC to the most commonly used two-arm parallel-group design. More specifically, let $x_1 = (x_{11}, \cdots, x_{n_1 1})$ and $x_2 = (x_{12}, \cdots, x_{n_2 2})$ be two independent sample obtained under two different treatments. Furthermore, it is assumed that $x_{ij}, i = 1, \cdots, n_j$ are independent and identically distributed normal random variables with mean $\mu_j$ and a common precision $\lambda$ within each treatment. Similar to the one-sample problem, we assume a conjugate prior distribution for the common precision, i.e.,

$$\lambda \sim \Gamma(v, \beta),$$

for some $v$ and $\beta$. That is, given $\lambda$, it is assumed that

$$\mu_j|\lambda \sim N(\mu_{0j}, n_{0j}\lambda) \text{ with } j = 1, 2.$$

Then, by treating the mean treatment difference $\theta = \mu_1 - \mu_2$ as the parameter of the interest, the methods of ACC, ALC, and WOC can be carried out in a similar manner as in the one-sample situation.

**Known Common Precision**

If the common precision $\lambda$ is known, then by conditioning on the observed data $x_1$ and $x_2$, the posterior distribution of the treatment difference $\theta$ is given by

$$\theta|x_1, x_2 \sim N\left\{\mu_{n_2 2} - \mu_{n_1 1}, \frac{\lambda(n_{01}+n_1)(n_{02}+n_2)}{n_1+n_2+n_{01}+n_{02}}\right\}, \quad (13.1.5)$$

where
$$\mu_{n_j j} = \frac{n_{0j}\mu_{0j} + n_j \bar{x}_j}{n_{0j} + n_j}, \quad j = 1, 2.$$

As it can be seen, the posterior variance of $\theta$ only depends on the data via the sample size $n_1$ and $n_2$. This situation is very similar to the one-sample case with known precision. Consequently, all of the three methods (i.e., ACC, ALC, and WOC) can be applied to obtain the desired sample size. For the case with equal sample size allocation (i.e., $n_1 = n_2$), the smallest sample size can be estimated by

$$n_1 = n_2 \geq \frac{-B + \sqrt{B^2 - 4AC}}{2A}, \tag{13.1.6}$$

where $A = \lambda^2$ and

$$B = \lambda^2(n_{01} + n_{02}) - 28z_{1-\alpha/2}^2/l^2$$
$$C = n_{01}n_{02}\lambda^2 - \frac{4(n_{01} + n_{02})\lambda z_{1-\alpha/2}^2}{l^2}.$$

In practice, it happens that $B^2 - 4AC \leq 0$, which implies that the prior information is sufficient and no additional sampling is needed.

As it can be seen from (13.1.5), if we fix the total information $n_1 + n_{01} + n_2 + n_{02}$, then the optimal sample size allocation, which can minimize the posterior variance, is given by $n_1 + n_{01} = n_2 + n_{02}$. In such a situation, the minimum sample size can be obtained by solving the following inequality

$$n_1 \geq \frac{8}{\lambda l^2} z_{1-\alpha/2}^2 - n_{01}, \tag{13.1.7}$$

with $n_2 = n_1 + n_{01} - n_{02}$. If $n_{01} = n_{02}$, then the sample size estimated by (13.1.6) and (13.1.7) reduce to the sample quantity.

**Unknown Common Precision**

In the situation where the two treatment groups share the same but unknown precision, the posterior distribution of $\theta$ can be derived based on the normal-gamma prior family as described above. More specifically,

$$\theta | x_1, x_2 \sim A + t_{2C}\sqrt{\frac{B}{2CD}},$$

where
$$A = E(\theta | x_1, x_2) = \frac{n_2 \bar{x}_2 + n_{02}\mu_{02}}{n_2 + n_{02}} = \frac{n_1 \bar{x}_1 + n_{01}\mu_{01}}{n_1 + n_{01}},$$
$$B = 2\beta + n_1 s_1^2 + n_2 s_2^2 + \frac{n_1 n_{01}}{n_1 + n_{01}}(\bar{x}_1 - \mu_{01})^2 + \frac{n_2 n_{02}}{n_2 + n_{02}}(\bar{x}_2 - \mu_{02})^2,$$

## 13.1. Posterior Credible Interval Approach

$$C = \frac{n_1 + n_2}{2} + v \quad \text{and} \quad D = \frac{(n_1 + n_{01})(n_2 + n_{02})}{n_1 + n_{01} + n_2 + n_{02}}.$$

Based on such a posterior distribution, the method of ACC, ALC, and WOC can be easily implemented, which are outlined below.

*Average Coverage Criterion.* As it has been shown by Joseph and Bélisle (1997), the sample size needed must satisfy the following inequality

$$\frac{(n_1 + n_{01})(n_2 + n_{02})}{n_1 + n_2 + n_{01} + n_{02}} \geq \frac{4\beta}{vl^2} t_{2v,1-\alpha/2}^2.$$

The above inequality can have an explicit solution if we adopt an equal sample size allocation strategy (i.e., $n_1 = n_2 = n$). In such a situation, the optimal sample size is given by

$$n \geq \frac{-B + \sqrt{B^2 - 4AC}}{2A},$$

where

$$A = \frac{vl^2}{4},$$

$$B = \frac{vl^2}{4}(n_{01} + n_{02}) - 2\beta t_{2v,1-\alpha/2}^2,$$

$$C = \frac{n_{01} n_{02} vl^2}{4} - \beta t_{2v,1-\alpha/2}^2 (n_{01} + n_{02}).$$

In the case where unequal sample allocation is allowed, how to minimize the expected posterior variance would be a reasonable criterion for an effective allocation of the sample sizes between treatment groups. Note that

$$\bar{x}_i \sim \mu_{0i} + t_{2v_i} \sqrt{\frac{\beta_i(n_i + n_{0i})}{v_i n_i n_{0i}}},$$

$$n_i s_i^2 \sim \Gamma - \Gamma\left(v_i, 2\beta_i, \frac{n_i - 1}{2}\right).$$

It can be verified that the expected variance of $\theta$ given the data is given by

$$\frac{1}{(n_1 + n_{01})(n_2 + n_{02})} \frac{n_1 + n_2 + n_{01} + n_{02}}{n_1 + n_2 + 2v - 2}$$

$$\times \left\{2\beta + \frac{(n_1 + n_2 - 2)\Gamma(v-1)}{\Gamma(v)} + \frac{2\beta}{v-1}\right\},$$

which implies that for a fixed total sample size $n_1 + n_2$, the minimum expected posterior variance is achieved if $n_1 + n_{01} = n_2 + n_{02}$.

*Average Length Criterion.* Similarly, the sample size selected by ALC can be obtained by solving the following inequality

$$2t_{n_1+n_2+2v,1-\alpha/2}\sqrt{\frac{2\beta(n_1+n_{01}+n_2+n_{02})}{(n_1+n_2+2v)(n_1+n_{01})(n_2+n_{02})}}$$

$$\times \frac{\Gamma\left(\frac{n_1+n_2+2v}{2}\right)\Gamma\left(\frac{2v-1}{2}\right)}{\Gamma\left(\frac{n_1+n_2+2v-1}{2}\right)\gamma\left(\frac{2v}{2}\right)} \leq 1.$$

In order to solve the above inequality, the standard bisectional search can be used. For unequal sample size situation, the constraint $n_1 + n_{10} = n_2 + n_{20}$ can be used.

*Worst Outcome Criterion.* The WOC selects the sample size $n_1$ and $n_2$ according to the following inequality

$$\frac{l^2(n_1+n_{01})(n_2+n_{02})}{8\beta(n_1+n_{01}+n_2+n_{02})}\frac{n_1+n_2+2v}{1+\{(n_1+n_2)/2v\}F_{n_1+n_2,2v,1-w}}$$

$$\geq t^2_{n_1+n_2+2v,1-\alpha/2}.$$

Again the simple bisectional search algorithm can be used to find the solution effectively.

*Mixed Bayesian-Likelihood.* For the mixed Bayesian-Likelihood method, there exists no exact solution. Therefore, appropriate simulation method has to be employed to estimate the desired sample size. Simply speaking, one can first generate $(\bar{x}_1, \bar{x}_2, n_1 s_1^2, n_2 s_2^2)$ vectors, then ACC, ALC, and WOC can be estimated via a standard bisectional search algorithm. Then, by averaging these estimated sample sizes or taking appropriate infimum, the desired sample size can be obtained. For a more detailed discussion, one can refer to Section 4.3 of Joseph and Bélisle (1997).

## 13.1.4 Two-Sample with Unequal Precisions

In this subsection, we consider the problem of two samples with unequal precisions. Similarly, we denote $x_1 = (x_{11}, \cdots, x_{n_1 1})$ and $x_2 = (x_{21}, \cdots, x_{n_2 1})$ independent samples obtained from the two different treatments. Furthermore, it is assumed that within each treatment group, the observation $x_{ij}$ is independent and identically distributed as a normal random variable with mean $\mu_j$ and precision $\lambda_j$. Once again the normal-gamma prior is used to reflect the prior information about the mean and the variance, i.e.,

$$\lambda_j \sim \Gamma(v_j, \beta_j)$$
$$\mu_j | \lambda_j \sim N(\mu_{0j}, n_{0j}\lambda_j).$$

## 13.1. Posterior Credible Interval Approach

Table 13.1.3: Two-Sample Sample Sizes with Unknown Common Precision ($n = n_1 = n_2$, $n_0 = n_{01} = n_{02}$, and $v = 2$)

| $\beta$ | $n_0$ | $l$ | $\alpha$ | FREQ | ACC | ALC | WOC(90%) | WOC(95%) |
|---|---|---|---|---|---|---|---|---|
| 2 | 10 | 0.2 | 0.20 | 329 | 461 | 506 | 1226 | 1840 |
|   |    |     | 0.10 | 542 | 899 | 840 | 2026 | 3037 |
|   |    |     | 0.05 | 769 | 1532 | 1198 | 2881 | 4315 |
|   |    |     | 0.01 | 1327 | 4230 | 2076 | 4983 | 7460 |
|   |    | 0.5 | 0.20 | 53 | 66 | 73 | 189 | 287 |
|   |    |     | 0.10 | 87 | 136 | 126 | 317 | 478 |
|   |    |     | 0.05 | 123 | 237 | 184 | 454 | 683 |
|   |    |     | 0.01 | 213 | 669 | 325 | 791 | 1187 |
|   | 50 | 0.2 | 0.20 | 329 | 421 | 466 | 1186 | 1800 |
|   |    |     | 0.10 | 542 | 859 | 800 | 1986 | 2996 |
|   |    |     | 0.05 | 769 | 1492 | 1158 | 2841 | 4275 |
|   |    |     | 0.01 | 1327 | 4190 | 2036 | 4943 | 7420 |
|   |    | 0.5 | 0.20 | 53 | 26 | 2 | 148 | 246 |
|   |    |     | 0.10 | 87 | 96 | 86 | 277 | 438 |
|   |    |     | 0.05 | 123 | 197 | 144 | 414 | 643 |
|   |    |     | 0.01 | 213 | 629 | 285 | 751 | 1147 |
| 5 | 10 | 0.2 | 0.20 | 329 | 1166 | 1280 | 3079 | 4613 |
|   |    |     | 0.10 | 542 | 2263 | 2115 | 5079 | 7605 |
|   |    |     | 0.05 | 769 | 3845 | 3008 | 7215 | 10801 |
|   |    |     | 0.01 | 1327 | 10589 | 5202 | 12468 | 18663 |
|   |    | 0.5 | 0.20 | 53 | 179 | 196 | 485 | 730 |
|   |    |     | 0.10 | 87 | 354 | 330 | 805 | 1209 |
|   |    |     | 0.05 | 123 | 607 | 473 | 1147 | 1721 |
|   |    |     | 0.01 | 213 | 1686 | 825 | 1988 | 2979 |
|   | 50 | 0.2 | 0.20 | 329 | 1126 | 1240 | 3039 | 4573 |
|   |    |     | 0.10 | 542 | 2223 | 2075 | 5039 | 7565 |
|   |    |     | 0.05 | 769 | 3805 | 2968 | 7175 | 10761 |
|   |    |     | 0.01 | 1327 | 10549 | 5162 | 12428 | 18623 |
|   |    | 0.5 | 0.20 | 53 | 139 | 156 | 445 | 690 |
|   |    |     | 0.10 | 87 | 314 | 290 | 765 | 1169 |
|   |    |     | 0.05 | 123 | 567 | 433 | 1107 | 1681 |
|   |    |     | 0.01 | 213 | 1646 | 785 | 1948 | 2939 |

Table 13.1.4: Two-Sample Sample Sizes with Unknown Common Precision ($n = n_1 = n_2$, $n_0 = n_{01} = n_{02}$, and $v = 2$)

| $\beta$ | $n_0$ | $l$ | $\alpha$ | FREQ | ACC | ALC | WOC(90%) | WOC(95%) |
|---|---|---|---|---|---|---|---|---|
| 2 | 10 | 0.2 | 0.20 | 329 | 141 | 141 | 260 | 324 |
|   |    |     | 0.10 | 542 | 253 | 241 | 436 | 540 |
|   |    |     | 0.05 | 769 | 388 | 349 | 623 | 771 |
|   |    |     | 0.01 | 1327 | 794 | 612 | 1083 | 1338 |
|   |    | 0.5 | 0.20 | 53 | 15 | 2 | 33 | 43 |
|   |    |     | 0.10 | 87 | 33 | 2 | 62 | 78 |
|   |    |     | 0.05 | 123 | 54 | 45 | 92 | 115 |
|   |    |     | 0.01 | 213 | 119 | 88 | 166 | 207 |
|   | 50 | 0.2 | 0.20 | 329 | 101 | 2 | 220 | 283 |
|   |    |     | 0.10 | 542 | 213 | 2 | 395 | 500 |
|   |    |     | 0.05 | 769 | 348 | 308 | 583 | 731 |
|   |    |     | 0.01 | 1327 | 754 | 572 | 1043 | 1298 |
|   |    | 0.5 | 0.20 | 53 | 0 | 2 | 2 | 2 |
|   |    |     | 0.10 | 87 | 0 | 2 | 20 | 37 |
|   |    |     | 0.05 | 123 | 14 | 2 | 51 | 75 |
|   |    |     | 0.01 | 213 | 79 | 2 | 126 | 167 |
| 5 | 10 | 0.2 | 0.20 | 329 | 367 | 373 | 666 | 824 |
|   |    |     | 0.10 | 542 | 648 | 623 | 1103 | 1364 |
|   |    |     | 0.05 | 769 | 983 | 890 | 1570 | 1941 |
|   |    |     | 0.01 | 1327 | 1999 | 1547 | 2719 | 3359 |
|   |    | 0.5 | 0.20 | 53 | 51 | 48 | 98 | 123 |
|   |    |     | 0.10 | 87 | 96 | 89 | 169 | 210 |
|   |    |     | 0.05 | 123 | 149 | 132 | 244 | 303 |
|   |    |     | 0.01 | 213 | 312 | 238 | 428 | 530 |
|   | 50 | 0.2 | 0.20 | 329 | 327 | 332 | 625 | 784 |
|   |    |     | 0.10 | 542 | 608 | 583 | 1063 | 1324 |
|   |    |     | 0.05 | 769 | 943 | 850 | 1530 | 1901 |
|   |    |     | 0.01 | 1327 | 1959 | 1507 | 2679 | 3319 |
|   |    | 0.5 | 0.20 | 53 | 11 | 2 | 57 | 83 |
|   |    |     | 0.10 | 87 | 56 | 2 | 128 | 170 |
|   |    |     | 0.05 | 123 | 109 | 2 | 203 | 263 |
|   |    |     | 0.01 | 213 | 272 | 197 | 388 | 490 |

## 13.1. Posterior Credible Interval Approach

**Known Precision**

If the precisions $\lambda_1$ and $\lambda_2$ are known, then the posterior distribution of the treatment mean difference $\theta$ is given by

$$\theta | x_1, x_2 \sim N\left(\mu_{n_2 2} - \mu_{n_1 1}, \frac{\lambda_{n_1 1} \lambda_{n_2 2}}{\lambda_{n_1 1} + \lambda_{n_2 2}}\right),$$

where $\lambda_{ni} = \lambda_i (n_{0i} + n_i)$ and

$$\mu_{n_i i} = \frac{\lambda_i (n_{0i} \mu_{0i} + n_i \bar{x}_i)}{\lambda_{n_i i}} = \frac{n_{0i} \mu_{0i} + n_i \bar{x}_i}{n_{0i} + n_i}.$$

If we assume an equal sample size allocation (i.e., $n = n_1 = n_2$), then the sample sizes selected by ACC, ALC, and WOC are all given by

$$n \geq \frac{-B + \sqrt{B^2 - 4AC}}{2A},$$

where $A = \lambda_1 \lambda_2$ and

$$B = \lambda_1 n_{02} \lambda_2 + \lambda_2 n_{01} \lambda_1 - \frac{4 z_{1-\alpha/2}^2}{l^2} (\lambda_1 + \lambda_2),$$

$$C = n_{01} \lambda_1 n_{02} \lambda_2 - \frac{4 z_{1-\alpha/2}^2}{l^2} (n_{01} \lambda_1 + n_{02} \lambda_2).$$

If unequal sample size allocation is considered, then the optimal sample size is given by

$$n_1 + n_{01} \geq \frac{4}{l^2} z_{1-\alpha/2}^2 \left\{\frac{1}{\sqrt{\lambda_1 \lambda_2}} + \frac{1}{\lambda_1}\right\}$$

$$n_2 + n_{02} = \sqrt{\frac{\lambda_1}{\lambda_2}} (n_1 + n_{01}).$$

**Unknown Precisions**

When $\lambda_1 \neq \lambda_2$, the exact posterior distribution of $\theta$ could be complicated. It, however, can be approximated by

$$\theta | x_1, x_2 \approx N(\mu_{n1} - \mu_{n2}, \lambda^*),$$

where

$$\mu_{nj} = \frac{n_{0j} \mu_{0j} + n_j \bar{x}_j}{n_j + n_{0j}},$$

$$\lambda^* = \left\{\frac{2\beta_{n_1 1}}{(n_1 + n_{01})(2v_1 + n_1 - 2)} + \frac{2\beta_{n_2 2}}{(n_2 + n_{02})(2v_2 + n_2 - 2)}\right\}^{-1}.$$

Due to the fact that the posterior distribution of $\theta$ does not have a standard form, appropriate numerical methods are necessarily employed for obtaining the required sample size. In most applications, however, normal approximation usually provides adequate sample sizes. Note that

$$\bar{x}_j \sim \mu_{0j} + \sqrt{\frac{\beta_j(n_j + n_{0j})}{v_j n_j n_{0j}}} t_{2v_j}$$

$$n_j s_j^2 \sim \Gamma - \Gamma\left(v_j, 2\beta_j, \frac{n_j - 1}{2}\right),$$

which is minimized if and only if

$$n_2 + n_{02} = \sqrt{\frac{\beta_2(v_1 - 1)}{\beta_1(v_2 - 1)}}(n_1 + n_{01}).$$

As a result, the optimal sample size, which minimizes the posterior variance, can be obtained.

## 13.2 Posterior Error Approach

Recently, Lee and Zelen (2000) developed a simple and yet general Bayesian sample size determination theory. It is very similar but different from the traditional frequentist approach. More specifically, the traditional frequentist approach selects the minimum sample size so that the type I and type II error rates can be controlled at a pre-specified levels of significance, i.e., $\alpha$ and $\beta$. Lee and Zelen (2000), on the other hand, proposed to select the minimum sample size so that the posterior error rate is controlled. Consequently, it is essential to understand what is the posterior error rate and its relationship with the traditional type I and type II error rates. Under this framework, the Bayesian sample size calculation for comparing means and survival rates are illustrated.

### 13.2.1 Posterior Error Rate

Following the notations of Lee and Zelen (2000), Denote by $\delta$ the noncentrality parameter, which is usually a function of the clinically meaningful difference and the population standard deviation. From a traditional frequentist point of view, the objective of a clinical trial is to differentiate between the following two hypotheses

$$H_0 : \delta = 0 \text{ vs. } H_a : \delta \neq 0.$$

## 13.2. Posterior Error Approach

In order to utilize the Bayesian framework, we assign a non-degenerate probability $\theta > 0$ to the joint even $\delta > 0$ or $\delta < 0$. Then, the prior probability for the null hypothesis (i.e., no treatment effect) would be $(1-\theta)$ by definition.

Consequently, the parameter $\theta$ summarizes the prior confidence regarding which hypothesis is more likely to be true. When there is no clear preference between $H_0$ and $H_1$, $\theta = 0.5$ seems to be a reasonable choice. However, if one wishes to be more conservative in concluding the treatment effect, then one may consider a $\theta < 0.5$ (e.g., $\theta = 0.25$). Similarly, one may also use a $\theta > 0.5$ (e.g., $\theta = 0.75$) to reflect a better confidence about the treatment effect. Furthermore, equal probability $\theta/2$ is assigned to each possible alternative $\delta > 0$ and $\delta < 0$. The reason to assign equal probability to each possible alternative is that if the physician has prior belief that one treatment is better or worse than the other, then the physician cannot ethically enter the patient into the trial (Lee and Zelen, 2000). Consequently, it seems that equal probability $\theta/2$ for $\delta > 0$ and $\delta < 0$ is a natural choice.

To facilitate discussion, we further classify the outcomes of a clinical trial into positive or negative ones. A positive outcome refers to a clinical trial with conclusion $\delta \neq 0$, while a negative outcome refers to a trial with conclusion $\delta = 0$. For convenience purposes, we use a binary indicator $C = +$ or $C = -$ to represent positive or negative outcomes, respectively. On the other hand, we consider $T$ as a similar indicator but it refers to the true status of hypothesis. In other words, $T = +$ refers to the situation where the alternative hypothesis is actually true, while $T = -$ refers to the situation where the null hypothesis is in fact true. It follows immediately that $P(T = +) = \theta$.

For a pre-specified type I and type II error rates $\alpha$ and $\beta$, the traditional frequentist approach tries to find the minimum sample size so that

$$\alpha = P(C = +|T = -),$$
$$\beta = P(C = -|T = +).$$

Similarly, from a Bayesian perspective, Lee and Zelen (2000) suggest to find the minimum sample size so that the posterior error rates are controlled as

$$\alpha^* = P(T = -|C = +),$$
$$\beta^* = P(T = +|C = -).$$

Simply speaking, they are the posterior probabilities that the true situation is opposite to the outcome of the trial. As long as these posterior error rates are well controlled at given levels of $\alpha^*$ and $\beta^*$, we are able to accept any trial outcome (either positive or negative) at an acceptable confidence level.

The merit of Lee and Zelen's method is that their posterior error rates $\alpha^*$ and $\beta^*$ are closely related to the most commonly used type I and type

II error rates $\alpha$ and $\beta$ via the following simple formula

$$P_1 = 1 - \alpha^* = P(T = -|C = -) = \frac{(1-\theta)(1-\alpha)}{(1-\theta)(1-\alpha) + \theta\beta},$$

$$P_2 = 1 - \beta^* = P(T = +|C = +) = \frac{\theta(1-\beta)}{(1-\beta)\theta + \alpha(1-\theta)},$$

where $P_1$ and $P_2$ define the posterior probability that the true status of the hypothesis is indeed consistent with the clinical trial outcome. Then, we have

$$\alpha = \frac{(1-P_2)(\theta + P_1 - 1)}{(1-\theta)(P_1 + P_2 - 1)} \tag{13.2.1}$$

$$\beta = \frac{(1-P_1)(P_2 - \theta)}{\theta(P_1 + P_2 - 1)}. \tag{13.2.2}$$

Consequently, for a given $\theta$ and $(P_1, P_2)$, we can first compute the value of $\alpha$ and $\beta$. Then, the traditional frequentist sample size formula can be used to determine the needed sample size. Note that such a procedure is not only very simple but also free of model and testing procedures. Hence, it can be directly applied to essentially any type of clinical trial and any type of the testing procedures. For illustration purposes, we consider its usage for comparing means and survival in the next two subsections. Table 13.2.1 provides a number of most likely $(\theta, P_1, P_2)$ values and their associated $(\alpha, \beta)$ values.

## 13.2.2 Comparing Means

In this subsection, we show in detail how Lee and Zelen's Bayesian approach can be used to determine the sample size for comparing means. For illustration purpose, we consider only the most commonly used two-arm parallel design with equal sample size allocation. The situation with multiple arms and unequal sample size allocation can be similarly obtained.

Following the notations of Chapter 3, denote $x_{ij}$ the response observed from the $j$th subject in the $i$th treatment group, $j = 1, ..., n_i$, $i = 1, 2$. It is assumed that $x_{ij}$, $j = 1, ..., n_i$, $i = 1, 2$, are independent normal random variables with mean $\mu_i$ and variance $\sigma^2$. In addition, define

$$\bar{x}_{i\cdot} = \frac{1}{n_i} \sum_{j=1}^{n_i} x_{ij} \quad \text{and} \quad s^2 = \frac{1}{n_1 + n_2 - 2} \sum_{i=1}^{2} \sum_{j=1}^{n_i} (x_{ij} - \bar{x}_{i\cdot})^2.$$

Suppose that the objective of a clinical trial is to test whether there is a difference between the mean responses of the test drug and a placebo control or an active control agent. The following hypotheses are of interest:

$$H_0 : \epsilon = 0 \quad \text{versus} \quad H_a : \epsilon \neq 0.$$

## 13.2. Posterior Error Approach

Table 13.2.1: Type I and II Errors for Various $P_1$, $P_2$ and $\theta$ Values

| $\theta$ | $P_1$ | $P_2$ | $\alpha$ | $\beta$ | $P_1$ | $P_2$ | $\alpha$ | $\beta$ |
|---|---|---|---|---|---|---|---|---|
| 0.25 | 0.80 | 0.80 | 0.0222 | 0.7333 | 0.90 | 0.80 | 0.0571 | 0.3143 |
| | | 0.85 | 0.0154 | 0.7385 | | 0.85 | 0.0400 | 0.3200 |
| | | 0.90 | 0.0095 | 0.7429 | | 0.90 | 0.0250 | 0.3250 |
| | | 0.95 | 0.0044 | 0.7467 | | 0.95 | 0.0118 | 0.3294 |
| | 0.85 | 0.80 | 0.0410 | 0.5077 | 0.95 | 0.80 | 0.0711 | 0.1467 |
| | | 0.85 | 0.0286 | 0.5143 | | 0.85 | 0.0500 | 0.1500 |
| | | 0.90 | 0.0178 | 0.5200 | | 0.90 | 0.0314 | 0.1529 |
| | | 0.95 | 0.0083 | 0.5250 | | 0.95 | 0.0148 | 0.1556 |
| 0.50 | 0.80 | 0.80 | 0.2000 | 0.2000 | 0.90 | 0.80 | 0.2286 | 0.0857 |
| | | 0.85 | 0.1385 | 0.2154 | | 0.85 | 0.1600 | 0.0933 |
| | | 0.90 | 0.0857 | 0.2286 | | 0.90 | 0.1000 | 0.1000 |
| | | 0.95 | 0.0400 | 0.2400 | | 0.95 | 0.0471 | 0.1059 |
| | 0.85 | 0.80 | 0.2154 | 0.1385 | 0.95 | 0.80 | 0.2400 | 0.0400 |
| | | 0.85 | 0.1500 | 0.1500 | | 0.85 | 0.1688 | 0.0438 |
| | | 0.90 | 0.0933 | 0.1600 | | 0.90 | 0.1059 | 0.0471 |
| | | 0.95 | 0.0438 | 0.1688 | | 0.95 | 0.0500 | 0.0500 |
| 0.75 | 0.80 | 0.80 | 0.7333 | 0.0222 | 0.90 | 0.80 | 0.7429 | 0.0095 |
| | | 0.85 | 0.5077 | 0.0410 | | 0.85 | 0.5200 | 0.0178 |
| | | 0.90 | 0.3143 | 0.0571 | | 0.90 | 0.3250 | 0.0250 |
| | | 0.95 | 0.1467 | 0.0711 | | 0.95 | 0.1529 | 0.0314 |
| | 0.85 | 0.80 | 0.7385 | 0.0154 | 0.95 | 0.80 | 0.7467 | 0.0044 |
| | | 0.85 | 0.5143 | 0.0286 | | 0.85 | 0.5250 | 0.0083 |
| | | 0.90 | 0.3200 | 0.0400 | | 0.90 | 0.3294 | 0.0118 |
| | | 0.95 | 0.1500 | 0.0500 | | 0.95 | 0.1556 | 0.0148 |

When $\sigma^2$ is unknown, the null hypothesis $H_0$ is rejected at the $\alpha$ level of significance if

$$\left| \frac{\bar{x}_{1\cdot} - \bar{x}_{2\cdot}}{s\sqrt{\frac{1}{n_1} + \frac{1}{n_2}}} \right| > t_{\alpha/2, n_1+n_2-2}.$$

For given error rates $\alpha$ and $\beta$, as shown in Chapter 3, the minimum sample size needed can be estimated by

$$n_1 = n_2 = \frac{2(z_{\alpha/2} + z_\beta)^2 \sigma^2}{\epsilon^2}. \tag{13.2.3}$$

In order to implement the Bayesian approach, one need to first specify the value of $\theta$ to reflect the prior knowledge about the null and the alternative hypotheses. Furthermore, one needs to specify the value of $(P_1, P_2)$, which controls the posterior error rate. Based on these specifications, one can obtain the values of $(\alpha, \beta)$ according to (13.2.1) and (13.2.2). Then, use the resultant significance levels $(\alpha, \beta)$ and the formula (13.2.3) to obtain the desired sample size.

Consider Example 3.2.4 as given in Chapter 3, where a clinical trial is conducted to evaluate the effectiveness of a test drug on cholesterol in patients with coronary heart disease (CHD). It is assumed that the clinical meaning difference is given by $\epsilon = 5\%$ and the standard deviation is $\sigma = 10\%$. It has been demonstrated in Example 3.2.4, if we specify the Type I and Type II error rate to be $(\alpha, \beta) = (0.05, 0.20)$, respectively, then the resulting sample size from (13.2.3) is given by 63. However, if we uses the Bayesian approach and specify $(\alpha^*, \beta^*) = (0.05, 0.20)$ with $\theta = 0.50$, then according to (13.2.1) and (13.2.2) we have $(\alpha, \beta) = (0.24, 0.04)$. It follows that the sample size needed is given by

$$n_1 = n_2 = \frac{2(z_{\alpha/2} + z_\beta)^2 \sigma^2}{\epsilon^2} = \frac{2 \times 2.46^2 \times 0.10^2}{0.05^2} \approx 49.$$

Consequently, only 49 subjects per treatment group are needed.

It, however, should be noted that the resultant sample sizes 63 and 49 are not directly comparable, because they are controlling different error rates. The sample size 63 per treatment group is selected to control the type I and type II error rates at the levels of 0.05 and 0.20, respectively. On the other hand, the 49 subjects per treatment group is selected to control the two posterior error rates $\alpha^*$ and $\beta^*$ at the levels of 0.05 and 0.20, respectively, which correspond to the traditional type I and type II error rates at the levels of 0.04 and 0.24 according to our computation. Therefore, which sample size should be used depends on what statistical test will be used for testing the hypotheses. To provide a better understanding, various sample sizes needed at different posterior error configuration are summarized in Table 13.2.2.

## 13.3. The Bootstrap-Median Approach

Table 13.2.2: Sample Sizes under Different $\theta$ and $P = P_1 = P_2$ Specification

| $\theta$ | $P$ | $\alpha$ | $\beta$ | $(\epsilon/\sigma)$ | $n$ | $P$ | $\alpha$ | $\beta$ | $(\epsilon/\sigma)$ | $n$ |
|---|---|---|---|---|---|---|---|---|---|---|
| 0.25 | 0.80 | 0.0222 | 0.7333 | 0.1 | 554 | 0.90 | 0.0250 | 0.3250 | 0.1 | 1453 |
| | | | | 0.2 | 139 | | | | 0.2 | 364 |
| | | | | 0.3 | 62 | | | | 0.3 | 162 |
| | | | | 0.4 | 35 | | | | 0.4 | 91 |
| | | | | 0.5 | 23 | | | | 0.5 | 59 |
| 0.25 | 0.85 | 0.0286 | 0.5143 | 0.1 | 928 | 0.95 | 0.0148 | 0.1556 | 0.1 | 2381 |
| | | | | 0.2 | 232 | | | | 0.2 | 596 |
| | | | | 0.3 | 104 | | | | 0.3 | 265 |
| | | | | 0.4 | 58 | | | | 0.4 | 149 |
| | | | | 0.5 | 38 | | | | 0.5 | 96 |
| 0.50 | 0.80 | 0.2000 | 0.2000 | 0.1 | 902 | 0.90 | 0.1000 | 0.1000 | 0.1 | 1713 |
| | | | | 0.2 | 226 | | | | 0.2 | 429 |
| | | | | 0.3 | 101 | | | | 0.3 | 191 |
| | | | | 0.4 | 57 | | | | 0.4 | 108 |
| | | | | 0.5 | 37 | | | | 0.5 | 69 |
| 0.50 | 0.85 | 0.1500 | 0.1500 | 0.1 | 1227 | 0.95 | 0.0500 | 0.0500 | 0.1 | 2599 |
| | | | | 0.2 | 307 | | | | 0.2 | 650 |
| | | | | 0.3 | 137 | | | | 0.3 | 289 |
| | | | | 0.4 | 77 | | | | 0.4 | 163 |
| | | | | 0.5 | 50 | | | | 0.5 | 104 |
| 0.75 | 0.80 | 0.7333 | 0.0222 | 0.1 | 1106 | 0.90 | 0.3250 | 0.0250 | 0.1 | 1734 |
| | | | | 0.2 | 277 | | | | 0.2 | 434 |
| | | | | 0.3 | 123 | | | | 0.3 | 193 |
| | | | | 0.4 | 70 | | | | 0.4 | 109 |
| | | | | 0.5 | 45 | | | | 0.5 | 70 |
| 0.75 | 0.85 | 0.5143 | 0.0286 | 0.1 | 1305 | 0.95 | 0.1556 | 0.0148 | 0.1 | 2586 |
| | | | | 0.2 | 327 | | | | 0.2 | 647 |
| | | | | 0.3 | 145 | | | | 0.3 | 288 |
| | | | | 0.4 | 82 | | | | 0.4 | 162 |
| | | | | 0.5 | 53 | | | | 0.5 | 104 |

## 13.3 The Bootstrap-Median Approach

As indicated earlier, both methods based on the posterior credible interval and the posterior error rate are useful Bayesian approach for sample size calculation. The method of posterior credible interval approach explicitly takes into consideration the prior information. In practice, however, prior information is either not available or not reliable. In this case, the application of Joseph and Bélisle's method is limited. On the other hand, the method of posterior error rate does not suffer from this limitation. In practice, it is suggested that the posterior error rates $P_1$ and $P_2$ be chosen in such a way that they correspond to the type I and type II error rates from the frequentist point of view. This method, however, may not be widely used and accepted given the fact that the traditional testing procedure for controlling both type I and type II error rates have been widely used and accepted in practice.

As a result, two important questions are raised. First, if there is no reliable prior information available, is there still a need for Bayesian sample size calculation method? Second, if there is a need for Bayesian's method for sample size calculation, then how does one incorporate it into the framework that is accepted from the frequentist point of view? With an attempt to address these two questions, we will introduce an alternative method.

### 13.3.1 Background

As indicated in Chapter 1, a pre-study power analysis for sample size calculation is usually performed at the planning stage of an intended clinical trial. Sample size calculation is done under certain assumptions regarding the parameters (e.g., clinically important difference and standard deviation) of the target patient population. In practice, since the standard deviation of the target patient population is usually unknown, a typical approach is to use estimates from some pilot studies as the surrogate for the true parameters. We then treat these estimates as the true parameters to justify the sample size needed for the intended clinical trial. It should be noted that the parameter estimate obtained from the pilot study inevitably suffers from the sampling error, which causes the uncertainty (variation) about the true parameter. Consequently, it is likely to yield an unstable estimate of sample size for the intended clinical trial.

In order to fix the idea, we conduct a simple simulation study to examine the effect of the pilot study uncertainty. For illustration purposes, we consider a simple one-sample design with the type I and type II error rates given by 5% and 10%, respectively. Furthermore, we assume that the population standard deviation $\sigma = 1$ and the true mean response is $\epsilon = 25\%$. Then, according to (3.1.2), the sample size needed, if the true parameters

## 13.3. The Bootstrap-Median Approach

are known, are given by

$$n = \frac{(z_{\alpha/2} + z_\beta)^2 \sigma^2}{\epsilon^2} \approx 169.$$

However, in practice the true parameters are never known. Hence, it has to be estimated from some pilot studies (with small small sizes). In the simulation, 10,000 independent simulation runs are generated to examine the distribution of the sample size estimates, which are obtained based on the estimates of the parameters of the pilot study. The results are summarized in Table 13.3.1.

As it can be seen from Table 13.3.1, for a pilot study with sample size as large as 100, the resulting sample size estimates are still very unstable with a mean given by 10,302, which is much larger than the ideal sample size 169. In order to have a more reliable sample size estimate, we need to increase the size of the pilot study up to 500, which is much larger than the planned larger scale trial with only 169 subjects! Hence, we conclude that the uncertainty due to sampling error of the pilot study is indeed a very important source of risk for the planned clinical trial.

Table 13.3.1: The Effect of the Pilot Study Sample Size

| $n_0$ | Mean | S.D. | Minimum | Median | Maximum |
|---|---|---|---|---|---|
| 10 | 20060568 | 1824564572 | 2 | 122 | 181767638343 |
| 50 | 72746 | 2754401 | 10 | 163 | 225999504 |
| 100 | 10302 | 452841 | 22 | 168 | 38265202 |
| 500 | 188 | 87 | 56 | 168 | 1575 |
| 1000 | 177 | 49 | 66 | 168 | 594 |

### 13.3.2 A Bootstrap-Median Approach

Note that Table 13.3.1 reveals two important points. First, it clearly demonstrates that there is serious effect of the sample size estimation uncertainty due to the sampling error of the pilot study. Second, it seems to suggest that although the mean of the estimated sample size is very unstable, its median is more robust. To some extent, this is not a surprising finding. Let $\hat{\epsilon}$ and $\hat{\sigma}^2$ be the sample mean and variance obtained from the pilot study, respectively. Then, by applying (3.1.2), the estimated sample size would be given by

$$\hat{n} = \frac{(z_{\alpha/2} + z_\beta)^2}{\hat{\sigma}^2} \hat{\epsilon}^2.$$

If we assume that the sample is normally distributed, then we have $\hat{\epsilon}$ also follows some normal distribution. Hence, we know immediately that

$E(\hat{n}) = \infty$, which naturally explains why naïve sample size estimates based on pilot data could be extremely unstable. However, the median of $\hat{n}$ is always well defined and according to Table 13.3.1, it seems be able to approximate the true sample size with quite a satisfactory precision.

All the above discussion seems to suggest that if we are able to generate independent copy of the sample (i.e., bootstrap data set), then we are able to estimate the sample size based on each bootstrapped data set. Then, the median of the those bootstrap sample size estimates may provide a much more reliable approximate to the true sample size needed. More specifically, let $\mathcal{S}$ be the original sample, then the following simple bootstrap procedure can be considered:

(1) First generate the bootstrap data set $\mathcal{S}_h$ from $\mathcal{S}$. It is is generated by simple random sampling with replacement and has the same sample size as $\mathcal{S}$.

(2) Compute the sample size $n_h$ based on the bootstrap data set $\mathcal{S}_h$ and appropriate objective and formula.

(3) Repeat step (1) and (2) for a total of $B$ times, then take the median of the $n_h, h = 1, \cdots, B$ to be the final sample size estimate.

In order to evaluate the finite sample performance of the above bootstrap procedure, a simple simulation study is conducted. It is simulated according to same parameter configuration used in Table 13.3.1. The number of bootstrap iteration $B$ is fixed to be $B = 1,000$ and the total number of simulation iterations is fixed to be 100. The results are summarized in Table 13.3.2. As it can be seen, although the final estimate may still suffer from instability to some extend, it represents a dramatical improvement as compared with the results in Table 13.3.1. For detailed discussion about the bootstrap sample size calculation, we refer to Lee, Wang and Chow (2006).

Table 13.3.2: The Bootstrap Sample Size Estimation

| $n_0$ | Mean | S.D. | Minimum | Median | Maximum |
|---|---|---|---|---|---|
| 10 | 103 | 71 | 9 | 88 | 239 |
| 50 | 266 | 275 | 45 | 150 | 1175 |
| 100 | 363 | 448 | 28 | 192 | 2090 |
| 500 | 182 | 80 | 79 | 154 | 479 |
| 1000 | 180 | 51 | 84 | 174 | 408 |

## 13.4 Concluding Remarks

As indicated in Lee, Wang, and Chow (2006), power analysis for sample size calculation of a later phase clinical study based on limited information collected from a pilot study could lead to an extremely unstable estimate of sample size. Lee, Wang, and Chow (2006) proposed the use of bootstrap median approach and evaluated the instability of the estimated sample size by means of the population squared coefficient of variation, i.e., $CV = \sigma/\xi$, where $\xi$ and $\sigma$ are the population mean and standard deviation, respectively. Lee, Wang, and Chow (2006) considered the parameter $\theta = (\sigma^2 + \xi^2)/\xi^2$ and showed that

$$n_{0.5} = 1.5 n^{-1} \theta \left\{ 1 + o(1) \right\},$$

where $n_{0.5}$ satisfies

$$P\left(\hat{\theta} \leq \eta_{0.5}\right) = 0.5,$$

where $\eta_{0.5}$ is the squared median of sample coefficient of variation.

# Chapter 14

# Nonparametrics

In clinical trials, a parametric procedure is often employed for evaluation of clinical efficacy and safety of the test compound under investigation. A parametric procedure requires assumptions on the underlying population from which the data are obtained. A typical assumption on the underlying population is the normality assumption. Under the normality assumption, statistical inference regarding treatment effects can be obtained through appropriate parametric statistical methods such as the analysis of variance under valid study designs. In practice, however, the primary assumptions on the underlying population may not be met. As a result, parametric statistical methods may not be appropriate. In this case, alternatively, a nonparametric procedure is often considered. Nonparametric methods require few assumptions about the underlying populations, which are applicable in situations where the normal theory cannot be utilized. In this chapter, procedures for sample size calculation for testing hypotheses of interest are obtained under appropriate nonparametric statistical methods.

In the next section, the loss in power due to the violation of the normality assumption is examined. Nonparametric methods for testing differences in location are discussed for one-sample and two-sample problems, respectively, in Sections 14.2 and 14.3. Included in these sections are the corresponding procedures for sample size calculation. Nonparametric tests for independence and the corresponding procedure for sample size calculation are given in Section 14.4. Some practical issues are presented in the last section.

## 14.1 Violation of Assumptions

Under a parametric model, normality is probably the most commonly made assumption when analyzing data obtained from clinical trials. In practice, however, it is not uncommon that the observed data do not meet the normality assumption at the end of the trial. The most commonly seen violation of the normality assumption is that the distribution of the observed variable is skewed (either to the right or to the left). In this case, a log-transformation is usually recommended to remove the skewness before data analysis. For a fixed sample size selected based on the primary assumption of normality, it is then of interest to know how the power is affected if the primary assumption is seriously violated. For illustration purposes, in this section, we address this question for situations when comparing means. Other situations when comparing proportions or time-to-event data can be addressed in a similar manner.

Consider a randomized, parallel-group clinical trial comparing a treatment group and an active control agent. Let $x_{ij}$ be the observation from the $j$th subject in the $i$th treatment, $i = 1, 2$, $j = 1, ..., n$. It is assumed that $\log(x_{ij})$ follows a normal distribution with mean $\mu_i$ and variance $\sigma^2$. Let $\mu_i^* = E(x_{ij}) = e^{\mu_i + \sigma^2/2}$. The hypothesis of interest is to test

$$H_0 : \mu_1^* = \mu_2^* \quad \text{versus} \quad H_a : \mu_1^* \neq \mu_2^*,$$

which is equivalent to

$$H_0 : \mu_1 = \mu_2 \quad \text{versus} \quad H_a : \mu_1 \neq \mu_2.$$

At the planning stage of the clinical trial, sample size calculation is performed under the assumption of normality and the assumption that a two-sample t-test statistic will be employed. More specifically, the test statistic is given by

$$T_1 = \frac{\sqrt{n}(\bar{x}_1 - \bar{x}_2)}{\sqrt{2}s},$$

where $\bar{x}_i$ is the sample mean of the $i$th treatment group and $s^2$ is the pooled sample variance of $x_{ij}$'s. We reject the null hypothesis at the $\alpha$ level of significance if

$$|T_1| > z_{\alpha/2}.$$

Under the alternative hypothesis that $\mu_1 \neq \mu_2$, the power of the above testing procedure is given by

$$\Phi\left(\frac{\sqrt{n}|e^{\mu_1} - e^{\mu_2}|}{\sqrt{(e^{2\mu_1} + e^{2\mu_2})(e^{\sigma^2} - 1)}} - z_{\alpha/2}\right). \quad (14.1.1)$$

## 14.2. One-Sample Location Problem

At end of the trial, it is found that the observed data is highly skewed and hence a log-transformation is applied. After the log-transformation, the data appear to be normally distributed. As a result, it is of interest to compare the power of the two-sample t-test based on either the untransformed (raw) data or the log-transformed data to determine the impact of the violation of normality assumption on power with the fixed sample size $n$ selected under the normality assumption of the untransformed data. Let $y_{ij} = \log(x_{ij})$. The test statistic is given by

$$T_2 = \frac{\sqrt{n}(\bar{y}_1 - \bar{y}_2)}{2 s_y}, \qquad (14.1.2)$$

where $\bar{y}_i$ is the sample mean of the log-transformed response from the $i$th treatment group and $s_y^2$ the pooled sample variance based on the log-transformed data. The power of the above test is given by

$$\Phi\left(\frac{\sqrt{n}|\mu_1 - \mu_2|}{\sqrt{2}\sigma} - z_{\alpha/2}\right). \qquad (14.1.3)$$

From (14.1.1) and (14.1.3), the loss in power is

$$\Phi\left(\frac{\sqrt{n}|e^{\mu_1} - e^{\mu_2}|}{\sqrt{(e^{2\mu_1} + e^{2\mu_2})(e^{\sigma^2} - 1)}} - z_{\alpha/2}\right) - \Phi\left(\frac{\sqrt{n}|\mu_1 - \mu_2|}{\sqrt{2}\sigma} - z_{\alpha/2}\right).$$

It can be seen that the violation of the model assumption can certainly have an impact on the power of a trial with a fixed sample size selected under the model assumption. If the true power is below the designed power, the trial may fail to detect a clinically meaningful difference, when it truly exists. If the true power is above the designed power, then the trial is not cost-effective. This leads to a conclusion that incorrectly applying a parametric procedure to a data set, which does not meet the parametric assumption, may result in a significant loss in power and efficiency of the trial. As an alternative, a nonparametric method is suggested. In what follows, sample size calculations based on nonparametric methods for comparing means are provided.

## 14.2 One-Sample Location Problem

As discussed in Chapter 3, one-sample location problem concerns two types of data. The first type of data consists of paired replicates. In clinical research, it may represent pairs of pre-treatment and post-treatment observations. The primary interest is whether there is a shift in location due to the application of the treatment. The second type of data consists of observations from a single population. Statistical inference is made on the location of this population. For illustration purposes, in this section, we focus on nonparametric methods for paired replicates. Let $x_i$ and $y_i$ be the paired observations obtained from the $i$th subject before and after the application of treatment, $i = 1, ..., n$. Let $z_i = y_i - x_i$, $i = 1, ..., n$. Then, $z_i$ can be described by the following model:

$$z_i = \theta + e_i, \quad i = 1, ..., n,$$

where $\theta$ is the unknown location parameter (or treatment effect) of interest and the $e_i$'s are unobserved random errors having mean 0. It is assumed that (i) each $e_i$ has a continuous population (not necessarily the same one) that is symmetric about zero and (ii) the $e_i$'s are mutually independent. The hypotheses regarding the location parameter of interest are given by

$$H_0 : \theta = 0 \quad \text{versus} \quad H_a : \theta \neq 0.$$

To test the above hypotheses, a commonly employed nonparametric test is the Wilcoxon signed rank test. Consider the absolute differences $|z_i|, i = 1, ..., n$. Let $R_i$ denote the rank of $|z_i|$ in the joint ranking from least to greatest. Define

$$\psi_i = \begin{cases} 1 & \text{if } z_i > 0 \\ 0 & \text{if } z_i < 0 \end{cases} \quad i = 1, ..., n.$$

The statistic

$$T^+ = \sum_{i=1}^{n} R_i \psi_i$$

is the sum of the positive signed ranks. Based on $T^+$, the Wilcoxon signed rank test rejects the null hypothesis at the $\alpha$ level of significance if

$$T^+ \geq t(\alpha_2, n)$$

or

$$T^+ \leq \frac{n(n+1)}{2} - t(\alpha_1, n),$$

where $t(\alpha, n)$ satisfies

$$P(T^+ \geq t(\alpha, n)) = \alpha$$

under the null hypothesis and $\alpha = \alpha_1 + \alpha_2$. Values of $t(\alpha, n)$ are given in the most standard nonparametric references (e.g., Hollander and Wolfe, 1973). It should be noted that under the null hypothesis, the statistic

$$T^* = \frac{T^+ - E(T^+)}{\sqrt{\text{var}(T^+)}} = \frac{T^+ - n(n+1)/4}{\sqrt{n(n+1)(2n+1)/24}}$$

## 14.2. One-Sample Location Problem

has an asymptotic standard normal distribution. In other words, we may reject the null hypothesis at the $\alpha$ level of significance for large $n$ if

$$|T^*| \geq z_{\alpha/2}.$$

To derive a formula for sample size calculation, we note that

$$T^+ = \sum_{i=1}^n \sum_{j=1}^n I\{|z_i| \geq |z_j|\}\psi_i$$

$$= \sum_{i=1}^n \psi_i > + \sum_{i \neq j} I\{|z_i| \geq |z_j|\}\psi_i$$

$$= \sum_{i=1}^n \psi_i + \sum_{i<j} (I\{|z_i| \geq |z_j|\}\psi_i + I\{|z_j| \geq |z_i|\}\psi_j).$$

Hence, the variance of $T^+$ can be obtained as

$$\begin{aligned}
\mathrm{var}(T^+) &= n\mathrm{var}(\psi_i) \\
&\quad + \frac{n(n-1)}{2}\mathrm{var}(I\{|z_i| \geq |z_j|\}\psi_i + I\{|z_j| \geq |z_i|\}\psi_j) \\
&\quad + 2n(n-1)\mathrm{cov}(\psi_i, I\{|z_i| \geq |z_j|\}\psi_i + I\{|z_j| \geq |z_i|\}\psi_j) \\
&\quad + n(n-1)(n-2)\mathrm{cov}(I\{|z_i| \geq |z_{j_1}|\}\psi_i + I\{|z_{j_1}| \geq |z_i|\}\psi_{j_1}, \\
&\quad\quad I\{|z_i| \geq |z_{j_2}|\}\psi_i + I\{|z_{j_2}| \geq |z_i|\}\psi_{j_2}) \\
&= np_1(1-p_1) + n(n-1)(p_1^2 - 4p_1p_2 + 3p_2 - 2p_2^2) \\
&\quad + n(n-1)(n-2)(p_3 + 4p_4 - 4p_2^2),
\end{aligned}$$

where

$$\begin{aligned}
p_1 &= P(z_i > 0) \\
p_2 &= P(|z_i| \geq |z_j|, z_i > 0) \\
p_3 &= P(|z_i| \geq |z_{j_1}|, |z_i| \geq |z_{j_2}|, z_i > 0) \\
p_4 &= P(|z_{j_1}| \geq |z_i| \geq |z_{j_2}|, z_{j_1} > 0, z_i > 0).
\end{aligned}$$

It should be noted that the above quantities can be readily estimated based on data from pilot studies. More specifically, suppose that $z_1, ..., z_n$ are data from a pilot study. Then, the corresponding estimators can be obtained as

$$\hat{p}_1 = \frac{1}{n}\sum_{i=1}^n I\{z_i > 0\}$$

$$\hat{p}_2 = \frac{1}{n(n-1)}\sum_{i \neq j} I\{|z_i| \geq |z_j|, z_i > 0\}$$

$$\hat{p}_3 = \frac{1}{n(n-1)(n-2)} \sum_{i \neq j_1 \neq j_2} I\{|z_i| \geq |z_{j_1}|, |z_i| \geq |z_{j_2}|, z_i > 0\}$$

$$\hat{p}_4 = \frac{1}{n(n-1)(n-2)} \sum_{i \neq j_1 \neq j_2} I\{|z_{j_1}| \geq |z_i| \geq |z_{j_2}|\}, z_{j_1} > 0, z_i > 0\}.$$

Under the alternative hypothesis, $E(T^+) \neq \frac{n(n+1)}{4}$. $T^+$ can be approximated by a normal random variable with mean $E(T^+) = np_1 + n(n-1)p_2$ and variance $\text{var}(T^+)$. Without loss of generality, assume that $E(T^+) > n(n+1)/4$. Thus, the power of the test can be approximated by

$$\begin{aligned}
\text{Power} &= P(|T^*| > z_{\alpha/2}) \\
&\approx P(T^* > z_{\alpha/2}) \\
&= P\left(T^+ > z_{\alpha/2}\sqrt{n(n+1)(2n+1)/24} + \frac{n(n+1)}{4}\right) \\
&\approx 1 - \Phi\left(\frac{z_{\alpha/2}/\sqrt{12} + \sqrt{n}(1/4 - p_2)}{\sqrt{p_3 + 4p_4 - 4p_2^2}}\right).
\end{aligned}$$

The last approximation in the above equation is obtained by ignoring the lower order terms of $n$. Hence, the sample size required for achieving the desired power of $1 - \beta$ can be obtained by solving the following equation:

$$\frac{z_{\alpha/2}/\sqrt{12} + \sqrt{n}(1/4 - p_2)}{\sqrt{p_3 + 4p_4 - 4p_2^2}} = -z_\beta.$$

This leads to

$$n = \frac{(z_{\alpha/2}/\sqrt{12} + z_\beta\sqrt{p_3 + 4p_4 - 4p_2^2})^2}{(1/4 - p_2)^2}.$$

**Remark**

As indicated before, when there are no ties,

$$\text{var}(T^+) = \frac{1}{24}\left[n(n+1)(2n+1)\right].$$

When there are ties, $\text{var}(T^+)$ is given by

$$\text{var}(T^+) = \frac{1}{24}\left[n(n+1)(2n+1) - \frac{1}{2}\sum_{j=1}^{g} t_j(t_j - 1)(t_j + 1)\right],$$

where $g$ is the number of tied groups and $t_j$ is the size of tied group $j$. In this case, the above formula for sample size calculation is necessarily modified.

## An Example

To illustrate the use of sample size formula derived above, we consider the same example concerning a study of osteoporosis in post-menopausal women described in Chapter 3 for testing one-sample. Suppose a clinical trial is planned to investigate the effect of a test drug on the prevention of the progression to osteoporosis in women with osteopenia. Suppose that a pilot study with 5 subjects was conducted. According to the data from the pilot study, it was estimated that $p_2 = 0.30$, $p_3 = 0.40$, and $p_4 = 0.05$. Hence, the sample size needed in order to achieve an 80% power for detection of such a clinically meaningful improvement can be estimated by

$$n = \frac{(z_{\alpha/2}/\sqrt{12} + z_\beta\sqrt{p_3 + 4p_4 - 4p_2^2})^2}{(1/4 - p_2)^2}$$

$$= \frac{(1.96/\sqrt{12} + 0.84\sqrt{0.4 + 4 \times 0.05 - 4 \times 0.3^2})^2}{(0.25 - 0.3)^2}$$

$$\approx 383.$$

Thus, a total of 383 subjects are needed in order to have an 80% power to confirm the observed post-treatment improvement.

## 14.3 Two-Sample Location Problem

Let $x_i$, $i = 1, ..., n_1$, and $y_j$, $j = 1, ..., n_2$, be two independent random samples, which are respectively from a control population and a treatment population in a clinical trial. Suppose that the primary objective is to investigate whether there is a shift of location, which indicates the presence of the treatment effect. Similar to the one-sample location problem, the hypotheses of interest are given by

$$H_0 : \theta = 0 \quad \text{versus} \quad H_a : \theta \neq 0,$$

where $\theta$ represents the treatment effect. Consider the following model:

$$x_i = e_i, \quad i = 1, ..., n_1,$$

and

$$y_j = \theta + e_{n_1+j}, \quad j = 1, ..., n_2,$$

where the $e_i$'s are random errors having mean 0. It is assumed that (i) each $e_i$ comes from the same continuous population and (ii) the $n_1 + n_2$ $e_i$'s are mutually independent. To test the above hypotheses, the Wilcoxon rank sum test is probably the most commonly used nonparametric test (Wilcoxon, 1945; Wilcoxon and Bradley, 1964; Hollander and Wolfe, 1973).

To obtain the Wilcoxon's rank sum test, we first order the $N = n_1 + n_2$ observations from least to greatest and let $R_j$ denote the rank of $y_j$ in this ordering. Let

$$W = \sum_{j=1}^{n} R_j,$$

which is the sum of the ranks assigned to the $y_j$'s. We then reject the null hypothesis at the $\alpha$ level of significance if

$$W \geq w(\alpha_2, n_2, n_1)$$

or

$$W \leq n_1(n_2 + n_1 + 1) - w(\alpha_1, n_2, n_1),$$

where $\alpha = \alpha_1 + \alpha_2$ and $w(\alpha, n_2, n_1)$ satisfies

$$P(W \geq w(\alpha, n_2, n_1)) = \alpha$$

under the null hypothesis. Values of $w(\alpha, n_2, n_1)$ are given in the most standard nonparametric references (e.g., Hollander and Wolfe, 1973). Under the null hypothesis, the test statistic

$$W^* = \frac{W - E(W)}{\sqrt{\text{var}(W)}} = \frac{W - \frac{1}{2}n_2(n_2 + n_1 + 1)}{\sqrt{\frac{1}{12}n_1 n_2(n_1 + n_2 + 1)}} \qquad (14.3.1)$$

is asymptotically distributed as a standard normal distribution. Thus, by normal theory approximation, we reject the null hypothesis at the $\alpha$ level of significance if $|W^*| \geq z_{\alpha/2}$.

Note that $W$ can be written as

$$W = \sum_{i=1}^{n_2} \left( \sum_{j=1}^{n_2} I\{y_i \geq y_j\} + \sum_{j=1}^{n_1} I\{y_i \geq x_j\} \right)$$

$$= \frac{n_2(n_2 + 1)}{2} + \sum_{i=1}^{n_2} \sum_{j=1}^{n_1} I\{y_i \geq x_j\}.$$

## 14.3. Two-Sample Location Problem

Hence, the variance of $W$ is given by

$$\text{var}(W) = \text{var}\left(\frac{n_2(n_2+1)}{2} + \sum_{i=1}^{n_2}\sum_{j=1}^{n_1} I\{y_i \geq x_j\}\right)$$

$$= \text{var}\left(\sum_{i=1}^{n_2}\sum_{j=1}^{n_1} I\{y_i \geq x_j\}\right)$$

$$= n_1 n_2 \text{var}(I\{y_i \geq x_j\}) + n_1 n_2 (n_1 - 1)\text{cov}(I\{y_i \geq x_{j_1}\},$$
$$I\{y_i \geq x_{j_2}\}) + n_1 n_2 (n_2 - 1)\text{cov}(I\{y_{i_1} \geq x_j\}, I\{y_{i_2} \geq x_j\})$$

$$= n_1 n_2 p_1 (1 - p_1) + n_1 n_2 (n_1 - 1)(p_2 - p_1^2)$$
$$+ n_1 n_2 (n_2 - 1)(p_3 - p_1^2)$$

where

$$p_1 = P(y_i \geq x_j)$$
$$p_2 = P(y_i \geq x_{j_1} \text{ and } y_i \geq x_{j_2})$$
$$p_3 = P(y_{i_1} \geq x_j \text{ and } y_{i_2} \geq x_j).$$

The above quantities can be estimated readily based on data from pilot studies. More specifically, assume that $x_1, ..., x_{n_1}$ and $y_1, ..., y_{n_2}$ are the data from a pilot study. The corresponding estimators can be obtained as

$$\hat{p}_1 = \frac{1}{n_1 n_2} \sum_{i=1}^{n_2}\sum_{j=1}^{n_1} I\{y_i \geq x_j\}$$

$$\hat{p}_2 = \frac{1}{n_1 n_2 (n_1 - 1)} \sum_{i=1}^{n_2}\sum_{j_1 \neq j_2} I\{y_i \geq x_{j_1} \text{ and } y_i \geq x_{j_2}\}$$

$$\hat{p}_3 = \frac{1}{n_1 n_2 (n_2 - 1)} \sum_{i_1 \neq i_2}\sum_{j=1}^{n_1} I\{y_{i_1} \geq x_j \text{ and } y_{i_2} \geq x_j\}.$$

Under the alternative hypothesis that $\theta \neq 0$, it can be shown that $p_1 \neq 1/2$,

$$E(W) = \frac{n_2(n_2+1)}{2} + n_1 n_2 p_1,$$

and that $W$ can be approximated by a normal random variable with mean

$$\mu_W = \frac{n_2(n_2+1)}{2} + n_1 n_2 p_1$$

and variance

$$\sigma_W^2 = n_1 n_2 p_1 (1 - p_1) + n_1 n_2 (n_1 - 1)(p_2 - p_1^2) + n_1 n_2 (n_2 - 1)(p_3 - p_1^2).$$

Without loss of generality, we assume that $p_1 > 1/2$. The power of the test can be approximated by

$$\begin{aligned}
\text{Power} &= P(|W^*| > z_{\alpha/2}) \\
&\approx P(W^* > z_{\alpha/2}) \\
&= P\left(\frac{W - n_2(n_2+1)/2 - n_1 n_2 p_1}{\sigma_W} > \right. \\
&\qquad \left. \frac{z_{\alpha/2}\sqrt{n_1 n_2(n_1+n_2+1)/12} + n_1 n_2(1/2 - p_1)}{\sigma_W}\right).
\end{aligned}$$

Under the assumption that $n_1/n_2 \to \kappa$, the above equation can be further approximated by

$$\text{Power} = 1 - \Phi\left(\frac{z_{\alpha/2} * \sqrt{\kappa(1+\kappa)/12} + \sqrt{n_2}\kappa(1/2 - p_1)}{\sqrt{\kappa^2(p_2 - p_1^2) + \kappa(p_3 - p_1^2)}}\right).$$

As a result, the sample size needed in order to achieve a desired power of $1 - \beta$ can be obtained by solving

$$\frac{z_{\alpha/2} * \sqrt{\kappa(1+\kappa)/12} + \sqrt{n_2}\kappa(1/2 - p_1)}{\sqrt{\kappa^2(p_2 - p_1^2) + \kappa(p_3 - p_1^2)}} = -z_\beta,$$

which leads to $n_1 = \kappa n_2$ and

$$n_2 = \frac{(z_{\alpha/2}\sqrt{\kappa(\kappa+1)/12} + z_\beta\sqrt{\kappa^2(p_2 - p_1^2) + \kappa(p_3 - p_1^2)})^2}{\kappa^2(1/2 - p_1)^2}.$$

**Remark**

As indicated in (14.3.1), when there are no ties,

$$\text{var}(W) = \frac{n_1 + n_2 + 1}{12}.$$

When there are ties among the $N$ observations,

$$\text{var}(W) = \frac{n_1 n_2}{12}\left[n_1 + n_2 + 1 - \frac{\sum_{j=1}^{g} t_j(t_j^2 - 1)}{(n_1 + n_2)(n_1 + n_2 - 1)}\right],$$

where $g$ is the number of tied groups and $t_j$ is the size of tied group $j$. In this case, the above formula for sample size calculation is necessary modified.

**An Example**

To illustrate the use of the sample size formula derived above, we consider the same example concerning a clinical trial for evaluation of the effect of a test drug on cholesterol in patients with coronary heart disease (CHD). Suppose the investigator is interested in comparing two cholesterol lowering agents for treatment of patients with CHD through a parallel design. The primary efficacy parameter is the LDL. The null hypothesis of interest is the one of no treatment difference. Suppose that a two-arm parallel pilot study was conducted. According to the data given in the pilot study, it was estimated that $p_2 = 0.70$, $p_3 = 0.80$, and $p_4 = 0.80$. Hence, the sample size needed in order to achieve an 80% power for detection of a clinically meaningful difference between the treatment groups can be estimated by

$$n = \frac{(z_{\alpha/2}/\sqrt{6} + z_\beta\sqrt{p_2 + p_3 - p_1^2})^2}{(1/2 - p_1)^2}$$
$$= \frac{(1.96/\sqrt{6} + 0.84\sqrt{0.80 + 0.80 - 2 \times 0.70^2})^2}{(0.50 - 0.70)^2}$$
$$\approx 54.$$

Hence, a total of 54 subjects is needed in order to have an 80% power to confirm the observed difference between the two treatment groups when such a difference truly exists.

## 14.4 Test for Independence

In many clinical trials, data collected may consist of a random sample from a bivariate population. For example, the baseline value and the post-treatment value. For such a data set, it is of interest to determine whether there is an association between the two variates (say $x$ and $y$) involved in the bivariate structure. In other words, it is of interest to test for independence between $x$ and $y$. Let $(x_i, y_i)$, $i = 1, ..., n$, be the $n$ bivariate observation from the $n$ subjects involved in a clinical trial. It is assumed that (i) $(x_i, y_i)$, $i = 1, ..., n$, are mutually independent and (ii) each $(x_i, y_i)$ comes from the same continuous bivariate population of $(x, y)$. To obtain a nonparametric test for independence between $x$ and $y$, define

$$\tau = 2P\{(x_1 - x_2)(y_1 - y_2) > 0\} - 1,$$

which is the so-called Kendall coefficient. Testing the hypothesis that $x$ and $y$ are independent, i.e.,

$$H_0 : P(x \leq a \text{ and } y \leq b) = P(x \leq a)P(y \leq b) \text{ for all } a \text{ and } b$$

is equivalent to testing the hypothesis that $\tau = 0$. A nonparametric test can be obtained as follows. First, for $1 \leq i < j \leq n$, calculate $\zeta(x_i, x_j, y_i, y_j)$, where

$$\zeta(a,b,c,d) = \begin{cases} 1 & \text{if } (a-b)(c-d) > 0 \\ -1 & \text{if } (a-b)(c-d) < 0. \end{cases}$$

For each pair of subscripts $(i,j)$ with $i < j$, $\zeta(x_i, x_j, y_i, y_j) = 1$ indicates that $(x_i - x_j)(y_i - y_j)$ is positive while $\zeta(x_i, x_j, y_i, y_j) = -1$ indicates that $(x_i - x_j)(y_i - y_j)$ is negative. Consider

$$K = \sum_{i=1}^{n-1} \sum_{j=i+1}^{n} \zeta(x_i, x_j, y_i, y_j).$$

We then reject the null hypothesis that $\tau = 0$ at the $\alpha$ level of significance if

$$K \geq k(\alpha_2, n) \text{ or } K \leq -k(\alpha_1, n),$$

where $k(\alpha, n)$ satisfies

$$P(K \geq k(\alpha, n)) = \alpha$$

and $\alpha = \alpha_1 + \alpha_2$. Values of $k(\alpha, n)$ are given in the most standard nonparametric references (e.g., Hollander and Wolfe, 1973). Under the null hypothesis,

$$K^* = \frac{K - E(K)}{\sqrt{\text{var}(K)}} = K \left[ \frac{n(n-1)(2n+5)}{18} \right]^{-1/2} \tag{14.4.1}$$

is asymptotically distributed as a standard normal. Hence, we would reject the null hypothesis at the $\alpha$ level of significance for large samples if $|K^*| \geq z_{\alpha/2}$. It should be noted that when there are ties among the $n$ $x$ observations or among the $n$ $y$ observations, $\zeta(a,b,c,d)$ should be replaced with

$$\zeta^*(a,b,c,d) = \begin{cases} 1 & \text{if } (a-b)(c-d) > 0 \\ 0 & \text{if } (a-b)(c-d) = 0 \\ -1 & \text{if } (a-b)(c-d) < 0. \end{cases}$$

## 14.4. Test for Independence

As a result, under $H_0$, $\text{var}(K)$ becomes

$$\text{var}(K) = \frac{1}{18}\left[n(n-1)(2n+5) - \sum_{i=1}^{g} t_i(t_i-1)(2t_i+5)\right.$$
$$\left. - \sum_{j=1}^{h} u_j(u_j-1)(2u_j+5)\right]$$
$$+ \frac{1}{9n(n-1)(n-2)}\left[\sum_{i=1}^{g} t_i(t_i-1)(t_i-2)\right]$$
$$\times \left[\sum_{j=1}^{h} u_j(u_j-1)(u_j-2)\right]$$
$$+ \frac{1}{2n(n-1)}\left[\sum_{j=1}^{g} t_i(t_i-1)\right]\left[\sum_{i=1}^{h} u_j(u_j-1)\right],$$

where $g$ is the number of tied $x$ groups, $t_i$ is the size of the tied $x$ group $i$, $h$ is the number of tied $y$ groups, and $u_j$ is the size of the tied $y$ group $j$.

A formula for sample size calculation can be derived base on test (14.4.1). Define

$$\zeta_{i,j} = \zeta(x_i, x_j, y_i, y_j).$$

It follows that

$$\text{var}(K) = \text{var}\left(\sum_{i=1}^{n-1}\sum_{j=i+1}^{n} \zeta_{i,j}\right)$$
$$= \frac{n(n-1)}{2}\text{var}(\zeta_{i,j}) + n(n-1)(n-2)\text{cov}(\zeta_{i,j_1}, \zeta_{i,j_2})$$
$$= \frac{n(n-1)}{2}[1 - (1-2p_1)^2]$$
$$+ n(n-1)(n-2)[2p_2 - 1 - (1-2p_1)^2],$$

where

$$p_1 = P((x_1 - x_2)(y_1 - y_2) > 0)$$
$$p_2 = P((x_1 - x_2)(y_1 - y_2)(x_1 - x_3)(y_1 - y_3) > 0).$$

The above quantities can be readily estimated based on data from pilot studies. More specifically, let $(x_1, y_1), ..., (x_n, y_n)$ be the data from a pilot study, the corresponding estimators can be obtained by

$$\hat{p}_1 = \frac{1}{n(n-1)} \sum_{i \neq j} I\{(x_i - x_j)(y_i - y_j) > 0\}$$

$$\hat{p}_2 = \frac{1}{n(n-1)(n-2)} \sum_{i \neq j_1 \neq j_2} I\{(x_i - x_{j_1})(y_i - y_{j_1})(x_i - x_{j_2})(y_i - y_{j_2}) > 0\}.$$

Under the alternative hypothesis, $K$ is approximately distributed as a normal random variable with mean

$$\mu_K = \frac{n(n-1)}{2}(2p_1 - 1)$$

and variance

$$\sigma_K^2 = \frac{n(n-1)}{2}[1 - (1 - 2p_1)^2] + n(n-1)(n-2)[2p_2 - 1 - (1 - 2p_1)^2].$$

Without loss of generality, we assume $p_1 > 1/2$. The power of test (14.4.1) can be approximated by

$$\begin{aligned}
\text{Power} &= P(|K^*| > z_{\alpha/2}) \\
&\approx P(K^* > z_{\alpha/2}) \\
&= P\left(\frac{K - n(n-1)(2p_1 - 1)/2}{\sigma_K} > \frac{z_{\alpha/2}\sqrt{n(n-1)(2n+5)/18} - n(n-1)(p_1 - 1/2)}{\sigma_K}\right) \\
&\approx 1 - \Phi\left(\frac{z_{\alpha/2}/3 - \sqrt{n}(p_1 - 1/2)}{\sqrt{2p_2 - 1 - (2p_1 - 1)^2}}\right).
\end{aligned}$$

Hence, the sample size needed in order to achieve a desired power of $1 - \beta$ can be obtained by solving the following equation:

$$\frac{z_{\alpha/2}/3 - \sqrt{n}(p_1 - 1/2)}{\sqrt{2p_2 - 1 - (2p_1 - 1)^2}} = -z_\beta.$$

This leads to

$$n = \frac{4(z_{\alpha/2}/3 + z_\beta \sqrt{2p_2 - 1 - (2p_1 - 1)^2})^2}{(2p_1 - 1)^2}.$$

**An Example**

In a pilot study, it is observed that a larger $x$ value resulted in a larger value of $y$. Thus, it is of interest to conduct a clinical trial to confirm such an association between two primary responses, $x$ and $y$, truly exists. Suppose that a two-arm parallel pilot study was conducted. Based on the data from the pilot study, it was estimated that $p_1 = 0.60$ and $p_2 = 0.70$. Hence, the sample size required for achieving an 80% power is

$$\begin{aligned} n &= \frac{(z_{\alpha/2}/3 + z_\beta \sqrt{2p_2 - 1 - (2p_1 - 1)^2})^2}{(p_1 - 0.5)^2} \\ &= \frac{(1.96/3 + 0.84\sqrt{2 \times 0.70 - 1 - (1.20 - 1.00)^2})^2}{(0.6 - 0.5)^2} \\ &\approx 135. \end{aligned}$$

Thus, a total of 135 subjects is needed in order to achieve an 80% power to confirm the observed association in the pilot study.

## 14.5 Practical Issues

### 14.5.1 Bootstrapping

When a nonparametric method is used, a formula for sample size calculation may not be available or may not exist a closed form, especially when the study design/objective is rather complicated. In this case, the technique of bootstrapping may be applied. For more details, see Shao and Tu (1999).

### 14.5.2 Comparing Variabilities

In practice, it is often of interest to compare variabilities between treatments observed from the trials. Parametric methods for comparing variabilities is examined in Chapter 9. Nonparametric methods for comparing variabilities between treatment groups, however, are much more complicated and require further research.

### 14.5.3 Multiple-Sample Location Problem

When there are more than two treatment groups, the method of analysis of variance is usually considered. The primary hypothesis is that there are no treatment differences across the treatment groups. Let $x_{ij}$ be the observation from the $i$th subject receiving the $j$th treatment, where $i = 1, ..., n_j$ and $j = 1, ..., k$. Similar to the analysis of variance model for the parametric case, we consider the following model:

$$x_{ij} = \mu + \tau_j + e_{ij}, \quad i = 1, ..., n_j, j = 1, ..., k,$$

where $\mu$ is the unknown overall mean, $\tau_j$ is the unknown $j$th treatment effect and $\sum_{j=1}^{k} \tau_j = 0$. It is assumed that (i) each $e_i$ comes from the same continuous population with mean 0 and (ii) the $e_i$'s are mutually independent. The hypotheses of interest are

$$H_0 : \tau_1 = \cdots = \tau_k \quad \text{versus} \quad H_a : \tau_i \neq \tau_j \text{ for some } i \neq j.$$

To test the above hypotheses, the following Kruskal-Wallis test is useful (Kruskal and Wallis, 1952). We first rank all $N = \sum_{j=1}^{k} n_j$ observations jointly from least to greatest. Let $R_{ij}$ denote the rank of $x_{ij}$ in this joint ranking, $R_j = \sum_{i=1}^{n_j} R_{ij}$, $R_{\cdot j} = R_j/n_j$, and $R_{\cdot \cdot} = \frac{N+1}{2}$, $j = 1, ..., k$. Note that $R_j$ is the sum of the ranks received by treatment $j$ and $R_{\cdot j}$ is the average rank obtained by treatment $j$. Based on $R_j$, $R_{\cdot j}$ and $R_{\cdot \cdot}$, the Kruskal-Wallis test statistic for the above hypotheses can be obtained as

$$H = \frac{12}{N(N+1)} \sum_{j=1}^{k} n_j (R_{\cdot j} - R_{\cdot \cdot})^2$$

$$= \left( \frac{12}{N(N+1)} \sum_{j=1}^{k} \frac{R_j^2}{n_j} \right) - 3(N+1).$$

We reject the null hypothesis at the $\alpha$ level of significance if

$$H \geq h(\alpha, k, n_1, \cdots, n_k),$$

where $h(\alpha, k, n_1, \cdots, n_k)$ satisfies

$$P(H \geq h(\alpha, k, n_1, \cdots, n_k)) = \alpha$$

under the null hypothesis. Values of $h(\alpha, k, (n_1, \cdots, n_k))$ are given in the most standard nonparametric references (e.g., Hollander and Wolfe, 1973). Note that under the null hypothesis, $H$ has an asymptotic chi-square distribution with $k-1$ degrees of freedom (Hollander and Wolfe, 1973). Thus, we may reject the null hypothesis at the $\alpha$ level of significance for large samples if $H \geq \chi^2_{\alpha, k-1}$, where $\chi^2_{\alpha, k-1}$ is the upper $\alpha$th percentile of a chi-square distribution with $k-1$ degrees of freedom.

Unlike the parametric approach, formulae or procedures for sample size calculation for testing difference in multiple-sample locations using nonparametric methods are much more complicated. Further research is needed.

### 14.5.4 Testing Scale Parameters

In clinical trials, the reproducibility of subjects' medical status in terms of intra-subject variability is often assessed. If the intra-subject variability is much larger than that of the standard therapy (or control), safety of the test product could be a concern. In practice, a replicate crossover design or a parallel-group design with replicates is usually recommended for comparing intra-subject variability. Although nonparametric methods for testing scale parameters are available in the literature (see, e.g., Hollander and Wolfe, 1973), powers of these tests under the alternative hypothesis are not fully studied. As a result, further research in this area is necessary.

# Chapter 15

# Sample Size Calculation in Other Areas

As indicated earlier, sample size calculation is an integral part of clinical research. It is undesirable to observe positive results with insufficient power. Sample size calculation should be performed based on the primary study endpoint using appropriate statistical methods under a valid study design with correct hypotheses, which can reflect the study objectives. In the previous chapters, we have examined formulas or procedures for sample size calculation based on various primary study endpoints for comparing means, proportions, variabilities, functions of means and variance components, and time-to-event data. In this chapter, in addition, we discuss several procedures for sample size calculation based on different study objectives and/or hypotheses using different statistical methods, which are not covered in the previous chapters.

In the next section, sample size calculations for QT/QTc studies with time-dependent replicates are examined. Sample size calculation based on propensity score analysis for non-randomized studies is given in Section 15.2. Section 15.3 discusses sample size calculation under an analysis of variance (ANOVA) model with repeated measures. Section 15.4 discusses sample size calculation for assessment of quality of life (QOL) under a time series model. In Section 15.5, the concept of reproducibility and sensitivity index for bridging studies is introduced. Also included in this section is a proposed method for assessing similarity of bridging studies, which is used for derivation of a procedure for sample size calculation. Statistical methods and the corresponding procedure for sample size calculation for vaccine clinical trials are briefly outlined in Section 15.6.

## 15.1 QT/QTc Studies with Time-Dependent Replicates

In clinical trials, a 12-lead electrocardiogram (ECG) is usually conducted for assessment of potential cardiotoxicity induced by the treatment under study. On an ECG tracing, the QT interval is measured from the beginning of the Q wave to the end of the T wave. QT interval is often used to indirectly assess the delay in cardiac repolarization, which can pre-dispose to the development of life threatening cardiac arrhythmias such as torsade de pointes (Moss, 1993). QTc interval is referred to as the QT interval corrected by heart rate. In clinical practice, it is recognized that the prolongation of the QT/QTc interval is related to increased risk of cardiotoxicity such as a life threatening arrhythmia (Temple 2003). Thus it is suggested that a careful evaluation of potential QT/QTc prolongation be assessed for potential drug-induced cardiotoxicity.

For development of a new pharmaceutical entity, most regulatory agencies such as the United States Food and Drug Administration (FDA) require the evaluation of pro-arrhythmic potential (see, e.g., CPMP, 1997; FDA/TPD, 2003; ICH, 2003). As a result, a draft guidance on the clinical evaluation of QT/QTc interval prolongation and proarrhythmic potential for non-antiarrhythmic drugs is being prepared by the ICH (ICH E14). This draft guidance calls for a placebo-controlled study in normal healthy volunteers with a positive control to assess cardiotoxicity by examining QT/QTc prolongation. Under a valid study design (e.g., a parallel-group design or a crossover design), ECG's will be collected at baseline and at several time points post-treatment for each subject. Malik and Camm (2001) recommend that it would be worthwhile to consider 3 to 5 replicate ECGs at each time point within 2 to 5 minute period. Replicate ECGs are then defined as single ECG recorded within several minutes of a nominal time (PhRMA QT Statistics Expert Working Team, 2003). Along this line, Strieter, et al (2003) studied the effect of replicate ECGs on QT variability in healthy subjects. In practice, it is then of interest to investigate the impact of recording replicates on power and sample size calculation in routine QT studies.

In clinical trials, a pre-study power analysis for sample size calculation is usually performed to ensure that the study will achieve a desired power (or the probability of correctly detecting a clinically meaningful difference if such a difference truly exists). For QT studies, the following information is necessarily obtained prior to the conduct of the pre-study power analysis for sample size calculation. These information include (i) the variability associated with the primary study endpoint such as the QT intervals (or the QT interval endpoint change from baseline) and (ii) the clinically meaning-

## 15.1. QT/QTc Studies with Time-Dependent Replicates

ful difference in QT interval between treatment groups. Under the above assumption, the procedures as described in Longford (1993) and Chow, Shao and Wang (2003c) can then be applied for sample size calculation under the study design (e.g., a parallel-group design or a crossover design).

In what follows, commonly used study designs such as a parallel-group design or a crossover design for routine QT studies with recording replicates are briefly described. Power analyses and the corresponding sample size calculations under a parallel-group design and a crossover design are derived. Extensions to the designs with covariates (PK responses) are also considered.

### 15.1.1 Study Designs and Models

A typical study design for QT studies is either a parallel-group design or a crossover design depending upon the primary objectives of the study. Statistical models under a parallel-group design and a crossover design are briefly outlined below.

Under a parallel-group design, qualified subjects will be randomly assigned to receive either treatment A or treatment B. ECG's will be collected at baseline and at several time points post-treatment. Subjects will fast at least 3 hours and rest at least 10 minutes prior to scheduled ECG measurements. Identical lead-placement and same ECG machine will be used for all measurements. As recommended by Malik and Camm (2001), 3 to 5 recording replicate ECGs at each time point will be obtained within a 2 to 5 minute period.

Let $y_{ijk}$ be the QT interval observed from the $k$th recording replicate of the $j$th subject who receives treatment $i$, where $i = 1, 2, j = 1, \ldots, n$ and $k = 1, \ldots, K$. Consider the following model

$$y_{ijk} = \mu_i + e_{ij} + \epsilon_{ijk}, \qquad (15.1.1)$$

where $e_{ij}$ are independent and identically distributed as a normal with mean 0 and variance $\sigma_s^2$ (between subject or inter-subject variability) and $\epsilon_{ijk}$ are independent and identically distributed as a normal with mean 0 and variance $\sigma_e^2$ (within subject or intra-subject variability or measurement error variance). Thus, we have $\text{Var}(y_{ijk}) = \sigma_s^2 + \sigma_e^2$.

Under a crossover design, qualified subjects will be randomly assigned to receive one of the two sequences of test treatments under study. In other words, subjects who are randomly assigned to sequence 1 will receive treatment 1 first and then be crossed over to receive treatment 2 after a sufficient period of washout. Let $y_{ijkl}$ be the QT interval observed from the $k$th recording replicate of the $j$th subject in the $l$th sequence who receives the $i$th treatment, where $i = 1, 2, j = 1, \ldots, n, k = 1, \ldots, K$, and $l = 1, 2$.

We consider the following model

$$y_{ijkl} = \mu_i + \beta_{il} + e_{ijl} + \epsilon_{ijkl}, \qquad (15.1.2)$$

where $\beta_{il}$ are independent and identically distributed normal random period effects (period uniquely determined by sequence $l$ and treatment $i$) with mean 0 and variance $\sigma_p^2$, $e_{ijl}$ are independent and identically distributed normal subject random effects with mean 0 and variance $\sigma_s^2$, and $\epsilon_{ijkl}$ are independent and identically distributed normal random errors with mean 0 and variance $\sigma_e^2$. Thus, $\text{Var}(y_{ijkl}) = \sigma_p^2 + \sigma_s^2 + \sigma_e^2$.

To have a valid comparison between the parallel design and the crossover design, we assume that $\mu_i, \sigma_s^2$, and $\sigma_e^2$ are the same as those given in (15.1.1) and (15.1.2) and consider an extra variability $\sigma_p^2$, which is due to the random period effect for the crossover design.

### 15.1.2  Power and Sample Size Calculation

#### Parallel Group Design

Under the parallel-group design as described in the previous section, to evaluate the impact of recording replicates on power and sample size calculation, for simplicity, we will consider only one time point post treatment. The results for recording replicates at several post-treatment intervals can be similarly obtained. Under model (15.1.1), consider sample mean of QT intervals of the $j$th subject who receives the $i$th treatment then $\text{Var}(\bar{y}_{ij.}) = \sigma_s^2 + \frac{\sigma_e^2}{K}$. The hypotheses of interest regarding treatment difference in QT interval are given by

$$H_0: \mu_1 - \mu_2 = 0, \quad \text{versus} \quad H_1: \mu_1 - \mu_2 = d, \qquad (15.1.3)$$

where $d \neq 0$ is a difference of clinically importance. Under the null hypothesis of no treatment difference, the following statistic can be derived

$$T = \frac{\bar{y}_{1..} - \bar{y}_{2..}}{\sqrt{\frac{2}{n}\left(\hat{\sigma}_s^2 + \frac{\hat{\sigma}_e^2}{K}\right)}},$$

where

$$\hat{\sigma}_e^2 = \frac{1}{2n(K-1)} \sum_{i=1}^{2} \sum_{j=1}^{n} \sum_{k=1}^{K} (y_{ijk} - \bar{y}_{ij.})^2,$$

and

$$\hat{\sigma}_s^2 = \frac{1}{2(n-1)} \sum_{i=1}^{2} \sum_{j=1}^{n} (\bar{y}_{ij.} - \bar{y}_{i..})^2 - \frac{1}{2nK(K-1)} \sum_{i=1}^{2} \sum_{j=1}^{n} \sum_{k=1}^{K} (y_{ijk} - \bar{y}_{ij.})^2.$$

## 15.1. QT/QTc Studies with Time-Dependent Replicates

Under the null hypothesis in (15.1.3), $T$ has a central t-distribution with $2n - 2$ degrees of freedom. Let $\sigma^2 = \text{Var}(y_{ijk}) = \sigma_s^2 + \sigma_e^2$ and $\rho = \frac{\sigma_s^2}{\sigma_s^2 + \sigma_e^2}$, then under the alternative hypothesis in (15.1.3), the power of the test can be obtained as follows

$$1 - \beta \approx 1 - \Phi\left(z_{\alpha/2} - \frac{\delta}{\sqrt{\frac{2}{n}\left(\rho + \frac{1-\rho}{K}\right)}}\right) +$$

$$\Phi\left(-z_{\alpha/2} - \frac{\delta}{\sqrt{\frac{2}{n}\left(\rho + \frac{1-\rho}{K}\right)}}\right), \quad (15.1.4)$$

where $\delta = d/\sigma$ is the relative effect size and $\Phi$ is the cumulative distribution of a standard normal. To achieve the desired power of $1 - \beta$ at the $\alpha$ level of significance, the sample size needed per treatment is

$$n = \frac{2(z_{\alpha/2} + z_\beta)^2}{\delta^2}\left(\rho + \frac{1-\rho}{K}\right). \quad (15.1.5)$$

**Crossover Design**

Under a crossover model (15.1.2), it can be verified that $\bar{y}_{i...}$ is an unbiased estimator of $\mu_i$ with variance $\frac{\sigma_p^2}{2} + \frac{\sigma_s^2}{2n} + \frac{\sigma_e^2}{2nK}$. Thus, we used the following test statistic to test the hypotheses in (15.1.3)

$$T = \frac{\bar{y}_{1...} - \bar{y}_{2...}}{\sqrt{\hat{\sigma}_p^2 + \frac{1}{n}\left(\hat{\sigma}_s^2 + \frac{\hat{\sigma}_e^2}{K}\right)}},$$

where

$$\hat{\sigma}_e^2 = \frac{1}{4n(K-1)}\sum_{i=1}^{2}\sum_{j=1}^{n}\sum_{k=1}^{K}\sum_{l=1}^{2}(y_{ijkl} - \bar{y}_{ij.l})^2,$$

$$\hat{\sigma}_s^2 = \frac{1}{4(n-1)}\sum_{i=1}^{2}\sum_{j=1}^{n}\sum_{l=1}^{2}(\bar{y}_{ij.l} - \bar{y}_{i..l})^2$$

$$- \frac{1}{4nK(K-1)}\sum_{i=1}^{2}\sum_{j=1}^{n}\sum_{k=1}^{K}\sum_{l=1}^{2}(y_{ijkl} - \bar{y}_{ij.l})^2,$$

and

$$\hat{\sigma}_p^2 = \frac{1}{2}\sum_{i=1}^{2}\sum_{l=1}^{2}(\bar{y}_{i..l} - \bar{y}_{....})^2 - \frac{1}{4n(n-1)}\sum_{i=1}^{2}\sum_{j=1}^{n}\sum_{l=1}^{2}(\bar{y}_{ij.l} - \bar{y}_{i..l})^2.$$

Under the null hypothesis in (15.1.3), $T$ has a central t-distribution with $2n - 4$ degrees of freedom. Let $\sigma^2$ and $\rho$ be defined as in the previous section, and $\gamma = \sigma_p^2/\sigma^2$, then $\text{Var}(y_{ijkl}) = \sigma^2(1+\gamma)$. Under the alternative hypothesis in (15.1.3), the power of the test can be obtained as follows

$$1 - \beta \approx 1 - \Phi\left(z_{\alpha/2} - \frac{\delta}{\sqrt{\gamma + \frac{1}{n}\left(\rho + \frac{1-\rho}{K}\right)}}\right)$$

$$+ \Phi\left(-z_{\alpha/2} - \frac{\delta}{\sqrt{\gamma + \frac{1}{n}\left(\rho + \frac{1-\rho}{K}\right)}}\right), \qquad (15.1.6)$$

where $\delta = d/\sigma$. To achieve the desired power of $1 - \beta$ at the $\alpha$ level of significance, the sample size needed per treatment is

$$n = \frac{(z_{\alpha/2} + z_\beta)^2}{\delta^2 - \gamma(z_{\alpha/2} + z_\beta)^2}\left(\rho + \frac{1-\rho}{K}\right). \qquad (15.1.7)$$

**Remarks**

Let $n_{\text{old}}$ be the sample size with $K = 1$ (i.e., there is single measure for each subject). Then, we have $n = \rho n_{\text{old}} + (1-\rho) n_{\text{old}}/K$. Thus, sample size (with recording replicates) required for achieving the desired power is a weighted average of $n_{\text{old}}$ and $n_{\text{old}}/K$. Note that this relationship holds under both a parallel and a crossover design. Table 15.1.1 provides sample sizes required under a chosen design (either parallel or crossover) for achieving the same power with single recording ($K = 1$), three recording replicates ($K = 3$), and five recording replicates ($K = 5$).

Note that if $\rho$ closes to 0, then these repeated measures can be treated as independent replicates. As it can be seen from the above, if $\rho \approx 0$, then $n \approx n_{\text{old}}/K$. In other words, sample size is indeed reduced when the correlation coefficient between recording replicates is close to 0 (in this case, the recording replicates are almost independent). Table 15.1.2 shows the sample size reduction for different values of $\rho$ under the parallel design. However, in practice, $\rho$ is expected to be close to 1. In this case, we have $n \approx n_{\text{old}}$. In other words, there is not much gain for considering recording replicates in the study.

In practice it is of interest to know whether the use of a crossover design can further reduce the sample size when other parameters such as $d, \sigma^2$, and $\rho$, remain the same. Comparing formulas (15.1.5) and (15.1.7), we conclude that the sample size reduction by using a crossover design depends upon the parameter $\gamma = \sigma_p^2/\sigma^2$, which is a measure of the relative magnitude

## 15.1. QT/QTc Studies with Time-Dependent Replicates

of period variability with respect to the within period subject marginal variability. Let $\theta = \frac{\gamma}{(z_{\alpha/2}+z_\beta)^2}$, then by (15.1.5) and (15.1.7) the sample size $n_{\text{cross}}$ under the crossover design and the sample size $n_{\text{parallel}}$ under the parallel group design satisfy $n_{\text{cross}} = \frac{n_{\text{parallel}}}{2(1-\theta)}$. When the random period effect is negligible, that is, $\gamma \approx 0$ and hence $\theta \approx 0$, then we have $n_{\text{cross}} = \frac{n_{\text{parallel}}}{2}$. This indicates that the use of a crossover design could further reduce the sample size by half as compared to a parallel group design when the random period effect is negligible (based on the comparison of the above formula and the formula given in (15.1.5)). However, when the random period effect is not small, the use of a crossover design may not result in sample size reduction. Table 15.1.3 shows the sample size under different values of $\gamma$. It is seen that the possibility of sample size reduction under a crossover design depends upon whether the carryover effect of the QT intervals could be avoided. As a result, it is suggested a sufficient length of washout be applied between dosing periods to wear off the residual (or carryover) effect from one dosing period to another. For a fixed sample size, the possibility of power increase by crossover design also depends on parameter $\gamma$.

Table 15.1.1: Sample Size for Achieving the Same Power with $K$ Recording Replicates.

| $\rho$ | 1 | $K$ 3 | 5 |
|---|---|---|---|
| 1.0 | $n$ | $1.00n$ | $1.00n$ |
| 0.9 | $n$ | $0.93n$ | $0.92n$ |
| 0.8 | $n$ | $0.86n$ | $0.84n$ |
| 0.7 | $n$ | $0.80n$ | $0.76n$ |
| 0.6 | $n$ | $0.73n$ | $0.68n$ |
| 0.5 | $n$ | $0.66n$ | $0.60n$ |
| 0.4 | $n$ | $0.60n$ | $0.52n$ |
| 0.3 | $n$ | $0.53n$ | $0.44n$ |
| 0.2 | $n$ | $0.46n$ | $0.36n$ |
| 0.1 | $n$ | $0.40n$ | $0.28n$ |
| 0.0 | $n$ | $0.33n$ | $0.20n$ |

Table 15.1.2: Sample Sizes Required Under a Parallel-Group Design.

| | power = 80% | | | | | power = 90% | | | | |
|---|---|---|---|---|---|---|---|---|---|---|
| | $\rho$ | | | | | $\rho$ | | | | |
| $(K, \delta)$ | 0.2 | 0.4 | 0.6 | 0.8 | 1.0 | 0.2 | 0.4 | 0.6 | 0.8 | 1.0 |
| (3, 0.3) | 81 | 105 | 128 | 151 | 174 | 109 | 140 | 171 | 202 | 233 |
| (3, 0.4) | 46 | 59 | 72 | 85 | 98 | 61 | 79 | 96 | 114 | 131 |
| (3, 0.5) | 29 | 38 | 46 | 54 | 63 | 39 | 50 | 64 | 73 | 84 |
| (5, 0.3) | 63 | 91 | 119 | 147 | 174 | 84 | 121 | 159 | 196 | 233 |
| (5, 0.4) | 35 | 51 | 67 | 82 | 98 | 47 | 68 | 89 | 110 | 131 |
| (5, 0.5) | 23 | 33 | 43 | 53 | 63 | 30 | 44 | 57 | 71 | 84 |

Table 15.1.3: Sample Sizes Required Under a Crossover Design With $\rho = 0.8$.

| | power = 80% | | | | |
|---|---|---|---|---|---|
| | $\gamma$ | | | | |
| $(K, \delta)$ | 0.000 | 0.001 | 0.002 | 0.003 | 0.004 |
| (3, 0.3) | 76 | 83 | 92 | 102 | 116 |
| (3, 0.4) | 43 | 45 | 47 | 50 | 53 |
| (3, 0.5) | 27 | 28 | 29 | 30 | 31 |
| (5, 0.3) | 73 | 80 | 89 | 99 | 113 |
| (5, 0.4) | 41 | 43 | 46 | 48 | 51 |
| (5, 0.5) | 26 | 27 | 28 | 29 | 30 |
| | power = 90% | | | | |
| | $\gamma$ | | | | |
| $(K, \delta)$ | 0.000 | 0.001 | 0.002 | 0.003 | 0.004 |
| (3, 0.3) | 101 | 115 | 132 | 156 | 190 |
| (3, 0.4) | 57 | 61 | 66 | 71 | 77 |
| (3, 0.5) | 36 | 38 | 40 | 42 | 44 |
| (5, 0.3) | 98 | 111 | 128 | 151 | 184 |
| (5, 0.4) | 55 | 59 | 64 | 69 | 75 |
| (5, 0.5) | 35 | 37 | 39 | 40 | 42 |

## 15.1.3 Extension

In the previous section, we consider models without covariates. In practice, additional information such as some pharmacokinetic (PK) responses, e.g.,

## 15.1. QT/QTc Studies with Time-Dependent Replicates

area under the blood or plasma concentration time curve (AUC) and the maximum concentration ($C_{\max}$), which are known to be correlated to the QT intervals may be available. In this case, models (15.1.1) and (15.1.2) are necessarily modified to include the PK responses as covariates for a more accurate and reliable assessment of power and sample size calculation (Cheng and Shao, 2005).

### Parallel Group Design

After the inclusion of the PK response as covariate, model (15.1.1) becomes

$$y_{ijk} = \mu_i + \eta x_{ij} + e_{ij} + \epsilon_{ijk},$$

where $x_{ij}$ is the PK response for subject $j$. The least square estimate of $\eta$ is given by

$$\hat{\eta} = \frac{\sum_{i=1}^{2} \sum_{j=1}^{n} (\bar{y}_{ij.} - \bar{y}_{i..})(x_{ij} - \bar{x}_{i.})}{\sum_{i=1}^{2} \sum_{j=1}^{n} (x_{ij} - \bar{x}_{i.})^2}.$$

Then $(\bar{y}_{1..} - \bar{y}_{2..}) - \hat{\eta}(\bar{x}_{1.} - \bar{x}_{2.})$ is an unbiased estimator of $\mu_1 - \mu_2$ with variance

$$\left[ \frac{(\bar{x}_{1.} - \bar{x}_{2.})^2}{\sum_{ij}(x_{ij} - \bar{x}_{i.})^2/n} + 2 \right] \left( \rho + \frac{1-\rho}{K} \right) \frac{\sigma^2}{n},$$

which can be approximated by

$$\left[ \frac{(\nu_1 - \nu_2)^2}{\tau_1^2 + \tau_2^2} + 2 \right] \left( \rho + \frac{1-\rho}{K} \right) \frac{\sigma^2}{n},$$

where $\nu_i = \lim_{n \to \infty} \bar{x}_{i.}$, and $\tau_i^2 = \lim_{n \to \infty} \sum_{j=1}^{n} (x_{ij} - \bar{x}_{i.})^2/n$. Similarly, to achieve the desired power of $1 - \beta$ at the $\alpha$ level of significance, the sample size needed per treatment group is given by

$$n = \frac{(z_{\alpha/2} + z_\beta)^2}{\delta^2} \left[ \frac{(\nu_1 - \nu_2)^2}{\tau_1^2 + \tau_2^2} + 2 \right] \left( \rho + \frac{1-\rho}{K} \right). \qquad (15.1.8)$$

In practice, $\nu_i$ and $\tau_i^2$ are estimated by the corresponding sample mean and sample variance from the pilot data. Note that if there are no covariates or the PK responses are balanced across treatments (i.e., $\nu_1 = \nu_2$), then formula (15.1.8) reduces to (15.1.5).

### Crossover Design

After taken the PK response into consideration as a covariate, model (15.1.2) becomes

$$y_{ijkl} = \mu_i + \eta x_{ijl} + \beta_{il} + e_{ijl} + \epsilon_{ijkl}.$$

Then $(\bar{y}_{1...} - \bar{y}_{2...}) - \hat{\eta}(\bar{x}_{1..} - \bar{x}_{2..})$ is an unbiased estimator of $\mu_1 - \mu_2$ with variance

$$\left[\gamma + \left(\frac{(\bar{x}_{1..} - \bar{x}_{2..})^2}{\sum_{ijl}(x_{ijl} - \bar{x}_{i..})^2/n} + 1\right)\left(\rho + \frac{1-\rho}{K}\right)\right]\sigma^2,$$

which can be approximated by

$$\left[\gamma + \left(\frac{(\nu_1 - \nu_2)^2}{\tau_1^2 + \tau_2^2} + 1\right)\left(\rho + \frac{1-\rho}{K}\right)\right]\sigma^2,$$

where $\nu_i = \lim_{n \to \infty} \bar{x}_{i..}$, and $\tau_i^2 = \lim_{n \to \infty} \sum_{jl}(x_{ijl} - \bar{x}_{i..})^2/n$. To achieve the desired power of $1 - \beta$ at the $\alpha$ level of significance, the sample size required per treatment group is

$$n = \frac{(z_{\alpha/2} + z_\beta)^2}{\delta^2 - \gamma(z_{\alpha/2} + z_\beta)^2}\left[\frac{(\nu_1 - \nu_2)^2}{\tau_1^2 + \tau_2^2} + 1\right]\left(\rho + \frac{1-\rho}{K}\right). \quad (15.1.9)$$

When there are no covariates or PK responses satisfy $\nu_1 = \nu_2$, formula (15.1.9) reduces to (15.1.7).

Formulas (15.1.8) and (15.1.9) indicate that under either a parallel group or a crossover design, a larger sample size is required to achieve the same power if the covariate information is to be incorporated.

### 15.1.4 Remarks

Under a parallel group design, the possibility of whether the sample size can be reduced depends upon the parameter $\rho$, the correlation between the QT recording replicates. As indicated earlier, when $\rho$ closes to 0, these recording repeats can be viewed as (almost) independent replicates. As a result, $n \approx n_{\text{old}}/K$. When $\rho$ is close to 1, we have $n \approx n_{\text{old}}$. Thus, there is not much gain for considering recording replicates in the study. On the other hand, assuming that all other parameters remain the same, the possibility of further reducing the sample size by a crossover design depends upon the parameter $\gamma$, which is a measure of the magnitude of the relative period effect.

When analyzing QT intervals with recording replicates, we may consider change from baseline. It is, however, not clear which baseline should be used when there are also recording replicates at baseline. Strieter et al (2003) proposed the use of the so-called time-matched change from baseline, which is defined as measurement at a time point on the post-baseline day minus measurement at same time point on the baseline. The statistical properties of this approach, however, are not clear. In practice, it may be of interest to investigate relative merits and disadvantages among the approaches using

(i) the most recent recording replicates, (ii) the mean recording replicates, or (iii) time-matched recording replicates as the baseline. This requires further research.

## 15.2 Propensity Analysis in Non-Randomized Studies

As indicated in Yue (2007), the use of propensity analysis in non-randomized trials has received much attention, especially in the area of medical device clinical studies. In non-randomized study, patients are not randomly assigned to treatment groups with equal probability. Instead, the probability of assignment varies from patient to patient depending on patient's baseline covariates. This often results in non-comparable treatment groups due to imbalance of the baseline covariates and consequently invalid the standard methods commonly employed in data analysis. To overcome this problem, Yue (2007) recommends the method of propensity score developed by Rosenbaum and Rubin (1983, 1984) be used.

In her review article, Yue (2007) described some limitations for use of propensity score. For example, propensity score method can only adjust or observed covariates and not for unobserved ones. As a result, it is suggested that a sensitivity analysis be conducted for possible hidden bias. In addition, Yue (2007) also posted several statistical and regulatory issues for propensity analysis in non-randomized trials including sample size calculation. In this discussion, our emphasis will be placed on the issue of sample size calculation in the context of propensity scores. We propose a procedure for sample size calculation based on weighted Mantel-Haenszel test with different weights across score subclasses.

In the next section, a proposed weighted Mantel-Haenszel test, the corresponding formula for sample size calculation, and a formula for sample size calculation ignoring strata are briefly described. Subsequent subsections summarize the results of several simulation studies conducted for evaluation of the performance of the proposed test in the context of propensity analysis. A brief concluding remark is given in the last section.

### 15.2.1 Weighted Mantel-Haenszel Test

Suppose that the propensity score analysis defines $J$ strata. Let $n$ denote the total sample size, and $n_j$ the sample size in stratum $j$ ($\sum_{j=1}^{J} n_j = n$). The data on each subject comprise of the response variable $x = 1$ for response and 0 for no response; $j$ and $k$ for the stratum and treatment group, respectively, to which the subject is assigned ($1 \leq j \leq J; k = 1, 2$).

We assume that group 1 is the control. Frequency data in stratum $j$ can be described as follows:

|          | Group |          |          |
|----------|-------|----------|----------|
| Response | 1     | 2        | Total    |
| Yes      | $x_{j11}$ | $x_{j12}$ | $x_{j1}$ |
| No       | $x_{j21}$ | $x_{j22}$ | $x_{j2}$ |
| Total    | $n_{j1}$  | $n_{j2}$  | $n_j$    |

Let $O_j = x_{j11}$, $E_j = n_{j1}x_{j1}/n_j$, and

$$V_j = \frac{n_{j1}n_{j2}x_{j1}x_{j2}}{n_j^2(n_j-1)}.$$

Then, the weighted Mantel-Haenszel (WMH) test is given by

$$T = \frac{\sum_{j=1}^{J}\hat{w}_j(O_j - E_j)}{\sqrt{\sum_{j=1}^{J}\hat{w}_j^2 V_j}},$$

where the weights $\hat{w}_j$ converges to a constant $w_j$ as $n \to \infty$. The weights are $\hat{w}_j = 1$ for the original Mantel-Haenszel (MH) test and $\hat{w}_j = \hat{q}_j = x_{j2}/n_j$ for the statistic proposed by Gart (1985).

Let $a_j = n_j/n$ denote the allocation proportion for stratum $j$ ($\sum_{j=1}^{J} a_j = 1$), and $b_{jk} = n_{jk}/n_j$ denote the allocation proportion for group $k$ within stratum $j$ ($b_{j1} + b_{j2} = 1$). Let $p_{jk}$ denote the response probability for group $k$ in stratum $j$ and $q_{jk} = 1 - p_{jk}$. Under $H_0: p_{j1} = p_{j2}, 1 \leq j \leq J$, $T$ is approximately $N(0,1)$. The optimal weights maximizing the power depend on the allocation proportions $\{(a_j, b_{1j}, b_{2j}), j = 1, ..., J\}$ and effect sizes $(p_{j1} - p_{j2}, 1, ..., J)$ under $H_1$.

## 15.2.2 Power and Sample Size

In order to calculate the power of WMH, we have to derive the asymptotic distribution of $\sum_{j=1}^{J} \hat{w}_j(O_j - E_j)$ and the limit of $\sum_{j=1}^{J} \hat{w}_j^2 V_j$ under $H_1$. We assume that the success probabilities $(p_{jk}, 1 \leq j \leq J, j = 1, 2)$ satisfy $p_{j2}q_{j1}/(p_{j1}q_{j2}) = \phi$ for $\phi \neq 1$ under $H_1$. Note that a constant odds ratio across strata holds if there exists no interaction between treatment and the propensity score when the binary response is regressed on the treatment indicator and the propensity score using a logistic regression. Following

## 15.2. Propensity Analysis in Non-Randomized Studies

derivations are based on $H_1$. It can be verified that

$$
\begin{aligned}
O_j - E_j &= \frac{n_{j1}n_{j2}}{n_j}(\hat{p}_{j1} - \hat{p}_{j2}) \\
&= \frac{n_{j1}n_{j2}}{n_j}(\hat{p}_{j1} - p_{j1} - \hat{p}_{j2} + p_{j2}) + \frac{n_{j1}n_{j2}}{n_j}(p_{j1} - p_{j2}) \\
&= na_j b_{j1} b_{j2}(\hat{p}_{j1} - p_{j1} - \hat{p}_{j2} + p_{j2}) + na_j b_{j1} b_{j2}(p_{j1} - p_{j2}).
\end{aligned}
$$

Thus, under $H_1$, $\sum_{j=1}^{J} \hat{w}_j(O_j - E_j)$ is approximately normal with mean $n\delta$ and variance $n\sigma_1^2$, where

$$
\begin{aligned}
\delta &= \sum_{j=1}^{J} w_j a_j b_{j1} b_{j2}(p_{j1} - p_{j2}) \\
&= (1 - \phi) \sum_{j=1}^{J} w_j a_j b_{j1} b_{j2} \frac{p_{j1} q_{j1}}{q_{j1} + \phi p_{j1}}
\end{aligned}
$$

and

$$
\begin{aligned}
\sigma_1^2 &= n^{-1} \sum_{j=1}^{J} w_j^2 \frac{n_{j1}^2 n_{j2}^2}{n_j^2} \left( \frac{p_{j1} q_{j1}}{n_{j1}} + \frac{p_{j2} q_{j2}}{n_{j2}} \right) \\
&= \sum_{j=1}^{J} w_j^2 a_j b_{j1} b_{j2} (b_{j2} p_{j1} q_{j1} + b_{j1} p_{j2} q_{j2}).
\end{aligned}
$$

Also, under $H_1$, we have

$$
\sum_{j=1}^{J} w_j^2 V_j = n\sigma_0^2 + o_p(n),
$$

where

$$
\sigma_0^2 = \sum_{j=1}^{J} w_j^2 a_j b_{j1} b_{j2} (b_{j1} p_{j1} + b_{j2} p_{j2})(b_{j1} q_{j1} + b_{j2} q_{j2}).
$$

Hence, the power of WMH is given as

$$
\begin{aligned}
1 - \beta &= P(|T| > z_{1-\alpha/2} | H_1) \\
&= P(\frac{\sigma_1}{\sigma_0} Z + \sqrt{n} \frac{|\delta|}{\sigma_0} > z_{1-\alpha/2}) \\
&= \bar{\Phi}\left( \frac{\sigma_0}{\sigma_1} z_{1-\alpha/2} - \sqrt{n} \frac{|\delta|}{\sigma_1} \right),
\end{aligned}
$$

where $Z$ is a standard normal random variable and $\bar{\Phi}(z) = P(Z > z)$. Thus, sample size required for achieving a desired power of $1 - \beta$ can be

obtained as
$$n = \frac{(\sigma_0 z_{1-\alpha/2} + \sigma_1 z_{1-\beta})^2}{\delta^2}. \tag{1}$$

Following the steps as described in Chow, Shao and Wang (2003c), the sample size calculation for the weighted Mantel-Haenszel test can be carried out as follows:

1. Specify the input variables

   - Type I and II error probabilities, $(\alpha, \beta)$.
   - Success probabilities for group 1 $p_{11}, ..., p_{J1}$, and the odds ratio $\phi$ under $H_1$. Note that $p_{j2} = \phi p_{j1}/(q_{j1} + \phi p_{j1})$.
   - Incidence rates for the strata, $(a_j, j = 1, ..., J)$. (Yue proposes to use $a_j \approx 1/J$.)
   - Allocation probability for group 1 within each stratum, $(b_{j1}, j = 1, ..., J)$.

2. Calculate $n$ by
$$n = \frac{(\sigma_0 z_{1-\alpha/2} + \sigma_1 z_{1-\beta})^2}{\delta^2},$$
where
$$\delta = \sum_{j=1}^{J} a_j b_{j1} b_{j2} (p_{j1} - p_{j2})$$
$$\sigma_1^2 = \sum_{j=1}^{J} a_j b_{j1} b_{j2} (b_{j2} p_{j1} q_{j1} + b_{j1} p_{j2} q_{j2})$$
$$\sigma_0^2 = \sum_{j=1}^{J} a_j b_{j1} b_{j2} (b_{j1} p_{j1} + b_{j2} p_{j2})(b_{j1} q_{j1} + b_{j2} q_{j2}).$$

**Sample Size Calculation Ignoring Strata**

We consider ignoring strata and combining data across $J$ strata. Let $n_k = \sum_{j=1}^{J} n_{jk}$ denote the sample size in group $k$. Ignoring strata, we may estimate the response probabilities by $\hat{p}_k = n_k^{-1} \sum_{j=1}^{J} x_{j1k}$ for group $k$ and $\hat{p} = n^{-1} \sum_{j=1}^{J} \sum_{k=1}^{2} x_{j1k}$ for the pooled data. The WHM ignoring strata reduces to
$$\tilde{T} = \frac{\hat{p}_1 - \hat{p}_2}{\sqrt{\hat{p}\hat{q}(n_1^{-1} + n_2^{-1})}},$$
where $\hat{q} = 1 - \hat{p}$.

## 15.2. Propensity Analysis in Non-Randomized Studies

Noting that $n_{jk} = na_j b_{jk}$, we have

$$\mathrm{E}(\hat{p}_k) \equiv p_k = \sum_{j=1}^{J} a_j b_{jk} p_{jk} / \sum_{j=1}^{J} a_j b_{jk} \qquad (2)$$

and $\mathrm{E}(\hat{p}) \equiv p = \sum_{j=1}^{J} a_j (b_{j1} p_{j1} + b_{j2} p_{j2})$. So, under $H_1$, $\hat{p}_1 - \hat{p}_2$ is approximately normal with mean $\tilde{\delta} = p_1 - p_2$ and variance $n^{-1}\tilde{\sigma}_1^2$, where $\tilde{\sigma}_1^2 = p_1 q_1 / b_1 + p_2 q_2 / b_2$, $q_k = 1 - p_k$ and $b_k = \sum_{j=1}^{J} a_j b_{jk}$. Also under $H_1$, $\hat{p}\hat{q}(n_1^{-1} + n_2^{-1}) = n^{-1}\tilde{\sigma}_0^2 + o_p(n^{-1})$, where $\tilde{\sigma}_0^2 = pq(b_1^{-1} + b_2^{-1})$. Hence, the sample size ignoring strata is given as

$$\tilde{n} = \frac{(\tilde{\sigma}_0 z_{1-\alpha/2} + \tilde{\sigma}_1 z_{1-\beta})^2}{(p_1 - p_2)^2}. \qquad (3)$$

Analysis based on propensity score is to adjust for possible unbalanced baseline covariates between groups. Under balanced baseline covariates (or propensity score), we have $b_{11} = \cdots = b_{J1}$, and, from (2), $p_1 = p_2$ when $H_0 : p_{j1} = p_{j2}, 1 \leq j \leq J$ is true. Hence, under balanced covariates, the test statistic $\tilde{T}$ ignoring strata will be valid too. However, by not adjusting for the covariates (or, propensity), it will have a lower power than the stratified test statistic $T$, see Nam (1998) for Gart's test statistic. On the other hand, if the distribution of covariates is unbalanced, we have $p_1 \neq p_2$ even under $H_0$, and the test statistic $\tilde{T}$ ignoring strata will not be valid.

**Remarks**

For non-randomized trials, the sponsors usually estimate sample size in the same way as they do in randomized trials. As a result, the United States Food and Drug Administration (FDA) usually gives a warning and requests sample size justification (increase) based on the consideration of the degree of overlap in the propensity score distribution. When there exists an imbalance in covariate distribution between arms, a sample size calculation ignoring strata is definitely biased. The use of different weights will have an impact on statistical power but will not affect the consistency of the proposed weighted Mantel-Haenszel test. Note that the sample size formula by Nam (1998) based on the test statistic proposed by Gart (1985) is a special case of the sample size given in (1) where $\hat{w}_j = \hat{q}_j$ and $w_j = 1 - b_{j1} p_{j1} - b_{j2} p_{j2}$.

### 15.2.3 Simulations

Suppose that we want to compare the probability of treatment success between control ($k = 1$) and new ($k = 2$) device. We consider partitioning the combined data into $J = 5$ strata based on propensity score, and the allocation proportions are projected as $(a_1, a_2, a_3, a_4, a_5) = (.15, .15, .2, .25, .25)$ and $(b_{11}, b_{21}, b_{31}, b_{41}, b_{51}) = (.4, .4, .5, .6, .6)$. Also, suppose that the response probabilities for control device are given as $(p_{11}, p_{21}, p_{31}, p_{41}, p_{51}) = (.5, .6, .7, .8, .9)$, and we want to calculate the sample size required for a power of $1 - \beta = 0.8$ to detect an odds ratio of $\phi = 2$ using two-sided $\alpha = 0.05$. For $\phi = 2$, the response probabilities for the new device are given as $(p_{12}, p_{22}, p_{32}, p_{42}, p_{52}) = (.6667, .7500, .8235, .8889, .9474)$. Under these settings, we need $n = 447$ for MH.

In order to evaluate the performance of the sample size formula, we conduct simulations. In each simulation, $n = 447$ binary observations are generate under the parameters (allocation proportions and the response probabilities) for sample size calculation. MH test with $\alpha = 0.05$ is applied to each simulation sample. Empirical power is calculated as the proportion of the simulation samples that reject $H_0$ out of $N = 10,000$ simulations. The empirical power is obtained as 0.7978, which is very close to the nominal $1 - \beta = 0.8$.

If we ignore the strata, we have $\tilde{p}_1 = 0.7519$ and $\tilde{p}_2 = 0.8197$ by (2) and the odds ratio is only $\tilde{\phi} = 1.5004$ which is much smaller than $\phi = 2$. For $(\alpha, 1 - \beta) = (.05, .8)$, we need $\tilde{n} = 1151$ by (3). With $n = 422$, $\tilde{T}$ with $\alpha = .05$ rejected $H_0$ for only 41.4% of simulation samples.

The performance of the test statistics, $T$ and $\tilde{T}$, are evaluated by generating simulation samples of size $n = 447$ under

$$H_0 : (p_{11}, p_{21}, p_{31}, p_{41}, p_{51}) = (p_{12}, p_{22}, p_{32}, p_{42}, p_{52}) = (.1, .3, .5, .7, .9).$$

Other parameters are specified at the same values as above. For $\alpha = 0.05$, the empirical type I error is obtained as 0.0481 for $T$ with MH scores and 0.1852 for $\tilde{T}$. While the empirical type I error of the MH stratified test is close to the nominal $\alpha = 0.05$, the unstratified test is severely inflated. Under this $H_0$, we have $\tilde{p}_1 = 0.7953$ and $\tilde{p}_1 = 0.7606$ ($\tilde{\phi} = 0.8181$), which are unequal due to the unbalanced covariate distribution between groups.

Now, let's consider a balanced allocation case, $b_{11} = \cdots = b_{J1} = 0.3$, with all the other parameter values the same as in the above simulations. Under above $H_1 : \phi = 2$, we need $n = 499$ for $T$ and $\tilde{n} = 542$ for $\tilde{T}$. Note that the unstratified test $\tilde{T}$ requires a slightly larger sample size due to loss of efficiency. From $N = 10,000$ simulation samples of size $n = 499$, we obtained an empirical power of 0.799 for $T$ and only 0.770 for $\tilde{T}$. From similar simulations under $H_0$, we obtained an empirical type I error of 0.0470 for $T$ with MH scores and 0.0494 for $\tilde{T}$. Note that both tests control the type I error very accurately in this case. Under $H_0$, we have $\tilde{p}_1 = \tilde{p}_2 = 0.78$ ($\tilde{\phi} = 1$).

### 15.2.4 Concluding Remarks

Sample size calculation plays an important role in clinical research when designing a new medical study. Inadequate sample size could have a significant impact on the accuracy and reliability of the evaluation of treatment effect especially in medical device clinical studies, which are often conducted in a non-randomized fashion (although the method of propensity score may have been employed to achieve balance in baseline covariates). We propose a unified sample size formula for weighted Mantel-Haenszel tests based on large-sample assumption. We found through simulations that our sample size formula accurately maintains the power. When the distribution of the covariates is unbalanced between groups, an analysis ignoring the strata could be severely biased.

## 15.3 ANOVA with Repeated Measures

In clinical research, it is not uncommon to have multiple assessments in a parallel-group clinical trial. The purpose of such a design is to evaluate the performance of clinical efficacy and/or safety over time during the entire study course. Clinical data collected from such a design is usually analyzed by means of the so-called analysis of variance (ANOVA) with repeated measures. In this section, formulas for sample size calculation under the design with multiple assessments is derived using the method of analysis of variance with repeated measures.

### 15.3.1 Statistical Model

Let $B_{ij}$ and $H_{ijt}$ be the illness score at baseline and the illness score at time $t$ for the $j$th subject in the $i$th treatment group, $t = 1, ..., m_{ij}$, $j = 1, ..., n_i$, and $i = 1, ..., k$. Then, $Y_{ijt} = H_{ijt} - B_{ij}$, the illness scores adjusted for baseline, can be described by the following statistical model (see, e.g., Longford, 1993; Chow and Liu, 2000):

$$Y_{ijt} = \mu + \alpha_i + S_{ij} + b_{ij}t + e_{ijt},$$

where $\alpha_i$ is the fixed effect for the $i$th treatment ( $\sum_{i=1}^{k} \alpha_i = 0$), $S_{ij}$ is the random effect due to the $j$th subject in the $i$th treatment group, $b_{ij}$ is the coefficient of the $j$th subject in the $i$th treatment group and $e_{ijt}$ is the random error in observing $Y_{ijt}$. In the above model, it is assumed that (i) $S_{ij}$'s are independently distributed as $N(0, \sigma_S^2)$, (ii) $b_{ij}$'s are independently distributed as $N(0, \sigma_\beta^2)$, and (iii) $e_{ijt}$'s are independently distributed as $N(0, \sigma^2)$. For any given subject $j$ within treatment $i$, $Y_{ijt}$ can be described by a regression line with slope $b_{ij}$ conditioned on $S_{ij}$, i.e.,

$$Y_{ijt} = \mu_{ij} + b_{ij}t + e_{ijt}, \quad t = 1, ..., m_{ij},$$

where $\mu_{ij} = \mu + \alpha_i + S_{ij}$. When conditioned on $S_{ij}$, i.e., it is considered as fixed, unbiased estimators of the coefficient can be obtained by the method of ordinary least squares (OLS), which are given by

$$\hat{\mu}_{ij} = \frac{\sum_{i=1}^{k} Y_i \sum_{i=1}^{k} t_i^2 - \sum_{i=1}^{k} t_i \sum_{i=1}^{k} Y_i t_i}{m_{ij} \sum_{i=1}^{k} t_i^2 - (\sum_{i=1}^{k} t_i)^2}$$

$$\hat{b}_{ij} = \frac{m_{ij} \sum_{i=1}^{k} Y_i t_i - \sum_{i=1}^{k} Y_i \sum_{i=1}^{k} t_i}{m_{ij} \sum_{i=1}^{k} t_i^2 - (\sum_{i=1}^{k} t_i)^2}.$$

The sum of squared error for the $j$th subject in the $i$th treatment group, denoted by $SSE_{ij}$, is distributed as $\sigma^2 \chi^2_{m_{ij}-2}$. Hence, an unbiased estimator of $\sigma^2$, the variation due to the repeated measurements, is given by

$$\hat{\sigma}^2 = \frac{\sum_{i=1}^{k} \sum_{j=1}^{n_i} SSE_{ij}}{\sum_{i=1}^{k} \sum_{j=1}^{n_i} (m_{ij} - 2)}.$$

Since data from subjects are independent, $\sum_{i=1}^{k} \sum_{j=1}^{n_i} SSE_{ij}$ is distributed as $\sigma^2 \chi^2_{n^*}$, where $n^* = \sum_{i=1}^{k} \sum_{j=1}^{n_i} (m_{ij} - 2)$. Conditioning on $S_{ij}$ and $b_{ij}$, we have

$$\hat{\mu}_{ij} \sim N\left(\mu_{ij}, \frac{\sigma^2 \sum_{i=1}^{k} t_i^2}{m_{ij} \sum_{i=1}^{k} t_i^2 - (\sum_{i=1}^{k} t_i)^2}\right),$$

$$\hat{b}_{ij} \sim N\left(b_{ij}, \frac{\sigma^2 m_{ij}}{m_{ij} \sum_{i=1}^{k} t_i^2 - (\sum_{i=1}^{k} t_i)^2}\right).$$

Thus, unconditionally,

$$\hat{\mu}_{ij} \sim N\left(\mu + \alpha_i, \sigma_S^2 + \sigma^2 \frac{\sum_{i=1}^{k} t_i^2}{m_{ij} \sum_{i=1}^{k} t_i^2 - (\sum_{i=1}^{k} t_i)^2}\right),$$

$$\hat{b}_{ij} \sim N\left(\beta_{ij}, \sigma_\beta^2 + \sigma^2 \frac{m_{ij}}{m_{ij} \sum_{i=1}^{k} t_i^2 - (\sum_{i=1}^{k} t_i)^2}\right).$$

When there is an equal number of repeated measurements for each subject, i.e., $m_{ij} = m$ for all $i, j$, the inter-subject variation, $\sigma_S^2$, can be estimated by

$$\hat{\sigma}_S^2 = \frac{\sum_{i=1}^{k} \sum_{j=1}^{n_i} (\mu_{ij} - \mu_{i.})^2}{\sum_{i=1}^{k} (n_i - 1)} - \hat{\sigma}^2 \frac{\sum_{i=1}^{k} t_i^2}{m \sum_{i=1}^{k} t_i^2 - (\sum_{i=1}^{k} t_i)^2},$$

where
$$\hat{\mu}_{i.} = \frac{1}{n_i} \sum_{j=1}^{n_i} \hat{\mu}_{ij}.$$

An estimator of the variation of $b_{ij}$ can then be obtained as
$$\hat{\sigma}_\beta^2 = \frac{\sum_{i=1}^k \sum_{j=1}^{n_i}(b_{ij} - b_{i.})^2}{\sum_{i=1}^k (n_i - 1)} - \hat{\sigma}^2 \frac{m}{m \sum_{i=1}^k t_i^2 - (\sum_{i=1}^k t_i)^2},$$

where
$$\hat{b}_{i.} = \frac{1}{n_i} \sum_{j=1}^{n_i} \hat{b}_{ij}.$$

Similarly, $\beta_i$ can be estimated by
$$\hat{\beta}_i = \frac{1}{n_i} \sum_{j=1}^{n_i} b_{ij} \sim N(\beta_i, \delta^2),$$

where
$$\delta^2 = \sigma_\beta^2 + \frac{\sigma^2}{n_i} \frac{m}{m \sum_{i=1}^k t_i^2 - (\sum_{i=1}^k t_i)^2}.$$

### 15.3.2 Hypotheses Testing

Since the objective is to compare the treatment effect on the illness scores, it is of interest to test the following hypotheses:
$$H_0 : \alpha_i = \alpha_{i'} \quad \text{versus} \quad H_a : \alpha_i \neq \alpha_{i'}.$$

The above hypotheses can be tested by using the statistic
$$T_1 = \sqrt{\frac{n_i n_{i'}}{n_i n_{i'}}} \left( \frac{\hat{\mu}_{i.} - \hat{\mu}_{i'.}}{\sum_{i=1}^k \sum_{j=1}^{n_i}(\hat{\mu}_{ij} - \hat{\mu}_{i.})^2 / \sum_{i=1}^k (n_i - 1)} \right).$$

Under the null hypotheses of no difference in the illness score between two treatment groups, $T_1$ follows a t distribution with $\sum_{i=1}^k (n_i - 1)$ degrees of freedom. Hence, we reject the null hypothesis at the $\alpha$ level of significance if
$$|T_1| > t_{\alpha/2, \sum_{i=1}^k (n_i - 1)}.$$

Furthermore, it is also of interest to test the following null hypothesis of equal slopes (i.e., rate of change in illness scores over the repeated measurement)
$$H_0 : \beta_i = \beta_{i'} \quad \text{versus} \quad H_a : \beta_i \neq \beta_{i'}.$$

The above hypotheses can be tested using the following statistic

$$T_2 = \sqrt{\frac{n_i n_{i'}}{n_i n_{i'}}} \left( \frac{\hat{b}_{i.} - \hat{b}_{i'.}}{\sum_{i=1}^{k} \sum_{j=1}^{n_i} (\hat{b}_{ij} - \hat{b}_{i.})^2 / \sum_{i=1}^{k} (n_i - 1)} \right).$$

Under the null hypotheses, $T_2$ follows a t distribution with $\sum_{i=1}^{k}(n_i - 1)$ degrees of freedom. Hence, we would reject the null hypotheses of no difference in rate of change in illness scores between treatment groups at the $\alpha$ level of significance if

$$|T_2| > t_{\alpha/2, \sum_{i=1}^{k}(n_i - 1)}.$$

### 15.3.3 Sample Size Calculation

Since the above tests are based on a standard t test, the sample size per treatment group required for detection of a clinically meaningful difference, $\Delta$, with a desired power of $1 - \beta$ at the $\alpha$ level of significance is given by

$$n \geq \frac{2\sigma^{*2}(z_{\alpha/2} + z_\beta)^2}{\Delta^2},$$

where $\sigma^{*2}$ is the sum of the variance components. When the null hypothesis $H_0 : \alpha_i = \alpha_{i'}$ is tested,

$$\sigma^{*2} = \sigma_\alpha^2 = \sigma_S^2 + \frac{\sigma^2 \sum_{i=1}^{k} t_i^2}{m_{ij} \sum_{i=1}^{k} t_i^2 - (\sum_{i=1}^{k} t_i)^2},$$

which can be estimated by

$$\hat{\sigma}_1^2 = \frac{\sum_{i=1}^{k} \sum_{j=1}^{n_i} (\hat{\mu}_{ij} - \hat{\mu}_{i.})^2}{\sum_{i=1}^{k} (n_i - 1)}.$$

When the null hypothesis $H_0 : \beta_i = \beta_{i'}$ is tested,

$$\sigma^{*2} = \sigma_\beta^2 + \sigma^2 \frac{m_{ij}}{m_{ij} \sum_{i=1}^{k} t_i^2 - (\sum_{i=1}^{k} t_i)^2},$$

which can be estimated by

$$\hat{\sigma}_2^2 = \frac{\sum_{i=1}^{k} \sum_{j=1}^{n_i} (\hat{\beta}_{ij} - \hat{\beta}_{i.})^2}{\sum_{i=1}^{k} (n_i - 1)}.$$

## 15.3.4 An Example

Suppose a sponsor is planning a randomized, parallel-group clinical trial on mice with multiple sclerosis (MS) for evaluation of a number of doses of an active compound, an active control, and/or a vehicle control. In practice, experimental autoimmune encephalomyelitis (EAE) is usually induced in susceptible animals following a single injection of central nervous system extract emulsified in the adjuvant. The chronic forms of EAE reflect many of pathophysiologic steps in MS. This similarity has initiated the usage of EAE models for development of MS therapies. Clinical assessment of the illness for the induction of EAE in mice that are commonly used is given in Table 15.3.1. Illness scores of mice are recorded between Day 10 and Day 19 before dosing regardless of the onset or the remission of the attack. Each mouse will receive a dose from Day 20 to Day 33. The post-inoculation performance of each mouse is usually assessed up to Day 34. Sample size calculation was performed using the analysis of variance model with repeated measures based on the assumptions that

1. the primary study endpoint is the illness scores of mice;

2. the scientifically meaningful difference in illness score is considered to be 1.0 or 1.5 (note that changes of 1.0 and 1.5 over the time period between Day 19 and Day 34 are equivalent to 0.067 and 0.1 changes in slope of the illness score curve);

3. the standard deviation for each treatment group is assumed to be same (various standard deviations such as 0.75, 0.80, 0.85, 0.90, 0.95, 1.0, 1.05, 1.1, 1.15, 1.2, or 1.25 are considered);

4. the null hypothesis of interest is that there is no difference in the profile of illness scores, which is characterized between baseline (at dosing) and a specific time point after dosing, among treatment groups;

5. the probability of committing a type II error is 10% or 20%, i.e., the power is respectively 90%, or 80%;

6. the null hypothesis is tested at the 5% level of significance;

7. Bonferroni's adjustment for $\alpha$ significant level for multiple comparisons were considered.

Under the one-way analysis of variance model with repeated measures, the formula for the sample size calculation given in the previous subsection can be used.

Table 15.3.1: Clinical Assessment of Induction of EAE in Mice

| | |
|---|---|
| Stage 0: | Normal |
| Stage 0.5: | Partial limp tail |
| Stage 1: | Complete limp tail |
| Stage 2: | Impaired righting reflex |
| Stage 2.5: | Righting reflex is delayed (Not weak enough to be stage 3) |
| Stage 3: | Partial hind limb paralysis |
| Stage 3.5: | One leg is completely paralyzed, and one leg is partially paralyzed |
| Stage 4: | Complete hind limb paralysis |
| Stage 4.5: | Legs are completely paralyzed and moribund |
| Stage 5: | Death due to EAE |

Table 15.3.2 provides sample sizes required for three-arm, four-arm, and five-arm studies with $\alpha$ adjustment for multiple comparisons, respectively. For example, a sample size of 45 subjects (i.e., 15 subjects per treatment group) is needed to maintain an 80% power for detection of a decrease in illness score by $\Delta = 1.5$ over the active treatment period between treatment groups when $\sigma^*$ is 1.25.

## 15.4 Quality of Life

In clinical research, it has been a concern that the treatment of disease or survival may not be as important as the improvement of quality of life (QOL), especially for patients with a chronic or life-threatening disease. Enhancement of life beyond absence of illness to enjoyment of life may be considered more important than the extension of life. QOL not only provides information as to how the patients feel about drug therapies, but also appeals to the physician's desire for the best clinical practice. It can be used as a predictor of compliance of the patient. In addition, it may be used to distinguish between therapies that appear to be equally efficacious and equally safe at the stage of marketing strategy planning. The information can be potentially used in advertising for the promotion of the drug therapy. As a result, in addition to the comparison of hazard rates, survival function, or median survival time, QOL is often assessed in survival trials.

QOL is usually assessed by a questionnaire, which may consist of a number of questions (items). We refer to such a questionnaire as a QOL instrument. A QOL instrument is a very subjective tool and is expected to have a

Table 15.3.2: Sample Size Calculation with $\alpha$ Adjustment for Multiple Comparisons

|  |  | Sample Size Per Arm | | | | | |
|---|---|---|---|---|---|---|---|
|  |  | Three Arms | | Four Arms | | Five Arms | |
| Power | $\sigma^*$ | $\Delta=1.0$ | $\Delta=1.5$ | $\Delta=1.0$ | $\Delta=1.5$ | $\Delta=1.0$ | $\Delta=1.5$ |
| 80% | 0.75 | 12 | 6 | 14 | 7 | 15 | 7 |
|  | 0.80 | 14 | 6 | 16 | 7 | 17 | 8 |
|  | 0.85 | 16 | 7 | 18 | 8 | 20 | 9 |
|  | 0.90 | 17 | 8 | 20 | 9 | 22 | 10 |
|  | 0.95 | 19 | 9 | 22 | 10 | 25 | 11 |
|  | 1.00 | 21 | 10 | 25 | 11 | 27 | 12 |
|  | 1.05 | 24 | 11 | 27 | 12 | 30 | 14 |
|  | 1.10 | 26 | 12 | 30 | 14 | 33 | 15 |
|  | 1.15 | 28 | 13 | 33 | 15 | 36 | 16 |
|  | 1.20 | 31 | 14 | 35 | 16 | 39 | 17 |
|  | 1.25 | 33 | 15 | 38 | 17 | 42 | 19 |
| 90% | 0.75 | 16 | 7 | 18 | 8 | 19 | 9 |
|  | 0.80 | 18 | 8 | 20 | 9 | 22 | 10 |
|  | 0.85 | 20 | 9 | 23 | 10 | 25 | 11 |
|  | 0.90 | 22 | 10 | 25 | 12 | 28 | 13 |
|  | 0.95 | 25 | 11 | 28 | 13 | 31 | 14 |
|  | 1.00 | 28 | 13 | 31 | 14 | 34 | 15 |
|  | 1.05 | 30 | 14 | 34 | 16 | 37 | 17 |
|  | 1.10 | 33 | 15 | 38 | 17 | 41 | 18 |
|  | 1.15 | 36 | 16 | 41 | 19 | 45 | 20 |
|  | 1.20 | 39 | 18 | 45 | 20 | 49 | 22 |
|  | 1.25 | 43 | 19 | 49 | 22 | 53 | 24 |

large variation. Thus, it is a concern whether the adopted QOL instrument can accurately and reliably quantify patients' QOL. In this section, we provide a comprehensive review of the validation of a QOL instrument, the use of QOL scores, statistical methods for assessment of QOL, and practical issues that are commonly encountered in clinical trials. For the assessment of QOL, statistical analysis based on subscales, composite scores, and/or overall score are often performed for an easy interpretation. For example, Tandon (1990) applied a global statistic to combine the results of the univariate analysis of each subscale. Olschewski and Schumacher (1990), on the other hand, proposed to use composite scores to reduce the dimensions of QOL. However, due to the complex correlation structure among subscales, optimal statistical properties may not be obtained. As an alternative, to account for the correlation structure, the following time series model proposed by Chow and Ki (1994) may be useful.

### 15.4.1 Time Series Model

For a given subscale (or component), let $x_{ijt}$ be the response of the $j$th subject to the $i$th question (item) at time $t$, where $i = 1, ..., k$, $j = 1, ..., n$, and $t = 1, ..., T$. Consider the average score over $k$ questions:

$$Y_{jt} = \bar{x}_{jt} = \frac{1}{k} \sum_{j=1}^{k} x_{ijt}.$$

Since the average scores $y_{j1}, ..., y_{jT}$ are correlated, the following autoregressive time series model may be an appropriate statistical model for $y_{jt}$:

$$y_{jt} = \mu + \psi(y_{j(t-1)} - \mu) + e_{jt}, \ j = 1, ..., n, \ t = 1, ..., T,$$

where $\mu$ is the overall mean, $|\psi| < 1$ is the autoregressive parameter, and $e_{jt}$ are independent identically distributed random errors with mean 0 and variance $\sigma_e^2$. It can be verified that

$$E(e_{jt} y'_{jt}) = 0 \ \text{ for all } t' < t.$$

The autoregressive parameter $\psi$ can be used to assess the correlation of consecutive responses $y_{jt}$ and $y_{j(t+1)}$. From the above model, it can be shown that the autocorrelation of responses with $m$ lag times is $\psi^m$, which is negligible when $m$ is large. Based on the observed average scores on the $j$th subject, $y_{j1}, ..., y_{jT}$, we can estimate the overall mean $\mu$ and the autoregressive parameter $\psi$. The ordinary least-square estimators of $\mu$ and $\psi$ can be approximated by

$$\hat{\mu}_j = \bar{y}_{j.} = \frac{1}{T} \sum_{t=1}^{T} y_{jt}$$

and
$$\hat{\psi}_j = \frac{\sum_{t=2}^{T}(y_{jt} - \bar{y}_{j.})(y_{j(t-1)} - \bar{y}_{j.})}{\sum_{t=2}^{T}(y_{jt} - \bar{y}_{j.})^2},$$

which are the sample mean and sample autocorrelation of consecutive observations. Under the above model, it can be verified that $\hat{\mu}_j$ is unbiased and that the variance of $\hat{\mu}_j$ is given by

$$\text{Var}(\bar{y}_{j.}) = \frac{\gamma_{j0}}{T}\left(1 + 2\sum_{t=1}^{T-1}\frac{T-t}{T}\psi^t\right),$$

where $\gamma_{j0} = \text{Var}(y_{jt})$. The estimated variance of $\hat{\mu}_j$ can be obtained by replacing $\psi$ with $\hat{\psi}_j$ and $\gamma_{j0}$ with

$$c_{j0} = \sum_{t=1}^{T}\frac{(y_{jt} - \bar{y}_{j.})^2}{T-1}.$$

Suppose that the $n$ subjects are from the same population with the same variability and autocorrelation. The QOL measurements of these subjects can be used to estimate the mean average scores $\mu$. An intuitive estimator of $\mu$ is the sample mean

$$\hat{\mu} = \bar{y}_{..} = \frac{1}{n}\sum_{j=1}^{n}\bar{y}_{j.}.$$

Under the time series model, the estimated variance of $\hat{\mu}$ is given by

$$s^2(\bar{y}_{..}) = \frac{c_0}{nT}\left(1 + 2\sum_{t=1}^{T-1}\frac{T-t}{T}\hat{\psi}^t\right),$$

where

$$c_0 = \frac{1}{n(T-1)}\sum_{j=1}^{n}\left[\sum_{t=1}^{T}(y_{jt} - \bar{y}_{j.})^2\right]$$

and

$$\hat{\psi} = \frac{1}{n}\sum_{j=1}^{n}\hat{\psi}_j.$$

An approximate $(1-\alpha)100\%$ confidence interval for $\mu$ has limits

$$\bar{y}_{..} \pm z_{1-\alpha/2}s(\bar{y}_{..}),$$

where $z_{1-\alpha/2}$ is the $(1-\alpha/2)$th quantile of a standard normal distribution.

Under the time series model, the method of confidence interval approach described above can be used to assess difference in QOL between treatments. Note that the assumption that all the QOL measurements over time are independent is a special case of the above model with $\psi = 0$. In practice, it is suggested that the above time series model be used to account for the possible positive correlation between measurements over the time period under study.

## 15.4.2 Sample Size Calculation

Under the time series model, Chow and Ki (1996) derived some useful formulas for determination of sample size based on normal approximation. For a fixed precision index $1 - \alpha$, to ensure a reasonable high power index $\delta$ for detecting a meaningful difference $\epsilon$, the sample size per treatment group should not be less than

$$n_\delta = \frac{c(z_{1-1/2\alpha} + z_\delta)^2}{\epsilon^2} \quad \text{for } \delta > 0.5,$$

where

$$c = \frac{\gamma_y}{T}\left(1 + 2\sum_{t=1}^{T-1}\frac{T-t}{T}\psi_y^t\right) + \frac{\gamma_u}{T}\left(1 + 2\sum_{t=1}^{T-1}\frac{T-t}{T}\psi_u^t\right).$$

For a fixed precision index $1 - \alpha$, if the acceptable limit for detecting an equivalence between two treatment means is $(-\Delta, \Delta)$, to ensure a reasonable high power $\phi$ for detecting an equivalence when the true difference in treatment means is less than a small constant $\eta$, the sample size for each treatment group should be at least

$$n_\phi = \frac{c}{(\Delta - \eta)^2}(z_{1/2+1/2\phi} + z_{1-1/2\alpha})^2.$$

If both treatment groups are assumed to have the same variability and autocorrelation coefficient, the constant $c$ can be simplified as

$$c = \frac{2\gamma}{T}\left(1 + 2\sum_{t=1}^{T-1}\frac{T-t}{T}\psi^t\right).$$

When $n = \max(n_\phi, n_\delta)$, it ensures that the QOL instrument will have precision index $1 - \alpha$ and power of no less than $\delta$ and $\phi$ in detecting a difference and an equivalence, respectively. It, however, should be noted that the required sample size is proportional to the variability of the average scores considered. The higher the variability, the larger the sample size that would be required. Note that the above formulas can also be applied to many clinical based research studies with time-correlated outcome measurements, e.g., 24-hour monitoring of blood pressure, heart rates, hormone levels, and body temperature.

## 15.4.3 An Example

To illustrate the use of the above sample size formulas, consider QOL assessment in two independent groups A and B. Suppose a QOL instrument containing 11 questions is to be administered to subjects at week 4, 8, 12, and 16. Denote the mean of QOL score of the subjects in group A and B by $y_{it}$ and $u_{jt}$, respectively. We assume that $y_{it}$ and $u_{jt}$ have distributions that follow the time series model described in the previous section with common variance $\gamma = 0.5$ sq. unit and have moderate autocorrelation between scores at consecutive time points, say $\psi = 0.5$. For a fixed 95% precision index, 87 subjects per group will provide a 90% power for detection of a difference of 0.25 unit in means. If the chosen acceptable limits are $(-0.35, 0.35)$, then 108 subjects per group will have a power of 90% that the 95% confidence interval of difference in group means will correctly detect an equivalence with $\eta = 0.1$ unit. If sample size is chosen to be 108 per group, it ensures that the power indices for detecting a difference of 0.25 unit or an equivalence are not less than 90%.

## 15.5 Bridging Studies

In the pharmaceutical industry, the sponsors are often interested in bringing their drug products from one region (e.g., the United States of America) to another region (e.g., Asian Pacific) to increase the exclusivity of the drug products in the marketplace. However, it is a concern whether the clinical results can be extrapolated from the target patient population in one region to a similar but different patient population in a new region due to a possible difference in ethnic factors. The International Conference on Harmonization (ICH) recommends that a bridging study may be conducted to extrapolate the clinical results between regions. However, little or no information regarding the criterion for determining whether a bridging study is necessary based on the evaluation of the complete clinical data package is provided by the ICH. Furthermore, no criterion on the assessment of similarity of clinical results between regions is given. In this section, we propose the use of a sensitivity index as a possible criterion for regulatory authorities in the new region to evaluate whether a bridging clinical study should be conducted and the sample size of such a bridging clinical study.

### 15.5.1 Sensitivity Index

Suppose that a randomized, parallel-group, placebo-controlled clinical trial is conducted for evaluation of a test compound as compared to a placebo control in the original region. The study protocol calls for a total of $n$

subjects with the disease under study. These $n = n_1 + n_2$ subjects are randomly assigned to receive either the test compound or a placebo control. Let $x_{ij}$ be the response observed from the $j$th subject in the $i$th treatment group, where $j = 1, ..., n_i$ and $i = 1, 2$. Assume that $x_{ij}$'s are independent and normally distributed with means $\mu_i$, $i = 1, 2$, and a common variance $\sigma^2$. Suppose the hypotheses of interest are

$$H_0: \mu_1 - \mu_2 = 0 \quad \text{versus} \quad H_a: \mu_1 - \mu_2 \neq 0.$$

Note that the discussion for a one-sided $H_a$ is similar. When $\sigma^2$ is unknown, we reject $H_0$ at the 5% level of significance if

$$|T| > t_{n-2},$$

where $t_{\alpha, n-2}$ is the $100(1 - \alpha/2)$th percentile of a t distribution with $n - 2$ degrees of freedom, $n = n_1 + n_2$,

$$T = \frac{\bar{x}_1 - \bar{x}_2}{\sqrt{\frac{(n_1-1)s_1^2 + (n_2-1)s_2^2}{n-2}} \sqrt{\frac{1}{n_1} + \frac{1}{n_2}}}, \quad (15.5.1)$$

and $\bar{x}_i$ and and $s_i^2$ are the sample mean and variance, respectively, based on the data from the $i$th treatment group. The power of $T$ is given by

$$p(\theta) = P(|T| > t_{n-2}) = 1 - \mathcal{T}_{n-2}(t_{n-2}|\theta) + \mathcal{T}_{n-2}(-t_{n-2}|\theta), \quad (15.5.2)$$

where

$$\theta = \frac{\mu_1 - \mu_2}{\sigma \sqrt{\frac{1}{n_1} + \frac{1}{n_2}}}$$

and $\mathcal{T}_{n-2}(\cdot|\theta)$ denotes the cumulative distribution function of the non-central t distribution with $n - 2$ degrees of freedom and the non-centrality parameter $\theta$.

Let $\boldsymbol{x}$ be the observed data from the first clinical trial and $T(\boldsymbol{x})$ be the value of $T$ based on $\boldsymbol{x}$. Replacing $\theta$ in the power function in (15.5.2) by its estimate $T(\boldsymbol{x})$, the estimated power can be obtained as follows

$$\hat{P} = p(T(\boldsymbol{x})) = 1 - \mathcal{T}_{n-2}(t_{n-2}|T(\boldsymbol{x})) + \mathcal{T}_{n-2}(-t_{n-2}|T(\boldsymbol{x})).$$

Note that Shao and Chow (2002) refer to $\hat{P}$ as the reproducibility probability for the second clinical trial with the same patient population. However, a different and more sensible way of defining a reproducibility probability is to define reproducibility probability as the posterior mean of $p(\theta)$, i.e.,

$$\tilde{P} = P(|T(\boldsymbol{y})| > t_{n-2}|\boldsymbol{x}) = \int p(\theta)\pi(\theta|\boldsymbol{x})d\theta,$$

## 15.5. Bridging Studies

where $y$ denotes the data set from the second trial and $\pi(\theta|x)$ is the posterior density of $\theta$, given $x$. When the non-informative prior $\pi(\mu_1, \mu_2, \sigma^2) = \sigma^{-2}$ is used, Shao and Chow (2002) showed that

$$\tilde{P} = E_{\delta,u}\left[1 - \mathcal{T}_{n-2}\left(t_{n-2}\left|\frac{\delta}{u}\right.\right) - \mathcal{T}_{n-2}\left(-t_{n-2}\left|\frac{\delta}{u}\right.\right)\right],$$

where $E_{\delta,u}$ is the expectation with respect to $\delta$ and $u$, $u^{-2}$ has the gamma distribution with the shape parameter $(n-2)/2$ and the scale parameter $2/(n-2)$, and given $u$, $\delta$ has the normal distribution $N(T(x), u^2)$.

When the test compound is applied to a similar but different patient population in the new region, it is expected that the mean and variance of the response would be different. Chow, Shao, and Hu (2002) proposed the following concept of sensitivity index for evaluation of the change in patient population due to ethnic differences. Suppose that in the second clinical trial conducted in the new region, the population mean difference is changed to $\mu_1 - \mu_2 + \varepsilon$ and the population variance is changed to $C^2\sigma^2$, where $C > 0$. If $|\mu_1 - \mu_2|/\sigma$ is the signal-to-noise ratio for the population difference in the original region, then the signal-to-noise ratio for the population difference in the new region is

$$\frac{|\mu_1 - \mu_2 + \varepsilon|}{C\sigma} = \frac{|\Delta(\mu_1 - \mu_2)|}{\sigma},$$

where

$$\Delta = \frac{1 + \varepsilon/(\mu_1 - \mu_2)}{C} \qquad (15.5.3)$$

is a measure of change in the signal-to-noise ratio for the population difference, which is the sensitivity index of population differences between regions. For most practical problems, $|\varepsilon| < |\mu_1 - \mu_2|$ and, thus, $\Delta > 0$. By (15.5.2), the power for the second trial conducted in the new region is $p(\Delta\theta)$.

As indicated by Chow, Shao, and Hu (2002), there are two advantages of using $\Delta$ as a sensitivity index, instead of $\varepsilon$ (changes in mean) and $C$ (changes in standard deviation). First, the result is easier to interpret when there is only one index. Second, the reproducibility probability is a strictly decreasing function of $\Delta$, whereas an increased population variance (or a decreased population difference) may or may not result in a decrease in the reproducibility probability.

If $\Delta$ is known, then the reproducibility probability

$$\hat{P}_\Delta = p(\Delta T(x))$$

can be used to assess the probability of generalizability between regions.

For the Bayesian approach, the generalizability probability is

$$\tilde{P}_\Delta = E_{\delta,u}\left[1 - \mathcal{T}_{n-2}\left(t_{n-2}\left|\frac{\Delta\delta}{u}\right.\right) - \mathcal{T}_{n-2}\left(-t_{n-2}\left|\frac{\Delta\delta}{u}\right.\right)\right].$$

In practice, the value of $\Delta$ is usually unknown. We may either consider a maximum possible value of $|\Delta|$ or a set of $\Delta$-values to carry out a sensitivity analysis (see Table 15.5.1). For the Bayesian approach, we may also consider the average of $\tilde{P}_\Delta$ over a prior density $\pi(\Delta)$, i.e.,

$$\tilde{P} = \int \tilde{P}_\Delta \pi(\Delta) d\Delta.$$

Table 15.5.1 provides a summary of reproducibility probability $\hat{P}_\Delta$ for various sample sizes, respectively. For example, a sample size of 30 will give an 80.5% of reproducibility provided that $\Delta T = 2.92$.

### 15.5.2 Assessment of Similarity

**Criterion for Similarity**

Let $x$ be a clinical response of interest in the original region. Here, $x$ could be either the response of the primary study endpoint from a test compound under investigation or the difference of responses of the primary study endpoint between a test drug and a control (e.g., a standard therapy or placebo). Let $y$ be similar to $x$ but is a response in a clinical bridging study conducted in the new region. Using the criterion for assessment of population and individual bioequivalence (FDA, 2001), Chow, Shao, and Hu (2002) proposed the following measure of similarity between $x$ and $y$:

$$\theta = \frac{E(x-y)^2 - E(x-x')^2}{E(x-x')^2/2}, \qquad (15.5.4)$$

where $x'$ is an independent replicate of $x$ and $y$, $x$, and $x'$ are assumed to be independent. Note that $\theta$ in (15.5.4) assesses not only the difference between the population means $E(x)$ and $E(y)$ but also the population variation of $x$ and $y$ through a function of mean squared differences. Also, $\theta$ is a relative measure, i.e., the mean squared difference between $x$ and $y$ is compared with the mean squared difference between $x$ and $x'$. It is related to the so-called *population difference ratio* (PDR), i.e.,

$$PDR = \sqrt{\frac{\theta}{2} + 1},$$

where

$$PDR = \sqrt{\frac{E(x-y)^2}{E(x-x')^2}}.$$

Table 15.5.1: Sensitivity Analysis of Reproducibility Probability $\hat{P}_\Delta$

| $\Delta T$ | \multicolumn{8}{c}{$n$} | | | | | | | |
|---|---|---|---|---|---|---|---|---|
| | 10 | 20 | 30 | 40 | 50 | 60 | 100 | $\infty$ |
| 1.96 | 0.407 | 0.458 | 0.473 | 0.480 | 0.484 | 0.487 | 0.492 | 0.500 |
| 2.02 | 0.429 | 0.481 | 0.496 | 0.504 | 0.508 | 0.511 | 0.516 | 0.524 |
| 2.08 | 0.448 | 0.503 | 0.519 | 0.527 | 0.531 | 0.534 | 0.540 | 0.548 |
| 2.14 | 0.469 | 0.526 | 0.542 | 0.550 | 0.555 | 0.557 | 0.563 | 0.571 |
| 2.20 | 0.490 | 0.549 | 0.565 | 0.573 | 0.578 | 0.581 | 0.586 | 0.594 |
| 2.26 | 0.511 | 0.571 | 0.588 | 0.596 | 0.601 | 0.604 | 0.609 | 0.618 |
| 2.32 | 0.532 | 0.593 | 0.610 | 0.618 | 0.623 | 0.626 | 0.632 | 0.640 |
| 2.38 | 0.552 | 0.615 | 0.632 | 0.640 | 0.645 | 0.648 | 0.654 | 0.662 |
| 2.44 | 0.573 | 0.636 | 0.654 | 0.662 | 0.667 | 0.670 | 0.676 | 0.684 |
| 2.50 | 0.593 | 0.657 | 0.675 | 0.683 | 0.688 | 0.691 | 0.697 | 0.705 |
| 2.56 | 0.613 | 0.678 | 0.695 | 0.704 | 0.708 | 0.711 | 0.717 | 0.725 |
| 2.62 | 0.632 | 0.698 | 0.715 | 0.724 | 0.728 | 0.731 | 0.737 | 0.745 |
| 2.68 | 0.652 | 0.717 | 0.735 | 0.743 | 0.747 | 0.750 | 0.756 | 0.764 |
| 2.74 | 0.671 | 0.736 | 0.753 | 0.761 | 0.766 | 0.769 | 0.774 | 0.782 |
| 2.80 | 0.690 | 0.754 | 0.771 | 0.779 | 0.783 | 0.786 | 0.792 | 0.799 |
| 2.86 | 0.708 | 0.772 | 0.788 | 0.796 | 0.800 | 0.803 | 0.808 | 0.815 |
| 2.92 | 0.725 | 0.789 | 0.805 | 0.812 | 0.816 | 0.819 | 0.824 | 0.830 |
| 2.98 | 0.742 | 0.805 | 0.820 | 0.827 | 0.831 | 0.834 | 0.839 | 0.845 |
| 3.04 | 0.759 | 0.820 | 0.835 | 0.842 | 0.846 | 0.848 | 0.853 | 0.860 |
| 3.10 | 0.775 | 0.834 | 0.849 | 0.856 | 0.859 | 0.862 | 0.866 | 0.872 |
| 3.16 | 0.790 | 0.848 | 0.862 | 0.868 | 0.872 | 0.874 | 0.879 | 0.884 |
| 3.22 | 0.805 | 0.861 | 0.874 | 0.881 | 0.884 | 0.886 | 0.890 | 0.895 |
| 3.28 | 0.819 | 0.873 | 0.886 | 0.892 | 0.895 | 0.897 | 0.901 | 0.906 |
| 3.34 | 0.832 | 0.884 | 0.897 | 0.902 | 0.905 | 0.907 | 0.911 | 0.916 |
| 3.40 | 0.844 | 0.895 | 0.907 | 0.912 | 0.915 | 0.917 | 0.920 | 0.925 |
| 3.46 | 0.856 | 0.905 | 0.916 | 0.921 | 0.924 | 0.925 | 0.929 | 0.932 |
| 3.52 | 0.868 | 0.914 | 0.925 | 0.929 | 0.932 | 0.933 | 0.936 | 0.940 |
| 3.58 | 0.879 | 0.923 | 0.933 | 0.937 | 0.939 | 0.941 | 0.943 | 0.947 |
| 3.64 | 0.889 | 0.931 | 0.940 | 0.944 | 0.946 | 0.947 | 0.950 | 0.953 |
| 3.70 | 0.898 | 0.938 | 0.946 | 0.950 | 0.952 | 0.953 | 0.956 | 0.959 |
| 3.76 | 0.907 | 0.944 | 0.952 | 0.956 | 0.958 | 0.959 | 0.961 | 0.965 |
| 3.82 | 0.915 | 0.950 | 0.958 | 0.961 | 0.963 | 0.964 | 0.966 | 0.969 |
| 3.88 | 0.923 | 0.956 | 0.963 | 0.966 | 0.967 | 0.968 | 0.970 | 0.973 |
| 3.94 | 0.930 | 0.961 | 0.967 | 0.970 | 0.971 | 0.972 | 0.974 | 0.977 |

In assessing population bioequivalence (or individual bioequivalence), the similarity measure $\theta$ is compared with a population bioequivalence (or individual bioequivalence) limit $\theta_U$ set by the FDA. For example, with log-transformed responses, FDA (2001) suggests

$$\theta_U = \frac{(\log 1.25)^2 + \epsilon}{\sigma_0^2},$$

where $\sigma_0^2 > 0$ and $\epsilon \geq 0$ are two constants given in the FDA guidance which depend upon the variability of the drug product.

Since a small value of $\theta$ indicates that the difference between $x$ and $y$ is small (relative to the difference between $x$ and $x'$), similarity between the new region and the original region can be claimed if and only if $\theta < \theta_U$, where $\theta_U$ is a similarity limit. Thus, the problem of assessing similarity becomes a hypothesis testing problem with hypotheses

$$H_0 : \theta \geq \theta_U \quad \text{versus} \quad H_a : \theta < \theta_U. \quad (15.5.5)$$

Let $k = 0$ indicate the original region and $k = 1$ indicate the new region. Suppose that there are $m_k$ study centers and $n_k$ responses in each center for a given variable of interest. Here, we first consider the balanced case where centers in a given region have the same number of observations. Let $z_{ijk}$ be the $i$th observation from the $j$th center of region $k$, $b_{jk}$ be the between-center random effect, and $e_{ijk}$ be the within-center measurement error. Assume that

$$z_{ijk} = \mu_k + b_{jk} + e_{ijk}, \quad i = 1, ..., n_k \ j = 1, ..., m_k, k = 0, 1, \quad (15.5.6)$$

where $\mu_k$ is the population mean in region $k$, $b_{jk} \sim N(0, \sigma_{Bk}^2)$, $e_{ijk} \sim N(0, \sigma_{Wk}^2)$, and $b_{jk}$'s and $e_{ijk}$'s are independent. Under model (15.5.6), the parameter $\theta$ in (15.5.4) becomes

$$\theta = \frac{(\mu_0 - \mu_1)^2 + \sigma_{T1}^2 - \sigma_{T0}^2}{\sigma_{T0}^2},$$

where $\sigma_{Tk}^2 = \sigma_{Bk}^2 + \sigma_{Wk}^2$ is the total variance (between center variance plus within center variance) in region $k$. The hypotheses in (15.5.5) are equivalent to

$$H_0 : \zeta \geq 0 \quad \text{versus} \quad H_a : \zeta < 0, \quad (15.5.7)$$

where

$$\zeta = (\mu_0 - \mu_1)^2 + \sigma_{T1}^2 - (1 + \theta_U)\sigma_{T0}^2. \quad (15.5.8)$$

## Statistical Methods

A statistical test of significance level 5% can be obtained by using a 95% upper confidence bound $\hat{\zeta}_U$ for $\zeta$ in (15.5.8), i.e., we reject $H_0$ in (15.5.7) if and only if $\hat{\zeta}_U < 0$.

Under model (15.5.6), an unbiased estimator of the population mean in region $k$ is

$$\bar{z}_k \sim N\left(\mu_k, \frac{\sigma_{Bk}^2}{m_k} + \frac{\sigma_{Wk}^2}{N_k}\right),$$

where $N_k = m_k n_k$ and $\bar{z}_k$ is the average of $z_{ijk}$'s over $j$ and $i$ for a fixed $k$. To construct a 95% upper confidence bound for $\zeta$ in (15.5.8) using the approach in Hyslop, Hsuan, and Holder (2000), which is proposed for testing individual bioequivalence, we need to find independent, unbiased, and chi-square distributed estimators of $\sigma_{Tk}^2$, $k = 0, 1$. These estimators, however, are not available when $n_k > 1$. Note that

$$\sigma_{Tk}^2 = \sigma_{Bk}^2 + n_k^{-1}\sigma_{Wk}^2 + (1 - n_k^{-1})\sigma_{Wk}^2, \quad k = 0, 1;$$

$\sigma_{Bk}^2 + n_k^{-1}\sigma_{Wk}^2$ can be unbiasedly estimated by

$$s_{Bk}^2 = \frac{1}{m_k - 1}\sum_{j=1}^{m_k}(\bar{z}_{jk} - \bar{z}_k)^2 \sim \frac{(\sigma_{Bk}^2 + n_k^{-1}\sigma_{Wk}^2)\chi_{m_k-1}^2}{m_k - 1},$$

where $\bar{z}_{jk}$ is the average of $z_{ijk}$'s over $i$ and $\chi_l^2$ denotes a random variable having the chi-square distribution with $l$ degrees of freedom; $\sigma_{Wk}^2$ can be estimated by

$$s_{Wk}^2 = \frac{1}{N_k - m_k}\sum_{j=1}^{m_k}\sum_{i=1}^{n_k}(z_{ijk} - \bar{z}_{jk})^2 \sim \frac{\sigma_{Wk}^2 \chi_{N_k-m_k}^2}{N_k - m_k};$$

and $\bar{z}_k$, $s_{Bk}^2$, $s_{Wk}^2$, $k = 0, 1$, are independent. Thus, an approximate 95% upper confidence bound for $\zeta$ in (15.5.8) is

$$\hat{\zeta}_U = (\bar{z}_0 - \bar{z}_1)^2 + s_{B1}^2 + (1 - n_1^{-1})s_{W1}^2$$
$$- (1 + \theta_U)[s_{B0}^2 + (1 - n_0^{-1})s_{W0}^2] + \sqrt{U},$$

where $U$ is the sum of the following five quantities:

$$\left[\left(|\bar{z}_0 - \bar{z}_1| + 1.645\sqrt{\frac{s_{B0}^2}{m_0} + \frac{s_{B1}^2}{m_1}}\right)^2 - (\bar{z}_0 - \bar{z}_1)^2\right]^2,$$

$$s_{B1}^4\left(\frac{m_1 - 1}{\chi_{0.05;m_1-1}^2} - 1\right)^2,$$

$$(1-n_1^{-1})^2 s_{W1}^4 \left(\frac{N_1-m_1}{\chi^2_{0.05;N_1-m_1}}-1\right)^2,$$

$$(1+\theta_U)^2 s_{B0}^4 \left(\frac{m_0-1}{\chi^2_{0.95;m_0-1}}-1\right)^2,$$

$$(1+\theta_U)^2(1-n_0^{-1})^2 s_{W0}^4 \left(\frac{N_0-m_0}{\chi^2_{0.95;N_0-m_0}}-1\right)^2,$$

and $\chi^2_{a;l}$ is the 100$a$th percentile of the chi-square distribution with $l$ degrees of freedom.

Thus, the null hypothesis $H_0$ in (15.5.7) can be rejected at approximately 5% significance level if $\hat{\zeta}_U < 0$. Similar to population bioequivalence testing (FDA, 2001), we conclude that the similarity between two regions (in terms of the given variable of interest) if and only if $H_0$ in (15.5.7) is rejected and the observed mean difference $\bar{z}_0 - \bar{z}_1$ is within the limits of $\pm 0.233$.

Consider now the situation where centers contain different numbers of observations in a given region, i.e., the $j$th center in region $k$ contains $n_{jk}$ observations. We have the following recommendations.

1. If all $n_{jk}$'s are large, then the previous described procedure is still approximately valid, provided that $N_k$ is defined to be $n_{1k}+\cdots+n_{m_k k}$ and $(1-n_k^{-1})s_{Wk}^2$ is replaced by

$$\tilde{s}_{Wk}^2 = \frac{1}{N_k-m_k}\sum_{j=1}^{m_k}\sum_{i=1}^{n_{jk}}(z_{ijk}-\bar{z}_{jk})^2.$$

2. If $n_{jk}$ are not very different (e.g., unequal sample sizes among centers are caused by missing values due to reasons that are not related to the variable of interest), then we may apply the Satterthwaite method (Johnson and Kotz, 1972) as follows. First, replace $s_{Wk}^2$ with $\tilde{s}_{Wk}^2$. Second, replace $n_k$ with

$$n_{0k} = \frac{1}{m_k-1}\left(N_k - \frac{1}{N_k}\sum_{j=1}^{m_k} n_{jk}^2\right).$$

Third, replace $s_{Bk}^2$ with

$$\tilde{s}_{Bk}^2 = \frac{1}{(m_k-1)n_{0k}}\sum_{j=1}^{m_k} n_{jk}(\bar{z}_{jk}-\bar{z}_k)^2.$$

Then, approximately,

$$\tilde{s}^2_{Bk} \sim \frac{(\sigma^2_{Bk} + n^{-1}_{0k}\sigma^2_{Wk})\chi^2_{d_k}}{m_k - 1}$$

with

$$d_k = \frac{(m_k - 1)(\hat{\rho}^{-1}_k + n_{0k})^2}{(\hat{\rho}^{-1}_k + n_{0k})^2 + v_k},$$

where

$$\hat{\rho}_k = \frac{\tilde{s}^2_{Bk}}{\tilde{s}^2_{Wk}} - \frac{1}{n_{0k}}$$

and

$$v_k = \frac{1}{m_k - 1}\left[\sum_{j=1}^{m_k} n^2_{jk} - \frac{m_k}{N_k}\sum_{j=1}^{m_k} n^3_{jk} + \frac{1}{N^2_k}\left(\sum_{j=1}^{m_k} n^2_{jk}\right)^2 - n^2_{0k}\right].$$

Finally, replace $m_k - 1$ with $d_k$.

**Sample Size Calculation**

Chow, Shao, and Hu (2002) proposed a procedure for determination of sample sizes $m_1$ and $n_1$ in the new region to achieve a desired power for establishment similarity between regions. The procedure is briefly outlined below. We first assume that sample sizes $m_0$ and $n_0$ in the original region have already been determined. Let $\psi = (\mu_0 - \mu_1, \sigma^2_{B1}, \sigma^2_{B0}, \sigma^2_{W1}, \sigma^2_{W0})$ be the vector of unknown parameters and let $U$ be given in the definition of $\hat{\zeta}_U$ and $U_\beta$ be the same as $U$ but with 5% and 95% replaced by $1 - \beta$ and $\beta$, respectively, where $\beta$ is a given desired power of the similarity test. Let $\tilde{U}$ and $\tilde{U}_\beta$ be $U$ and $U_\beta$, respectively, with $(\bar{z}_0 - \bar{z}_k, s^2_{BT}, s^2_{BR}, s^2_{WT}, s^2_{WR})$ replaced by $\tilde{\psi}$, an initial guessing value for which the value of $\zeta$ (denoted by $\tilde{\zeta}$) is negative. Then, the sample sizes $m_1$ and $n_1$ should be chosen so that

$$\tilde{\zeta} + \sqrt{\tilde{U}} + \sqrt{\tilde{U}_\beta} \leq 0 \tag{15.5.9}$$

holds. We may start with some initial values of $m_1$ and $n_1$ and gradually increase them until (15.5.9) holds.

### 15.5.3 Remarks

In the assessment of sensitivity, regulatory guidance/requirement for determining whether a clinical bridging study is critical as to (i) whether a bridging study is recommended for providing substantial evidence in the new region based on the clinical results observed in the original region, and (ii) what sample size of the clinical bridging study is needed for extrapolating the clinical results to the new region with desired reproducibility probability. It is suggested the therapeutic window and intra-subject variability of the test compound must be taken into consideration when choosing the criterion and setting regulatory requirements. A study of historical data related to the test compound is strongly recommended before a regulatory requirement is implemented.

The criterion for assessment of similarity proposed by Chow, Shao, and Hu (2002) accounts for the average and variability of the response of the primary study endpoint. This aggregated criterion, however, suffers the following disadvantages: (i) the effects of individual components cannot be separated and (ii) the difference in averages may be offset by the reduction in variability (Chow, 1999). As a result, it is suggested that an additional constraint be placed on the difference in means between two regions (FDA, 2001). An alternative to this aggregated criterion is to consider a set of disaggregate criteria on average and variability of the primary study endpoint (Chow and Liu, 2000). This approach, however, is not favored by the regulatory agency due to some practical considerations. For example, we will never be able to claim the new region is similar to the original region if the variability of the response of the primary endpoint is significantly lower than that in the original region.

The FDA recommends the use of PDR for selection of $\theta_U$. In practice, the determination of the maximum allowable PDR should depend upon the therapeutic window and intra-subject variability to reflect the variability from drug product to drug product and from patient population to patient population.

## 15.6 Vaccine Clinical Trials

Similar to clinical development of drug products, there are four phases of clinical trials in vaccine development. Phase I trials are referred to early studies with human subjects. The purpose of phase I trials is to explore the safety and immunogenicity of multiple dose levels of the vaccine under investigation. Phase I trials are usually on small scales. Phase II trials are to assess the safety, immunogenicity, and early efficacy of selected dose levels of the vaccine. Phase III trials, which are usually large in scale, are to confirm the efficacy of the vaccine in the target population. Phase III trials are usually conducted for collecting additional information regarding long-term safety, immuogenicity, or efficacy of the vaccine to fulfill regulatory requirements and/or marketing objectives after regulatory approval of the vaccine.

## 15.6.1 Reduction in Disease Incidence

As indicated in Chan, Wang, and Heyse (2003), one of the most critical steps of evaluation of a new vaccine is to assess the protective efficacy of the vaccine against the target disease. An efficacy trial is often conducted to evaluate whether the vaccine can prevent the disease or reduce the incidence of the disease in the target population. For this purpose, prospective, randomized, placebo-controlled trials are usually conducted. Subjects who meet the inclusion/exclusion criteria are randomly assigned to receive either the test vaccine (T) or placebo control (C). Let $p_T$ and $p_C$ be the true disease incidence rates of the $n_T$ vaccinees and $n_C$ controls randomized in the trial, respectively. Thus, the relative reduction in disease incidence for subjects in the vaccine group as compared to the control groups is given by

$$\pi = \frac{p_C - p_T}{p_C} = 1 - \frac{p_T}{p_C} = 1 - R.$$

In most vaccine clinical trials, $\pi$ has been widely used and is accepted as a primary measure of vaccine efficacy. Note that a vaccine is considered 100% efficacious (i.e., $\pi = 1$) if it prevents the disease completely (i.e., $P_T = 0$). On the other hand, it has no efficacy (i.e., $\pi = 0$) if $p_T = p_C$. Let $x_T$ and $x_C$ be the number of observed diseases for treatment and control groups, respectively. It follows that the natural estimators for $p_T$ and $p_C$ are given by

$$\hat{p}_T = \frac{x_T}{n_T} \quad \text{and} \quad \hat{p}_C = \frac{x_C}{n_C}.$$

Let $\beta = p_T/p_C$, which can be estimated by

$$\hat{\beta} = \frac{\hat{p}_T}{\hat{p}_C}.$$

By Taylor's expansion and the Central Limit Theorem (CLT), $\log(\hat{\beta})$ is asymptotically distributed as a normal random variable with mean $\log(\beta)$ and variance given by

$$\sigma^2 = \frac{1 - p_T}{n_T p_T} + \frac{1 - p_C}{n_C p_C}. \quad (15.6.1)$$

For a given confidence level of $1 - \alpha$, a $(1 - \alpha)$ confidence interval of $\log(\beta)$ is given by

$$(\log(\hat{\beta}) - z_{\alpha/2}\hat{\sigma}, \log(\hat{\beta}) + z_{\alpha/2}\hat{\sigma}),$$

where $\hat{\sigma}$ is obtained according to (15.6.1) by replacing $p_T$ and $p_C$ by $\hat{p}_T$ and $\hat{p}_C$, respectively. In practice, sample size is usually determined by specifying the half length ($d$) of the confidence interval of $\beta$. Assuming that $n = n_T = n_C$, it follows that

$$z_{\alpha/2}\sqrt{\frac{1-p_T}{np_T} + \frac{1-p_C}{np_C}} = d.$$

This leads to

$$n = \frac{z_{\alpha/2}^2}{d^2}\left(\frac{1-p_T}{p_T} + \frac{1-p_C}{p_C}\right).$$

### An Example

An investigator is interested in obtaining a 95% confidence interval for $\pi$ where it is expected that $p_T = 0.01$ and $p_C = 0.02$. It is desirable to have a confidence interval in log-scale with half length of 0.20 ($d = 0.20$). The sample size needed is then given by

$$n = \left(\frac{1.96}{0.2}\right)^2 \left(\frac{1-0.01}{0.01} + \frac{1-0.02}{0.02}\right) \approx 14214.$$

## 15.6.2 The Evaluation of Vaccine Efficacy with Extremely Low Disease Incidence

In many cases, the disease incidence rate is extremely low. In this case, a much larger scale of study is required to demonstrate vaccine efficacy as described in the previous subsection. For sufficiently large sample sizes and small incidence rates, the numbers of cases in the vaccine groups and the control groups approximately have the Poisson distribution with rate parameters $\lambda_T (\approx n_T p_T)$ and $\lambda_C (\approx n_C p_C)$, respectively. As a result, the number of cases in the vaccine group given the total number of cases (denoted by $S$) is distributed as a binomial random variable with parameter $\theta$, i.e., $b(S, \theta)$, where

$$\theta = \frac{\lambda_T}{\lambda_C + \lambda_T} = \frac{n_T p_T}{n_T p_T + n_C p_C} = \frac{R}{R+u} = \frac{1-\pi}{1-\pi+u}$$

and $u = n_C/n_T$. Since $\theta$ is a decreasing function in $\pi$, testing hypotheses that

$$H_0 : \pi \leq \pi_0 \quad \text{versus} \quad H_a : \pi > \pi_0$$

is equivalent to testing the following hypotheses:

$$H_0 : \theta \geq \theta_0 \quad \text{versus} \quad H_a : \theta < \theta_0,$$

where

$$\theta_0 = \frac{1-\pi_0}{1-\pi_0+u}.$$

## 15.6. Vaccine Clinical Trials

Let $x_T$ and $x_C$ be the number of the observed diseases for the treatment and control, respectively. A natural estimator for $\theta$ is given by $\hat{\theta} = x_T/(x_T + x_C)$. The test statistic is given by

$$T = \frac{\sqrt{x_T + x_C}(\hat{\theta} - \theta_0)}{\sqrt{\theta_0(1 - \theta_0)}}.$$

Under the null hypothesis, $T$ is asymptotically distributed as a standard normal random variable. Hence, we reject the null hypothesis at $\alpha$ level of significance if $T > z_\alpha$. Under the alternative hypothesis, the power of the above test can be approximated by

$$1 - \Phi\left(\frac{z_\alpha\sqrt{\theta_0(1 - \theta_0)} + \sqrt{x_T + x_C}(\theta_0 - \theta)}{\sqrt{\theta(1 - \theta)}}\right).$$

In order to achieve a desired power $1 - \beta$, the total number of diseases needed can be obtained by solving

$$\frac{z_\alpha\sqrt{\theta_0(1 - \theta_0)} + (\theta_0 - \theta)}{\sqrt{\theta(1 - \theta)}} = -z_\beta.$$

This leads to

$$x_T + x_C = \frac{[z_\alpha\sqrt{\theta_0(1 - \theta_0)} + z_\beta\sqrt{\theta(1 - \theta)}]^2}{(\theta - \theta_0)^2}.$$

Under the assumption that $n = n_T = n_C$, it follows that

$$n = \frac{[z_\alpha\sqrt{\theta_0(1 - \theta_0)} + z_\beta\sqrt{\theta(1 - \theta)}]^2}{(p_T + p_C)(\theta - \theta_0)^2}.$$

**An Example**

Suppose the investigator is interested in conducting a two-arm parallel trial with equal sample size ($u = 1$) to compare a study vaccine with a control in terms of controlling the disease rates. It is expected that the disease rate for the treatment group is 0.001 and the disease rate for the control group is 0.002. The hypotheses of interest are given by

$$H_0 : \theta \leq 0.5 \quad \text{versus} \quad H_a : \theta > 0.5.$$

Hence, $\theta_0 = 0.5$. It can be obtained that

$$\theta = \frac{0.001}{0.001 + 0.002} = \frac{1}{3}.$$

As a result, the sample size needed in order to achieve an 80% ($\beta = 0.20$) power at the 5% ($\alpha = 0.05$) level of significance is given by

$$n = \frac{[1.64\sqrt{0.5(1-0.5)} + 0.84\sqrt{1/3(1-1/3)}]^2}{(0.001 + 0.002)(1/3 - 1/2)^2} \approx 17837.$$

Thus, 17837 subjects per arm is needed in order to detect such a difference with an 80% power.

### 15.6.3 Relative Vaccine Efficacy

In vaccine trials, when the control is a licensed vaccine (an active control), the relative efficacy $\pi$ can be evaluated through the relative risk (i.e., $R = P_T/P_C$) based on the relationship $\pi = 1 - R$. If the absolute efficacy of the control (i.e., $\pi_C$) has been established, one can estimate the absolute efficacy of the test vaccine by

$$\pi_T = 1 - R(1 - \pi_C).$$

For a comparative vaccine trial, it is often designed as a non-inferiority trial by testing the following hypotheses:

$$H_0 : R \geq R_0 \quad \text{versus} \quad H_a : R < R_0,$$

where $R_0 > 1$ is a pre-specified non-inferiority margin or a threshold for relative risk. In practice, the hypotheses regarding relative risk are most often performed based on log-scale. In other words, instead of testing the above hypotheses, we usually consider the following hypotheses:

$$H_0 : \log(R) \geq \log(R_0) \quad \text{versus} \quad H_a : \log(R) < \log(R_0).$$

As it can be seen, this becomes the two-sample problem for relative risk, which has been discussed in Section 4.6. Hence, detailed discussion is omitted.

### 15.6.4 Composite Efficacy Measure

As indicated by Chang et al. (1994), in addition to the prevention of the disease infection, a test vaccine may also reduce the severity of the target disease as well. As a result, it is suggested that a composite efficacy measure be considered to account for both incidence and severity of the disease when evaluating the efficacy of the test vaccine. Chang et al. (1994) proposed the so-called burden-of-illness composite efficacy measure.

Suppose $n_T$ subjects were assigned to receive treatment while $n_C$ subjects were assigned to receive control (placebo). Let $x_T$ and $x_C$ be the

## 15.6. Vaccine Clinical Trials

number of cases observed in treatment and control group, respectively. Without loss of generality, we assume the first $x_T$ subjects in the treatment group and $x_C$ subjects in the control group experienced the events. Let $s_{ij}, i = T, C; j = 1, ..., x_i$ be the severity score associated with the $j$th case in the $i$th treatment group. For a fixed $i = T$ or $C$, it is assumed that $s_{ij}$ are independent and identically distributed random variables with mean $\mu_i$ and variance $\sigma_i^2$. Let $p_i$ be the true event rate of the $i$th treatment group. The hypotheses of interest is given by

$$H_0: p_T = p_C \quad \text{and} \quad \mu_T = \mu_C \quad \text{versus} \quad H_a: p_T \neq p_C \quad \text{or} \quad \mu_T \neq \mu_C.$$

Let

$$\bar{s}_i = \frac{1}{n_i} \sum_{j=1}^{x_i} s_{ij},$$

$$\bar{x} = \frac{n_T \bar{s}_T + n_C \bar{s}_C}{n_T + n_C},$$

$$s_i^2 = \frac{1}{n_i - 1} \sum_{j=1}^{n_i} (s_{ij} - \bar{s}_i)^2.$$

The test statistic is given by

$$T = \frac{\bar{s}_T - \bar{s}_C}{\sqrt{\bar{x}^2 \hat{p}(1-\hat{p})(1/n_T + 1/n_C) + \hat{p}(s_0^2/n_T + s_1^2/n_C)}}.$$

Under the null hypothesis, Chang et al. (1994) showed that $T$ is asymptotically distributed as a standard normal random variable. Hence, we would reject the null hypothesis if $|T| > z_{\alpha/2}$. Assume that $n = n_T = n_C$ and under the alternative hypothesis, it can be shown that

$$\bar{x} \to_{a.s.} (\mu_T + \mu_C)/2 = \mu_*$$

$$\hat{p} \to_{a.s.} (p_T + p_C)/2 = p_*.$$

Without loss of generality, we assume $p_T \mu_T > p_C \mu_C$ under the alternative hypothesis. Thus, the power of the above test can be approximated by

$$1 - \Phi\left(\frac{z_{\alpha/2}\sqrt{2\mu_*^2(p_*(1-p_*)) + 2p_*(\sigma_T^2 + \sigma_C^2)} - (\mu_T p_T - \mu_R p_R)}{\sqrt{p_T(\sigma_T^2 + \mu_T^2(1-p_T)) + p_R(\sigma_R^2 + \mu_R^2(1-p_R))}}\right).$$

Hence, the sample size needed in order to achieve a desired power of $1 - \beta$ can be obtained by solving

$$\frac{z_{\alpha/2}\sqrt{2\mu_*^2 p_*(1-p_*) + 2p_*(\sigma_T^2 + \sigma_C^2)} - \sqrt{n}(\mu_T p_T - \mu_R p_R)}{\sqrt{p_T(\sigma_T^2 + \mu_T^2(1-p_T)) + p_R(\sigma_R^2 + \mu_R^2(1-p_R))}} = -z_\beta.$$

This leads to

$$n = \frac{1}{(\mu_T p_T - \mu_R p_R)^2} \left[ z_{\alpha/2}\sqrt{2\mu_*^2 p_*(1-p_*) + 2p_*(\sigma_T^2 + \sigma_C^2)} \right.$$
$$\left. + z_\beta\sqrt{p_T(\sigma_T^2 + \mu_T^2(1-p_T)) + p_R(\sigma_R^2 + \mu_R^2(1-p_R))} \right]^2.$$

It should be noted that the above formula is slightly different from the one derived by Chang et al. (1994), which is incorrect.

**An Example**

Consider a clinical trial with $\mu_T = 0.20$, $\mu_C = 0.30$, $p_T = 0.10$, $p_R = 0.20$ and $\sigma_T^2 = \sigma_C^2 = 0.15$. The sample size needed in order to have an 80% ($\beta = 0.20$) power for detecting such a difference at the 5% ($\alpha = 0.05$) level of significance is given by

$$n = \frac{1}{(0.2 \times 0.1 - 0.3 \times 0.2)^2} \left[ 1.96\sqrt{2 \times 0.25^2 \times 0.15 \times 0.85 + 2 \times 0.15 \times 0.3} \right.$$
$$\left. + 0.84\sqrt{0.1(0.15^2 + 0.2 \times 0.9) + 0.2(0.15^2 + 0.3 \times 0.8)} \right]^2$$
$$\approx 468.$$

As a result, 468 subjects per treatment group are required for achieving an 80% power for detecting such a difference in the burden-of-illness score.

### 15.6.5 Remarks

In the previous subsections, procedures for sample size calculation in vaccine clinical trials were discussed based on a primary efficacy study endpoint using parametric approach. Durham et al. (1998) considered a nonparametric survival method to estimate the long-term efficacy of a cholera vaccine in the presence of warning protection. For evaluation of long-term vaccine efficacy, as indicated by Chan, Wang, and Heyse (2003), the analysis of time-to-event may be useful for determining whether breakthrough rates among vaccinees change over time. However, it should be noted that sample size calculation may be different depending upon the study objectives, the hypotheses of interest, and the corresponding appropriate statistical tests.

Clinical development for vaccine has recently received much attention both from regulatory agencies such as the US. FDA and the pharmaceutical industry. For example, Ellenberg and Dixon (1994) discussed some important statistical issues of vaccine trials (related to HIV vaccine trials). O'Neill (1988) and Chan and Bohida (1998) gave asymptotic and exact formulas for sample size and power calculations for vaccine efficacy studies, respectively. Chan, Wang, and Heyse (2003) provided a comprehensive review of vaccine clinical trials and statistical issues that are commonly encountered in vaccine clinical trials.

# Tables of Quantiles

Upper Quantiles of the Central t Distribution

| df | $\alpha$ | | | | |
|---|---|---|---|---|---|
| | 0.100 | 0.050 | 0.025 | 0.010 | 0.005 |
| 1 | 3.0777 | 6.3138 | 12.7062 | 31.8205 | 63.6567 |
| 2 | 1.8856 | 2.9200 | 4.3027 | 6.9646 | 9.9248 |
| 3 | 1.6377 | 2.3534 | 3.1824 | 4.5407 | 5.8409 |
| 4 | 1.5332 | 2.1318 | 2.7764 | 3.7470 | 4.6041 |
| 5 | 1.4759 | 2.0150 | 2.5706 | 3.3649 | 4.0322 |
| 6 | 1.4398 | 1.9432 | 2.4469 | 3.1427 | 3.7074 |
| 7 | 1.4149 | 1.8946 | 2.3646 | 2.9980 | 3.4995 |
| 8 | 1.3968 | 1.8595 | 2.3060 | 2.8965 | 3.3554 |
| 9 | 1.3830 | 1.8331 | 2.2622 | 2.8214 | 3.2498 |
| 10 | 1.3722 | 1.8125 | 2.2281 | 2.7638 | 3.1693 |
| 11 | 1.3634 | 1.7959 | 2.2010 | 2.7181 | 3.1058 |
| 12 | 1.3562 | 1.7823 | 2.1788 | 2.6810 | 3.0545 |
| 13 | 1.3502 | 1.7709 | 2.1604 | 2.6503 | 3.0123 |
| 14 | 1.3450 | 1.7613 | 2.1448 | 2.6245 | 2.9768 |
| 15 | 1.3406 | 1.7531 | 2.1314 | 2.6025 | 2.9467 |
| 16 | 1.3368 | 1.7459 | 2.1199 | 2.5835 | 2.9208 |
| 17 | 1.3334 | 1.7396 | 2.1098 | 2.5669 | 2.8982 |
| 18 | 1.3304 | 1.7341 | 2.1009 | 2.5524 | 2.8784 |
| 19 | 1.3277 | 1.7291 | 2.0930 | 2.5395 | 2.8609 |
| 20 | 1.3253 | 1.7247 | 2.0860 | 2.5280 | 2.8453 |
| 21 | 1.3232 | 1.7207 | 2.0796 | 2.5176 | 2.8314 |
| 22 | 1.3212 | 1.7171 | 2.0739 | 2.5083 | 2.8188 |
| 23 | 1.3195 | 1.7139 | 2.0687 | 2.4999 | 2.8073 |
| 24 | 1.3178 | 1.7109 | 2.0639 | 2.4922 | 2.7969 |
| 25 | 1.3163 | 1.7081 | 2.0595 | 2.4851 | 2.7874 |
| 26 | 1.3150 | 1.7056 | 2.0555 | 2.4786 | 2.7787 |
| 27 | 1.3137 | 1.7033 | 2.0518 | 2.4727 | 2.7707 |
| 28 | 1.3125 | 1.7011 | 2.0484 | 2.4671 | 2.7633 |
| 29 | 1.3114 | 1.6991 | 2.0452 | 2.4620 | 2.7564 |
| 30 | 1.3104 | 1.6973 | 2.0423 | 2.4573 | 2.7500 |

## Upper Quantiles of the $\chi^2$ Distribution

| df | \multicolumn{5}{c}{$\alpha$} |
|---|---|---|---|---|---|
|    | 0.100 | 0.050 | 0.025 | 0.010 | 0.005 |
| 1  | 2.7055  | 3.8415  | 5.0239  | 6.6349  | 7.8794  |
| 2  | 4.6052  | 5.9915  | 7.3778  | 9.2103  | 10.5966 |
| 3  | 6.2514  | 7.8147  | 9.3484  | 11.3449 | 12.8382 |
| 4  | 7.7794  | 9.4877  | 11.1433 | 13.2767 | 14.8603 |
| 5  | 9.2364  | 11.0705 | 12.8325 | 15.0863 | 16.7496 |
| 6  | 10.6446 | 12.5916 | 14.4494 | 16.8119 | 18.5476 |
| 7  | 12.0170 | 14.0671 | 16.0128 | 18.4753 | 20.2777 |
| 8  | 13.3616 | 15.5073 | 17.5345 | 20.0902 | 21.9550 |
| 9  | 14.6837 | 16.9190 | 19.0228 | 21.6660 | 23.5894 |
| 10 | 15.9872 | 18.3070 | 20.4832 | 23.2093 | 25.1882 |
| 11 | 17.2750 | 19.6751 | 21.9200 | 24.7250 | 26.7568 |
| 12 | 18.5493 | 21.0261 | 23.3367 | 26.2170 | 28.2995 |
| 13 | 19.8119 | 22.3620 | 24.7356 | 27.6882 | 29.8195 |
| 14 | 21.0641 | 23.6848 | 26.1189 | 29.1412 | 31.3193 |
| 15 | 22.3071 | 24.9958 | 27.4884 | 30.5779 | 32.8013 |
| 16 | 23.5418 | 26.2962 | 28.8454 | 31.9999 | 34.2672 |
| 17 | 24.7690 | 27.5871 | 30.1910 | 33.4087 | 35.7185 |
| 18 | 25.9894 | 28.8693 | 31.5264 | 34.8053 | 37.1565 |
| 19 | 27.2036 | 30.1435 | 32.8523 | 36.1909 | 38.5823 |
| 20 | 28.4120 | 31.4104 | 34.1696 | 37.5662 | 39.9968 |
| 21 | 29.6151 | 32.6706 | 35.4789 | 38.9322 | 41.4011 |
| 22 | 30.8133 | 33.9244 | 36.7807 | 40.2894 | 42.7957 |
| 23 | 32.0069 | 35.1725 | 38.0756 | 41.6384 | 44.1813 |
| 24 | 33.1962 | 36.4150 | 39.3641 | 42.9798 | 45.5585 |
| 25 | 34.3816 | 37.6525 | 40.6465 | 44.3141 | 46.9279 |
| 26 | 35.5632 | 38.8851 | 41.9232 | 45.6417 | 48.2899 |
| 27 | 36.7412 | 40.1133 | 43.1945 | 46.9629 | 49.6449 |
| 28 | 37.9159 | 41.3371 | 44.4608 | 48.2782 | 50.9934 |
| 29 | 39.0875 | 42.5570 | 45.7223 | 49.5879 | 52.3356 |
| 30 | 40.2560 | 43.7730 | 46.9792 | 50.8922 | 53.6720 |

## Upper Quantiles of the F Distribution ($\alpha = 0.100$)

| df2 | df1=1 | 2 | 3 | 4 | 5 | 6 | 7 | 8 |
|---|---|---|---|---|---|---|---|---|
| 2 | 8.5263 | 9.0000 | 9.1618 | 9.2434 | 9.2926 | 9.3255 | 9.3491 | 9.3668 |
| 3 | 5.5383 | 5.4624 | 5.3908 | 5.3426 | 5.3092 | 5.2847 | 5.2662 | 5.2517 |
| 4 | 4.5448 | 4.3246 | 4.1909 | 4.1072 | 4.0506 | 4.0097 | 3.9790 | 3.9549 |
| 5 | 4.0604 | 3.7797 | 3.6195 | 3.5202 | 3.4530 | 3.4045 | 3.3679 | 3.3393 |
| 6 | 3.7759 | 3.4633 | 3.2888 | 3.1808 | 3.1075 | 3.0546 | 3.0145 | 2.9830 |
| 7 | 3.5894 | 3.2574 | 3.0741 | 2.9605 | 2.8833 | 2.8274 | 2.7849 | 2.7516 |
| 8 | 3.4579 | 3.1131 | 2.9238 | 2.8064 | 2.7264 | 2.6683 | 2.6241 | 2.5893 |
| 9 | 3.3603 | 3.0065 | 2.8129 | 2.6927 | 2.6106 | 2.5509 | 2.5053 | 2.4694 |
| 10 | 3.2850 | 2.9245 | 2.7277 | 2.6053 | 2.5216 | 2.4606 | 2.4140 | 2.3772 |
| 11 | 3.2252 | 2.8595 | 2.6602 | 2.5362 | 2.4512 | 2.3891 | 2.3416 | 2.3040 |
| 12 | 3.1765 | 2.8068 | 2.6055 | 2.4801 | 2.3940 | 2.3310 | 2.2828 | 2.2446 |
| 13 | 3.1362 | 2.7632 | 2.5603 | 2.4337 | 2.3467 | 2.2830 | 2.2341 | 2.1953 |
| 14 | 3.1022 | 2.7265 | 2.5222 | 2.3947 | 2.3069 | 2.2426 | 2.1931 | 2.1539 |
| 15 | 3.0732 | 2.6952 | 2.4898 | 2.3614 | 2.2730 | 2.2081 | 2.1582 | 2.1185 |
| 16 | 3.0481 | 2.6682 | 2.4618 | 2.3327 | 2.2438 | 2.1783 | 2.1280 | 2.0880 |
| 17 | 3.0262 | 2.6446 | 2.4374 | 2.3077 | 2.2183 | 2.1524 | 2.1017 | 2.0613 |
| 18 | 3.0070 | 2.6239 | 2.4160 | 2.2858 | 2.1958 | 2.1296 | 2.0785 | 2.0379 |
| 19 | 2.9899 | 2.6056 | 2.3970 | 2.2663 | 2.1760 | 2.1094 | 2.0580 | 2.0171 |
| 20 | 2.9747 | 2.5893 | 2.3801 | 2.2489 | 2.1582 | 2.0913 | 2.0397 | 1.9985 |
| 21 | 2.9610 | 2.5746 | 2.3649 | 2.2333 | 2.1423 | 2.0751 | 2.0233 | 1.9819 |
| 22 | 2.9486 | 2.5613 | 2.3512 | 2.2193 | 2.1279 | 2.0605 | 2.0084 | 1.9668 |
| 23 | 2.9374 | 2.5493 | 2.3387 | 2.2065 | 2.1149 | 2.0472 | 1.9949 | 1.9531 |
| 24 | 2.9271 | 2.5383 | 2.3274 | 2.1949 | 2.1030 | 2.0351 | 1.9826 | 1.9407 |
| 25 | 2.9177 | 2.5283 | 2.3170 | 2.1842 | 2.0922 | 2.0241 | 1.9714 | 1.9292 |
| 26 | 2.9091 | 2.5191 | 2.3075 | 2.1745 | 2.0822 | 2.0139 | 1.9610 | 1.9188 |
| 27 | 2.9012 | 2.5106 | 2.2987 | 2.1655 | 2.0730 | 2.0045 | 1.9515 | 1.9091 |
| 28 | 2.8938 | 2.5028 | 2.2906 | 2.1571 | 2.0645 | 1.9959 | 1.9427 | 1.9001 |
| 29 | 2.8870 | 2.4955 | 2.2831 | 2.1494 | 2.0566 | 1.9878 | 1.9345 | 1.8918 |
| 30 | 2.8807 | 2.4887 | 2.2761 | 2.1422 | 2.0492 | 1.9803 | 1.9269 | 1.8841 |

## Upper Quantiles of the F Distribution ($\alpha = 0.100$)

| df2 | \multicolumn{7}{c}{df1} |
|---|---|---|---|---|---|---|---|
|  | 9 | 10 | 11 | 12 | 16 | 20 | 25 | 30 |
| 2  | 9.3805 | 9.3916 | 9.4006 | 9.4081 | 9.4289 | 9.4413 | 9.4513 | 9.4579 |
| 3  | 5.2400 | 5.2304 | 5.2224 | 5.2156 | 5.1964 | 5.1845 | 5.1747 | 5.1681 |
| 4  | 3.9357 | 3.9199 | 3.9067 | 3.8955 | 3.8639 | 3.8443 | 3.8283 | 3.8174 |
| 5  | 3.3163 | 3.2974 | 3.2816 | 3.2682 | 3.2303 | 3.2067 | 3.1873 | 3.1741 |
| 6  | 2.9577 | 2.9369 | 2.9195 | 2.9047 | 2.8626 | 2.8363 | 2.8147 | 2.8000 |
| 7  | 2.7247 | 2.7025 | 2.6839 | 2.6681 | 2.6230 | 2.5947 | 2.5714 | 2.5555 |
| 8  | 2.5612 | 2.5380 | 2.5186 | 2.5020 | 2.4545 | 2.4246 | 2.3999 | 2.3830 |
| 9  | 2.4403 | 2.4163 | 2.3961 | 2.3789 | 2.3295 | 2.2983 | 2.2725 | 2.2547 |
| 10 | 2.3473 | 2.3226 | 2.3018 | 2.2841 | 2.2330 | 2.2007 | 2.1739 | 2.1554 |
| 11 | 2.2735 | 2.2482 | 2.2269 | 2.2087 | 2.1563 | 2.1230 | 2.0953 | 2.0762 |
| 12 | 2.2135 | 2.1878 | 2.1660 | 2.1474 | 2.0938 | 2.0597 | 2.0312 | 2.0115 |
| 13 | 2.1638 | 2.1376 | 2.1155 | 2.0966 | 2.0419 | 2.0070 | 1.9778 | 1.9576 |
| 14 | 2.1220 | 2.0954 | 2.0729 | 2.0537 | 1.9981 | 1.9625 | 1.9326 | 1.9119 |
| 15 | 2.0862 | 2.0593 | 2.0366 | 2.0171 | 1.9605 | 1.9243 | 1.8939 | 1.8728 |
| 16 | 2.0553 | 2.0281 | 2.0051 | 1.9854 | 1.9281 | 1.8913 | 1.8603 | 1.8388 |
| 17 | 2.0284 | 2.0009 | 1.9777 | 1.9577 | 1.8997 | 1.8624 | 1.8309 | 1.8090 |
| 18 | 2.0047 | 1.9770 | 1.9535 | 1.9333 | 1.8747 | 1.8368 | 1.8049 | 1.7827 |
| 19 | 1.9836 | 1.9557 | 1.9321 | 1.9117 | 1.8524 | 1.8142 | 1.7818 | 1.7592 |
| 20 | 1.9649 | 1.9367 | 1.9129 | 1.8924 | 1.8325 | 1.7938 | 1.7611 | 1.7382 |
| 21 | 1.9480 | 1.9197 | 1.8956 | 1.8750 | 1.8146 | 1.7756 | 1.7424 | 1.7193 |
| 22 | 1.9327 | 1.9043 | 1.8801 | 1.8593 | 1.7984 | 1.7590 | 1.7255 | 1.7021 |
| 23 | 1.9189 | 1.8903 | 1.8659 | 1.8450 | 1.7837 | 1.7439 | 1.7101 | 1.6864 |
| 24 | 1.9063 | 1.8775 | 1.8530 | 1.8319 | 1.7703 | 1.7302 | 1.6960 | 1.6721 |
| 25 | 1.8947 | 1.8658 | 1.8412 | 1.8200 | 1.7579 | 1.7175 | 1.6831 | 1.6589 |
| 26 | 1.8841 | 1.8550 | 1.8303 | 1.8090 | 1.7466 | 1.7059 | 1.6712 | 1.6468 |
| 27 | 1.8743 | 1.8451 | 1.8203 | 1.7989 | 1.7361 | 1.6951 | 1.6602 | 1.6356 |
| 28 | 1.8652 | 1.8359 | 1.8110 | 1.7895 | 1.7264 | 1.6852 | 1.6500 | 1.6252 |
| 29 | 1.8568 | 1.8274 | 1.8024 | 1.7808 | 1.7174 | 1.6759 | 1.6405 | 1.6155 |
| 30 | 1.8490 | 1.8195 | 1.7944 | 1.7727 | 1.7090 | 1.6673 | 1.6316 | 1.6065 |

## Upper Quantiles of the F Distribution ($\alpha = 0.050$)

| df2 | df1 1 | 2 | 3 | 4 | 5 | 6 | 7 | 8 |
|---|---|---|---|---|---|---|---|---|
| 2 | 18.5128 | 19.0000 | 19.1643 | 19.2468 | 19.2964 | 19.3295 | 19.3532 | 19.3710 |
| 3 | 10.1280 | 9.5521 | 9.2766 | 9.1172 | 9.0135 | 8.9406 | 8.8867 | 8.8452 |
| 4 | 7.7086 | 6.9443 | 6.5914 | 6.3882 | 6.2561 | 6.1631 | 6.0942 | 6.0410 |
| 5 | 6.6079 | 5.7861 | 5.4095 | 5.1922 | 5.0503 | 4.9503 | 4.8759 | 4.8183 |
| 6 | 5.9874 | 5.1433 | 4.7571 | 4.5337 | 4.3874 | 4.2839 | 4.2067 | 4.1468 |
| 7 | 5.5914 | 4.7374 | 4.3468 | 4.1203 | 3.9715 | 3.8660 | 3.7870 | 3.7257 |
| 8 | 5.3177 | 4.4590 | 4.0662 | 3.8379 | 3.6875 | 3.5806 | 3.5005 | 3.4381 |
| 9 | 5.1174 | 4.2565 | 3.8625 | 3.6331 | 3.4817 | 3.3738 | 3.2927 | 3.2296 |
| 10 | 4.9646 | 4.1028 | 3.7083 | 3.4780 | 3.3258 | 3.2172 | 3.1355 | 3.0717 |
| 11 | 4.8443 | 3.9823 | 3.5874 | 3.3567 | 3.2039 | 3.0946 | 3.0123 | 2.9480 |
| 12 | 4.7472 | 3.8853 | 3.4903 | 3.2592 | 3.1059 | 2.9961 | 2.9134 | 2.8486 |
| 13 | 4.6672 | 3.8056 | 3.4105 | 3.1791 | 3.0254 | 2.9153 | 2.8321 | 2.7669 |
| 14 | 4.6001 | 3.7389 | 3.3439 | 3.1122 | 2.9582 | 2.8477 | 2.7642 | 2.6987 |
| 15 | 4.5431 | 3.6823 | 3.2874 | 3.0556 | 2.9013 | 2.7905 | 2.7066 | 2.6408 |
| 16 | 4.4940 | 3.6337 | 3.2389 | 3.0069 | 2.8524 | 2.7413 | 2.6572 | 2.5911 |
| 17 | 4.4513 | 3.5915 | 3.1968 | 2.9647 | 2.8100 | 2.6987 | 2.6143 | 2.5480 |
| 18 | 4.4139 | 3.5546 | 3.1599 | 2.9277 | 2.7729 | 2.6613 | 2.5767 | 2.5102 |
| 19 | 4.3807 | 3.5219 | 3.1274 | 2.8951 | 2.7401 | 2.6283 | 2.5435 | 2.4768 |
| 20 | 4.3512 | 3.4928 | 3.0984 | 2.8661 | 2.7109 | 2.5990 | 2.5140 | 2.4471 |
| 21 | 4.3248 | 3.4668 | 3.0725 | 2.8401 | 2.6848 | 2.5727 | 2.4876 | 2.4205 |
| 22 | 4.3009 | 3.4434 | 3.0491 | 2.8167 | 2.6613 | 2.5491 | 2.4638 | 2.3965 |
| 23 | 4.2793 | 3.4221 | 3.0280 | 2.7955 | 2.6400 | 2.5277 | 2.4422 | 2.3748 |
| 24 | 4.2597 | 3.4028 | 3.0088 | 2.7763 | 2.6207 | 2.5082 | 2.4226 | 2.3551 |
| 25 | 4.2417 | 3.3852 | 2.9912 | 2.7587 | 2.6030 | 2.4904 | 2.4047 | 2.3371 |
| 26 | 4.2252 | 3.3690 | 2.9752 | 2.7426 | 2.5868 | 2.4741 | 2.3883 | 2.3205 |
| 27 | 4.2100 | 3.3541 | 2.9604 | 2.7278 | 2.5719 | 2.4591 | 2.3732 | 2.3053 |
| 28 | 4.1960 | 3.3404 | 2.9467 | 2.7141 | 2.5581 | 2.4453 | 2.3593 | 2.2913 |
| 29 | 4.1830 | 3.3277 | 2.9340 | 2.7014 | 2.5454 | 2.4324 | 2.3463 | 2.2783 |
| 30 | 4.1709 | 3.3158 | 2.9223 | 2.6896 | 2.5336 | 2.4205 | 2.3343 | 2.2662 |

## Upper Quantiles of the F Distribution ($\alpha = 0.050$)

| df2 | \multicolumn{7}{c}{df1} |
|---|---|---|---|---|---|---|---|
| | 9 | 10 | 11 | 12 | 16 | 20 | 25 | 30 |
| 2 | 19.3848 | 19.3959 | 19.4050 | 19.4125 | 19.4333 | 19.4458 | 19.4558 | 19.4624 |
| 3 | 8.8123 | 8.7855 | 8.7633 | 8.7446 | 8.6923 | 8.6602 | 8.6341 | 8.6166 |
| 4 | 5.9988 | 5.9644 | 5.9358 | 5.9117 | 5.8441 | 5.8025 | 5.7687 | 5.7459 |
| 5 | 4.7725 | 4.7351 | 4.7040 | 4.6777 | 4.6038 | 4.5581 | 4.5209 | 4.4957 |
| 6 | 4.0990 | 4.0600 | 4.0274 | 3.9999 | 3.9223 | 3.8742 | 3.8348 | 3.8082 |
| 7 | 3.6767 | 3.6365 | 3.6030 | 3.5747 | 3.4944 | 3.4445 | 3.4036 | 3.3758 |
| 8 | 3.3881 | 3.3472 | 3.3130 | 3.2839 | 3.2016 | 3.1503 | 3.1081 | 3.0794 |
| 9 | 3.1789 | 3.1373 | 3.1025 | 3.0729 | 2.9890 | 2.9365 | 2.8932 | 2.8637 |
| 10 | 3.0204 | 2.9782 | 2.9430 | 2.9130 | 2.8276 | 2.7740 | 2.7298 | 2.6996 |
| 11 | 2.8962 | 2.8536 | 2.8179 | 2.7876 | 2.7009 | 2.6464 | 2.6014 | 2.5705 |
| 12 | 2.7964 | 2.7534 | 2.7173 | 2.6866 | 2.5989 | 2.5436 | 2.4977 | 2.4663 |
| 13 | 2.7144 | 2.6710 | 2.6347 | 2.6037 | 2.5149 | 2.4589 | 2.4123 | 2.3803 |
| 14 | 2.6458 | 2.6022 | 2.5655 | 2.5342 | 2.4446 | 2.3879 | 2.3407 | 2.3082 |
| 15 | 2.5876 | 2.5437 | 2.5068 | 2.4753 | 2.3849 | 2.3275 | 2.2797 | 2.2468 |
| 16 | 2.5377 | 2.4935 | 2.4564 | 2.4247 | 2.3335 | 2.2756 | 2.2272 | 2.1938 |
| 17 | 2.4943 | 2.4499 | 2.4126 | 2.3807 | 2.2888 | 2.2304 | 2.1815 | 2.1477 |
| 18 | 2.4563 | 2.4117 | 2.3742 | 2.3421 | 2.2496 | 2.1906 | 2.1413 | 2.1071 |
| 19 | 2.4227 | 2.3779 | 2.3402 | 2.3080 | 2.2149 | 2.1555 | 2.1057 | 2.0712 |
| 20 | 2.3928 | 2.3479 | 2.3100 | 2.2776 | 2.1840 | 2.1242 | 2.0739 | 2.0391 |
| 21 | 2.3660 | 2.3210 | 2.2829 | 2.2504 | 2.1563 | 2.0960 | 2.0454 | 2.0102 |
| 22 | 2.3419 | 2.2967 | 2.2585 | 2.2258 | 2.1313 | 2.0707 | 2.0196 | 1.9842 |
| 23 | 2.3201 | 2.2747 | 2.2364 | 2.2036 | 2.1086 | 2.0476 | 1.9963 | 1.9605 |
| 24 | 2.3002 | 2.2547 | 2.2163 | 2.1834 | 2.0880 | 2.0267 | 1.9750 | 1.9390 |
| 25 | 2.2821 | 2.2365 | 2.1979 | 2.1649 | 2.0691 | 2.0075 | 1.9554 | 1.9192 |
| 26 | 2.2655 | 2.2197 | 2.1811 | 2.1479 | 2.0518 | 1.9898 | 1.9375 | 1.9010 |
| 27 | 2.2501 | 2.2043 | 2.1655 | 2.1323 | 2.0358 | 1.9736 | 1.9210 | 1.8842 |
| 28 | 2.2360 | 2.1900 | 2.1512 | 2.1179 | 2.0210 | 1.9586 | 1.9057 | 1.8687 |
| 29 | 2.2229 | 2.1768 | 2.1379 | 2.1045 | 2.0073 | 1.9446 | 1.8915 | 1.8543 |
| 30 | 2.2107 | 2.1646 | 2.1256 | 2.0921 | 1.9946 | 1.9317 | 1.8782 | 1.8409 |

## Upper Quantiles of the F Distribution ($\alpha = 0.025$)

| df2 | \ df1 \ 1 | 2 | 3 | 4 | 5 | 6 | 7 | 8 |
|---|---|---|---|---|---|---|---|---|
| 2 | 38.5063 | 39.0000 | 39.1655 | 39.2484 | 39.2982 | 39.3315 | 39.3552 | 39.3730 |
| 3 | 17.4434 | 16.0441 | 15.4392 | 15.1010 | 14.8848 | 14.7347 | 14.6244 | 14.5399 |
| 4 | 12.2179 | 10.6491 | 9.9792 | 9.6045 | 9.3645 | 9.1973 | 9.0741 | 8.9796 |
| 5 | 10.0070 | 8.4336 | 7.7636 | 7.3879 | 7.1464 | 6.9777 | 6.8531 | 6.7572 |
| 6 | 8.8131 | 7.2599 | 6.5988 | 6.2272 | 5.9876 | 5.8198 | 5.6955 | 5.5996 |
| 7 | 8.0727 | 6.5415 | 5.8898 | 5.5226 | 5.2852 | 5.1186 | 4.9949 | 4.8993 |
| 8 | 7.5709 | 6.0595 | 5.4160 | 5.0526 | 4.8173 | 4.6517 | 4.5286 | 4.4333 |
| 9 | 7.2093 | 5.7147 | 5.0781 | 4.7181 | 4.4844 | 4.3197 | 4.1970 | 4.1020 |
| 10 | 6.9367 | 5.4564 | 4.8256 | 4.4683 | 4.2361 | 4.0721 | 3.9498 | 3.8549 |
| 11 | 6.7241 | 5.2559 | 4.6300 | 4.2751 | 4.0440 | 3.8807 | 3.7586 | 3.6638 |
| 12 | 6.5538 | 5.0959 | 4.4742 | 4.1212 | 3.8911 | 3.7283 | 3.6065 | 3.5118 |
| 13 | 6.4143 | 4.9653 | 4.3472 | 3.9959 | 3.7667 | 3.6043 | 3.4827 | 3.3880 |
| 14 | 6.2979 | 4.8567 | 4.2417 | 3.8919 | 3.6634 | 3.5014 | 3.3799 | 3.2853 |
| 15 | 6.1995 | 4.7650 | 4.1528 | 3.8043 | 3.5764 | 3.4147 | 3.2934 | 3.1987 |
| 16 | 6.1151 | 4.6867 | 4.0768 | 3.7294 | 3.5021 | 3.3406 | 3.2194 | 3.1248 |
| 17 | 6.0420 | 4.6189 | 4.0112 | 3.6648 | 3.4379 | 3.2767 | 3.1556 | 3.0610 |
| 18 | 5.9781 | 4.5597 | 3.9539 | 3.6083 | 3.3820 | 3.2209 | 3.0999 | 3.0053 |
| 19 | 5.9216 | 4.5075 | 3.9034 | 3.5587 | 3.3327 | 3.1718 | 3.0509 | 2.9563 |
| 20 | 5.8715 | 4.4613 | 3.8587 | 3.5147 | 3.2891 | 3.1283 | 3.0074 | 2.9128 |
| 21 | 5.8266 | 4.4199 | 3.8188 | 3.4754 | 3.2501 | 3.0895 | 2.9686 | 2.8740 |
| 22 | 5.7863 | 4.3828 | 3.7829 | 3.4401 | 3.2151 | 3.0546 | 2.9338 | 2.8392 |
| 23 | 5.7498 | 4.3492 | 3.7505 | 3.4083 | 3.1835 | 3.0232 | 2.9023 | 2.8077 |
| 24 | 5.7166 | 4.3187 | 3.7211 | 3.3794 | 3.1548 | 2.9946 | 2.8738 | 2.7791 |
| 25 | 5.6864 | 4.2909 | 3.6943 | 3.3530 | 3.1287 | 2.9685 | 2.8478 | 2.7531 |
| 26 | 5.6586 | 4.2655 | 3.6697 | 3.3289 | 3.1048 | 2.9447 | 2.8240 | 2.7293 |
| 27 | 5.6331 | 4.2421 | 3.6472 | 3.3067 | 3.0828 | 2.9228 | 2.8021 | 2.7074 |
| 28 | 5.6096 | 4.2205 | 3.6264 | 3.2863 | 3.0626 | 2.9027 | 2.7820 | 2.6872 |
| 29 | 5.5878 | 4.2006 | 3.6072 | 3.2674 | 3.0438 | 2.8840 | 2.7633 | 2.6686 |
| 30 | 5.5675 | 4.1821 | 3.5894 | 3.2499 | 3.0265 | 2.8667 | 2.7460 | 2.6513 |

## Upper Quantiles of the F Distribution ($\alpha = 0.025$)

| df2 | \multicolumn{8}{c}{df1} | | | | | | | |
|---|---|---|---|---|---|---|---|---|
| | 9 | 10 | 11 | 12 | 16 | 20 | 25 | 30 |
| 2 | 39.3869 | 39.3980 | 39.4071 | 39.4146 | 39.4354 | 39.4479 | 39.4579 | 39.4646 |
| 3 | 14.4731 | 14.4189 | 14.3742 | 14.3366 | 14.2315 | 14.1674 | 14.1155 | 14.0805 |
| 4 | 8.9047 | 8.8439 | 8.7935 | 8.7512 | 8.6326 | 8.5599 | 8.5010 | 8.4613 |
| 5 | 6.6811 | 6.6192 | 6.5678 | 6.5245 | 6.4032 | 6.3286 | 6.2679 | 6.2269 |
| 6 | 5.5234 | 5.4613 | 5.4098 | 5.3662 | 5.2439 | 5.1684 | 5.1069 | 5.0652 |
| 7 | 4.8232 | 4.7611 | 4.7095 | 4.6658 | 4.5428 | 4.4667 | 4.4045 | 4.3624 |
| 8 | 4.3572 | 4.2951 | 4.2434 | 4.1997 | 4.0761 | 3.9995 | 3.9367 | 3.8940 |
| 9 | 4.0260 | 3.9639 | 3.9121 | 3.8682 | 3.7441 | 3.6669 | 3.6035 | 3.5604 |
| 10 | 3.7790 | 3.7168 | 3.6649 | 3.6209 | 3.4963 | 3.4185 | 3.3546 | 3.3110 |
| 11 | 3.5879 | 3.5257 | 3.4737 | 3.4296 | 3.3044 | 3.2261 | 3.1616 | 3.1176 |
| 12 | 3.4358 | 3.3736 | 3.3215 | 3.2773 | 3.1515 | 3.0728 | 3.0077 | 2.9633 |
| 13 | 3.3120 | 3.2497 | 3.1975 | 3.1532 | 3.0269 | 2.9477 | 2.8821 | 2.8372 |
| 14 | 3.2093 | 3.1469 | 3.0946 | 3.0502 | 2.9234 | 2.8437 | 2.7777 | 2.7324 |
| 15 | 3.1227 | 3.0602 | 3.0078 | 2.9633 | 2.8360 | 2.7559 | 2.6894 | 2.6437 |
| 16 | 3.0488 | 2.9862 | 2.9337 | 2.8890 | 2.7614 | 2.6808 | 2.6138 | 2.5678 |
| 17 | 2.9849 | 2.9222 | 2.8696 | 2.8249 | 2.6968 | 2.6158 | 2.5484 | 2.5020 |
| 18 | 2.9291 | 2.8664 | 2.8137 | 2.7689 | 2.6404 | 2.5590 | 2.4912 | 2.4445 |
| 19 | 2.8801 | 2.8172 | 2.7645 | 2.7196 | 2.5907 | 2.5089 | 2.4408 | 2.3937 |
| 20 | 2.8365 | 2.7737 | 2.7209 | 2.6758 | 2.5465 | 2.4645 | 2.3959 | 2.3486 |
| 21 | 2.7977 | 2.7348 | 2.6819 | 2.6368 | 2.5071 | 2.4247 | 2.3558 | 2.3082 |
| 22 | 2.7628 | 2.6998 | 2.6469 | 2.6017 | 2.4717 | 2.3890 | 2.3198 | 2.2718 |
| 23 | 2.7313 | 2.6682 | 2.6152 | 2.5699 | 2.4396 | 2.3567 | 2.2871 | 2.2389 |
| 24 | 2.7027 | 2.6396 | 2.5865 | 2.5411 | 2.4105 | 2.3273 | 2.2574 | 2.2090 |
| 25 | 2.6766 | 2.6135 | 2.5603 | 2.5149 | 2.3840 | 2.3005 | 2.2303 | 2.1816 |
| 26 | 2.6528 | 2.5896 | 2.5363 | 2.4908 | 2.3597 | 2.2759 | 2.2054 | 2.1565 |
| 27 | 2.6309 | 2.5676 | 2.5143 | 2.4688 | 2.3373 | 2.2533 | 2.1826 | 2.1334 |
| 28 | 2.6106 | 2.5473 | 2.4940 | 2.4484 | 2.3167 | 2.2324 | 2.1615 | 2.1121 |
| 29 | 2.5919 | 2.5286 | 2.4752 | 2.4295 | 2.2976 | 2.2131 | 2.1419 | 2.0923 |
| 30 | 2.5746 | 2.5112 | 2.4577 | 2.4120 | 2.2799 | 2.1952 | 2.1237 | 2.0739 |

## Upper Quantiles of the F Distribution ($\alpha = 0.010$)

| df2 | \multicolumn{8}{c}{df1} | | | | | | | |
|---|---|---|---|---|---|---|---|---|
|  | 1 | 2 | 3 | 4 | 5 | 6 | 7 | 8 |
| 2 | 98.5025 | 99.0000 | 99.1662 | 99.2494 | 99.2993 | 99.3326 | 99.3564 | 99.3742 |
| 3 | 34.1162 | 30.8165 | 29.4567 | 28.7099 | 28.2371 | 27.9107 | 27.6717 | 27.4892 |
| 4 | 21.1977 | 18.0000 | 16.6944 | 15.9770 | 15.5219 | 15.2069 | 14.9758 | 14.7989 |
| 5 | 16.2582 | 13.2739 | 12.0600 | 11.3919 | 10.9670 | 10.6723 | 10.4555 | 10.2893 |
| 6 | 13.7450 | 10.9248 | 9.7795 | 9.1483 | 8.7459 | 8.4661 | 8.2600 | 8.1017 |
| 7 | 12.2464 | 9.5466 | 8.4513 | 7.8466 | 7.4604 | 7.1914 | 6.9928 | 6.8400 |
| 8 | 11.2586 | 8.6491 | 7.5910 | 7.0061 | 6.6318 | 6.3707 | 6.1776 | 6.0289 |
| 9 | 10.5614 | 8.0215 | 6.9919 | 6.4221 | 6.0569 | 5.8018 | 5.6129 | 5.4671 |
| 10 | 10.0443 | 7.5594 | 6.5523 | 5.9943 | 5.6363 | 5.3858 | 5.2001 | 5.0567 |
| 11 | 9.6460 | 7.2057 | 6.2167 | 5.6683 | 5.3160 | 5.0692 | 4.8861 | 4.7445 |
| 12 | 9.3302 | 6.9266 | 5.9525 | 5.4120 | 5.0643 | 4.8206 | 4.6395 | 4.4994 |
| 13 | 9.0738 | 6.7010 | 5.7394 | 5.2053 | 4.8616 | 4.6204 | 4.4410 | 4.3021 |
| 14 | 8.8616 | 6.5149 | 5.5639 | 5.0354 | 4.6950 | 4.4558 | 4.2779 | 4.1399 |
| 15 | 8.6831 | 6.3589 | 5.4170 | 4.8932 | 4.5556 | 4.3183 | 4.1415 | 4.0045 |
| 16 | 8.5310 | 6.2262 | 5.2922 | 4.7726 | 4.4374 | 4.2016 | 4.0259 | 3.8896 |
| 17 | 8.3997 | 6.1121 | 5.1850 | 4.6690 | 4.3359 | 4.1015 | 3.9267 | 3.7910 |
| 18 | 8.2854 | 6.0129 | 5.0919 | 4.5790 | 4.2479 | 4.0146 | 3.8406 | 3.7054 |
| 19 | 8.1849 | 5.9259 | 5.0103 | 4.5003 | 4.1708 | 3.9386 | 3.7653 | 3.6305 |
| 20 | 8.0960 | 5.8489 | 4.9382 | 4.4307 | 4.1027 | 3.8714 | 3.6987 | 3.5644 |
| 21 | 8.0166 | 5.7804 | 4.8740 | 4.3688 | 4.0421 | 3.8117 | 3.6396 | 3.5056 |
| 22 | 7.9454 | 5.7190 | 4.8166 | 4.3134 | 3.9880 | 3.7583 | 3.5867 | 3.4530 |
| 23 | 7.8811 | 5.6637 | 4.7649 | 4.2636 | 3.9392 | 3.7102 | 3.5390 | 3.4057 |
| 24 | 7.8229 | 5.6136 | 4.7181 | 4.2184 | 3.8951 | 3.6667 | 3.4959 | 3.3629 |
| 25 | 7.7698 | 5.5680 | 4.6755 | 4.1774 | 3.8550 | 3.6272 | 3.4568 | 3.3239 |
| 26 | 7.7213 | 5.5263 | 4.6366 | 4.1400 | 3.8183 | 3.5911 | 3.4210 | 3.2884 |
| 27 | 7.6767 | 5.4881 | 4.6009 | 4.1056 | 3.7848 | 3.5580 | 3.3882 | 3.2558 |
| 28 | 7.6356 | 5.4529 | 4.5681 | 4.0740 | 3.7539 | 3.5276 | 3.3581 | 3.2259 |
| 29 | 7.5977 | 5.4204 | 4.5378 | 4.0449 | 3.7254 | 3.4995 | 3.3303 | 3.1982 |
| 30 | 7.5625 | 5.3903 | 4.5097 | 4.0179 | 3.6990 | 3.4735 | 3.3045 | 3.1726 |

## Upper Quantiles of the F Distribution ($\alpha = 0.010$)

| df2 | \multicolumn{8}{c}{df1} |
|---|---|---|---|---|---|---|---|---|

| df2 | 9 | 10 | 11 | 12 | 16 | 20 | 25 | 30 |
|---|---|---|---|---|---|---|---|---|
| 2 | 99.3881 | 99.3992 | 99.4083 | 99.4159 | 99.4367 | 99.4492 | 99.4592 | 99.4658 |
| 3 | 27.3452 | 27.2287 | 27.1326 | 27.0518 | 26.8269 | 26.6898 | 26.5790 | 26.5045 |
| 4 | 14.6591 | 14.5459 | 14.4523 | 14.3736 | 14.1539 | 14.0196 | 13.9109 | 13.8377 |
| 5 | 10.1578 | 10.0510 | 9.9626 | 9.8883 | 9.6802 | 9.5526 | 9.4491 | 9.3793 |
| 6 | 7.9761 | 7.8741 | 7.7896 | 7.7183 | 7.5186 | 7.3958 | 7.2960 | 7.2285 |
| 7 | 6.7188 | 6.6201 | 6.5382 | 6.4691 | 6.2750 | 6.1554 | 6.0580 | 5.9920 |
| 8 | 5.9106 | 5.8143 | 5.7343 | 5.6667 | 5.4766 | 5.3591 | 5.2631 | 5.1981 |
| 9 | 5.3511 | 5.2565 | 5.1779 | 5.1114 | 4.9240 | 4.8080 | 4.7130 | 4.6486 |
| 10 | 4.9424 | 4.8491 | 4.7715 | 4.7059 | 4.5204 | 4.4054 | 4.3111 | 4.2469 |
| 11 | 4.6315 | 4.5393 | 4.4624 | 4.3974 | 4.2134 | 4.0990 | 4.0051 | 3.9411 |
| 12 | 4.3875 | 4.2961 | 4.2198 | 4.1553 | 3.9724 | 3.8584 | 3.7647 | 3.7008 |
| 13 | 4.1911 | 4.1003 | 4.0245 | 3.9603 | 3.7783 | 3.6646 | 3.5710 | 3.5070 |
| 14 | 4.0297 | 3.9394 | 3.8640 | 3.8001 | 3.6187 | 3.5052 | 3.4116 | 3.3476 |
| 15 | 3.8948 | 3.8049 | 3.7299 | 3.6662 | 3.4852 | 3.3719 | 3.2782 | 3.2141 |
| 16 | 3.7804 | 3.6909 | 3.6162 | 3.5527 | 3.3720 | 3.2587 | 3.1650 | 3.1007 |
| 17 | 3.6822 | 3.5931 | 3.5185 | 3.4552 | 3.2748 | 3.1615 | 3.0676 | 3.0032 |
| 18 | 3.5971 | 3.5082 | 3.4338 | 3.3706 | 3.1904 | 3.0771 | 2.9831 | 2.9185 |
| 19 | 3.5225 | 3.4338 | 3.3596 | 3.2965 | 3.1165 | 3.0031 | 2.9089 | 2.8442 |
| 20 | 3.4567 | 3.3682 | 3.2941 | 3.2311 | 3.0512 | 2.9377 | 2.8434 | 2.7785 |
| 21 | 3.3981 | 3.3098 | 3.2359 | 3.1730 | 2.9931 | 2.8796 | 2.7850 | 2.7200 |
| 22 | 3.3458 | 3.2576 | 3.1837 | 3.1209 | 2.9411 | 2.8274 | 2.7328 | 2.6675 |
| 23 | 3.2986 | 3.2106 | 3.1368 | 3.0740 | 2.8943 | 2.7805 | 2.6856 | 2.6202 |
| 24 | 3.2560 | 3.1681 | 3.0944 | 3.0316 | 2.8519 | 2.7380 | 2.6430 | 2.5773 |
| 25 | 3.2172 | 3.1294 | 3.0558 | 2.9931 | 2.8133 | 2.6993 | 2.6041 | 2.5383 |
| 26 | 3.1818 | 3.0941 | 3.0205 | 2.9578 | 2.7781 | 2.6640 | 2.5686 | 2.5026 |
| 27 | 3.1494 | 3.0618 | 2.9882 | 2.9256 | 2.7458 | 2.6316 | 2.5360 | 2.4699 |
| 28 | 3.1195 | 3.0320 | 2.9585 | 2.8959 | 2.7160 | 2.6017 | 2.5060 | 2.4397 |
| 29 | 3.0920 | 3.0045 | 2.9311 | 2.8685 | 2.6886 | 2.5742 | 2.4783 | 2.4118 |
| 30 | 3.0665 | 2.9791 | 2.9057 | 2.8431 | 2.6632 | 2.5487 | 2.4526 | 2.3860 |

# Bibliography

Adcock, C.J. (1988). A Bayesian approach to calculating sample size. *Statistician*, 37, 433–439.

Alizadeh, A.A. and Staudt, L.M. (2000). Genomic-scale gene expression profiling of normal and malignant immune cells. *Curr. Opin. Immunol.* 12(2), 219–225.

Anderson, S. and Hauck, W.W. (1990). Considerations of individual bioequivalence. *Journal of Pharmacokinetics and Biopharmaceutics*, 8, 259-273.

Armitage, P. (1955). Tests for linear trends in proportions and frequencies, Biometrics, 11, 375-386.

Armitage, P. and Berry, G. (1987). *Statistical Methods in Medical Research*. Blackwell Scientific Publications, London, UK.

Armitage, P., McPherson, C.K., and Rowe, B.C. (1969). Repeated significance tests on accumulating data. *Journal of Royal Statistical Society*, A, 132, 235-244.

Babb, J.S. and Rogatko, A. (2004). Bayesian methods for cancer phase I clinical trials, In *Advances in Clinical Trial Biostatistics*, Ed. by Nancy L. Geller, Marcel Dekker, Inc, New York, NY.

Bailar, J.C. and Mosteller, F. (1986). *Medical Uses of Statistics*. Massachusetts Medical Society, Waltham, MA.

Barry, M.J., Fowler, F.J. Jr., O'Leary, M.P., Bruskewitz, R.C., Holtgrewe, H.L., Mebust, W.K., and Cockett, A.T. (1992). The American Urological Association Symptom Index for Benign Prostatic Hyperplasia. *Journal of Urology*, 148, 1549-1557.

Bauer, P. (1989). Multistage testing with adaptive designs (with discussion). *Biometrie und Informatik in Medizin und Biologie*, 20, 130-148.

Bauer, P. and Rohmel, J. (1995). An adaptive method for establishing a dose-response relationship. *Statistics in Medicine*, 14, 1595-1607.

Becker, M.P. and Balagtas, C.C. (1993). Marginal modeling of binary cross-over data. *Biometrics*, 49, 997-1009.

Benjamini, Y. and Hochberg, Y. (1995). Controlling the false discovery rate: A practical and powerful approach to multiple testing. *Journal of the Royal Statistical Society* B, 57(1), 289–300.

Benjamini, Y. and Yekutieli D. (2001) The control of the false discovery rate in multiple testing under dependency. *Annals of Statistics* 29(4):1165–1188.

Berger, R.L. and Hsu, J.C. (1996). Bioequivalence trials, intersection-union tests and equivalence confidence sets. *Statistical Science*, 11, 283-302.

Berger, J.O., Boukai, B., and Wang, Y. (1997). Unified frequentist and Bayesian testing of a precision hypothesis. *Statistical Science*, 12, 133–160.

Berry, D.A. (1990). *Statistical Methodology in the Pharmaceutical Science*. Marcel Dekker, Inc., New York, NY.

Biswas, N., Chan, I.S.F., and Ghosh, K. (2000). Equivalence trials: statistical issues. Lecture note for the one-day short course at Joint Statistical Meetings, Indianapolis, IN.

Black, M.A. and Doerge, R.W. (2002). Calculation of the minimum number of replicate spots required for detection of significant gene expression fold change in microarray experiments. *Bioinformatics* 18(12), 1609–1616.

Blackwelder, W.C. (1982). Proving the null hypothesis in clinical trials. *Controlled Clinical Trials*, 3, 345-353.

Bretz, F. and Hothorn, L.A. (2002). Detecting dose-response using contrasts: asymptotic power and sample size determination for binary data. *Statistics in Medicine*, 21, 3325-3335.

Breslow, N.E. and Day, N.E. (1980). *Statistical Methods in Cancer Research, Vol.1: The Analysis of Case-Control Studies*. Oxford University Press, New York, NY.

Breslow, N.E. and Day, N.E. (1987). *Statistical Methods in Cancer Research, Vol.2: The Analysis of Cohort Studies*. Oxford University Press, New York, NY.

Bryant, J. and Day, R. (1995). Incorporating toxicity considerations into the design of two-stage phase II clinical trials. *Biometrics*, 51, 1372-1383.

Buncher, C.R. and Tsay, J.Y. (1994). *Statistics in Pharmaceutical Industry*, 2nd Edition, Marcel Dekker, Inc., New York, NY.

Buyse, M.E., Staquet, M.J., and Sylvester, R.J. (1984). *Cancer Clinical Trials: Methods and Practice.* Oxford Medical Publications, New York, NY.

Capizzi, T. and Zhang, J. (1996). Testing the hypothesis that matters for multiple primary endpoints. *Drug Information Journal*, 30, 349-356.

CAST (1989). Cardiac Arrhythmia Supression Trial. Preliminary report: effect of encainide and flecainide on mortality in a randomized trial of arrhythmia supression after myocardial infarction. *New England Journal of Medicine*, 321, 406-412.

Chan, I.S.F., Wang, W., and Heyse, J.F. (2003). Vaccine clinical trials. In Encyclopedia of Biopharmaceutical Statistics, 2nd Edition. Chow, S.C., Marcel Dekker, Inc., New York, NY.

Chan, I.S.F. and Bohida, N.R. (1998). Exact power and sample size for vaccine efficacy studies. *Communications in Statistics*, A, 27, 1305-1322.

Chang, M.N. (1989). Confidence intervals for a normal mean following group sequential test. *Biometrics*, 45, 247-254.

Chang, M.N. (2004). Power and sample size calculations for dose response studies, Dose-Response Trial Design Workshop, November 15, 2004, Philadelphia, PA.

Chang, M. and Chow, S.C. (2005). A hybrid Bayesian adaptive design for dose response trials. *Journal of Biopharmaceutical Statistics*, 15, 677-691.

Chang, M. and Chow, S.C. (2006). Power and sample size for dose response studies. In *Dose Finding in Drug Development*, Ed. Ting, N., Springer, New York, NY.

Chang, M.N. and O'Brien, P.C. (1986). Confidence interval following group sequential test. *Controlled Clinical Trials*, 7, 18-26.

Chang, M.N., Guess, H.A., and Heyse, J.F. (1994). Reduction in burden of illness: A review efficacy measure for prevention trials. *Statistics in Medicine*, 13, 1807-1814.

Chang, M.N., Wieand, H.S., and Chang, V.T. (1989). The bias of the sample proportion following a group sequential phase II trial. *Statistics in Medicine*, 8, 563-570.

Channon, E.J. (2000). Equivalence testing in dose-reponse study. *Drug Information Journal*, 34.

Chen, K.W., Li, G., and Chow, S.C. (1997). A note on sample size determination for bioequivalence studies with higher-order crossover designs. *Journal of Pharmacokinetics and Biopharmaceutics*, 25, 753-765.

Chen, J.J., Tsong, Y. and Kang S. (2000). Tests for equivalence or non-inferiority between two proportions. *Drug Information Journal*, 34.

Chen, M.L. (1997). Individual bioequivalence - a regulatory update. *Journal of Biopharmaceutical Statistics*, 7, 5-11.

Chen, T.T. (1997). Optimal three-stage designs for phase II cancer clinical trials. *Statistics in Medicine*, 16, 2701-2711.

Chen, T.T. and Ng, T.H. (1998). Optimal flexible designs in phase II clinical trials. *Statistics in Medicine*, 17, 2301-2312.

Cheng, B, Chow, S.C., and Wang, H. (2006). Test for departure from dose linearity under a crossover design: a slope approach. Submitted.

Cheng, B. and Shao, J. (2005), Exact tests for negligible interaction in two-way linear models. *Statistica Sinica*, To appear.

Chinchilli, V.M. and Esinhart, J.D. (1996). Design and analysis of intra-subject variability in cross-over experiments. *Statistics in Medicine*, 15, 1619-1634.

Chow, S.C. (1999). Individual bioequivalence - a review of FDA draft guidance. *Drug Information Journal*, 33, 435-444.

Chow, S.C. (2000). *Encyclopedia of Biopharmaceutical Statistics*. Marcel Dekker, Inc., New York, NY.

Chow, S.C. and Ki, F.Y.C. (1994). On statistical characteristics of quality of life assessment. *Journal of Biopharmaceutical Statistics*, 4, 1-17.

Chow, S.C. and Ki, F.Y.C. (1996). Statistical issues in quality of life assessment. *Journal of Biopharmaceutical Statistics*, 6, 37-48.

Chow, S.C. and Liu, J.P. (1992). *Design and Analysis of Bioavailability and Bioequivalence Studies*. Marcel Dekker, Inc., New York, NY.

Chow, S.C. and Liu, J.P. (1995). *Statistical Design and Analysis in Pharmaceutical Science.* Marcel Dekker, Inc., New York, NY.

Chow, S.C. and Liu, J.P. (1998). *Design and Analysis of Clinical Trials.* John Wiley and Sons, New York, NY.

Chow, S.C. and Liu, J.P. (2000). *Design and Analysis of Bioavailability and Bioequivalence Studies*, 2nd Edition, Marcel Dekker, Inc., New York, NY.

Chow, S.C. and Liu, J.P. (2003). *Design and Analysis of Clinical Trials, 2nd Edition,* John Wiley & Sons, New York, NY.

Chow, S.C. and Shao, J. (1988). A new procedure for the estimation of variance components. *Statistics and Probability Letters*, 6, 349-355.

Chow, S.C. and Shao, J. (2002). *Statistics in Drug Research - Methodology and Recent Development.* Marcel Dekker, Inc., New York, NY.

Chow, S.C. and Shao, J. (2004). Analysis of clinical data with breached blindness. *Statistics in Medicine*, 23, 1185-1193.

Chow, S.C., Shao, J. and Hu, O.Y.P. (2002). Assessing sensitivity and similarity in bridging studies. *Journal of Biopharmaceutical Statistics*, 12, 269-285.

Chow, S.C., Shao, J. and Wang, H. (2002). Individual bioequivalence testing under $2 \times 3$ crossover designs. *Statistics in Medicine*, 21, 629-648.

Chow, S.C., Shao, J. and Wang, H. (2003a). Statistical tests for population bioequivalence. *Statistica Sinica*, 13, 539-554.

Chow, S.C., Shao, J. and Wang, H. (2003b). In vitro bioequivalence testing. *Statitics in Medicine*, 22, 55-68.

Chow, S.C., Shao, J. and Wang, H. (2003c). Sample Size Calculations in Clinical Reserach. Marcel Dekker, New York, NY.

Chow, S.C. and Tse, S.K. (1990). A related problem in bioavailability/bioequivalence studies—estimation of intra-subject variability with a common CV. *Biometrical Journal*, 32, 597-607.

Chow, S.C. and Tse, S.K. (1991). On variance estimation in assay validation. *Statistics in Medicine*, 10, 1543-1553.

Chow, S.C. and Wang, H. (2001). On sample size calculation in bioequivalence trials. *Journal of Pharmacokinetics and Pharmacodynamics*, 28, 155-169.

Chuang-Stein, C. and Agresti, A. (1997). A review of tests for detecting a monotone dose-response relationship with ordinal response data. *Statistics in Medicine*, 16, 2599-2618.

Cochran, W.G. (1954). Some methods for stengthening the common chi-square tests. *Biometrics*, 10, 417-451.

Colton, T. (1974). *Statistics in Medicine.* Little, Brown and Company, Boston, MA.

Conaway, M.R. and Petroni, G.R. (1996). Designs for phase II trials allowing for a trade-off between response and toxicity. *Biometrics*, 52, 1375-1386.

Cornfield, J. (1956). A statistical problem arising from retrospective studies. In J. Neyman ed. Proc. Third Berkeley Symposium on Mathematical Statistics and Probability, 4, 135-148.

Cox, D.R. (1952). A note of the sequential estimation of means. *Proc. Camb. Phil. Soc.*, 48, 447-450.

CPMP (1997). Points to consider: The assessment of the potential for QT interval prolongation by non-cardiovascular products.

Crawford, E.D., Eisenberg, M.A., Mcleod, D.G., Spaulding, J.T., Benson, R., Dorr, A., Blumenstein, B.A., Davis, M.A., and Goodman, P.J. (1989). A controlled trial of Leuprolide with and without flutamide in prostatic carcinoma. *New England Journal of Medicine*, 321, 419-424.

Crowley, J. (2001). *Handbook of Statistics in Clinical Oncology*, Marcel Dekker, Inc., New York, NY.

CTriSoft Intl. (2002). Clinical Trial Design with ExpDesign Studio, www.ctrisoft.net., CTriSoft Intl., Lexington, MA.

Cui, X. and Churchill, G.A. (2003). How many mice and how many arrays? Replication in mouse cDNA microarray experiments. Methods of Microarray Data Analysis II, edited by Kimberly F. Johnson and Simon M. Lin. Norwell, MA: Kluwer Academic Publishers, 139–154.

DeMets, D. and Lan, K.K.G. (1994). Interim analysis: the alpha spending function approach. *Statistics in Medicine*, 13, 1341-1352.

Dixon, D.O. and Simon, R. (1988). Sample size consideration for studies comparing survial curves using historical controls. *Journal of Clinical Epidemiology*, 41, 1209-1213.

Dubey, S.D. (1991). Some thoughts on the one-sided and two-sided tests. *Journal of Biopharmaceutical Statistics*, 1, 139-150.

Dudoit, S., Shaffer, J.P., and Boldrick, J.C. (2003). Multiple hypothesis testing in microarray experiments. *Statistical Science* 18, 71–103.

Dudoit, S, Yang, Y.H., Callow, M.J., and Speed, T.P. (2002). Statistical methods for identifying differentially expressed genes in replicated cDNA microarray experiments. *Statistica Sinica* 12, 111–139.

Dunnett, C.W. and Gent, M. (1977). Significance testing to establish equivalence between treatments with special reference to data in the form of 2x2 tables. *Biometrics*, 33, 593-602.

Durham, S.D., Flourney, N., and Li, W. (1998). A sequential design for maximizing the probability of a favorable response. *Canadian Journal of Statistics*, 26, 479-495.

EAST (2000). Software for the design and interim monitoring of group sequential clinical trials. CYTEL Software Corportation.

Ellenberg, S.S. and Dixon, D.O. (1994). Statistical issues in designing clinical trials of AIDS treatments and vaccines. *Journal of Statistical Planning and Inference*, 42, 123-135.

EMEA (2002). Point to Consider on Methodological Issues in Confirmatory Clinical Trials with Flexible Design and Analysis Plan. The European Agency for the Evaluation of Medicinal Products Evaluation of Medicines for Human Use. CPMP/EWP/2459/02, London, UK.

Emrich, L.J. (1989). Required duration and power determinations for historically controlled studies of survival times. *Statistics in Medicine*, 8, 153-160.

Ensign, L.G., Gehan, E.A., Kamen, D.S., and Thall, P.F. (1994). An optimal three-stage design for phase II clinical trials. *Statistics in Medicine*, 13, 1727-1736.

Esinhart, J.D. and Chinchilli, V.M. (1994). Extension to the use of tolerance intervals for assessment of individual bioequivalence. *Journal of Biopharmaceutical Statistics*, 4, 39-52.

Fairweather, W.R. (1994). Statisticians, the FDA and a time of transition. Presented at Pnarmaceutical Manufacturers Association Education and Research Institute Training Course in Non-Clinical Statistics, Georgetown University Conference Center, February 6-8, 1994, Washington, D.C.

Farrington, C.P. and Manning, G. (1990). Test statistics and sample size formulae for comparative binomial trials with null hypothesis of non-zero risk difference or non-unity relative risk. *Statistics in Medicine*, 9, 1447-1454.

FDA (1988). Guideline for the Format and Content of the Clinical and Statistical Section of New Drug Application, U.S. Food and Drug Administration, Rockville, MD.

FDA (1992). Guidance on Statistical Procedures for Bioequivalence Studies Using a Standard Two-Treatment Crossover Design. Office of Generic Drugs, Center for Drug Evaluation and Research, Food and Drug Administration, Rockville, MD.

FDA (1998). Guidance for Industry on Providing Clinical Evidence of Effectiveness for Human Drug and Biological Products. Food and Drug Administration, Rockville, MD.

FDA (1999a). Average, Population, and Individual Approaches to Establishing Bioequivalence. Center for Drug Evaluation and Research, Food and Drug Administration, Rockville, MD.

FDA (1999b). Guidance for Industry on Bioavailability and Bioequivalence Studies for Nasal Aerosols and Nasal Sprays for Local Action. Center for Drug Evaluation and Research, Food and Drug Administration, Rockville, MD.

FDA (2000). Guidance for Industry: Bioavailability and Bioequivalence Studies for Orally Administered Drug Products - General Considerations. Center for Drug Evaluation and Research, Food and Drug Administration, Rockville, MD.

FDA (2001). Guidance for Industry on Statistical Approaches to Establishing Bioequivalence. Center for Drug Evaluation and Research, Food and Drug Administration, Rockville, MD.

FDA/TPD (2003). Preliminary concept paper: The clinical evaluation of QT/QTc interval prolongation and proarrhythmic potential for non-arrhythmic drug products. Released on November 15, 2005. Revised on February 6, 2003.

Feigl, P., Blumestein, B., Thompson, I., Crowley, J., Wolf, M., Kramer, B.S., Coltman, C.A. Jr., Brawley, O.W., Ford, L.G. (1995). Design of the Prostate Cancer Prevention Trial (PCPT). *Controlled Clinical Trials*, 16, 150-163.

Feinstein, A.R. (1977). *Clinical Biostatistics*. The Mosby Company, St. Louis, MO.

Fine, G.D. (1997). A formula for determing sample size to study dose-response. *Drug Information Journal*, 31, 911-916.

Fisher, L. (1990). *Biostatistics: Methodology for the Health Sciences*. John Wiley and Sons, New York, NY.

Fleiss, J.L. (1986). *The Design and Analysis of Clinical Experiments*. John Wiley and Sons, New York, NY.

Fleming, T.R. (1990). Evaluation of active control trials in AIDS. *Journal of Acquired Immune Deficiency Syndromes*, 3 (suppl. 2), 582-587.

Fleming, T.R. and Harrington, D.R. (1991). *Counting Process and Survival Analysis*. John Wiley and Sons, New York, NY.

Freedman, L.S. (1982). Tables of the number of patients required in clinical trials using logrank test. *Statistics in Medicine*, 1, 121-129.

Frick, M.H., Elo, O., Haapa, K., Heinonen, O.P., Heinsalmi, P., Helo, P. Huttunen, J.K., Kaitaniemi, P., Koskinen, P., Manninen, V., Maenpaa, H., Malkonen, M., Manttari, M., Norola, S., Pasternack, A., Pikkarainen, J., Romo, M., Sjoblom, T., and Nikkila, E.A. (1987). Helsikini heart study: primary-prevention trial with gemfibrozil in middle-aged men with dyslipidemia. *New England Journal of Medicine*, 317, 1237-1245.

Friedman, L.M., Furberg, C.D., and DeMets, D.L. (1981). *Fundamentals of Clinical Trials*. John Wiley and Sons, New York, NY.

Gadbury, G.L., Page, G.P., Edwards, J., Kayo, T,. Prolla, T.A., Weindruch, R., Permana, P.A., Mountz, J.D., and Allison, D.B. (2004) Power and sample size estimation in high dimensional biology. *Statistical Methods in Medical Research* 13:325–338.

Gail, M.H. (1985). Applicability of sample size calculations based on a comparison of proportions for use with the logrank test. *Controlled Clinical Trials*, 6, 112-119.

Gail, M.H. and Simon, R. (1985). Testing for qualitative interactions between treatment effects and patient subjects. *Biometrics*, 71, 431-444.

Gart (1985). Approximate tests and interval estimation of the common relative risk in the combination of $2 \times 2$ tables. *Biometrika*, 72, 673-677.

Gasprini, M. and Eisele, J. (2000). A curve-free method for phase I clinical trials. Biometrics, 56, 609-615.

Gastwirth, J.L. (1995). The use of maximum efficiency robust tests in combining contingency tables and survival analysis. *Journal of American Statistical Association*, 80, 380-384.

Ge, Y., Dudoit, S. and Speed, T.P. (2003). Resampling-based multiple testing for microarray data analysis. *TEST* 12(1), 1–44.

Geller, N.L. (1994). Discussion of interim analysis: the alpha spending function approach. *Statistics in Medicine*, 13, 1353-1356.

Genovese, C., and Wasserman, L. (2002) Operating characteristics and extensions of the false discovery rate procedure. *Journal of the Royal Statistical Society, Series B* 64(3):499–517.

George, S.L. and Desu, M.M. (1973). Planning the size and duration of a clinical trial studying the time to some critical event. *Journal of Chronic Diseases*, 27, 15-24.

Gilbert, G.S. (1992). *Drug Safety Assessment in Clinical Trials*. Marcel Dekker, Inc., New York, NY.

Glantz, S.A. (1987). *Primer of Biostatistics*, 2nd Edition, McGraw-Hill, Inc., New York, NY.

Golub, T.R., Slonim, D.K., Tamayo, P., Huard, C., Gaasenbeek, M., Mesirov, J.P., Coller, H., Loh, M.L., Downing, J.R., Caligiuri, M.A., Bloomfield, C.D., and Lander, E.S. (1999). Molecular classification of cancer: Class discovery and class prediction by gene expression monitoring. *Science* 286(15), 531–537.

Gould, A.L. (1995). Planning and revision the sample size for a trial. *Statistics in Medicine*, 14, 1039-1051.

Graybill, F. and Wang, C.M. (1980). Confidence intervals on nonnegative linear combinations of variances. *Journal of American Statistical Association*, 75, 869-873.

Green, S. J. and Dahlberg, S. (1992). Planned versus attained designs in phase II clinical trials. *Statistics in Medicine*, 11, 853-862.

GUSTO (1993). An investigational randomized trial comparing four thrombolytic strategies for acute myocardial infarction. The GUSTO Investigators. *The New England Journal of Medicine*, 329, 673-682.

Haaland, P.D. (1989). *Experiemntal Design in Biotechnology*. Marcel Dekker, Inc., New York, NY.

Hamasaki, T., Isomura, T., and etc. (2000), Statistical approaches to detecting dose-response relationship. *Drug Information Journal*, 34.

Haybittle, J.L. (1971). Repeated assessment of results in clinical trials of cancer treatment. *British Journal of Radiology*, 44, 793-797.

Harris, E.K. and Albert, A. (1990). *Survivorship Analysis for Clinical Studies*. Marcel Dekker, Inc., New York, NY.

Heart Special Project Committee (1988). Organization, review and administration of cooperative studies (Greenberg report): A report from the Heart Special Project Committee to the National Advisory Council. *Controlled Clinical Trials*, 9, 137-148.

Hochberg, Y. (1988). A sharper Bonferroni procedure for multiple tests of significance. *Biometrika* 75, 800–802.

Hochberg, Y. and Tamhane, A.C. (1987). *Multiple Comparison Procedure*. John Wiley and Sons, New York, NY.

Hollander, M. and Wolfe, D.A. (1973). *Nonparametric Statistical Methods*. John Wiley and Sons, New York, NY.

Holm, S. (1979). A simple sequentially rejective multiple test procedure. *Scand. J. Statist.* 6, 65–70.

Hothorn, L. A. (2000). Evaluation of animal carcinogenicity studies: Cochran-Armitage trend test vs. multiple contrast tests. *Biometrical Journal*, 42, 553-567.

Howe, W.G. (1974). Approximate confidence limits on the mean of $X+Y$ where $X$ and $Y$ are two tabled independent random variables. *Journal of American Statistical Association*, 69, 789-794.

Hughes, M.D. (1993). Stopping guidelines for clinical trials with multiple treatments. *Statistics in Medicine*, 12, 901-913.

Hughes, M.D., and Pocock, S.J. (1988). Stopping rules and estimation problems in clinical trias. *Statistics in Medicine*, 7, 1231-1242.

Huque, M.F. and Dubey, S. (1990). Design and analysis for therapeutic equivalence clinical trials with binary clinical endpoints. Proceedings of Biopharmaceutical Section of the American Statistical Association, Alexandria, VA, 91-97.

Hyslop, T., Hsuan, F. and Holder, D.J. (2000). A small sample confidence interval approach to assess individual bioequivalence. *Statistics in Medicine*, 19, 2885-2897.

ICH (1998a). Ethnic Factors in the Acceptability of Foreign Clinical Data. Tripartite International Conference on Harmonization Guideline, E5.

ICH (1998b). Statistical Principles for Clinical Trials. Tripartite International Conference on Harmonization Guideline, E9.

ICH (1999). Choice of Control Group in Clinical Trials. Tripartite International Conference on Harmonization Guideline, E10.

ICH (2003). ICH E14 Guidance on The Clinical Evaluation of QT/QTc Interval Prolongation and Proarrhythmic Potential for Non-Antiarrhythmic Drugs.

Jennison, C., and Turnbull, B. (1989). Interim analysis: the repeated confidence interval approach (with discussion). *Journal of Royal Statistical Society*, B, 51, 305-361.

Jennison, C. and Turnbull, B.W. (1990). Statistical approaches to interim monitoring of medical trials: A review and cormmentary. *Statistics in Medicine*, 5, 299-317.

Jennison, C. and Turnbull, B. (1993). Sequential equivalence testing and repeated confidence intervals, with application to normal and binary response. *Biometrics*, 49, 31-34.

Jennison, C. and Turnbull B. (2000). *Group Sequential Methods with Applications to Clinical Trials*. Chapman and Hall, New York, NY.

Johnson, N.L. and Kotz, S. (1972). *Distribution in Statistics*. Houghton Mifflin Company, Boston, MA.

Jones, B. and Kenward, M.G. (1989). *Design and Analysis of Cross-over Trials*. Chapman and Hall, New York, NY.

Joseph, L. and Belisle, P. (1997). Bayesian sample size determination for normal means and differences between normal means. *Statistician*, 44, 209–226.

Joseph, L., Wolfson, D.B., and Berger, R.D. (1995). Sample size calculations for binomial proportions via highest posterior density intervals (with discussion). *Journal of the Royal Statistical Society*, Series D (The Statistician), 44, 143-154.

Jung, S.H. (2005). Sample size for FDR-control in microarray data analysis. Bioinformatics, 21, 3097-3104.

Jung S.H., Bang, H., and Young, S.S. (2005) Sample size calculation for multiple testing in microarray data analysis. *Biostatics* **6**(1):157–169.

Jung, S.H., Chow, S.C., and Chi, E.M. (2007). On sample size calculation based on propensity analysis in non-randomized trials. *Journal of Biopharmaceutical Statistics*, 17, 35-41.

Kessler, D.A. (1989). The regulation of investigational drugs. *New England Journal of Medicine*, 320, 281-288.

Kessler, D.A. and Feiden, K.L. (1995). Faster evaluation of vital drugs. *Scientific American*, 272, 48-54.

Kim, K. and DeMets, D.L. (1987). Confidence intervals following group sequential tests in clinical trials. *Biometrics*, 43, 857-864.

Kim, K. (1989). Point estimation following group sequential tests. *Biometrics*, 45, 613-617.

Kruskal, W.H. and Wallis, W.A. (1952). Use of ranks in one-criterion variance analysis. *Journal of American Statistical Association*, 47, 583-621.

Lachin, J.M. (1981). Introduction to sample size determination and power analysis for clinical trials. *Controlled Clinical Trials*, 2, 93-113.

Lachin, J.M. and Foulkes, M.A. (1986). Evaluation of sample size and power for analysis of survival with allowance for nonuniform patient entry, losses to follow-up, noncompliance, and stratification. *Biometrics*, 42, 507-519.

Lakatos, E. (1986). Sample size determination in clinical trials with time-dependent rates of losses and noncompliance. *Controlled Clinical Trials*, 7, 189-199.

Lakatos, E. (1988). Sample sizes based on the log-rank statistic in complex clinical trials. *Biometrics*, 44, 229-241.

Lan, K.K.G. and DeMets, D.L. (1983). Discrete sequential boundaries for clinical trials. *Biometrika*, 70, 659-663.

Lan, K.K.G. and Wittes, J. (1988). The B-value: A tool of monitoring data. *Biometrics*, 44, 579-585.

Landis, J.R., Heyman, E.R., and Koch, G.G. (1976). Average partial association in three-way contingency tables: a review and discussion of alternative tests. *International Statistical Review*, 46, 237-254.

Laubscher, N.F. (1960). Normalizing the noncentral t and F distribution. *Annals of Mathematical Statistics*, 31, 1105-1112.

Lee, M.L.T. and Whitmore, G.A. (2002). Power and sample size for DNA microarray studies. *Statistics in Medicine*, 21, 3543–3570.

Lee, S.J. and Zelen, M. (2000). Clinical trials and sample size considerations: another prespective. *Statistical Science*, 15, 95-110.

Lee, Y., Shao, J., and Chow, S.C. (2004). The modified large sample confidence intervals for linear combinations of variance components: extension, theory, and application. *Journal of the American Statistical Association*, 99, 467-478.

Lee, Y., Shao, J., Chow, S.C., and Wang, H. (2002). Test for inter-subject and total variabilities under crossover design. *Journal of Biopharmaceutical Statistics*, 12, 503-534.

Lin, Y. and Shih W. J. (2001). Statistical properties of the traditional algorithm-based designs for phase I cancer clinical trials, *Biostatistics*, 2, 203-215.

Lindley, D.V. (1997). The choice of sample size. *Statistician*, 44, 167–171.

Liu, G. and Liang, K.Y. (1995). Sample size calculations for studies with correlated observations. Unpublished manuscript.

Liu, J.P. and Chow, S.C. (1992). Sample size determination for the two one-sided tests procedure in bioequivalence. *Journal of Pharmacokinetics and Biopharmaceutics*, 20, 101-104.

Liu, K.J. (2001). Letter to the editor: a flexible design for multiple armed screening trials. *Statistics in Medicine*, 20, 1051-1060.

Liu, Q. (1998). An order-directed score test for trend in ordered 2xK Tables. *Biometrics*, 54, 1147-1154.

Liu, Q., Proschan, M.A., and Pledger, G.W. (2002). A unified theory of two-stage adaptive designs. *Journal of American Statistical Association*, 97, 1034-1041.

Longford, N.T. (1993). Regression analysis of multilevel data with measurement error. *British Journal of Mathematical and Statistical Psychology*, 46, 301-312.

Longford, N. T. (1993). *Random Coefficient Models*. Oxford University Press Inc., New York, NY.

Malik, M. and Camm, A. J. (2001). Evaluation of drug-induced QT interval prolongation. *Drug Safety*, 24, 323-351.

Mantel, N. and Haenzsel, W. (1959). Statistical aspects of the analysis of data from retrospective studies of disease. *Journal of National Cancer Institute*, 22, 719-748.

Margolies, M.E. (1994). Regulations of combination products. *Applied Clinical Trials*, 3, 50-65.

Marcus, R., Peritz, E., and Gabriel, K.R. (1976). On closed testing procedures with special reference to ordered analysis of variance. *Biometrika*, 63, 655-660.

McCullagh, P. and Nelder, J.A. (1983). Quasi-likelihood functions. *Annals of Statistics*, 11, 59-67.

Mehrotra, D.V. and Railkar, R. (2000). Minimum risk weights for comparing treatments in stratified binomial trials. *Statistics in Medicine*, 19, 811-825.

Meier, P. (1989). The biggest public health experiment ever, the 1954 field trial of the Salk poliomyelitis vaccine. In Statistics: A Guide to the Unknown, ed. by Tanur, J.M., Mosteller, F., and Kruskal, W.H., 3rd ed. Wadsworth, Belmont, CA, 3-14.

Meinert, C.L. (1986). *Clinical Trials: Design, Conduct, and Analysis*. Oxford University Press, New York, NY.

Miettinen, O. and Nurminen, M. (1985). Comparative analysis of two rates. *Statistics in Medicine*, 4, 213-226.

Mike, V. and Stanley, K.E. (1982). *Statistics in Medical Research: Methods and Issues, with Applications in Cancer Research*. John Wiley and Sons, New York, NY.

Miller R.G. (1997). Jr. *Beyond ANOVA, Basics of Applied Statistics*, 2nd Edition. Springer-Verlag, New York, NY.

Moses, L.E. (1992). Statistical concepts fundamental to investigations. In Medical Uses of Statistics, ed. by Bailar, J.C. and Mosteller, F., New England Journal of Medicine Books, Boston, MA. 5-26.

Moss, A. J. (1993). Measurement of the QT interval and the risk associated with QT interval prolongation. *American Journal of Cardiology*, 72, 23B-25B.

Müller, P.,. Parmigiani, G., Robert, C., and Rousseau, J. (2004) Optimal sample size for multiple testing: The case of gene expression microarrays. *Journal of the American Statistical Association* 99, 990–1001.

Mutter, G.L., Baak, J.P.A., Fitzgerald, J.T., Gray, R., Neuberg, D., Kust, G.A., Gentleman, R., Gallans, S.R., Wei, L.J., and Wilcox, M. (2001). Global express changes of constitutive and hormonally regulated genes during endometrial neoplastic transformation. *Gynecologic Oncology* 83, 177–185.

Nam, J.M. (1987). A simple approximation for calculating sample sizes for detecting linear trend in proportions. *Biometrics*, 43, 701-705.

Nam, J.M. (1998). Power and sample size for stratified prospective studies using the score method for testign relative risk. *Biometrics*, 54, 331-336.

Neuhauser, M., and Hothorn, L. (1999). An exact Cochran-Armitage test for trend when dose-response shapes are a priori unknown. Computational Statistics and Data Analysis, 30, 403-412.

O'Brien, P.C. and Fleming, T.R. (1979). A multiple testing procedure for clinical trials. *Biometrics*, 35, 549-556.

Olkin, I. (1995). Meta-analysis: reconciling the results of independent studies. *Statistics in Medicine*, 14, 457-472.

Olschewski, M. and Schumacher, M. (1990). Statistical analysis of quality of life data in cancer clinical trials. *Statistics in Medicine*, 9, 749-763.

O'Neill, R.T. (1988). Assessment of safety. In Biopharmaceutical Statistics for Drug Development, ed. by Peace, K., Marcel Dekker, Inc., New York, NY.

O'Quigley, J., Pepe, M., and Fisher, L. (1990). Continual reassessment method: A practical design for phase I clinical trial in cancer. Biometrics, 46, 33-48.

O'Quigley, J., and Shen, L. (1996). Continual reassessment method: A likelihood approach. Biometrics, 52, 673-684.

Pagana, K.D. and Pagana, T.J. (1998). *Manual of Dignostic and Laboratory Tests*. Mosby, Inc., St. Louis, MO.

Pan, W. (2002). A comparative review of statistical methods for discovering differentially expressed genes in replicated microarray experiments. *Bioinformatics*, 18(4), 546–554.

Pan, W., Lin, J., and Le, C.T. (2002). How many replicated of arrays are required to detect gene expression changes in microarray experiments? A mixture model approach. *Genome Biology*, 3(5), 1–10.

Patulin Clinical Trials Committee (of the Medical Research Council) (1944). Clinical trial of Patulin in the common cold. *Lancet*, 2, 373-375.

Pawitan, Y. and Hallstrom, A. (1990). Statistical interim monitoring of the cardiac arrhythmia suppression trial. *Statistics in Medicine*, 9, 1081-1090.

Peace, K.E. (1987). *Biopharmaceutical Statistics for Drug Development.* Marcel Dekker, Inc., New York, NY.

Peace, K.E. (1990). *Statistical Issues in Drug Research and Development.* Marcel Dekker, Inc., New York, NY.

Peto, R., Pike, M.C., Armitage, P., Breslow, N.E., Cox, D.R., Howard, S.V., Mantel, N., McPherson, K., Peto, J. and Smith, P.G. (1976). Design and analysis of randomized clinical trials requiring prolonged observation of each patient. *British Journal of Cancer,* 34, 585-612.

Petricciani, J.C. (1981). An overview of FDA, IRBs and regulations. *IRB,* 3, p1.

Pham-Gia, T.G. (1997). On Bayesian analysis, Bayesian decision theory and the sample size problem. *Statistician,* 46, 139–144.

Phillips, K.F. (1990). Power of the two one-sided tests procedure in bioequivalence. *Journal of Pharmacokinetics and Biopharmaceutics,* 18, 137-144.

PhRMA (2003). Investigating drug-induced QT and QTc prolongation in the clinic: statistical design and analysis considerations. Report from the Pharmaceutical Research and Manufacturers of America QT Statistics Expert Team, August 14, 2003.

PHSRG (1989). Steering Committee of the Physician's Health Study Research Group. Final report of the aspirin component of the ongoing physicians' health study. *New England Journal of Medicine,* 321, 129-135.

PMA (1993). PMA Biostatistics and Medical Ad Hoc Committee on Interim Analysis. Interim analysis in the pharmaceutical industry. *Controlled Clinical Trials,* 14, 160-173.

Pocock, S.J. (1977). Group sequential methods in the design and analysis of clinical trials. *Biometrika,* 64, 191-199.

Pocock, S.J. (1983). *Clinical Trials: A Practical Approach.* John Wiley and Sons, New York, NY.

Pocock, S.J. and Hughes, M.D. (1989). Practical problems in interim analyses with particular regard to estimation. *Controlled Clinical Trials,* 10, S209-S221.

Podgor, M.J., Gastwirth, J.L., and Mehta, C.R. (1996). Efficiency robust tests of independence in contingency tables with ordered classifications. *Statistics in Medicine,* 15, 2095-2105.

Portier, C. and Hoel, D. (1984). Type I error of trend tests in proportions and design of cancer screens. *Communications in Statistics*, 13, 1-14.

Press, W.H., Teukolsky, S.A., Vetterling, W.T., and Flannery, B.P. (1996). *Numerical Recipes in Fortran 90*. Cambridge University Press, New York, NY.

Proschan, M.A., Follmann, D.A., and Geller, N.L. (1994). Monitoring multi-armed trials. *Statistics in Medicine*, 13, 1441-1452.

Quan and Shih (1996). Assessing reproducibility by the within-subject coefficient of variation with random effects models. *Biometrics*, 52, 1195-1203.

Rosenbaum, P.R. and Rubin, D.B. (1983). The central role of the propensity score in observational studies for causal effects. *Biometrika*, 70, 41-55.

Rosenbaum, P.R. and Rubin, D.B. (1984). Reducing bias in observational studies using subclassification on the propensity score. *Journal of American Statistical Association*, 95, 749-759.

Rosenberger, W., and Lachin, J. (2003). Randomization in Clinical Trials, John Wiley and Sons, New York, NY.

Ruberg, S.J. (1995a). Dose response studies: I. Some design considerations. *Journal of Biopharmaceutical Statistics*, 5, 1-14.

Ruberg, S.J. (1995b). Dose response studies: II. Analysis and interpretation. *Journal of Biopharmaceutical Statistics*, 5, 15-42.

Rubinstein, L.V., Gail, M. H., and Santner, T.J. (1981). Planning the duration of a comparative clinical trial with loss to follow-up and a period of continued observation. *Journal of Chronic Diseases*, 34, 469-479.

Sander, C. (2000). Genomic medicine and the future of health care. *Science*, 287(5460), 1977–1978.

Sargent, D. and Goldberg, R. (2001). A flexible design for multiple armed screening trials. *Statistics in Medicine*, 20, 1051-1060.

Schall, R. and Luus, H.G. (1993). On population and individual bioequivalence, *Statistics in Medicine*, 12, 1109-1124.

Schoenfeld, D. (1981). Table, life; test, logmark; test, Wilcoxon: The asymptotic properties of nonparametric tests for comparing survival distributions. *Biometrika*, 68, 316-319.

Schuirmann, D.J. (1987). A comparison of the two one-sided tests procedure and the power approach for assessing the equivalence of average bioequivalence. *Journal of Pharmacokinetics and Biopharmaceutics*, 15, 657-680.

Self, S. and Mauritsen, R. (1988). Power/sample size calculations for generalized linear models. *Biometrics*, 44, 79-86.

Self, S., Mauritsen, R. and Ohara, J. (1992). Power calculations for likelihood ratio tests in generalized linear models. *Biometrics*, 48, 31-39.

Self, S., Prentice, R., Iverson, D., Henderson, M., Thompson, D., Byar, D., Insull, W., Gorbach, S.L., Clifford, C., Goldman, S., Urban, N., Sheppard, L., and Greenwald, P. (1988). Statistical design of the women's health trial. *Controlled Clinical Trials*, 9, 119-136.

SERC (1993). EGRET SIZ: sample size and power for nonlinear regression models. Reference Manual, Version 1. Statistics and Epidemiology Research Corporation.

Shaffer, J.P. (2002). Multiplicity, directional (Type III) errors, and the null hypothesis. *Psychological Methods*, 7, 356–369.

Shao, J. and Chow, S.C. (1990). Test for treatment effect based on binary data with random sample sizes. *Australian Journal of Statistics*, 32, 53-70.

Shao, J. and Chow, S.C. (2002). Reproducibility probability in clinical trials. *Statistics in Medicine*, 21, 1727-1742.

Shao, J. and Tu, D. (1999). *The Jackknife and Bootstrap*. Springer-Verlag, New York, NY.

Shapiro, S.H. and Louis, T.A. (1983). *Clinical Trials, Issues and Approaches*. Marcel Dekker, Inc, New York, NY.

Sheiner, L.B. (1992). Bioequivalence revisited. *Statistics in Medicine*, 11, 1777-1788.

Shih, J.H. (1995). Sample size calculation for complex clinical trials with survival endpoints. *Controlled Clinical Trials*, 16, 395-407.

Shih, W.J. (1993). Sample size re-estimation for triple blind clinical trials. *Drug Information Journal*, 27, 761-764.

Shih, W.J. and Zhao, P.L. (1997). Design for sample size re-estimation with interim data for double-blind clinical trials with binary outcomes. *Statistics in Medicine*, 16, 1913-1923.

Shirley, E. (1977). A non-parametric equivalent of William' test for contrasting increasing dose levels of treatment. *Biometrics*, 33, 386-389.

Simon, R. (1989). Optimal two-stage designs for phase II clinical trials. *Controlled Clinical Trials*, 10, 1-10.

Simon, R., Radmacher, M.D., and Dobbin, K. (2002). Design of studies with DNA microarrays. *Genetic Epidemiology*, 23, 21–36.

Spiegelhalter, D.J. and Freedman L.S. (1986). A predictive approach to selecting the size of a clinical trial, based on subjective clinical opinion. *Statistics in Medicine*, 5, 1-13.

Spilker, B. (1991). *Guide to Clinical Trials*. Raven Press, New York, NY.

Spriet, A. and Dupin-Spriet, T. (1992). *Good Practice of Clinical Trials*. Karger, S. Karger, AG, Medical and Scientific Publication, Basel.

Stewart, W. and Ruberg, S. J. (2000). Detecting dose response with contrasts. Statistics in Medicine, 19, 913-921.

Storey, J.D. (2002). A direct approach to false discovery rates. *Journal of the Royal Statistical Society* B, 64(1), 479–498.

Storey, J.D. (2003) The positive false discovery rate: a Bayesian interpretation and the q-value. *Annals of Statistics*, 31(6), 2013–2035.

Storey, J.D., Taylor, J.E., Siegmund, D. (2004) Strong control, conservative point estimation and simultaneous conservative consistency of false discovery rates: a unified approach. *Journal of the Royal Statistical Society, Series B*, 66(1), 187–205.

Storey, J.D., and Tibshirani, R. (2001) Estimating false discovery rates under dependence, with applications to DNA microarrays. Technical Report 2001-28, Department of Statistics, Stanford University.

Storey, J.D., and Tibshirani, R. (2003) SAM thresholding and false discovery rates for detecting differential gene expression in DNA microarrays. In The Analysis of Gene Expression Data: Methods and Software, by G Parmigiani, ES Garrett, RA Irizarry and SL Zeger (editors). Springer, New York.

Strieter, D., Wu, W., and Agin, M. (2003). Assessing the effects of replicate ECGs on QT variability in healthy subjects. Presented at Midwest Biopharmaceutical Workshop, May 21, 2003.

Stuart, A. (1955). A test for homogeneity of the marginal distributions in a two-way classification. *Biometrika*, 42, 412-416.

Tandon, P.K. (1990). Applications of global statistics in analyzing quality of life data. *Statistics in Medicine*, 9, 819-827.

Temple, R. (1993). Trends in pharmaceutical development. *Drug Information Journal*, 27, 355-366.

Temple, R. (2003). Presentation at Drug Information Agency/FDA Workshop.

Tessman, D.K., Gipson, B., and Levins, M. (1994). Cooperative fast-track development: the fludara story. *Applied Clinical Trials*, 3, 55-62.

Thall, P.F., Simon, R.M., and Estey, E.H. (1995). Baysian sequential monitoring designs for single-arm clinical trials with multiple outcomes. *Statistics in Medicine*, 14, 357-379.

Thall, P.F., Simon, R.M., and Estey, E.H. (1996). New statistical strategy for monitoring safety and efficacy in single-arm clinical trials. *Journal of Clinical Oncology*, 14, 296-303.

Thomas, J.G., Olson, J.M., Tapscott, S.J., and Zhao, L.P. (2001). An efficient and robust statistical modeling approach to discover differentially expressed genes using genomic expression profiles. *Genome Research*, 11, 1227–1236.

Ting, N., Burdick, R.K., Graybill, F.A., Jeyaratnam, S., Lu, T.C. (1990). *Journal of Statistical Computation and Simulation*, 35, 135-143.

Troendle, J.F., Korn, E.L., and McShane, L.M. (2004). An example of slow convergence of the bootstrap in high dimensions. *American Statistician*, 58, 25–29.

Tsai, A.A., Rosner, G.L., and Mehta, C.R. (1984). Exact confidence interval following a group sequential test. *Biometrics*, 40, 797-803.

Tsiatis, A.A, Rosner, G.L., and Mehta, C.R. (1984). Exact confidence interval for following a group sequential test. *Biometrics*, 40, 797-803.

Tu, D. (1997). Two one-sided tests procedures in establishing therapeutic equivalence with binary clinical endpoints: fixed sample performances and sample size determination. *Journal of Statistical Computation and Simulation*, 59, 271-290.

Tukey, J.W., and Heyse, J.F. (1985). Testing the statistical certainty of a response to increasing doses of a drug. *Biometrics*, 41, 295-301.

Tygstrup, N., Lachin, J.M., and Juhl, E. (1982). *The Randomized Clinical Trials and Therapeutic Decisions.* Marcel Dekker, Inc., New York, NY.

van den Oord E.J.C.G. and Sullivan, P.F. (2003) A framework for controlling false discovery rates and minimizing the amount of genotyping in gene-finding studies. *Human Heredity,* 56(4), 188–199.

Wang, H. and Chow, S.C. (2002). A practical approach for parallel trials without equal variance assumption. *Statistics in Medicine,* 21, 3137-3151.

Wang, H., Chow, S.C. and Chen, M. (2005). A Bayesian approach on sample size calculation for comparing means. *Journal of Biopharmaceutical Statistics,* 15, 799-807.

Wang, S.K. and Tsiatis, A.A. (1987). Approximately optimal one-parameter boundaries for group sequential trials. *Biometrics,* 43, 193-200.

West, M., Blanchette, C., Dressman, H., Huang, E., Ishida, S., Sprang, R., Zuzan, H., Olson, J., Marks, J., and Nevins, J. (2001). Predicting the clinical status of human breast cancer by using gene expression profiles. *Proc. Natl. Acad. Sci.,* 98, 11462–11467.

Westfall, P.H. and Young, S.S. (1989). P-value adjustments for multiple tests in multivariate binomial models. *Journal of the American Statistical Association,* 84, 780–786.

Westfall, P.H. and Young, S.S. (1993). *Resampling-based Multiple Testing: Examples and Methods for P-value Adjustment.* Wiley, New York, NY.

Westfall, P.H. and Wolfinger, R.D. (1997). Multiple tests with discrete distributions. *American Statistician,* 51, 3–8.

Westfall, P.H., Zaykin, D.V. AND Young, S.S. (2001). Multiple tests for genetic effects in association studies: Methods in Molecular Biology. In Biostatistical Methods, S. Looney (ed.). Toloway, New Jersey: Humana Press, 143–168.

Whitehead, J (1993). Sample size calculation for ordered categorical data. Statistics in Medicine, 12, 2257-2271.

Whitehead, J. (1997). Bayesian decision procedures with application to dose-finding studies. *International Journal of Pharmaceutical Medicine,* 11, 201-208.

Wiens, B.L., Heyse, J.F., and Matthews (1996). Similarity of three treatments, with application to vaccine development. Proceedings of the Biopharmaceutical Section of the American Statistical Association, 203-206.

Wilcoxon, F. (1945). Individual comparisons by ranking methods. *Biometrics*, 1, 80-83.

Wilcoxon, F. and Bradley, R.A. (1964). A note on the paper "Two sequential two-sample grouped rank tests with application to screening experiments." *Biometrics*, 20, 892-895.

Williams, D.A. (1971). A test for differences between treatment means when several doses are compared with a zero dose control. *Biometrics*, 27, 103-118.

Williams, D.A. (1972). The comparison of several dose levels with a zero dose control. *Biometrics*, 28, 519-531.

Witte, J.S., Elston, R.C., and Cardon, L.R. (2000). On the relative sample size required for multiple comparisons. *Statistics in Medicine*, 19, 369–372.

Wolfinger, R.D., Gibson, G., Wolfinger, E.D., Bennett, L., Hamadeh, H., Bushel, P., Afshari, C., and Paules, R.S. (2001). Assessing gene significance from cDNA microarray expression data via mixed models. *Journal of Computational Biology*, 8(6), 625–637.

Wooding, W.M. (1993). *Planning Pharmaceutical Clinical Trials: Basic Statistical Principles*. John Wiley and Sons, New York, NY.

Wu, M., Fisher, M. and DeMets, D. (1980). Sample sizes of long-term medical trials with time-dependent noncompliance and event rates. *Controlled Clinical Trials*, 1, 109-121.

Yue, L. (2007). Statistical and regulatory issues with the application of propensity score analysis to non-randomized medical device clinical studies. *Journal of Biopharmaceutical Statistics*, 17, 1-13.

# Index

## A

Alpha spending function, group sequential method, 204—206
Analysis of variance. *See* ANOVA
ANOVA, with repeated measures, 389—394
    example, 393—394
    hypotheses testing, 391—392
    sample size calculation, 392
    statistical model, 389—391
Asymptotic tests, large sample, for proportions, 111—112
Average bioequivalence, 259—263
    example, 262—263

## B

Bayesian sample size calculation, 327—354
    bootstrap-median approach, 350—352
        background, 350—351
        bootstrap-median approach, 351—352
    posterior credible interval approach, 328—344
        one sample, 331—337
            known precision, 331—332
            mixed Bayesian likelihood, 336—337
            unknown precision, 332—335
                average coverage criterion, 332
                average length criterion, 333
                worst outcome criterion, 333
            three selection criteria, 329—331
                average coverage criterion, 330
                average length criterion, 330
                worst outcome criterion, 331
        two-sample with common precision, 337—340
            known common precision, 337—338
            unknown common precision, 338—340
        two-sample with unequal precisions, 340—344
            known precision, 343
            unknown precision, 343—344
    posterior error approach, 344—349
        comparing means, 346—349
        posterior error rate, 344—346
Binary dose response, 284
Binary variables, group sequential method, 201—202
    example, 201—202
    procedure, 201
Binomial test, for proportions, 117—121
    example, 121
    procedure, 118—120
Binomial *vs.* time-to-event, time-to-event data comparison, 185
Bioequivalence testing, 257—278
    average bioequivalence, 259—263
        example, 262—263
    bioequivalence criteria, 258—259
    individual bioequivalence, 265—271
        example, 271
    population bioequivalence, 263—265
        example, 265
    *in vitro* bioequivalence, 271—277
        example, 277
Bootstrap-median approach, Bayesian sample size calculation, 350—352
    background, 350—351
    bootstrap-median approach, 351—352
Bootstrapping, 369
Bridging studies, 399—408
    assessment of similarity, 402—407
        criterion for similarity, 402—404
        sample size calculation, 407

statistical methods, 405—407
sensitivity index, 399—402

## C

Carry-over effect test, 158—160
    example, 160
    test procedure, 158—160
Categorical shift, test for, 153—158
    examples, 157—158
        McNemar test, 157
        Stuart-Maxwell test, 157—158
    McNemar test, 153—155
    Stuart-Maxwell test, 155—157
Center imbalance, treatment of, 43—44
Central $t$ distribution, upper quantiles, 417
CFR. *See* Code of Federal Regulation
Clinically meaningful difference, 12—13
Cochran-Armitage test for trend, 293—296
Cochran-Mantel-Haenszel test, independence/multiple strata, 151—152
Code of Federal Regulation, 314.126 of 21 CFR, 3—4
Comparing inter-subject variabilities, 233—241
    example, 237
    parallel design with replicates, 234—237
    replicated crossover design, 237—241
        test for equality, 238—239
        test for non-inferiority/superiority, 239—240
    test for equality, 234—235
    test for non-inferiority/superiority, 235—236
Comparing intra-subject CVs, 224—233
    conditional random effects model, 228—233
        example, 232
        test for equality, 230—231
        test for non-inferiority/superiority, 231
        test for similarity, 232
    simple random effects model, 225—228
        example, 228
        test for equality, 226
        test for non-inferiority/superiority, 226—227
        test for similarity, 227—228
Comparing intra-subject variabilities, 216—224
    parallel design with replicates, 216—220
        example, 219—220
        test for equality, 217
        test for non-inferiority/superiority, 217—218
        test for similarity, 218—219
    replicated crossover design, 220—224
        example, 224
        test for equality, 221—222
        test for non-inferiority/superiority, 222—223
        test for similarity, 223—224
Comparing means, 49—82
    multiple-sample one-way ANOVA, 70—74
        example, 72—73
        pairwise comparison, 71
        simultaneous comparison, 71—72
    multiple-sample Williams design, 74—77
        example, 77
        test for equality, 75—76
        test for equivalence, 76—77
        test for non-inferiority/superiority, 76
    one-sample design, 50—57
        example, 55—57
        test for equivalence, 57

Index    453

test for non-inferiority, 56
test for equality, 50—52
test for equivalence, 54—55
test for non-inferiority/superiority, 52—54
one-sided vs. two-sided test, 78
parallel design vs. crossover design, 78—79
sensitivity analysis, 79—81
two-sample crossover design, 65—70
   example, 69
      non-inferiority, 69
      therapeutic equivalence, 69
   test for equality, 66—67
   test for equivalence, 67—68
   test for non-inferiority/superiority, 67
two-sample parallel design, 57—65
   example, 63—65
      test for equality, 63—64
      test for equivalence, 64
      test for non-inferiority, 64
   test for equality, 58—59
   test for equivalence, 61—63
   test for non-inferiority/superiority, 59—61
Comparing total variabilities, 241—254
   parallel design with replicates, 245—248
      example, 248
      test for equality, 245—246
      test for non-inferiority/superiority, 246—247
   parallel designs without replicates, 241—245
      example, 244—245
      test for equality, 242
      test for non-inferiority/superiority, 243
      test for similarity, 243—244
   replicated 2 x 2m crossover design, 251—254

      example, 254
      test for equality, 251—252
      test for non-inferiority/superiority, 253—254
   standard 2 x 2 crossover design, 248—251
      example, 251
      test for equality, 248—249
      test for non-inferiority/superiority, 250
Comparing variabilities, 369
Conditional power, group sequential method, 209—211
   comparing means, 209—210
   comparing proportions, 210—211
Conditional random effects model, intra-subject CVs comparison, 228—233
   example, 232
   test for equality, 230—231
   test for non-inferiority/superiority, 231
   test for similarity, 232
Confounding, 26
Confounding effects, defined, 26
Contingency tables, 145—162
Continuous dose response, 280—283
   linear contrast test, 281—283
      example, 282—283
Controlled clinical trials, regulation of, 3—4
Covariates, adjustment for, 39—40
Cox proportional hazards model, time-to-event data comparison, 174—179
   example, 178—179
      test for equality, 179
      test for equivalence, 179
      test for superiority, 179
   test for equality, 175—177
   test for equivalence, 178
   test for non-inferiority/superiority, 177—178
Crossover design vs. parallel design, 30—32

crossover design, 31—32
inter-subject variability, 30—31
intra-subject variability, 30—31
parallel design, 32

## D

Data transformation, 36—38
Dose escalation trials, 296—300
    A + B escalation design
        with dose de-escalation,
           299—300
        without dose de-escalation,
           297—298
Dose response studies, 279—302
    binary response, 284
    Cochran-Armitage test for trend,
        293—296
    continuous response, 280—283
        linear contrast test, 281—283
           example, 282—283
    dose escalation trials, 296—300
        A + B escalation design
           with dose de-escalation,
               299—300
           without dose de-escalation,
               297—298
    time-to-event endpoint, 285—291
        example, 285—287
    Williams test for minimum effective
        dose, 279, 287—293
        example, 288—293
Dropouts, adjustment for, 39—40

## E

Early stopping, multiple-stage design
    for, 45—46
Exact tests, large sample, for
    proportions, 111—112
Exact tests for proportions, 117—144
    binomial test, 117—121
        example, 121
        procedure, 118—120
    Fisher exact test, 121—124
        example, 124
        procedure, 122

multiple-arm trials, flexible designs
    for, 141—143
single arm trials, multiple-stage
    designs for, 124—141
    flexible two-stage designs,
        128—129
    optimal three-stage designs,
        129—141
    optimal two-stage designs,
        124—128
Exponential model, time-to-event data
    comparison, 166—174
    example, 171—173
        dropout, 174
        losses to follow-up, 174
        noncompliance, 174
        test for equality, 172
        test for equivalence, 172—173
        test for superiority, 172
        unconditional *vs.* conditional,
            173—174
    test for equality, 169—170
    test for equivalence, 171
    test for non-inferiority/superiority,
        170—171
Extremely low disease incidence,
    evaluation of vaccine efficacy
    with, vaccine clinical trials,
    410—412

## F

F distribution, upper quantiles, 419—426
False discovery rate control, microarray
    study, 305—315
    model/assumptions, 305—306
    sample size calculation, 307—315
        examples, 312
        one-sided tests
            constant effect sizes, 312
            varying effect sizes,
                312—313
        two-sided tests, constant
            effect sizes, 314
        lemma 12.2.1, 309—311
        $t$-distribution, formula based on,
            314—315

Index 455

two-sided tests, 313—314
Family-wise error rate control,
microarray study, 315—324
leukemia example, 322—324
multiple testing procedures,
316—319
single-step *vs.* multi-step,
316—319
sample size calculation, 319—322
algorithms for sample size
calculation, 319—321
FDA. *See* Food and Drug
Administration
FDR. *See* False discovery rate
Fisher exact test, for proportions,
121—124
example, 124
procedure, 122
Food and Drug Administration, 5
regulatory requirements, 2—6
Food and Drug and Cosmetics Act,
Kefauver-Harris amendments
to, 4
FWER. *See* Family-wise error rate

## G

Generalizability
defined, 5
provision of information regarding,
4
Goodness-of-fit, tests for, 146—148
example, 147—148
Pearson test, 146—147
Group sequential methods, 187—214
alpha spending function, 204—206
binary variables, 201—202
example, 201—202
procedure, 201
conditional power, 209—211
comparing means, 209—210
comparing proportions, 210—211
inner wedge test, 197—200
example, 199—200
procedure, 198—199
O'Brien and Fleming test, 192—193
example, 192—193

O'Brien-Fleming type stopping
rule, 193
procedure, 192
Pocock test, 188—191
example, 190—191
Pocock type stopping rule, 190
procedure, 188—190
sample size re-estimation, 206—209
example, 208—209
procedure, 206—208
time-to-event data, 202—203
example, 203
procedure, 202—203
Wang and Tsiatis test, 193—197
example, 196—197
procedure, 195—196

## H

Hazard function, time-to-event data
comparison, 165
Hypotheses, 9—11
test for equality, 10
test for equivalence, 11
test for non-inferiority, 10
test for superiority, 10—11

## I

*In vitro* bioequivalence, 271—277
example, 277
Independence, test for, 365—369
example, 368—369
Independence/multiple strata, test for,
151—153
Cochran-Mantel-Haenszel test,
151—152
example, 152—153
Independence/single stratum, test for,
148—151
example, 150—151
likelihood ratio test, 149—150
Pearson test, 148—149
Individual bioequivalence, 265—271
example, 271
Inner wedge test, 197—200
example, 199—200

procedure, 198—199
Inter-subject variabilities, comparing, 233—241
   example, 237
   parallel design with replicates, 234—237
   replicated crossover design, 237—241
      test for equality, 238—239
      test for non-inferiority/superiority, 239—240
   test for equality, 234—235
   test for non-inferiority/superiority, 235—236
Interaction, 27
Interaction effect between factors, defined, 27
Intra-subject CVs, comparing, 224—233
   conditional random effects model, 228—233
      example, 232
      test for equality, 230—231
      test for non-inferiority/superiority, 231
      test for similarity, 232
   simple random effects model, 225—228
      example, 228
      test for equality, 226
      test for non-inferiority/superiority, 226—227
      test for similarity, 227—228
Intra-subject CVs comparison, 224—233
Intra-subject variabilities, comparing, 216—224
   parallel design with replicates, 216—220
      example, 219—220
      test for equality, 217
      test for non-inferiority/superiority, 217—218
      test for similarity, 218—219
   replicated crossover design, 220—224
      example, 224
      test for equality, 221—222
      test for non-inferiority/superiority, 222—223
      test for similarity, 223—224

## K

Kefauver-Harris amendments, Food and Drug and Cosmetics Act, 4

## L

Large sample tests for proportions, 83—116
   asymptotic tests, 111—112
   exact tests, 111—112
   more than two proportions, equivalence test for, 115
   one-sample design, 84—88
      example, 87—88
         test for equality, 87
         test for equivalence, 88
         test for non-inferiority, 87
      test for equality, 84—85
      test for equivalence, 86—87
      test for non-inferiority/superiority, 85—86
   one-way analysis of variance, 99—101
      example, 100
      pairwise comparison, 99—100
   relative risk/crossover design, 109—111
      test for equality, 109—110
      test for equivalence, 111
      test for non-inferiority/superiority, 110—111
   relative risk/parallel design, 104—109
      example, 108—109
      test for equality, 108

# Index

test for equivalence, 108—109
test for superiority, 108
test for equality, 106
test for equivalence, 107
test for non-
   inferiority/superiority,
   106—107
stratified analysis, 113—114
two-sample crossover design, 95—99
  example, 97—98
    test for equality, 98
    test for equivalence, 98
    test for non-inferiority, 98
  test for equality, 96
  test for equivalence, 97
  test for non-
     inferiority/superiority,
     96—97
two-sample parallel design, 89—95
  example, 91—93
    test for equality, 92
    test for equivalence, 93
    test for non-inferiority, 92
    test for superiority, 93
  test for equality, 89
  test for equivalence, 90—91
  test for non-
     inferiority/superiority,
     90
variance estimates, 112—113
Williams design, 101—104
  example, 103—104
    test for equality, 104
    test for equivalence, 104
    test for superiority, 104
  test for equality, 102
  test for equivalence, 103
  test for non-
     inferiority/superiority,
     102
Likelihood ratio test, test for, 149—150
Linear contrast test, 281—283
Local alternative vs. fixed alternative,
   time-to-event data comparison,
   185

**M**

McNemar test, categorical shift,
   153—155
  examples, 157
Means comparison, 49—82
  multiple-sample one-way ANOVA,
     70—74
    example, 72—73
    pairwise comparison, 71
    simultaneous comparison, 71—72
  multiple-sample Williams design,
     74—77
    example, 77
    test for equality, 75—76
    test for equivalence, 76—77
    test for non-
       inferiority/superiority,
       76
  one-sample design, 50—57
    example, 55—57
      test for equivalence, 57
      test for non-inferiority, 56
    test for equality, 50—52
    test for equivalence, 54—55
    test for non-
       inferiority/superiority,
       52—54
  one-sided vs. two-sided test, 78
  parallel design vs. crossover design,
     78—79
  sensitivity analysis, 79—81
  two-sample crossover design, 65—70
    example, 69
      non-inferiority, 69
      therapeutic equivalence, 69
    test for equality, 66—67
    test for equivalence, 67—68
    test for non-
       inferiority/superiority,
       67
  two-sample parallel design, 57—65
    example, 63—65
      test for equality, 63—64
      test for equivalence, 64
      test for non-inferiority, 64
    test for equality, 58—59
    test for equivalence, 61—63

test for non-inferiority/superiority, 59—61
Median survival time, time-to-event data comparison, 165
Microarray studies, 303—326
  false discovery rate control, 305—315
    model/assumptions, 305—306
    sample size calculation, 307—315
      examples, 312
      one-sided tests
        constant effect sizes, 312
        varying effect sizes, 312—313
      two-sided tests, constant effect sizes, 314
      lemma 12.2.1, 309—311
      $t$-distribution, formula based on, 314—315
      two-sided tests, 313—314
  family-wise error rate control, 315—324
    leukemia example, 322—324
    multiple testing procedures, 316—319
    single-step *vs.* multi-step, 316—319
    sample size calculation, 319—322
      algorithms for sample size calculation, 319—321
Mixed-up randomization schedules, 40—43
Modernization Act, 5
More than two proportions, equivalence test for, large sample test, 115
Multiple-arm trials, for proportions, flexible designs for, 141—143
Multiple-sample location problem, 369—370
Multiple-sample one-way ANOVA, comparing means, 70—74
  example, 72—73
  pairwise comparison, 71
  simultaneous comparison, 71—72

Multiple-sample Williams design, comparing means, 74—77
  example, 77
  test for equality, 75—76
  test for equivalence, 76—77
  test for non-inferiority/superiority, 76
Multiple testing procedures, family-wise error rate control
  microarray study, 316—319
  single-step *vs.* multi-step, 316—319
Multiplicity, 44—45

## N

Nonparametrics, 355—372
  bootstrapping, 369
  comparing variabilities, 369
  multiple-sample location problem, 369—370
  one-sample location problem, 357—361
    example, 361
  test for independence, 365—369
    example, 368—369
  testing scale parameters, 370—371
  two-sample location problem, 361—365
    example, 364—365
  violation of assumptions, 356—357

## O

O'Brien and Fleming test, 192—193
  example, 192—193
  O'Brien-Fleming type stopping rule, 193
  procedure, 192
One-sample design
  comparing means, 50—57
    example, 55—57
      test for equivalence, 57
      test for non-inferiority, 56
    test for equality, 50—52
    test for equivalence, 54—55

Index    459

test for non-inferiority/superiority, 52—54
large sample test for proportions, 84—88
   example, 87—88
      test for equality, 87
      test for equivalence, 88
      test for non-inferiority, 87
   test for equality, 84—85
   test for equivalence, 86—87
   test for non-inferiority/superiority, 85—86
One-sample location problem, 357—361
   example, 361
One-sample *vs.* historical control, time-to-event data comparison, 185—186
One-sided test *vs.* two-sided test, 28—30
One-sided *vs.* two-sided test, comparing means, 78
One-way analysis of variance, large sample test for proportions, 99—101
   example, 100
   pairwise comparison, 99—100

## P

Parallel design, *vs.* crossover design, 30—32
   crossover design, 31—32
   inter-subject variability, 30—31
   intra-subject variability, 30—31
   parallel design, 32
Parallel design *vs.* crossover design, comparing means, 78—79
Parallel design with replicates
   intra-subject variabilities comparison, 216—220
      example, 219—220
      test for equality, 217
      test for non-inferiority/superiority, 217—218
      test for similarity, 218—219

total variabilities comparison, 245—248
   example, 248
   test for equality, 245—246
   test for non-inferiority/superiority, 246—247
Parallel designs without replicates, total variabilities comparison, 241—245
   example, 244—245
   test for equality, 242
   test for non-inferiority/superiority, 243
   test for similarity, 243—244
Pearson test
   goodness-of-fit, 146—147
   independence/single stratum, 148—149
Pocock test, 188—191
   example, 190—191
   Pocock type stopping rule, 190
   procedure, 188—190
Population bioequivalence, 263—265
   example, 265
Posterior credible interval approach, Bayesian sample size calculation, 328—344
   one sample, 331—337
      known precision, 331—332
      mixed Bayesian likelihood, 336—337
      unknown precision, 332—335
         average coverage criterion, 332
         average length criterion, 333
         worst outcome criterion, 333
   three selection criteria, 329—331
      average coverage criterion, 330
      average length criterion, 330
      worst outcome criterion, 331
   two-sample with common precision, 337—340
      known common precision, 337—338
      unknown common precision, 338—340

two-sample with unequal precisions, 340—344
    known precision, 343
    unknown precision, 343—344
Posterior error approach, Bayesian sample size calculation, 344—349
    comparing means, 346—349
    posterior error rate, 344—346
Power analysis, 16—17
Practical issues, 38—47
Precision analysis, 15—16
Primary study endpoint, 11—12
Prior to sample size calculation, 25—48
    center imbalance, treatment of, 43—44
    confounding, 26
    confounding effects, defined, 26
    crossover design vs. parallel design, 30—32
        crossover design, 31—32
        inter-subject variability, 30—31
        parallel design, 32
    data transformation, 36—38
    dropouts, 39—40
    early stopping, multiple-stage design for, 45—46
    interaction, 27
    interaction effect between factors, defined, 27
    mixed-up randomization schedules, 40—43
    multiplicity, 44—45
    one-sided test vs. two-sided test, 28—30
    practical issues, 38—47
    rare incidence rate, 46—47
    subgroup/interim analyses, 32—36
        alpha spending function, 35—36
        group sequential boundaries, 33—35
    unequal treatment allocation, 38—39
Probability, reproducibility, 19—20
Probability assessment, 18—19
Procedures for sample size calculation, 12—21
    power analysis, 16—17

precision analysis, 15—16
probability assessment, 18—19
reproducibility probability, 19—20
sample size re-estimation without unblinding, 20—21
type I error, 14
type II error, 14
Propensity analysis in non-randomized studies, 383—389
    power, sample size, 384—387
    sample size calculation ignoring strata, 386—387
    simulations, 387—388
    weighted Mantel-Haenszel test, 383—384
Proportions
    exact tests for, 117—144
        binomial test, 117—121
            example, 121
            procedure, 118—120
        Fisher exact test, 121—124
            example, 124
            procedure, 122
        multiple-arm trials, flexible designs for, 141—143
        single arm trials, multiple-stage designs for, 124—141
            flexible two-stage designs, 128—129
            optimal three-stage designs, 129—141
            optimal two-stage designs, 124—128
    large sample tests for, 83—116
        exact tests, 111—112
        more than two proportions, equivalence test for, 115
        one-sample design, 84—88
            example, 87—88
                test for equality, 87
                test for equivalence, 88
                test for non-inferiority, 87
            test for equality, 84—85
            test for equivalence, 86—87

# Index

test for non-inferiority/superiority, 85—86
one-way analysis of variance, 99—101
  example, 100
  pairwise comparison, 99—100
relative risk/crossover design, 109—111
  test for equality, 109—110
  test for equivalence, 111
  test for non-inferiority/superiority, 110—111
relative risk/parallel design, 104—109
  example, 108—109
    test for equality, 108
    test for equivalence, 108—109
    test for superiority, 108
  test for equality, 106
  test for equivalence, 107
  test for non-inferiority/superiority, 106—107
stratified analysis, 113—114
two-sample crossover design, 95—99
  example, 97—98
    test for equality, 98
    test for equivalence, 98
    test for non-inferiority, 98
  test for equality, 96
  test for equivalence, 97
  test for non-inferiority/superiority, 96—97
two-sample parallel design, 89—95
  example, 91—93
    test for equality, 92
    test for equivalence, 93
    test for non-inferiority, 92
    test for superiority, 93
  test for equality, 89
  test for equivalence, 90—91
  test for non-inferiority/superiority, 90
variance estimates, 112—113
Williams design, 101—104
  example, 103—104
    test for equality, 104
    test for equivalence, 104
    test for superiority, 104
  test for equality, 102
  test for equivalence, 103
  test for non-inferiority/superiority, 102

## Q

QT/QTc studies with time-dependent replicates, 374—383
  extension, 380—382
    crossover design, 381—382
    parallel group design, 381
  power, sample size calculation, 376—380
    crossover design, 377—378
    parallel group design, 376—377
  study designs, models, 375—376
Quality of life, 394—399
  example, 399
  sample size calculation, 398
  time series model, 396—398
Quantiles tables, 417—426

## R

Rare incidence rate, 46—47
Reduction in disease incidence, vaccine clinical trials, 409—410
  example, 410—412
Regulatory requirements, 2—7
Relative risk/crossover design, large sample test for proportions, 109—111
  test for equality, 109—110
  test for equivalence, 111

test for non-inferiority/superiority, 110—111
Relative risk/parallel design, large sample test for proportions, 104—109
  example, 108—109
    test for equality, 108
    test for equivalence, 108—109
    test for superiority, 108
  test for equality, 106
  test for equivalence, 107
  test for non-inferiority/superiority, 106—107
Relative vaccine efficacy, vaccine clinical trials, 412
Replicated 2 x $2m$ crossover design, total variabilities comparison, 251—254
  example, 254
  test for equality, 251—252
  test for non-inferiority/superiority, 253—254
Replicated crossover design, intra-subject variabilities comparison, 220—224
  example, 224
  test for equality, 221—222
  test for non-inferiority/superiority, 222—223
  test for similarity, 223—224
Reproducibility of results
  assurance of, 4
  defined, 4—5
Reproducibility probability, 19—20

## S

Sample size re-estimation, group sequential method, 206—209
  example, 208—209
  procedure, 206—208
Sample size re-estimation without unblinding, 20—21
Sensitivity analysis, comparing means, 79—81

Simple random effects model, intra-subject CVs comparison, 225—228
  example, 228
  test for equality, 226
  test for non-inferiority/superiority, 226—227
  test for similarity, 227—228
Single arm trials, for proportions, multiple-stage designs for, 124—141
  flexible two-stage designs, 128—129
  three-stage designs, 129—141
  two-stage designs, 124—128
Single trial, substantial evidence with, 5—6
Standard 2 x 2 crossover design, total variabilities comparison, 248—251
  example, 251
  test for equality, 248—249
  test for non-inferiority/superiority, 250
Stratified analysis, large sample test for proportions, 113—114
Stuart-Maxwell test, categorical shift, 155—157
  examples, 157—158
Study design, 8—9
Subgroup/interim analyses, 32—36
  alpha spending function, 35—36
  group sequential boundaries, 33—35
Survival function, time-to-event data comparison, 164

## T

$T$-distribution, central, upper quantiles, 417
$T$-distribution, exact formula based on, 314—315
$T$-distribution, upper quantiles, 417
Tables of quantiles, 417—426
Test for equality, 10
Test for equivalence, 11
Test for non-inferiority, 10
Test for superiority, 10—11

Time-to-event data, group sequential
    method, 202—203
  example, 203
  procedure, 202—203
Time-to-event data comparison,
    163—186
  binomial *vs.* time-to-event, 185
  Cox proportional hazards model,
      174—179
    example, 178—179
      test for equality, 179
      test for equivalence, 179
      test for superiority, 179
    test for equality, 175—177
    test for equivalence, 178
    test for non-
        inferiority/superiority,
        177—178
  example, 165—166
  exponential model, 166—174
    example, 171—173
      dropout, 174
      losses to follow-up, 174
      noncompliance, 174
      test for equality, 172
      test for equivalence, 172—173
      test for superiority, 172
      unconditional *vs.* conditional,
          173—174
    test for equality, 169—170
    test for equivalence, 171
    test for non-
        inferiority/superiority,
        170—171
  hazard function, 165
  local alternative *vs.* fixed alternative,
      185
  median survival time, 165
  one-sample *vs.* historical control,
      185—186
  practical issues, 185—186
  survival function, 164
  weighted log-rank test, 179—184
    example, 181—184
    Tarone-Ware test, 180—181
Time-to-event endpoint, dose response,
    285—291

  example, 285—287
Total variabilities, comparing, 241—254
  parallel design with replicates,
      245—248
    example, 248
    test for equality, 245—246
    test for non-
        inferiority/superiority,
        246—247
  parallel designs without replicates,
      241—245
    example, 244—245
    test for equality, 242
    test for non-
        inferiority/superiority,
        243
    test for similarity, 243—244
  replicated 2 x 2*m* crossover design,
      251—254
    example, 254
    test for equality, 251—252
    test for non-
        inferiority/superiority,
        253—254
  standard 2 x 2 crossover design,
      248—251
    example, 251
    test for equality, 248—249
    test for non-
        inferiority/superiority,
        250
Two clinical studies, requirement of,
    4—5
Two-sample crossover design
  comparing means, 65—70
    example, 69
      non-inferiority, 69
      therapeutic equivalence, 69
    test for equality, 66—67
    test for equivalence, 67—68
    test for non-
        inferiority/superiority,
        67
  large sample test for proportions,
      95—99
    example, 97—98
    test for equality, 98

test for equivalence, 98
test for non-inferiority, 98
test for equality, 96
test for equivalence, 97
test for non-inferiority/superiority, 96—97
Two-sample location problem, 361—365
   example, 364—365
Two-sample parallel design
   comparing means, 57—65
      example, 63—65
         test for equality, 63—64
         test for equivalence, 64
         test for non-inferiority, 64
      test for equality, 58—59
      test for equivalence, 61—63
      test for non-inferiority/superiority, 59—61
   large sample test for proportions, 89—95
      example, 91—93
         test for equality, 92
         test for equivalence, 93
         test for non-inferiority, 92
         test for superiority, 93
      test for equality, 89
      test for equivalence, 90—91
      test for non-inferiority/superiority, 90
Type I error, 14
Type II error, 14

## U

Unblinding, sample size re-estimation without, 20—21
Unequal treatment allocation, 38—39
Upper quantiles
   central $t$ distribution, 417
   F distribution, 419—426
   $X^2$ distribution, 418
Upper quantiles of central $t$ distribution, 417
Upper quantiles of F distribution, 419—426
Upper quantiles of $X^2$ distribution, 418
U.S. Food and Drug Administration, 5
   regulatory requirements, 2—6

## V

Vaccine clinical trials, 408—417
   composite efficacy measure, 412—414
      example, 414
   evaluation of vaccine efficacy with extremely low disease incidence, 410—412
   reduction in disease incidence, 409—410
      example, 410—412
   relative vaccine efficacy, 412
Variabilities comparison, 215—256
   inter-subject variabilities, comparing, 233—241
      example, 237
      parallel design with replicates, 234—237
      replicated crossover design, 237—241
         test for equality, 238—239
         test for non-inferiority/superiority, 239—240
      test for equality, 234—235
      test for non-inferiority/superiority, 235—236
   intra-subject CVs, comparing, 224—233
   conditional random effects model, 228—233
      example, 232
      test for equality, 230—231
      test for non-inferiority/superiority, 231
      test for similarity, 232
   simple random effects model, 225—228

Index 465

example, 228
test for equality, 226
test for non-inferiority/superiority, 226—227
test for similarity, 227—228
intra-subject variabilities, comparing, 216—224
parallel design with replicates, 216—220
example, 219—220
test for equality, 217
test for non-inferiority/superiority, 217—218
test for similarity, 218—219
replicated crossover design, 220—224
example, 224
test for equality, 221—222
test for non-inferiority/superiority, 222—223
test for similarity, 223—224
total variabilities, comparing, 241—254
parallel design with replicates, 245—248
example, 248
test for equality, 245—246
test for non-inferiority/superiority, 246—247
parallel designs without replicates, 241—245
example, 244—245
test for equality, 242
test for non-inferiority/superiority, 243
test for similarity, 243—244
replicated 2 x 2m crossover design, 251—254
example, 254
test for equality, 251—252
test for non-inferiority/superiority, 253—254
standard 2 x 2 crossover design, 248—251
example, 251
test for equality, 248—249
test for non-inferiority/superiority, 250
Variance estimates, large sample test for proportions, 112—113
Violation of assumptions, 356—357

## W

Wang and Tsiatis test, 193—197
example, 196—197
procedure, 195—196
Weighted log-rank test, time-to-event data comparison, 179—184
example, 181—184
Tarone-Ware test, 180—181
Well-controlled study, definition of, 3—4
Williams design, large sample test for proportions, 101—104
example, 103—104
test for equality, 104
test for equivalence, 104
test for superiority, 104
test for equality, 102
test for equivalence, 103
test for non-inferiority/superiority, 102
Williams test for minimum effective dose, 279, 287—293
example, 288—293

## X

$X^2$ distribution, upper quantiles, 418